Pathology

First, second and third edition authors:

Bethan Goodman Jones

Daniel J O'Connor

Atul Anand

Fourth edition author:

Philip Xiu

5th Edition

CRASH COURSE

SERIES EDITORS

Philip Xiu

MA, MB BChir, MRCP
GP Registrar
Yorkshire Deanery
Leeds, UK

Shreelata Datta

MD, MRCOG, LLM, BSc (Hons), MBBS
Honorary Senior Lecturer
Imperial College London
Consultant Obstetrician and Gynaecologist
King's College Hospital
London, UK

FACULTY ADVISOR

Hizbullah Shaikh

Pathology

Olivia McKinney

BA, MBBS, FRCPath
Consultant Histopathologist
Kings College Hospital
London, UK

Isabel Woodman

MA (Cantab), MSc, MBBS, FRCPath
Histopathology Registrar
Kent, Surrey, Sussex Deanery
London, UK

For additional online content visit StudentConsult.com

ELSEVIER

ELSEVIER

Content Strategist: Jeremy Bowes
Content Development Specialist: Alexandra Mortimer
Project Manager: Andrew Riley
Design: Christian Bilbow
Illustration Manager: Karen Giacomucci
Illustrator: MPS North America LLC
Marketing Manager: Deborah Watkins

First edition 1998

Notices

Practitioners and researchers must always rely on their own experience and knowledge in evaluating and using any information, methods, compounds or experiments described herein. Because of rapid advances in the medical sciences, in particular, independent verification of diagnoses and drug dosages should be made. To the fullest extent of the law, no responsibility is assumed by Elsevier, authors, editors or contributors for any injury and/or damage to persons or property as a matter of products liability, negligence or otherwise, or from any use or operation of any methods, products, instructions, or ideas contained in the material herein.

ISBN: 978-0-7020-7354-0
eISBN: 978-0-7020-7355-7

The publisher's policy is to use **paper manufactured from sustainable forests**

Last digit is the print number: 9 8 7 6 5 4 3 2 1

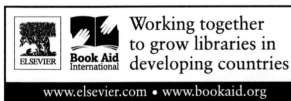

Dedication

To Nicola and Gordon: Thank you for being my personal cheerleaders, and always providing me with love, support…and food!

Olivia McKinney

To Robert and Phil for their infinite love and patience. You guys are my rocks and I could not have done this without you. Thank you with all my heart.

To Alex for providing sanity in the maëlstrom.

Isabel Woodman

Series Editors' foreword

The *Crash Course* series was conceived by Dr Dan Horton-Szar who as series editor presided over it for more than 15 years – from publication of the first edition in 1997, until publication of the fourth edition in 2011. His inspiration, knowledge and wisdom lives on in the pages of this book. As the new series editors, we are delighted to be able to continue developing each book for the twenty-first century undergraduate curriculum.

The flame of medicine never stands still, and keeping this all-new fifth series relevant for today's students is an ongoing process. Each title within this new fifth edition has been re-written to integrate basic medical science and clinical practice, after extensive deliberation and debate. We aim to build on the success of the previous titles by keeping the series up-to-date with current guidelines for best practice, and recent developments in medical research and pharmacology.

We always listen to feedback from our readers, through focus groups and student reviews of the *Crash Course* titles. For the fifth editions we have reviewed and re-written our self-assessment material to reflect today's 'single-best answer' and 'extended matching question' formats. The artwork and layout of the titles has also been largely re-worked and are now in colour, to make it easier on the eye during long sessions of revision. The new on-line materials supplement the learning process.

Despite fully revising the books with each edition, we hold fast to the principles on which we first developed the series. *Crash Course* will always bring you all the information you need to revise in compact, manageable volumes that still maintain the balance between clarity and conciseness, and provide sufficient depth for those aiming at distinction. The authors are junior doctors who have recent experience of the exams you are now facing, and the accuracy of the material is checked by a team of faculty editors from across the UK.

We wish you all the best for your future careers!

Philip Xiu and Shreelata Datta

Prefaces

Authors

Pathology is the heart of medicine, and it is much more than just microscopes and slides. When Elsevier first approached us about editing this edition of *Crash Course: Pathology* we were delighted – we wanted to try and bring pathology back to the forefront of medicine. We knew it would be difficult and challenging, but worthwhile.

This book has been in the making for the best part of two years during which time we have rotated to three hospitals, started three new jobs and sat four exams. We have extensively rewritten a large proportion of this book with the aim of providing a useful and succinct guide to key pathological topics and their clinical relevance. We have included new chapters on postmortems and death certification (topics that are often side-lined), and molecular pathology which heralds a new era in this age-old discipline.

If we instil an understanding and passion for pathology then we have been successful in our venture. Whether you are a medical student trying to pass a pathology exam or someone exploring the field in a little more depth we hope that you find this useful. Enjoy!

Olivia McKinney, Isabel Woodman

Faculty Advisor

This book is the product of a year of work by my colleagues Isabel, Olivia and myself.

We have thoroughly revised and edited the chapters of the previous edition to bring them up-to-date, and restructured part of the content to form new chapters on head and neck pathology and hepatopancreaticobiliary pathology. In addition, we have introduced brand new chapters on molecular pathology and postmortems, as well as new EMQs, SBAs and clinical scenarios on death certification.

Although the book is geared towards undergraduate and postgraduate medical students, we think it may also be a valuable resource for biomedical scientists and other healthcare workers with an interest in pathology.

We hope we have been successful in our goals and have peaked the interests of budding pathologists. We wish you happy studying!

Hizbullah Shaikh

Acknowledgements

We would like to personally thank everyone who has helped and supported us during the writing of this fifth edition, especially our families, friends and fellow trainees who have had numerous esoteric, random questions thrown at them at varying intervals.

We would also like to thank King's College Hospital Cellular Pathology Department for supporting us in this endeavour, especially Dr Hizbullah Shaikh. Special thanks go to Anthony and Ursula McKinney, Nicola McKinney, Gordon Summers, Dr Mojisola Giwa, Helena and David Woodman, Dr Philip Mairs, Dr Michael Coutts and Lauren Millar for their constant encouragement and support. Thank you.

Finally, we wish to thank all of those at Elsevier for this experience, their support and unwavering patience.

Series Editors' acknowledgements

We would like to thank the support of our colleagues who have helped in the preparation of this edition, namely the junior doctor contributors who helped write the manuscript as well as the faculty editors who check the veracity of the information.

We are extremely grateful for the support of our publisher, Elsevier, whose staffs' insight and persistence has maintained the quality that Dr Horton-Szar has set-out since the first edition. Jeremy Bowes, our commissioning editor, has been a constant support. Alex Mortimer and Barbara Simmons our development editors have managed the day-to-day work on this edition with extreme patience and unflappable determination to meet the ever looming deadlines, and we are ever grateful for Kim Benson's contribution to the online editions and additional online supplementary materials.

Contents

Introduction to pathology 1

DISEASES

A disease is an alteration from the normal function/structure of an organ or system, which manifests as a characteristic set of signs and symptoms.

PATHOLOGY

Pathology is the scientific study of disease. It is concerned with the causes and effects of disease, and the functional and structural changes that occur. Changes at the molecular and cellular level correlate with the clinical manifestations of the disease.

Understanding the processes of disease assists in the accurate recognition, diagnosis and treatment of diseases.

Divisions of pathology

Pathology is traditionally subdivided into seven main clinical disciplines:

1. Histopathology—the study of histological abnormalities of diseased cells and tissues.
2. Haematology—the study of primary diseases of the blood and the secondary effects of other diseases on the blood.
3. Chemical pathology—the study of biochemical abnormalities associated with disease.
4. Microbiology—the study of infectious diseases and the organisms that cause them.
5. Virology—the study of infections with viral aetiology.
6. Immunopathology—the study of diseases through the analysis of immune function.
7. Molecular pathology—the study of disease at a molecular level.

Classification of disease

The causes of disease are numerous and diverse. For convenience, diseases are often classified as either congenital or acquired disorders. Congenital diseases are present from birth and can be either genetic (e.g., cystic fibrosis) or non-genetic (e.g., thalidomide anomalies). Acquired disorders are incurred as a result of factors originating in the external environment. The Hints and Tips box shows a helpful mnemonic or 'surgical sieve' (VITAMIN C, D, E, F) for remembering disease classification.

HINTS AND TIPS

CLASSIFICATION OF DISEASE

The 'surgical sieve' gives an approach to differential diagnosis. Remember the mnemonic VITAMIN C, D, E, F

Vascular
Inflammatory/*i*nfectious
Trauma
Autoimmune
Metabolic
Iatrogenic/*i*diopathic
Neoplastic
Congenital
Drugs/*d*egenerative disorders
Endocrine disorders
Functional

Many, if not most, diseases arise from a combination of causes, and they are therefore said to have a multifactorial aetiology. Table 1.1 illustrates categories for analysing any disease.

Table 1.1 Characteristics of disease

Characteristic	Explanation
Definition	A clear, concise and accurate description
Demographics	What age, gender and ethnicity are prone to a disease
Aetiology	Cause of disease
Incidence	Number of new cases of disease occurring in a population of a defined size during a defined period
Prevalence	Total number of cases of disease to be found in a defined population at a stated time
Pathogenesis	Mechanism by which a disease is caused
Morphology	Form and structural changes
Treatment	Treatment regimens, effectiveness and side-effects
Prognosis	Expected outcome of the disease
Complications and sequelae	Secondary consequences of disease

HOW PATHOLOGY IS COVERED IN THIS BOOK

Part I: Principles of pathology

A limited number of tissue responses underlie all diseases. These responses are known as basic pathological responses. The first part of this book describes the principles of these in relation to our advancing knowledge of the molecular sciences.

Part II: Systemic pathology

As well as an understanding of the basic pathological responses, it is also necessary to understand how they affect organ systems. The second part of this book describes the common pathology of specific diseases as they affect individual organs or organ systems.

Chapter Summary

- Pathology is the scientific study of disease.
- Pathology is divided into histopathology, haematology, chemical pathology, microbiology, virology, immunology and molecular pathology.
- Diseases can be congenital or acquired.
- Pathology has unifying core concepts (e.g., inflammation and neoplasia), which form the basis of diseases occurring in different organ systems.
- Postmortems are an important part of pathology.

Postmortem pathology 2

POSTMORTEM AND INQUEST

What is a postmortem?

A postmortem or autopsy is the external and internal examination of a person to determine cause of death. There are two types of postmortems: hospital postmortems and coronial postmortems. Table 2.1 highlights the main differences between the two.

Postmortem procedure

Preparation for a postmortem examination requires reading any pertinent clinical history and the circumstances surrounding the death.

Table 2.1 Differences between hospital and coronial postmortems

	Hospital	Coroner
Requested by	Doctor involved in patient care or relatives	The coroner (following referral by doctor)
Circumstances requiring postmortem	• To answer a specific clinical question • At the family's request • For medical education when there is a natural death with a known cause of death	• Unknown cause of death • Unnatural death • Unexplained death • Patient not seen by a doctor in the 2 weeks prior to death • Intraoperative or postoperative (whilst still under anaesthesia) death
Consent	Next of kin (voluntary)	Coroner (mandatory)
Performed by	Pathologist	Pathologist
Inquest required?	No	Sometimes—the coroner may request an inquest depending on the cause of death (e.g., death in custody, unnatural death, unascertained cause of death after postmortem)

Before an examination can begin, the pathologist must prepare by putting on proper garb—personal protective equipment such as face mask, goggles, gown and boots. This protects the pathologist from blood and fluid splatter and any pathogens that he/she may be exposed to during the procedure. High-risk dissecting rooms are available for infectious cases.

The external examination begins by accurately identifying the deceased, followed by a thorough inspection of the body. As in life, a plethora of information can be obtained from a proper external examination.

The internal examination is started by an incision to the chest and abdomen. A number of different methods are commonly practised—the best known is the 'Y' incision. Removal of the internal organs is performed en bloc or by cavity, e.g., chest, abdomen and pelvis. Each system is examined, organs are washed (to remove blood and improve visualization) and each organ is weighed. Pertinent findings (including normal appearances) are recorded. Lastly, the cranial cap is opened and the brain removed and examined. Unless consent has been obtained, no specimens (e.g., histology or microbiology samples) are taken from the body—all contents are returned.

The final steps in a postmortem are composing a thorough and accurate report and writing a death certificate. Some cases may require the pathologist to attend an inquest.

CLINICAL NOTE

TOOLS OF THE TRADE

The tools of the trade include a scalpel, rib shears and bone saw.

The role of the inquest

An inquest is a hearing presided over by a coroner to determine the mode, manner and cause of death. The mode of death is the mechanism by which a person died (e.g., drowning) and the manner is how they died (e.g., accident, suicide or murder). The purpose of an inquest is not to assign blame, but to ascertain the circumstances surrounding a death and to provide a verdict (Box 2.1). Doctors at any level of training may be called upon to give evidence at an inquest.

BOX 2.1 OUTCOMES AT AN INQUEST

The usual verdicts of an inquest are:

- Natural death
- Accidental death
- Death by misadventure
- Suicide
- Murder
- Narrative
- Open

THE HUMAN TISSUE ACT

Since the introduction of the Human Tissue Act of 2004, which governs the storage and handling of tissue, pathologists in the UK require consent (from the coroner or next of kin) for retention of any human tissue taken at the time of autopsy (e.g., blood samples or histology samples).

DEATH CERTIFICATION

A medical certificate of cause of death (MCCD) or death certificate is issued by a doctor present during a patient's last illness. The following is a guide to MCCD structure.

Examples of medical certificate of cause of death

The MCCD is divided into two parts: part 1 and part 2.

Part 1 is further subdivided into immediate cause of death and any underlying causes; a causal sequence from last cause to the first (1a) should be clear.

Part 2 of the MCCD allows for documentation of conditions related to death but not directly causing death.

Example 1:

1a. Acute myocardial infarction in left lateral wall
1b. Circumflex artery thrombosis
1c. Hypertension

Interpretation: in this example, hypertension has led to development of coronary artery thrombosis, and thrombosis has led to acute myocardial infarction—there is causal progression from 1c to 1a (Fig. 2.1).

HINTS AND TIPS

When writing an accurate medical certificate of cause of death:

1. Try to be specific, e.g., provide the site (lateral wall) of an acute myocardial infarction.
2. Whenever possible, stay away from using mode of death in the certificate, e.g., avoid heart failure, respiratory failure, etc. If used, an underlying cause should be given.

Example 2:

1a. Haemoperitoneum
1b. Ruptured peptic ulcer
1c. Nonsteroidal antiinflammatory drugs (NSAID) use
1d. Previous myocardial infarction
2. Hypertension

Interpretation: in this example, the patient regularly took NSAIDs after his myocardial infarction. A peptic ulcer subsequently developed and eventually ruptured, leading to haemoperitoneum and exsanguination (note: exsanguination is a mode of death and hence is not used in 1a). The

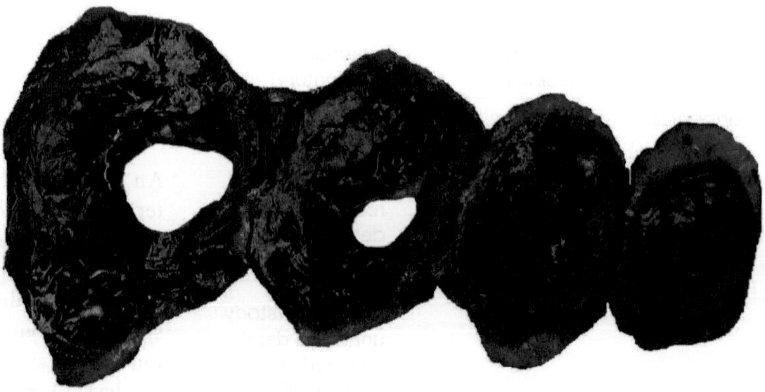

Fig. 2.1 Acute myocardial infarction. Postmortem photograph showing sequential slices of the heart with acute myocardial infarction in the wall of the left ventricle. This appears as a well demarcated red area upon the normal brown appearance of the cardiac muscle.

patient is known to have hypertension, which contributed to development of his initial infarction and would have exacerbated a ruptured peptic ulcer. However, this was not directly related to ulcer formation or haemoperitoneum and hence it is included in part 2.

Example 3:

1a. Subarachnoid haemorrhage
1b. Ruptured berry aneurysm
2. Hypertension

Example 4:

1a. Subarachnoid haemorrhage

Interpretation: in example 3, a clear sequential cause of death is demonstrated, but sometimes the underlying cause of death is not evident (as in example 4). A causal chain is not required in all cases (Fig. 2.2).

Example 5:

1a. Pulmonary thromboembolism
1b. Left leg deep vein thrombosis
1c. Immobility owing to fracture of the left femur (operated on 23 November 2017)

Interpretation: in this example, the death should be discussed with the coroner as a fracture is an accident, and an operation has been performed which is directly related to death. The date of surgery should always be provided in the death certificate (Fig. 2.3).

COMMON PITFALLS

EXAMPLE OF AN INCORRECT DEATH CERTIFICATE

An example of an incorrect medical certificate of cause of death is given below:

1a. Acute MI
1b. Hospital-acquired pneumonia
1c. Cirrhosis
2. Hepatitis C infection

Interpretation: this is incorrect as, although each condition may individually cause death, there is no clear causal link between them. Therefore, it is unclear which condition directly led to death. In addition, abbreviations (such as MI) are not permitted.

A more acceptable sequence would be:

1a. Hospital-acquired pneumonia
1b. Acute myocardial infarction
2. Cirrhosis secondary to hepatitis C infection

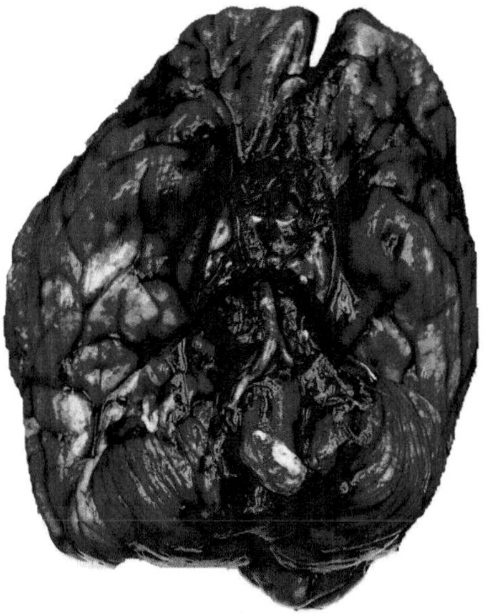

Fig. 2.2 Subarachnoid haemorrhage. Postmortem photograph showing subarachnoid haemorrhage over the base of the brain.

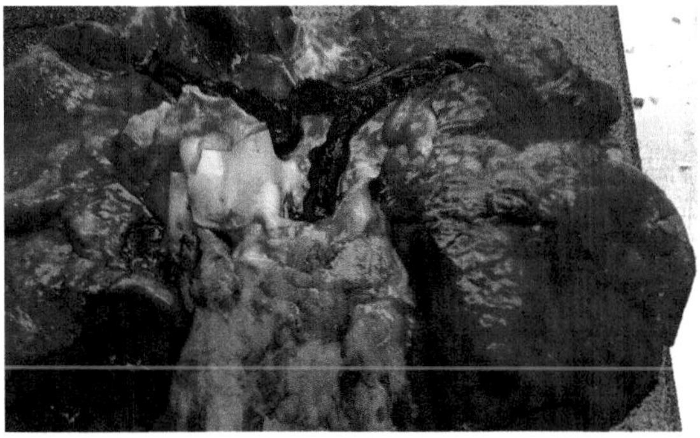

Fig. 2.3 Pulmonary thrombo embolism. Postmortem photograph showing a saddle pulmonary thromboembolus in the right and left pulmonary arteries.

THE POSTMORTEM IN MEDICAL EDUCATION

Autopsy room sessions can provide students with excellent opportunities to correlate gross histopathological features with clinical history and the natural history of a disease. Medical students should see at least one postmortem to understand the role of clinicopathological correlation and so that they can provide informed answers when obtaining familial consent for autopsy.

ADVANCES IN POSTMORTEM STUDIES

A number of recent advances have been made in autopsy services. Limited postmortems (e.g., thoracic cavity only) and noninvasive postmortems (e.g., computed tomographic- or magnetic resonance imaging-guided) are becoming increasingly common, especially in cases where there is hesitancy towards giving consent for autopsy on cultural or religious grounds.

Another change will be the introduction of National Medical Examiners in 2018. Their role is to review all deaths that are not referred directly to a coroner. The aim is to highlight substandard care of any patient at home, in a care facility or in hospital.

Chapter Summary

- There are two types of postmortems: hospital postmortems and coronial postmortems.
- The indications for performing a postmortem are varied.
- Postmortems involve several steps: obtaining clinical history, the external examination, the internal examination, interpreting findings, writing a report, and death certification.
- An inquest establishes (where possible) the mode, manner and cause of death.
- The Human Tissue Act was introduced in 2004 to provide a legal framework for retention and storage of all human tissue.
- A proper understanding of how to form a medical certificate of cause of death is a requirement for doctors.
- Postmortems are just as important today as they were historically to provide information about an individual's death and the natural history of disease.

Inflammation, repair and cell death

3

INFLAMMATION

Definition

Inflammation is the response of living tissues to cellular injury. It involves both innate and adaptive immune mechanisms.

PURPOSE

The purpose of inflammation is to localize and eliminate the causative agent, limit tissue injury and restore tissue to normality.

Inflammation can be divided into two types: acute and chronic. The division of inflammation is based according to the time course and cellular components involved. These categories are not mutually exclusive, and some overlap exists (Fig. 3.1; Table 3.1).

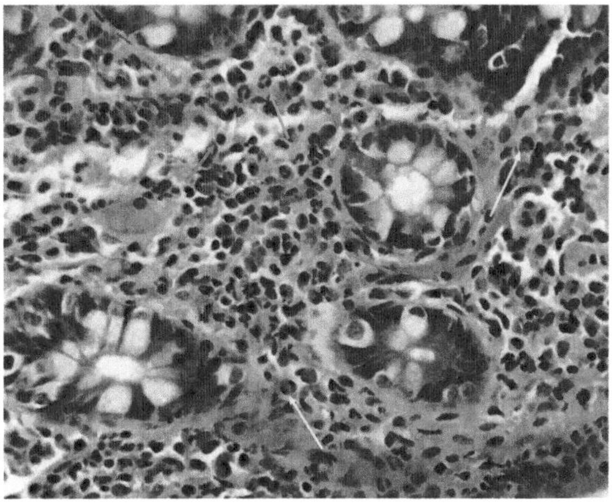

Fig. 3.1 Microscopic appearance of inflammatory cells. Mixed inflammatory cells within the colon. *Blue arrows,* neutrophils, identified by multilobated nuclei and pink cytoplasm; green arrows: lymphocytes, identified as round, dark nuclei with minimal cytoplasm; yellow arrows: eosinophils, identified by their bright orange/red cytoplasm and bilobed nuclei (tomatoes with sunglasses on).

Table 3.1 Comparison of acute and chronic inflammation

	Acute inflammation	Chronic inflammation
Response	Immediate reaction of tissue to injury	Persisting reaction of tissue to injury
Onset	Rapid	Slow
Immunity	Innate	Cell-mediated
Predominant cell type	Neutrophils	Lymphocytes, plasma cells, macrophages
Duration	Hours to weeks	Weeks/months/years
Vascular response	Prominent	Less important

Note that the acute and chronic categories are not mutually exclusive.

ACUTE INFLAMMATION

Causes of acute inflammation

The causes of acute inflammation are:

- physical agents, e.g., trauma, heat, cold, ultraviolet light, radiation
- irritant and corrosive chemical substances, e.g., acids, alkalis
- microbial infections, e.g., pyogenic bacteria
- immune-mediated hypersensitivity reactions, e.g., immune-mediated vasculitis, seasonal allergic rhinitis (hay fever)
- tissue necrosis, e.g., ischaemia resulting in myocardial infarction.

Classic signs of acute inflammation

The classic signs of acute inflammation are:

- rubor (redness)
- calor (heat)
- tumour (swelling)
- dolour (pain)
- functio laesa (loss of function).

These classical signs are produced by a rapid vascular response and cellular events characteristic of acute inflammation.

The main function of these events is to bring elements of the immune system to the site of injury and prevent further tissue damage.

Vascular response

Vasodilatation

Blood flow to the capillary bed is normally limited by the precapillary sphincters. In acute inflammation, vasodilatation occurs when the arterioles and precapillary sphincters relax. This results in increased blood flow to the injured area.

Increased vascular permeability

Endothelial intracellular proteins contract under the influence of chemical inflammatory mediators, such as histamine, bradykinin, nitric oxide and leukotriene B4. Endothelial contraction results in:

- increased fenestrations between endothelial cells
- increased permeability of vessels to plasma proteins.

Proteins leak out of the plasma into the interstitial spaces, leading to a decrease in the plasma oncotic pressure. These include includes circulating components such as immunoglobulins and coagulation factors.

Inflammatory oedema

The combined increase in hydrostatic pressure and the decreased oncotic pressure (from leakage of proteins into interstitial spaces) causes net fluid movement from plasma into tissues; this is inflammatory oedema.

Advantages of inflammatory oedema

- Fluid increase in the damaged tissue dilutes and modifies the action of toxins.
- Protein levels increase in the tissue—these include protective antibodies and fibrin.
- Nonspecific antibodies act as opsonins for neutrophil-mediated phagocytosis and function to neutralize toxins.
- The formation of a fibrin net acts as a scaffold for inflammatory cells and prevents the spread of microorganisms.
- Circulation of the exudate into the lymphatic system assists in antigen presentation and helps mount a specific immune response.

Cellular events

Extravasation

Neutrophils pass between endothelial cell junctions and invade damaged tissue to combat the effects of injury. The movement of leucocytes out of the vessel lumen is termed extravasation, and is achieved in five stages (Fig. 3.2):

1. Margination to the periphery. This is assisted by increased viscosity.
2. 'Rolling' of leucocytes owing to the repeated formation and destruction of transient adhesions with the endothelium.
3. Adhesion ('pavementing')—leucocytes eventually firmly adhere to the vascular endothelium because of the interaction of paired molecules on the leucocyte and endothelial cell surface, e.g., β_2-integrin and ICAM-1.
4. Transmigration (diapedesis)—leucocytes pass between the endothelial cell junctions, through the vessel wall into tissue spaces.
5. Chemotaxis—neutrophils migrate towards, and are possibly activated by, chemical substances (chemotaxins) released at sites of tissue injury. These chemotaxins are leukotrienes, complement components and bacterial products.

HINTS AND TIPS

CELLS OF ACUTE AND CHRONIC INFLAMMATION

The predominant cell type of acute inflammation is the neutrophil. Lymphocytes, plasma cells and macrophages are the cells found in chronic inflammation.

Phagocytosis and intracellular killing

Neutrophils and monocytes ingest debris and foreign particles at the site of injury (Fig. 3.3). Cellular pseudopodia engulf the foreign particle and fuse to produce a phagocytic vacuole or phagosome. Phagocytosis is assisted by opsonization with immunoglobulins and complement components.

Following phagocytosis, leucocytes attempt to destroy phagocytosed material by:

- discharge of lysosomal enzymes into the phagosome to form a phagolysosome
- oxygen-dependent mechanisms, such as H_2O_2, O_2^-, $OH^\bullet$ (free radicals)
- oxygen-independent mechanisms, such as lactoferrin, lysozyme and hydrolases.

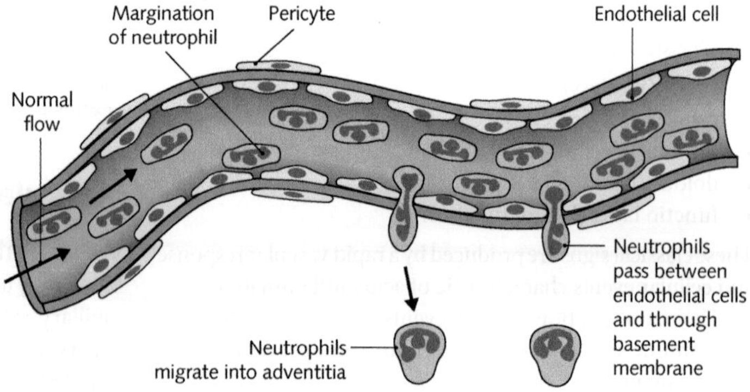

Fig. 3.2 Cellular events in acute inflammation. Neutrophils reach the injured tissues by margination, rolling, adhesion and transmigration.

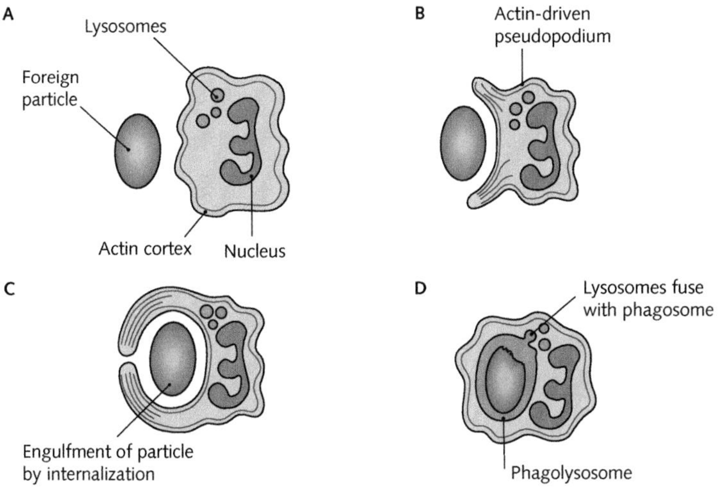

Fig. 3.3 Phagocytosis of a foreign particle by a leucocyte. (A) Attachment of foreign particle. (B) Pseudopodium engulfing particle. (C) and (D) Incorporation within the cell in a vacuole called a phagosome.

Chemical mediators of inflammation

Chemical mediators are derived either from cells or from plasma proteins in the blood and interact to produce and help coordinate the inflammatory response.

The complement system

This is a group of serum proteins (C1–C9) which sequentially activate each other in an enzymatic cascade, generating proteins that have various functions within the inflammatory response. This is a 'complementary' adjunct to the innate and adaptive immune systems.

Complement activation can be triggered through different pathways:

1. Alternative pathway: bacterial surface/cell wall molecules, e.g., lipopolysaccharide or endotoxin.
2. Classical pathway: antibody–antigen complexes via binding to C1.
3. Mannose-binding lectin pathway: mannose-binding protein binds to carbohydrates on pathogen surfaces, which activates C1.

The different activation routes converge to a common pathway that results in the generation of C3 convertase (C4bC2a) that splits C3 to C3a (anaphylatoxin) and C3b (opsonin). C5 convertase (C4bC2aC3b) is subsequently generated, splitting C5 to C5a and C5b, which ultimately leads to the formation of the membrane attack complex (MAC). The MAC is a protein pore formed from C5–C9 which inserts into the cell membrane causing cell lysis (Figs. 3.4 and 3.5).

Kinins

Kinins are small, vasoactive peptides derived from plasma proteins and are linked to the coagulation/fibrinolytic system. Bradykinin is the most well known and its production is stimulated by activated coagulation factor XII (the Hageman factor). Its action is similar to that of histamine, causing increased vascular permeability, vasodilatation and pain—the cardinal features of acute inflammation.

Arachidonic acid, prostaglandins and leukotrienes

Arachidonic acid (AA) is located within the membrane phospholipids and is liberated during acute inflammation by phospholipases. AAs are metabolized to form prostaglandins and leukotrienes, which act as chemical mediators during acute inflammation (Fig. 3.6).

The antiinflammatory action of drugs (e.g., aspirin) is attributable to their ability to inhibit prostaglandin production.

CLINICAL NOTE

ANTIINFLAMMATORY DRUGS

Antiinflammatory drugs act on the arachidonic acid pathway to reduce the effects of inflammation:

Nonsteroidal antiinflammatory drugs, e.g., ibuprofen, paracetamol, aspirin:
- COX1 and 2 inhibitors
- Selective COX2 inhibitors exist, but many have significant cardiac side-effects.

Corticosteroids, e.g., prednisolone:
- Reduce the action of phospholipase
- Judicious use is required due to side-effects associated with long-term use, e.g., osteoporosis, diabetes mellitus, hypertension and cataracts.

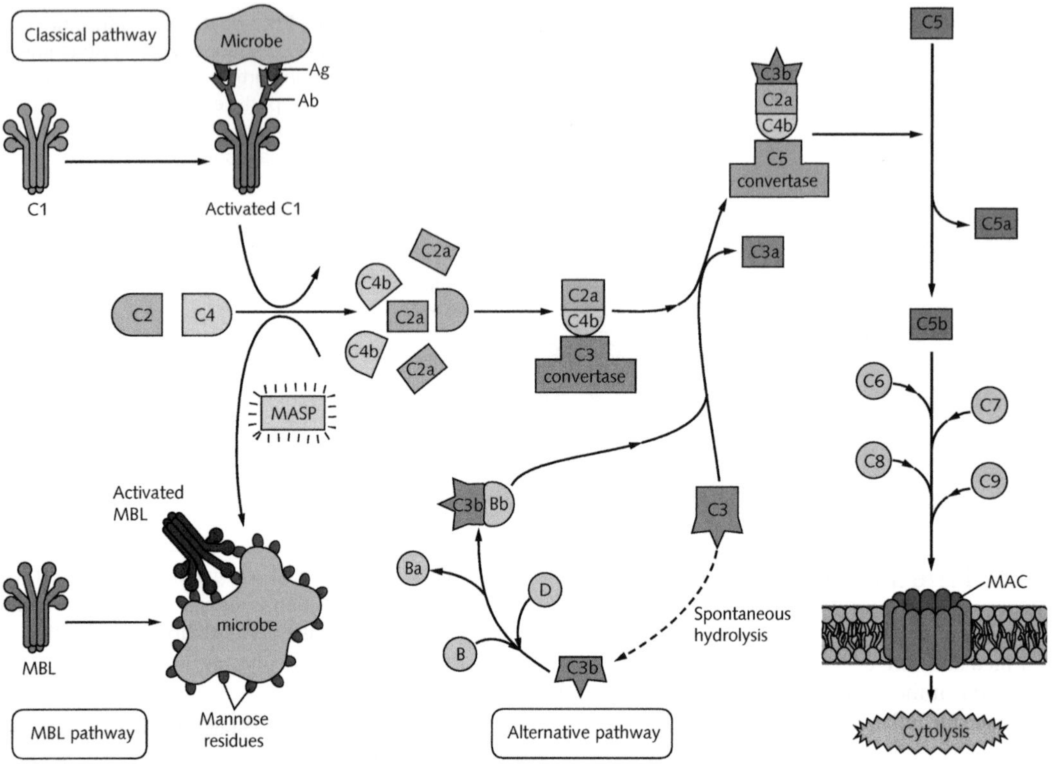

Fig. 3.4 Complement cascade. ***Classical pathway***: *C1* is activated by the binding of antigen *(Ag)*/antibody *(Ab)* complexes and enzymatically splits C2 and C4 to form C2a and C4b, which combine to form the C3 convertase.
Alternative pathway: spontaneous background hydrolysis of C3 occurs. C3b combines with factor B, which is cleaved by factor D to form an alternative C3 convertase C3bBb. This localizes to pathogen surfaces where it is stabilized and begins to cleave more C3.
Mannose-binding lectin (MBL) pathway: MBL binds to mannose residues on bacteria or viruses, causing the activation of *MASP* enzymes which cleave *C4* and *C2*. (MASP: MBL-associated serine proteases)
The C3 convertase hydrolyses C3 into C3a and C3b. C3b joins the C3 convertase to form *C5 convertase*, which cleaves C5 into C5a and C5b. A sequence of polymerization reactions is initiated by C5b, resulting in the formation of the membrane attack complex *(MAC)*, a protein pore which inserts into a pathogen's cell membrane causing hypotonic cytolysis.

Platelet activation factors

Platelet activation factors are released from mast cells and neutrophils during degranulation. They:

- induce platelet aggregation and degranulation
- increase vascular permeability
- induce leucocyte adhesion to the endothelium
- stimulate synthesis of arachidonic acid derivatives.

Vasoactive amines

These are preformed inflammatory mediators that can be rapidly released, causing vasodilatation and increased vascular permeability. These effects facilitate the influx of inflammatory cells and other inflammatory mediators to an area. Histamine and serotonin are notable examples. Histamine is released by mast cell degranulation and is also present in basophils and platelets. Serotonin is produced by platelets.

Cytokines

Cytokines are a family of chemical messengers that act over short distances to modulate and regulate cell function. This is achieved by binding to specific receptors on target cell surfaces. Cytokines include:

- Interleukins (ILs)—protein signals that act between cells of the immune system to influence their behaviour.
- Interferons (IFNs) interfere with viral replication within cells and influence major histocompatibility complex class I expression and antigen processing in cells. They are produced by natural killer (NK) cells and T-cells. There are three classes: alpha, beta and gamma.
- Tumour necrosis factors (TNFs) are a superfamily of proteins which can trigger apoptosis, cause cachexia by altering metabolism, act as pyrogens and cause cell proliferation and differentiation. They are mainly produced by macrophages.

TNF-α and IL-1 are key cytokines in acute inflammation (Table 3.2).

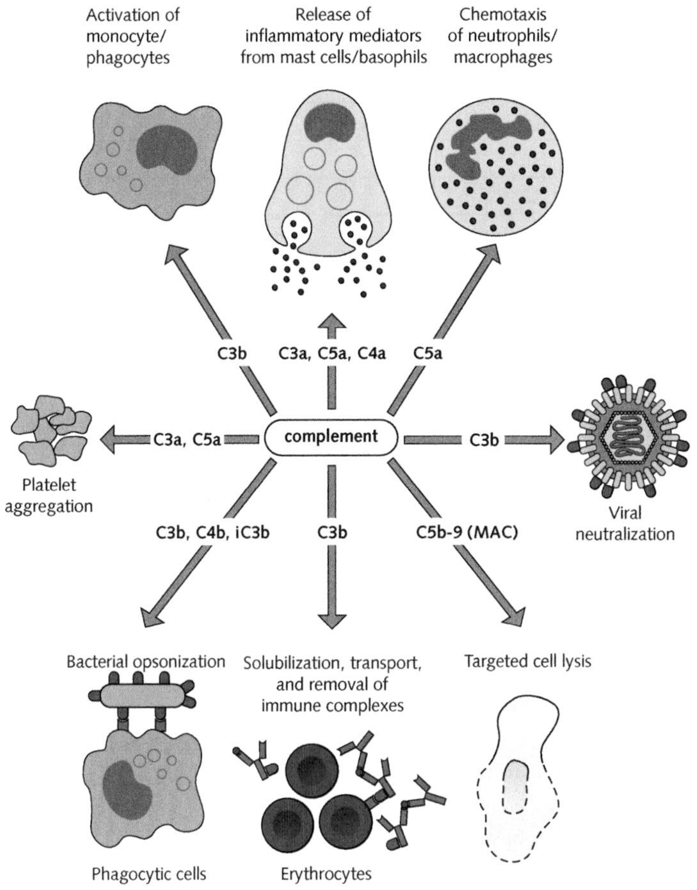

Fig. 3.5 The major functions of the complement system. *MAC,* Membrane attack complex.

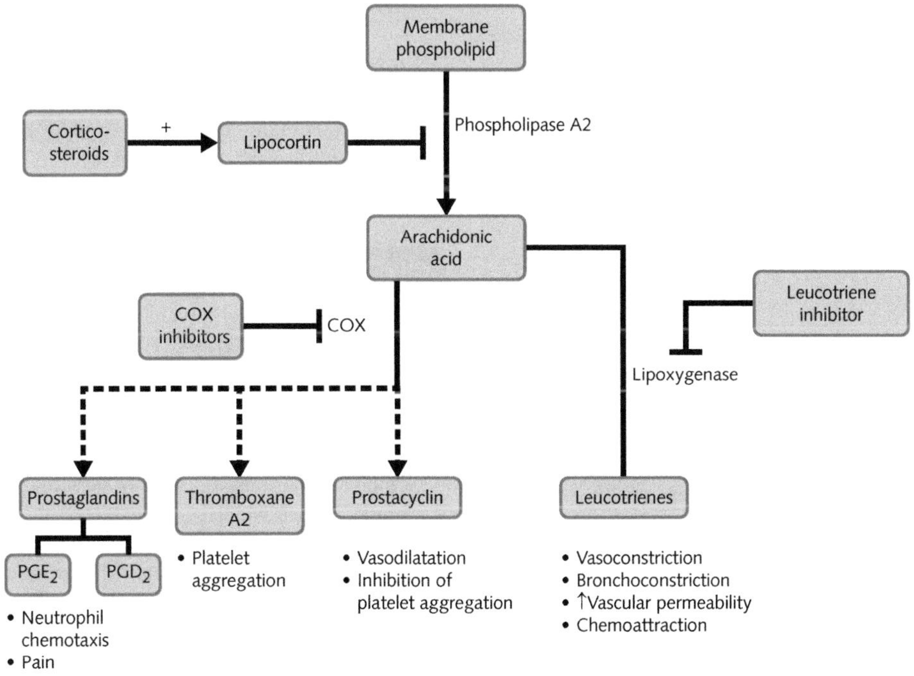

Fig. 3.6 Formation of arachidonic acid and its metabolites. *COX:* Cyclo-oxygenase; *PGE_2*, Prostaglandin E_2; *PGD_2*, Prostaglandin D_2.

Table 3.2 Key cytokines

Cytokine	Effect
IL-1	Pyrogen Induces expression of endothelial vascular adhesion molecules Stimulates cytokine production Activation of T-, B- and NK-cells Stimulates macrophages
IL-2	Activates T-cells
IL-4	Causes T_H2 development Helps B-cell Ig switching
IL-5	Growth and differentiation of eosinophils B-cell helps to produce IgA and IgM
IL-6	Terminally differentiates B-cells to plasma cells Stimulates liver to produce acute phase proteins
IL-10	Downregulation of immune responses
IL-12	Stimulates NK-cells Tc activation and T_H1 formation Innate and adaptive immunity against intracellular pathogens
TNF-α and -β	Pyrogens Clotting system activation Stimulates liver to produce acute phase proteins Act on neutrophils and endothelial cells Lyse tumour cells
IFN-α and β	Phagocyte activation Antiviral
IFN-γ	Antiviral Stimulates T_H1 differentiation Macrophage activation Induces MHC expression
TGF-β	Inhibits T-cell proliferation Increases IL-1 Proangiogenic factor

Ig, Immunoglobulin; IL, interleukin; IFN, interferon; MHC, major histocompatibility complex; NK, natural killer cells; Tc, cytotoxic T-cells; TGF β, transforming growth factor β; TH1, T-helper type 1 cells; TH2, T-helper type 2 cells; TNF, tumour necrosis factor.

HINTS AND TIPS

CYTOKINES VERSUS CHEMOKINES

Cytokines—chemical messengers that modulate the function of other cells.

Chemokines—a type of cytokine that acts as a chemoattractant for leucocytes.

Nitric oxide

Nitric oxide (NO) is a potent vasodilator that is released from endothelial cells and macrophages. NO acts as a regulator of inflammation, inhibiting leucocyte recruitment and actively reducing the effect of other proinflammatory mediators. It is also part of the innate immune system and has microbicidal properties.

Table 3.3 Acute-phase proteins

Proteins increased in concentration	Proteins decreased in concentration[a]
CRP	Albumin
SAA	Transferrin
C3, C4	Transthyretin
Haptoglobin	
Ceruloplasmin	
Fibrinogen	

[a] Decreasing the concentration of some proteins enables amino acids to become available for the synthesis of other proteins during the acute phase response.
CRP, C-reactive protein; SAA, serum amyloid A protein.

Acute-phase proteins

Proteins whose serum level dramatically increase or decrease during the acute-phase response are called acute-phase proteins (Table 3.3). These proteins are produced by the liver and are induced by proinflammatory cytokines such as IL-1, IL-6 and TNF-α, e.g., C-reactive protein (CRP). Their functions include:

- complement activation
- opsonization of microbes
- chemoattractants for inflammatory cells
- free radical scavengers.

CLINICAL NOTE

C-reactive protein can be measured in the serum as a non-specific marker of inflammation. Serial measurements can be used to monitor progress of an inflammatory disease over time.

CHRONIC INFLAMMATION

Causes of chronic inflammation

Chronic inflammation usually develops as a primary response to:

- microorganisms resistant to phagocytosis or intracellular killing mechanisms, e.g., Mycobacterium species
- foreign bodies, which can be endogenous (e.g., bone, adipose tissue, uric acid crystals) or exogenous (e.g., silica, suture materials, implanted prostheses)
- autoimmune diseases, e.g., Hashimoto thyroiditis, rheumatoid arthritis, contact hypersensitivity reactions
- primary granulomatous diseases, e.g., Crohn disease, sarcoidosis.

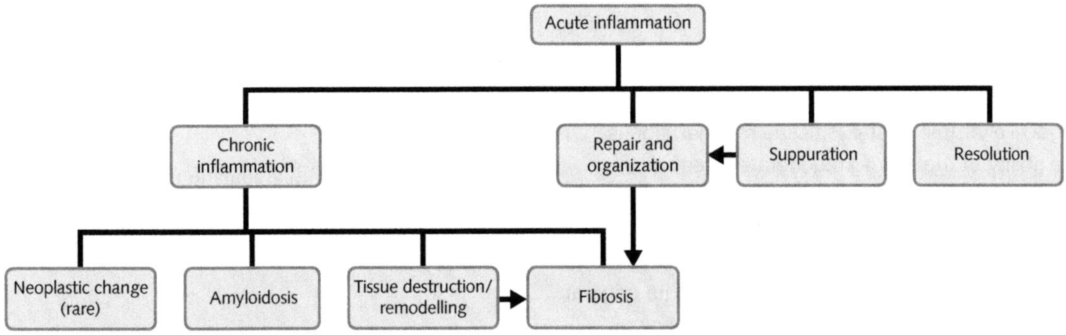

Fig. 3.7 Sequelae of inflammation.

Inflammation becomes chronic when it occurs over a prolonged period of time with simultaneous tissue destruction and attempted repair. It may occur secondary to acute inflammation owing to the persistence of the causative agent. Fig. 3.7 shows the sequelae of inflammation.

Mononuclear infiltration and granulation tissue

Chronic inflammation is dominated by:

- lymphocytes
- plasma cells (for antibody production)
- macrophages (for phagocytosis)—some macrophages fuse to form multinucleate giant cells.

Macrophages in inflamed tissue are transformed blood monocytes. The number of macrophages gradually increases during acute inflammation until they are the dominant cell type in chronic inflammation. These macrophages are activated by numerous stimuli, including IFN-γ, which is produced by activated lymphocytes.

The macrophages gradually remove damaged tissue by phagocytosis and produce growth factors to aid repair through fibrosis. This results in the slow replacement of damaged tissue with granulation tissue, which consists of new capillaries and new connective tissue formed from myofibroblasts and the collagen that they secrete.

The prolonged presence of activated macrophages in chronic inflammation leads to overproduction of biologically active products and therefore tissue damage (Fig. 3.8).

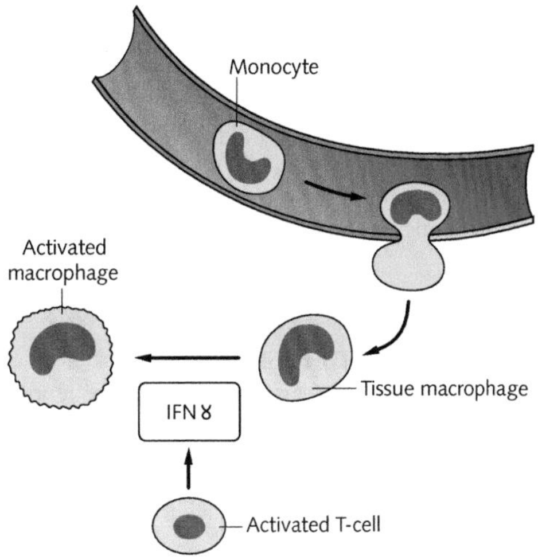

Fig. 3.8 Monocytes and macrophages in chronic inflammation.

> **HINTS AND TIPS**
>
> **CHRONIC INFLAMMATION IN IMPORTANT DISEASES**
>
> Chronic inflammation is a crucial process in many important diseases. Excellent examples are provided later in this book, including atherosclerosis (Chapter 9), tuberculosis (Chapter 10) and rheumatoid arthritis (Chapter 16).

WOUND HEALING

Nature of cells

The regenerative capacity of tissue can be categorized in three main ways: labile, stable and permanent:

- Labile tissue is constantly dividing, usually through stem cell division. This allows the replacement of tissue such as surface epithelia of the skin, gastrointestinal tract and uterus. Blood cells are derived from labile cells of the bone marrow.
- Stable tissues are in a state of quiescence, meaning that the cells slowly replicate to maintain tissue size. However, such tissue may rapidly regenerate if stimulated, e.g., liver.
- Permanent tissues consist of cells that have left the cell cycle and so are incapable of division. Neurones, cardiac and skeletal muscle cells are good examples.

CLINICAL NOTE

LIVER REGENERATION

A good example of stable tissue regeneration is the ability of the liver to regenerate after part of it is surgically removed (partial hepatectomy). In living-donor hepatic transplantations, one lobe of the donor's liver may be removed. Within weeks of the operation, the donor's liver returns to its original size by compensatory growth of the remaining tissue.

The ultimate consequence of tissue injury therefore depends on many factors. Although labile and stable cells may be capable of division, complex tissue architecture might not be replaced. The process of wound healing in the skin depends on the size of the injury; it occurs by two mechanisms.

1. Healing by primary intention

Apposed wound margins are joined by fibrin deposition, which is subsequently replaced by collagen and covered by epidermal growth (Fig. 3.9), e.g., surgical incision wound.

2. Healing by secondary intention

Healing by secondary intention (Fig. 3.10) involves the following:

- wound margins are unopposed, owing to extensive tissue damage
- tissue defect fills with granulation tissue
- epithelial regeneration covers the surface
- granulation tissue eventually contracts, resulting in scar formation.

CLINICAL NOTE

TYPES OF COLLAGEN

Types of collagen:

I Bone, skin, tendon
II Cartilage
III Reticulin fibres
IV Basement membrane
V Hair

Scar formation

Myofibroblasts within granulation tissue are attached to one another and to adjacent extracellular matrix. Their contraction draws together the surrounding matrix and thus reduces the size of the defect, but in doing so produces a scar.

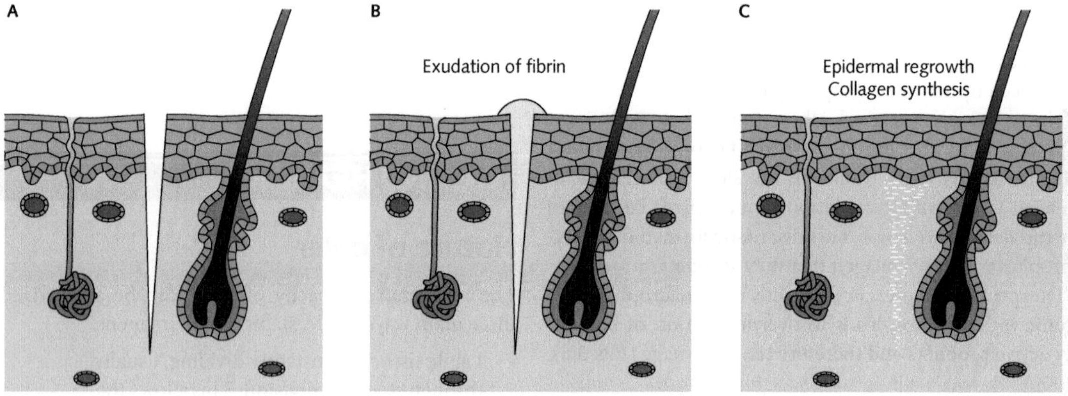

Fig. 3.9 Healing by primary intention. Skin incision healed by primary intention. (A) Incision. (B) Fibrin deposition (weak). (C) Collagen deposition (strong).

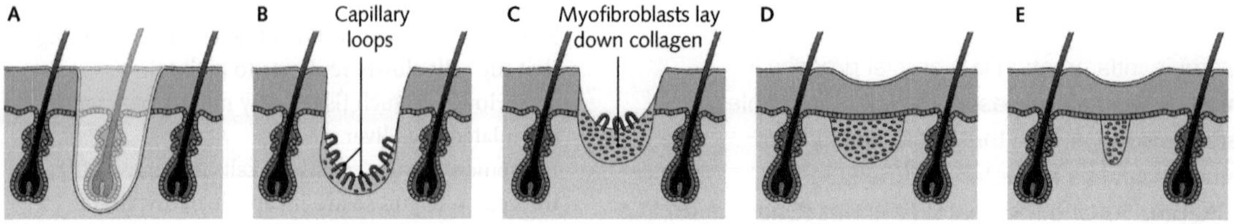

Fig. 3.10 Healing by secondary intention. Skin wound repaired by secondary intention. (A) Loss of tissue. (B) Granulation tissue. (C) Organization. (D) Early fibrous scar. (E) Scar contraction.

COMMON PITFALLS

HYPERTROPHIC SCAR VERSUS KELOID

Hypertrophic scars and keloids are both defined as abnormal scarring in response to trauma. However, hypertrophic scars do not grow beyond the boundaries of the initial wound, whereas keloids do.

PATTERNS OF INFLAMMATION

Fibrinous inflammation

Fibrinous inflammation is the deposition of increased amounts of fibrin on a tissue surface, e.g., in acute pleuritis secondary to acute lobar pneumonia.

If the fibrin is eventually removed, resolution is said to have occurred. However, if the fibrin persists, it may stimulate formation of scar tissue (known as organization).

Suppurative inflammation

Suppurative inflammation is characterized by the production of pus. This purulent inflammation contains neutrophils and is usually caused by infection with pyogenic bacteria such as *Staphylococcus aureus* and *Streptococcus pyogenes*. If it becomes localized by fibroblastic proliferation, it is called an abscess.

Haemorrhagic inflammation

If damage is severe, blood vessels within the area may rupture, e.g., haemorrhagic pneumonia, meningococcal septicaemia.

Granulomatous inflammation

Granulomatous inflammation is a form of chronic inflammation in which modified macrophages (termed epithelioid histiocytes) aggregate to form small clusters, or granulomas, surrounded by lymphoid cells. Granulomas may be necrotizing or non-necrotizing (Fig. 3.11). This type of inflammation usually occurs in response to indigestible particulate matter within macrophages. Causes of granulomatous inflammation include:

- microorganisms resistant to intracellular killing mechanisms, e.g., *Mycobacterium tuberculosis* and *Mycobacterium leprae*
- foreign bodies—endogenous (e.g., bone, adipose tissue, uric acid crystals) or exogenous (e.g., silica, suture materials, implanted prostheses)

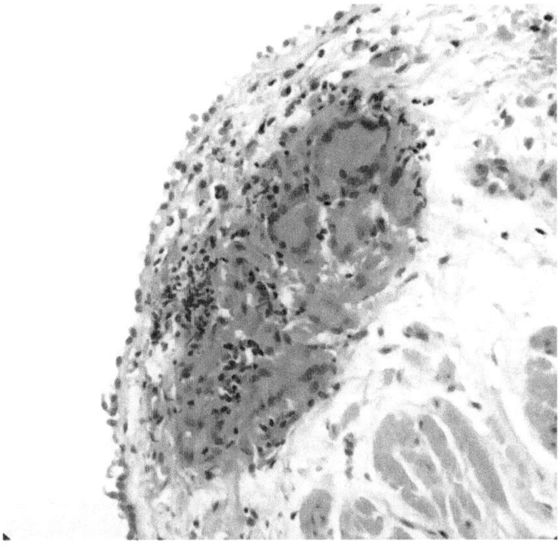

Fig. 3.11 Granuloma. Micrograph of a granuloma. Note the epithelioid histiocytes and multinucleated giant cells. Central necrosis is seen.

- idiopathic, e.g., in Crohn disease, sarcoidosis and granulomatosis with polyangiitis (formerly Wegener granulomatosis)
- drugs, e.g., allopurinol and sulfonamides can cause hepatic granulomas.

Granulomas are aggregates of epithelioid histiocytes. These histiocytes commonly fuse or divide without cytoplasmic separation to produce multinucleate giant cells. Examples include Langhans giant cells (typical in tuberculosis) and foreign-body giant cells (where indigestible foreign material is present).

CLINICAL NOTE

DIFFERENTIAL DIAGNOSES OF GRANULOMATOUS INFLAMMATION

Some causes of granulomatous inflammation include:

Tuberculosis
Fungal infection
Sarcoidosis
Crohn disease
Foreign body
Drugs
Hypersensitivity pneumonitis
Granulomatosis with polyangiitis
Toxoplasmosis
Cat-scratch disease
Note: this list is not exhaustive!

COMMON PITFALL

GRANULOMA VERSUS GRANULATION TISSUE

Commonly confused terms:

- *A granuloma* is an aggregation of epithelioid histiocytes. It is a feature of some chronic inflammatory diseases.
- *Granulation tissue* is the formation of new connective tissue with myofibroblasts and new capillary proliferation. It is a feature of wound healing.

SYSTEMIC EFFECTS OF INFLAMMATION

Both acute and chronic inflammation can produce a number of systemic effects, including:

- pyrexia—neutrophils and macrophages produce pyrogens (e.g., IL-1), which act on the hypothalamus;
- constitutional symptoms—malaise, nausea and anorexia;
- reactive hyperplasia of the mononuclear phagocyte system—enlargement of local and systemic lymph nodes;
- haematological changes—increased erythrocyte sedimentation rate, leucocytosis and acute-phase protein release (e.g., CRP);
- weight loss—occurs in severe chronic inflammation, such as tuberculosis.

CELL DEATH

Cells may be damaged either reversibly (sublethal damage) or irreversibly (lethal damage). This exists on a continuum with no absolute ultrastructural criteria by which reversible and irreversible cellular damage can be distinguished.

The type of damage depends on the:

- nature and duration of injury,
- type of cells affected,
- regenerative ability of tissues.

There are two types of cell death: necrosis and apoptosis. Necrosis tends to occur after severe cellular injury and is always pathological. Apoptosis can be a physiological process, e.g., post-lactational breast tissue involution, or a pathological process often following DNA damage and cell-cycle arrest.

Aetiology of cell death

Cell death can be caused by different mechanisms of injury, which are summarized in Fig. 3.12.

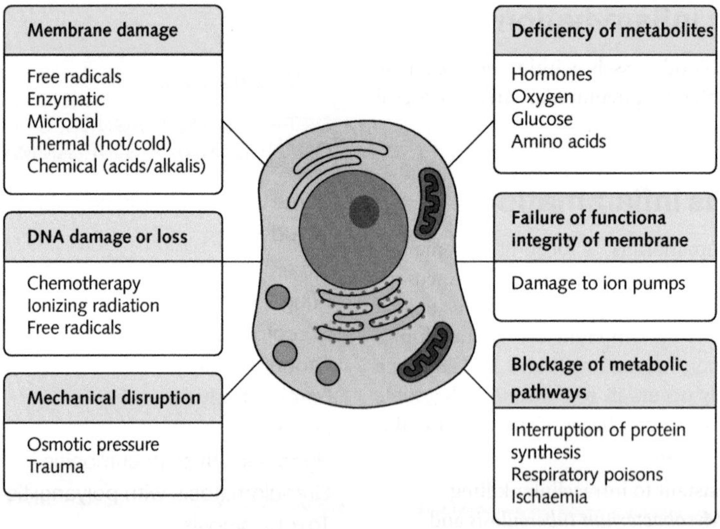

Fig. 3.12 Aetiology of cell death. Various cell and tissue types are differentially susceptible to various injurious agents, e.g., ischaemia.

Necrosis

Necrosis is the unregulated death of cells or tissues in a living organism. It is a pathological process following cellular injury that incites an inflammatory reaction. This is due to loss of plasma membrane integrity with rupture and leakage of cell contents into the surrounding tissues. The dead cells are degraded either by their own lysosomal content or that of other cells. It occurs in continuity with viable tissue.

Regardless of the aetiology of the cellular insult, necrosis occurs with:

- depletion of intracellular energy systems
- disruption of cytoplasmic organelles
- liberation of intracellular enzymes
- production of oxygen free radicals
- disintegration of the nucleus
- plasma membrane alterations, disruption or failure
- alteration in ionic transport mechanisms

Histological types of necrosis

Coagulative necrosis

This is the most common form of necrosis. Dead tissue is initially swollen and firm, but later becomes soft as a result of digestion by macrophages. Microscopically, the area of necrosis is demarcated adjacent to viable tissue. Tissue architecture is retained with the outlines of dead cells still visible but lacking nuclei ('ghost cells'). Coagulative necrosis is usually caused by ischaemia and is seen in the distribution of the affected vessel.

CLINICAL NOTE

COAGULATIVE NECROSIS AND MYOCARDIAL INFARCTION

Coagulative necrosis is the classic pattern seen in myocardial tissue following a myocardial infarction (MI). It takes several hours to develop. However, the loss of plasma membrane integrity in necrosis allows the leaking of cardiac enzymes into the bloodstream very quickly, making them useful as biochemical markers. The levels of these enzymes (e.g., troponin T/I) in the blood are routinely used to aid the diagnosis of a MI.

Liquefactive necrosis

This occurs in the central nervous system where necrotic neural tissue undergoes total liquefaction, e.g., following stroke/trauma, with a glial reaction at the periphery. A cystic cavity rather than a scar forms.

Caseous necrosis (caseation)

Macroscopically, the tissue appears soft, white and friable, reminiscent of cottage cheese, hence the term 'caseous' (cheese-like). Histologically, the tissue is amorphous with complete loss of architecture, appearing granular and eosinophilic, akin to pink mashed potatoes. Caseous necrosis is almost synonymous with tuberculosis and can be present at the core of granulomas.

Fibrinoid necrosis

This refers to a specific type of necrosis in blood vessel walls. Bright pink (eosinophilic) amorphous debris resembling fibrin is seen within the walls of blood vessels. Inflammation is inconspicuous. This occurs in malignant hypertension, autoimmune diseases, vasculitis and lupus.

CLINICAL NOTE

FAT NECROSIS

This is not a separate subtype of necrosis but is clinically important as it may mimic tumour, especially when located within the breast, as hard nodules are produced. There is not always an associated history of trauma. Fat necrosis is also seen with pancreatitis.

Apoptosis

Apoptosis is an energy-dependent mechanism of programmed cell death for the deletion of unwanted individual cells. The rate of apoptosis must be matched by the rate of cellular division to maintain a stable tissue size. Increased apoptosis results in net cell loss, e.g., tissue atrophy, and apoptosis inhibition results in cell accumulation, e.g., as seen in neoplasia (see Chapter 4). Apoptosis can be:

- physiological—such as in the maintenance of organ size, regulation of the immune system and the shedding of the endometrium at menstruation
- pathological—when cellular damage has occurred, often at the nuclear level (i.e., DNA damage) preventing the perpetuation of a genetically abnormal cell.

HINTS AND TIPS

APOPTOSIS VERSUS NECROSIS

Apoptosis is an energy-dependent process that does not result in an inflammatory response. Necrosis is an energy-independent process that causes inflammation.

Mechanisms of apoptosis

The execution of apoptosis is achieved by the activation of a cascade of proteases known as caspases (*c*ysteine-dependent *asp*artate-directed prote*ases*). The caspase cascade can be initiated by two pathways, each resulting in caspase-3 activation as the crucial final step (Fig. 3.13):

1. The extrinsic pathway—external 'death receptors' (e.g., TNF receptors/Fas receptors) are activated by an appropriate ligand.
2. The intrinsic pathway—pro-apoptotic molecules are released from mitochondria after the breakdown of normal anti-apoptotic signalling (e.g. Bcl-2 or DNA damage). This can occur by the loss of cellular signalling and exposure to radiation or toxins.

Morphologically, an apoptotic cell is characterized by:

- loss of membrane contact with neighbouring cells
- cell shrinkage owing to cytoskeletal breakdown
- nuclear chromatin condensation
- formation of apoptotic bodies with intact plasma membrane and organelles
- Blebbing.

These are eventually phagocytosed by adjacent cells and macrophages in the absence of inflammation.

A comparison of cell death by apoptosis and necrosis is given in Table 3.4.

MOLECULAR

P53

p53 is principally induced by DNA damage or conditions resulting in cellular stress. It has four main functions:

1. Cell cycle arrest:
   - Induces p21 expression.
2. Apoptosis:
   - Upregulates pro-apoptotic genes
   - Inhibition of anti-apoptotic genes
   - Induces FasR expression
   - Induces Bax causing cytochrome C release from mitochondria.
3. DNA repair:
   - Induces antioxidant proteins
   - Induces proteins involved in DNA repair.
4. Angiogenesis inhibition.

p53 mutations commonly occur in the DNA binding domain, resulting in transcriptional failure of downstream protein. One of these is MDM2, which facilitates p53 degradation. In cancer cells, mutated p53 accumulates as it can no longer initiate its own destruction.

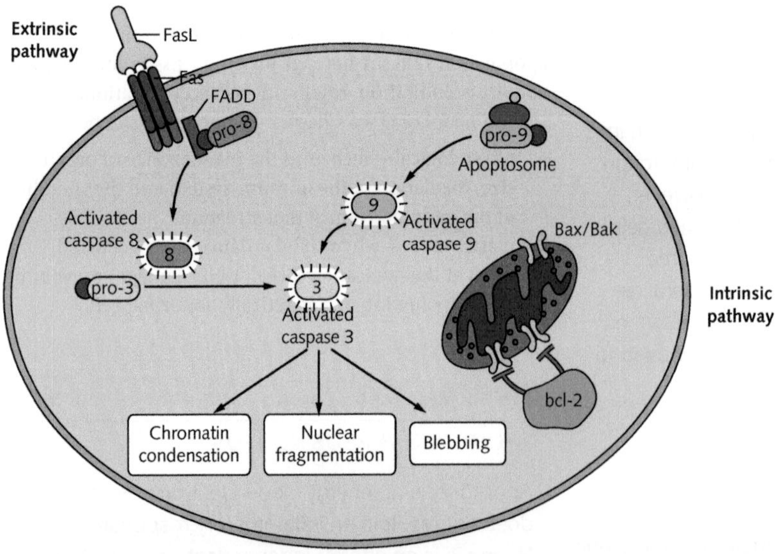

Fig. 3.13 Mechanism of apoptosis. The common caspase cascade may be triggered by the extrinsic ('death receptor') pathway or intrinsic (mitochondrial) pathway. *FasL,* Fas ligand, *FADD,* Fas-associated death domain protein.

Table 3.4 Comparison of cell death by necrosis and apoptosis

Feature	Necrosis	Apoptosis
Inducing stimulus	Pathological conditions	Pathological or physiological conditions
Number of cells	Groups of cells	Single cells
Plasma membrane	Loss of membrane integrity	Membrane remains intact
Morphology	Cell swelling and lysis Eosinophilia Nuclear disintegration	Cell shrinkage and nuclear fragmentation Pyknotic nuclei Chromatin condensation Blebbing Formation of characteristic apoptotic bodies Loss of contact with neighbouring cells/rounding up
Inflammation	Inflammatory response	No inflammatory response
Fate of cells	Phagocytosed by neutrophils and macrophages	Phagocytosed by neighbouring cells and macrophages
Biochemical mechanism	Energy-independent Loss of ion homeostasis Protein denaturation Lysosomal degradation	Energy-dependent Endonuclease activity

Chapter Summary

- The classic signs of acute inflammation are: rubor, calor, tumour, dolour and functio laesa.
- The neutrophil is the predominant inflammatory cell in acute inflammation.
- The five steps of leucocyte extravasation are: margination, rolling, adhesion, diapedesis and chemotaxis.
- Complement is a group of serum proteins that activate each other in an enzymatic cascade and are part of the innate immune system.
- The predominant chronic inflammatory cells are lymphocytes, plasma cells and macrophages.
- Wound healing is by primary intention, secondary intention and scar formation.
- Patterns of inflammation are fibrinous, suppurative, haemorrhagic and granulomatous.
- Apoptosis is programmed cell death/cell suicide and is an energy-dependent process.
- Necrosis is unregulated death of cells/tissue and is an energy-independent process.
- Types of necrosis include: coagulative, liquefactive, fibrinoid and caseous.
- Caseous necrosis is almost synonymous with tuberculosis.
- Apoptosis involves the activation of caspases.
- There are various groups of chemical mediators that help orchestrate the inflammatory response, e.g., bradykinin, histamine and interleukins (IL-1).

Cancer 4

DEFINITIONS AND NOMENCLATURE

Definitions

Tumour

A tumour can be defined as an abnormal mass of tissue resulting from autonomous disordered growth that persists after the initiating stimulus has been removed. A tumour results from genetic alteration and deregulated growth control mechanisms. There may be an inherited predisposition to tumour development (e.g., breast and ovarian cancer families), although this accounts for only a small proportion of tumours. Tumours are:

- Progressive—they are independent of normal growth control and continue to grow regardless of requirements and in the absence of any external stimuli.
- Purposeless—the abnormal mass serves no useful purpose.
- Parasitic—they are endogenous in origin but draw nourishment from the body while contributing nothing to its function.

All tumours have the suffix '-oma', which means a swelling.

Other related definitions are:

- neoplasm (i.e., new growth)—synonymous with tumour
- neoplasia—the process of tumour growth
- cancer—a malignant neoplasm
- anaplastic neoplasm— an undifferentiated neoplasm.

Anaplastic specimens highlight the typical changes of a malignant neoplasm: pleomorphism (variation in shape and size) of cells and nuclei, numerous abnormal mitoses, abnormal nuclear morphology and chromatin pattern and cellular disorganization (i.e., loss of cellular polarity).

Dysplasia

Dysplasia is the disordered maturation of cells resulting in an alteration in their size, shape and organization. It is regarded as a premalignant condition as it may precede neoplasia or proceed to invasion. It may, however, be reversible.

Metaplasia

Metaplasia is the reversible change in differentiation from one type of fully differentiated tissue to another. This is usually in response to chronic irritation, e.g., respiratory (columnar) epithelium to stratified squamous epithelium in the bronchi associated with cigarette smoking. Metaplasia therefore often represents an adaptive response to environmental stress.

Hyperplasia

This refers to an increase in the *number of cells* in a tissue or organ, which may result in an increase in the overall size, e.g., breast tissue during pregnancy.

Hypertrophy

Hypertrophy is an increase in tissue or organ size owing to an increase in the *size of cells*. Crucially, there is no increase in the number of cells in the tissue. Cells that are permanent (e.g., myocardial fibres) cannot divide and so undergo hypertrophy to increase tissue size (e.g., left ventricular hypertrophy as a response to hypertension).

> **COMMON PITFALLS**
>
> **HETEROTOPIA VERSUS HAMARTOMA**
>
> Heterotopia and hamartoma are terms that are commonly confused; they are not tumours:
>
> *Heterotopia:* Mature tissue of one type in an abnormal location, e.g., pancreatic tissue in a Meckel diverticulum, gastric epithelium in the duodenum (normal tissue; normal architecture; abnormal site).
>
> *Hamartoma:* A focal disorganized architectural mix of the normal tissue components belonging to that site, which can appear tumour-like, e.g., bile duct hamartoma (von Meyenburg complex), a collection of haphazardly arranged bile ducts within the liver forming a tumour-like mass (normal tissue; abnormal architecture; normal site).

Benign versus malignant

Tumours are classified as either benign or malignant according to their appearance and behaviour (Table 4.1). Benign tumours are usually well-differentiated, localized neoplasms that do not invade the surrounding tissues or metastasize to other organs. Metastasis is the process whereby malignant cells spread from their site of origin (a primary tumour) to distant sites and grow into secondary tumours.

Table 4.1 Characteristics of benign versus malignant tumours

Benign	Malignant
Macroscopic features	
• Localized	• Widespread
• No invasion	• Invasion
• No metastases	• Metastases
• Slow growth rate (usually)	• Rapid growth rate/ turnover (usually)
Microscopic features	
• Well-differentiated	• Poorly differentiated
• Few and normal mitoses	• Many and abnormal mitoses
• Normal nuclear chromatin	• Coarse, clumped hyperchromatic nuclear chromatin
• Uniform size cells	• Cells and nuclei vary in size (pleomorphism)
• Well circumscribed	• Infiltrative
• Compression of adjacent tissue	• Invasion and destruction of adjacent tissue

Malignant tumours are by definition able to invade and metastasize to distant sites. This distinction is crucial because metastatic disease is associated with significant morbidity and mortality.

Stage, grade and differentiation

These relate to various characteristics of a malignant tumour which help to predict behaviour and prognosis and help to guide treatment.

- ***Stage:*** An assessment of how far the tumour has spread from its primary site, i.e., like in a game of baseball - has it reached first base, second base, etc.?
  There are a variety of staging systems in use depending on the origin of the tumour, e.g., colon, endometrium. The most commonly used is the ***T****umour* ***N****odes* ***M****etastasis* (TNM) system. The specific criteria for T, N and M vary between organ systems and TNM editions; however, the overall principles are the same.
  'T' describes the primary tumour by a numerical value (usually from 1 to 4) which, depending on the type/ site of tumour, relates to a prognostic feature of the tumour, e.g., depth of invasion, overall size, adjacent organ/structures invasion or mitotic index. The higher the stage the more advanced the tumour and the worse the prognosis.
  'N' describes positive lymph nodes—i.e., those that contain metastatic tumour deposits. The number assigned to N, e.g., N1, is not a direct record of the number of positive lymph nodes but is defined separately for each tumour, e.g., N1 could equal 1–4 positive lymph nodes.
  'M' describes metastatic disease. This is commonly present (M1) or absent (M0); however, there are exceptions.
- ***Grade and differentiation:*** An assessment of how well the tumour resembles its tissue of origin. Grade can be described as high or low or be assigned a number based on a scoring system of features, e.g., G2 breast carcinoma. A tumour can be well-differentiated, moderately differentiated, poorly differentiated or undifferentiated, e.g., well-differentiated squamous cell carcinoma. The better the differentiation the more alike the tumour is to the tissue of origin. Grade and differentiation go hand-in-hand, such that high-grade tumours tend to be moderately to poorly differentiated and low-grade tumours are well differentiated.

HINTS AND TIPS

PREFIXES AND SUFFIXES TO TUMOUR NODES METASTASIS (TNM) SYSTEM

Some useful prefixes and suffixes for TNM system to remember:

'y' prefix e.g., yT yN: staging is postchemotherapy.
'p' prefix e.g., pT3 pN1: staging is pathological, i.e., histological assessment.
's' prefix e.g., sN: sentinel lymph node.
'x' suffix e.g., Nx Mx: not assessed.
'is' suffix e.g., Tis: tumour is in situ, i.e., no invasion has occurred.

HINTS AND TIPS

POORLY DIFFERENTIATED CANCER

The more poorly differentiated a tumour is, the poorer the prognosis. Stage is usually high and survival rate is low. Other independent features also predict a worse outcome, e.g., vascular invasion.

Nomenclature of tumours

Tumour nomenclature is an imperfect art based on tissue of origin and tumour behaviour (Table 4.2). Histology provides information about the type of cell from which the tumour has arisen, whereas behaviour provides information as to whether the cell is benign or malignant.

Table 4.2 Important tumour nomenclature

Histological type	Benign	Malignant
Epithelial		
Glandular	Adenoma	Adenocarcinoma
Non-glandular	Papilloma	Carcinoma
Connective tissue		
Adipose	Lipoma	Liposarcoma
Cartilage	Chondroma	Chondrosarcoma
Bone	Osteoma	Osteosarcoma
Smooth muscle	Leiomyoma	Leiomyosarcoma
Skeletal muscle	Rhabdomyoma	Rhabdomyosarcoma
Blood vessels	Angioma/haemangioma	Angiosarcoma
Nerve	Neurofibroma	Neurofibrosarcoma
Others		
Haemopoietic	[a]	Leukaemia
Lymphoreticular	[a]	Lymphoma
Melanocytes	[a]	Melanoma
Mesothelial	[a]	Mesothelioma
Germ cell	Benign teratoma	Malignant teratoma

[a] *These tumours are always malignant and do not have benign counterparts.*

HINTS AND TIPS

TUMOUR NAMING

A few simple rules to follow:

- '-oma' suffix for benign tumours, but there are some non-neoplastic '-omas' (e.g., granuloma) and some malignant '-omas' (e.g., mesothelioma and melanoma).
- Carcinomas—malignant tumours of epithelial origin; prefixed by tissue of origin. (e.g. squamous cell carcinoma).
- '-sarcoma' suffix for malignant tumours of mesenchymal (connective tissue) origin.

Classification of carcinomas

Carcinomas are malignant tumours of epithelial tissue. Carcinomas of non-glandular epithelium are prefixed by the name of the epithelial cell type, e.g., urothelial carcinoma. Malignant tumours of glandular epithelium are termed adenocarcinomas.

Intraepithelial neoplasia

Intraepithelial neoplasia describes dysplastic to neoplastic changes occurring within an epithelium. This covers the spectrum of changes short of invasive carcinoma:

- mild dysplasia
- moderate dysplasia
- severe dysplasia/carcinoma in situ.

CLINICAL NOTE

CERVICAL INTRAEPITHELIAL NEOPLASIA (CIN)

CIN is a premalignant condition categorized according to the thickness of dysplasia seen within the squamous epithelium of the cervical transformation zone. Three grades are observed:

- CIN I—mildly dysplastic
- CIN II—moderately dysplastic
- CIN III—severely dysplastic (carcinoma in situ at high risk of invasion).

CIN may exist for many years before cervical cancer develops. Ninety percent of CIN I lesions spontaneously regress, compared with CIN III lesions, which are more likely to progress to invasive disease (Fig 4.1).

Carcinoma in situ

This is an epithelial neoplasm with all the cellular features associated with malignancy, but which has not yet invaded through the epithelial basement membrane. The in-situ phase may not progress, or it may last for several years before invasion commences.

Invasive carcinoma

This is an epithelial neoplasm that invades through the basement membrane into the underlying stroma. The tumour can gain access to the vasculature and lymphatics and metastasize to distant tissues (Fig. 4.2).

EPIDEMIOLOGICAL ASPECTS OF CANCER

Cancer in the UK

Cancer is the biggest killer in the UK, accounting for 28% of all deaths; cardiovascular disease is the second, accounting for 26%.

- Almost one in three of the population will develop cancer during their lifetime.
- More than one in four of the population will die of cancer.
- Incidence of cancer varies between males and females.
- Half of cancers in the UK are diagnosed in people over 70 years of age.
- Smoking is the largest single preventable cause of cancer in the UK.
- Half of people with cancer survive >10 years.

Breast, prostate, bowel and lung are the most common types of cancer in both females and males. Fig. 4.3 shows the 10 commonest cancers in males and females.

Cancer worldwide

Lung cancer is the commonest cancer worldwide. The incidence of different cancers varies from country to country. This variation provides clues to the causes of cancers. For example, in Japan, gastric carcinoma is 30 times more common than in the UK, whereas pancreatic cancer is much rarer. However, migration of a subset of the Japanese population to different geographical areas (e.g., the United States, the UK) alters the incidence of these diseases within that population. These findings suggest that environmental factors (such as diet, occupation, social and geographic effects) rather than genetic causes account for most of the observed differences between countries.

Screening programmes

The purpose of a screening programme is to detect cancer at a preinvasive or early stage to increase the success of treatment and improve survival. Current screening programmes in the UK include cervical (25–64 years), breast (50–70 years) and bowel (60–74 years) cancer screening.

MOLECULAR BASIS OF CANCER

Oncogenes and tumour suppressor genes

Cell proliferation and division is usually tightly regulated by two sets of opposing functioning genes:

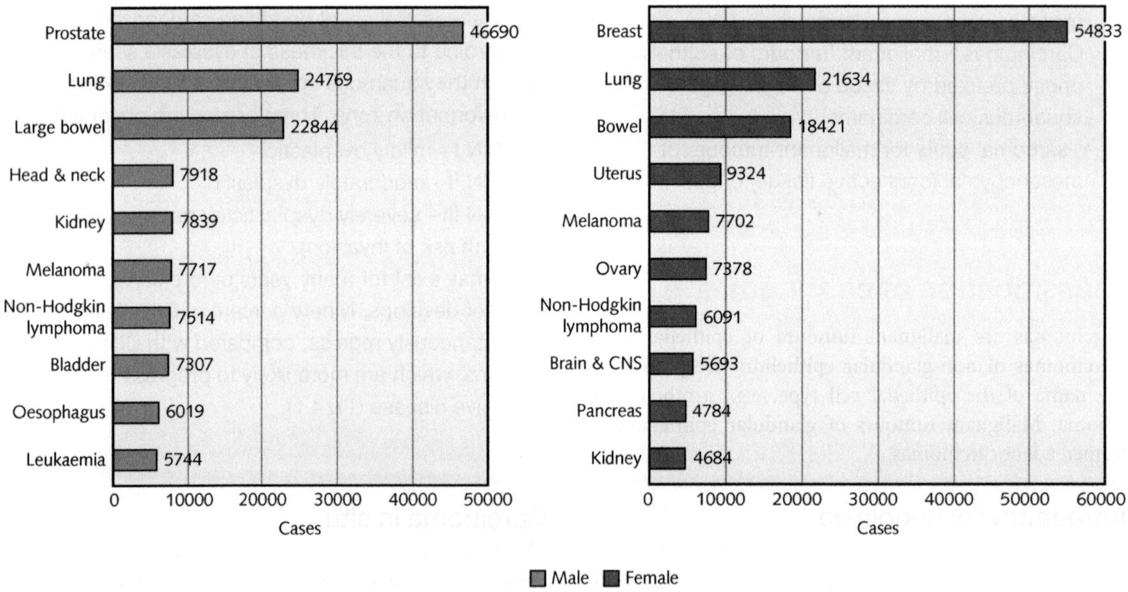

Fig. 4.3 Incidence of the 10 commonest types of cancer in the UK. (Data from Cancer Research UK 2014.)

1. Growth promoting genes, called proto-oncogenes.
2. Growth inhibiting genes, called tumour suppressor genes (TSGs).

Gain of function in proto-oncogenes and loss of function in TSGs can both lead to transformation of a normal cell into a neoplastic cell.

An in-depth discussion of the molecular basis of cancer can be found in Chapter 6, Molecular pathology.

Oncogenes

Oncogenes are the mutated versions of the proto-oncogenes that are normally expressed in cells to positively regulate growth and differentiation. Proto-oncogenes (Table 4.3) code for different components of the pathways that positively regulate growth, such as growth factors, transcription factors and receptor molecules. In healthy cells, the transcription of these genes is tightly controlled. Oncogenes produce oncoproteins, which lead to abnormal cell growth and survival. The mutations in oncogenes tend to be dominant, such that mutation in one allele is sufficient for gain of function to occur.

Normally functioning proto-oncogenes can become activated into cancer-causing oncogenes in two ways:

- *Mutation* can produce an oncoprotein that is functionally altered and abnormally active. For example, intracellular signalling is affected by the hyperactive mutant Ras protein.
- *Increased production*: a normal oncoprotein can be produced in abnormally large quantities owing to gene amplification (e.g., the *myc* oncogene in neuroblastomas) or enhanced transcription (formation of the Philadelphia chromosome from a translocation between chromosomes 9 and 22 in chronic myeloid leukaemia).

Table 4.3 Proto-oncogenes

Proto-oncogene[a]	Function	Examples of associated cancers
ras	Intracellular signal transduction by GTP/GDP binding	Colorectal carcinoma
*Erb*B2/HER2	Receptor tyrosine kinase	Breast carcinoma
c-myc	Transcription factor	Burkitt lymphoma, colorectal carcinoma, small cell–lung carcinoma
ret	Growth factor tyrosine kinase receptor	Papillary thyroid carcinoma, MEN2
b-raf	Kinase responsible for intracellular signal transduction	Melanoma
Bcl2	Apoptosis inhibitor	B-cell lymphomas

[a] These are a few examples of proto-oncogenes with some of their cancer associations, but it is in no way an exhaustive list.GTP/GDP; guanosine triphosphate/diphosphate; MEN, multiple endocrine neoplasia.

Oncogenes include genes that express:

- transcription factors, e.g., *c-myc*
- tyrosine kinase proteins, e.g., Src
- growth factors, e.g., platelet-derived growth factor
- receptors for growth factors, e.g., *c-erb*B2/HER2, which is a member of the epidermal growth factor receptor (EGFR) family
- guanosine triphosphate (GTP) binding signal-transduction proteins, e.g., Ras.

Expression of abnormal oncogene products confers the behaviour and appearance of transformed cells. These include:

- independence from the requirement of extrinsic growth factors
- production of proteases that assist tissue invasion
- reduced cell cohesiveness, which assists metastasis
- loss of contact inhibition, therefore they are able to grow at higher cell densities
- abnormal cellular orientation
- increased plasma membrane and cellular motility.

HINTS AND TIPS

SOMATIC VERSUS GERMLINE MUTATIONS

Mutations can be germline, i.e., encoded within a person's DNA from birth, or somatic, i.e., acquired during life. Germline mutations can cause cancer syndromes, with tumours being more numerous and occurring at a younger age, e.g., *ret* in MEN2 (multiple endocrine neoplasia 2) syndrome.

Tumour suppressor genes

TSGs (e.g., *p53* and *RB1*) maintain the integrity of the genome as they encode proteins that prevent or suppress the growth of cells. They cause cell-cycle arrest in abnormally dividing cells and repair DNA damage. They also promote apoptosis (see Chapter 3) in cells with sustained DNA damage. Examples of dysfunctional TSGs involved in human cancers are given in Table 4.4.

Inactivation of TSGs results in increased susceptibility to cancer formation. Unlike proto-oncogenes, mutations result in loss of function and both alleles are usually required to be mutated before an effect is seen. This is known as the Knudson two-hit hypothesis (Fig. 4.4); Knudson first proposed a genetically increased susceptibility to cancer formation after studying retinoblastoma in children.

Table 4.4 Tumour suppressor genes

Tumour suppressor gene	Function	Associated cancers (sporadic mutations)	Associated cancer syndromes (germline mutations)
APC	Regulates β-catenin involved in cell cycle and adhesion	Colorectal carcinomas	Familial adenomatous polyposis
MLH1, PMS2, MSH2, MSH6	DNA mismatch repair	Colorectal carcinomas	Lynch syndrome
NF1	Growth regulation	Neurofibromas, sarcomas	Neurofibromatosis type 1
RB1	Transcription regulator	Retinoblastoma, osteosarcoma	Familial retinoblastoma
BRCA1 and 2	DNA repair	Breast and ovarian carcinomas	Familial breast carcinoma
p53	Growth arrest, transcription regulation and apoptosis	Many tumours	Li–Fraumeni syndrome
PTEN	Phosphatase, and apoptosis initiator	Breast carcinoma, glioblastoma	Cowden syndrome

CLINICAL NOTE

RETINOBLASTOMA

Retinoblastoma is a rare malignant tumour of the retina. In familial cases (bilateral), a germline mutation in the *RB1* gene is present, meaning that only one further somatic mutation is required for tumour formation. Other cases of retinoblastoma are unilateral and sporadic, needing two somatic mutations on an initially fully functioning *RB1* gene. This requirement for separate mutations in both alleles of a tumour suppressor gene has been termed the 'two-hit' hypothesis of oncogenesis.

Loss of function of TSGs or their protein products can result in uncontrolled neoplastic cell growth. TSGs can lose their normal function by a variety of mechanisms:

- Mutations (hereditary or acquired).
- Binding of normal TSG protein to proteins encoded by viral genes, e.g., human papilloma virus proteins E6/E7.
- Complexing of normal TSG protein to mutant TSG protein in heterozygous cells.

One of the most studied TSGs is the *p53* gene, which is located at 17p; it is called 'the guardian of the genome' as it is involved in maintaining genetic integrity and preventing the accumulation of oncogenic mutations. *p53* is mutated or functionally altered in over 50% of all human cancers. In addition, a familial inherited mutation is found in Li–Fraumeni syndrome, in which there is an increased predisposition to several tumour types, e.g., sarcomas, breast carcinomas and brain tumours.

p53 is induced by cellular stress, such as hypoxia and DNA damage, and responds either through cell-cycle growth arrest at the G1 checkpoint or through the initiation of apoptosis. For example, the p53 protein product recognizes DNA damage (thymine dimers) caused by ultraviolet radiation and activates apoptotic pathways before the cell can divide and proliferate (Fig. 4.5).

HINTS AND TIPS

PROTO-ONCOGENES AND TUMOUR SUPPRESSOR GENES (TSGS)

Cellular proliferation is tightly regulated by two sets of opposing functioning genes. Proto-oncogenes are growth-promoting genes, whereas TSGs are growth-suppressing genes. Deregulated function of proto-oncogenes and TSGs leads to cell transformation and tumorigenesis.

Tumorigenesis

Tumorigenesis is a multistage process that results from accumulated mutations. Tumours arise from single cells, which proliferate to form a clone of cells with identical genetic abnormalities. As tumours develop, they undergo further somatic mutations, which cause abnormalities in other proto-oncogenes and/or TSGs. These additional mutations result in cells that are genetically different from each other, but which are part of the same tumour: this is heterogeneity.

Fast-growing, less-differentiated cells take over and eliminate the slower-growing, better-differentiated cells.

Chemotherapy will kill the majority of tumour cells. However, tumour cells that are resistant to chemotherapy will survive and be selected (because of ablation of competing, nonresistant cells), resulting in the regrowth of a tumour that is resistant to chemotherapy (Fig. 4.6). This

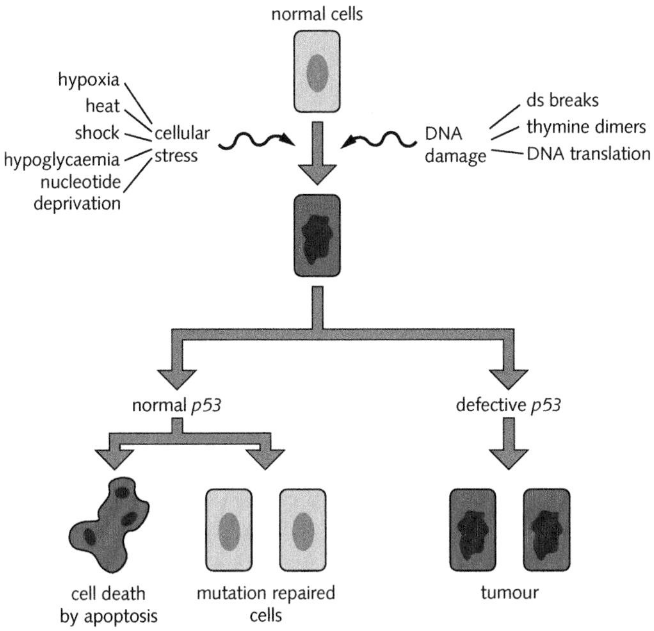

Fig. 4.5 Role of *p53*. Cellular stress ± DNA damage induces *p53* activation that results in transcription of various genes. As a result, cells either undergo G1 arrest and DNA repair or apoptotic death. If *p53* is defective, the genetic damage persists and oncogenic mutations are allowed to accumulate with eventual tumour generation. *ds*, Double strand. (Adapted from Underwood, 2009.)

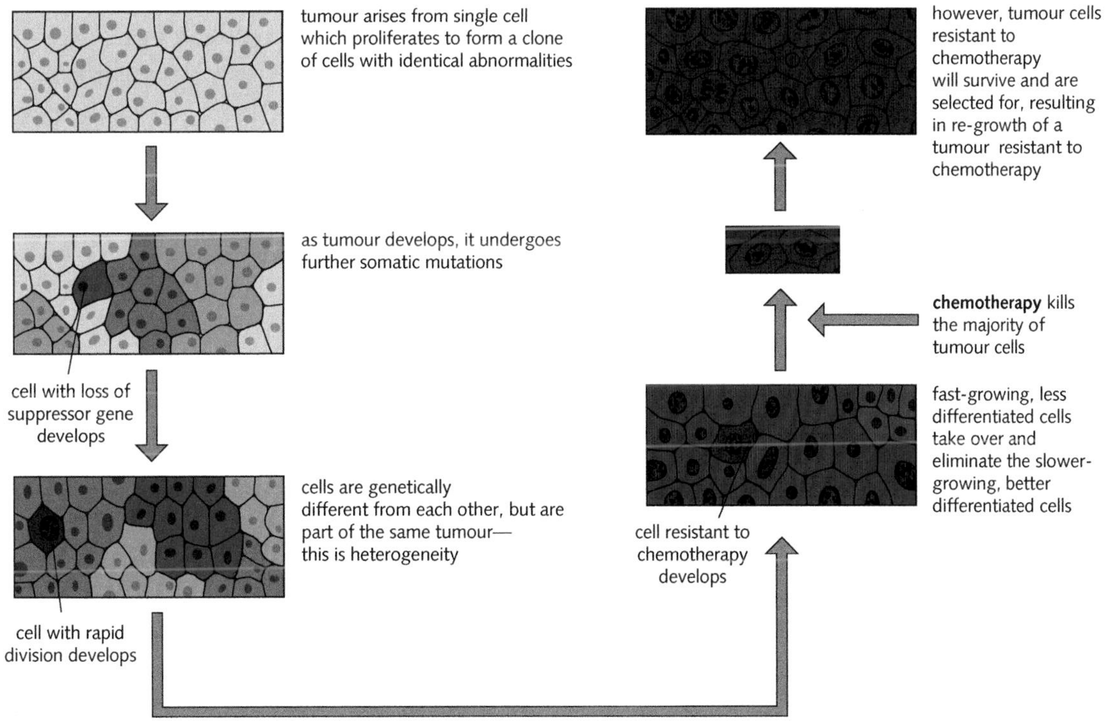

Fig. 4.6 Tumour progression and genetic heterogeneity.

highlights the concept of 'minimal residual disease', i.e., the small number of tumour cells that survive an intervention such as chemotherapy.

The progressive nature of tumorigenesis is clearly illustrated in Vogelstein's model of the development of colonic cancer. The accumulation over time of mutations in oncogenes such as *K-ras* and loss-of-function mutations in TSGs such as *APC* results in the eventual formation of colon carcinoma (Fig. 4.7).

TUMOUR GROWTH AND SPREAD

Kinetics of tumour growth and angiogenesis

Angiogenesis is the formation of new blood vessels and is an important physiological process in normal embryogenesis, the female reproductive cycle and wound healing. However, pathological angiogenesis is a key player in many disorders, including cancer. This is because a solid tumour cannot grow beyond a few millimetres in diameter without a blood supply to maintain nutrient and oxygen provision and remove metabolic waste.

In normal cells, angiogenesis is a highly regulated mechanism. In contrast, tumour cells can release proangiogenic factors, which induce unregulated vascular proliferation. This is sometimes called the 'angiogenic switch'. The angiogenic switch results in the production of proangiogenic molecules such as vascular endothelial growth factor.

Eventually, the tumour outgrows its blood supply and areas of necrosis may appear, resulting in slower growth but a more malignant phenotype. This is because only the strongest cells survive the hypoxic conditions.

Mechanisms and pathways of invasion and metastasis

Invasion

The ability to invade is the only absolute criterion for malignancy. Invading malignant cells have the following properties:

- Abnormal or increased cellular motility—owing to loss of contact inhibition.
- Altered cellular adhesion—owing to changes in surface adhesion molecules.
- Increased secretion of proteolytic enzymes, e.g., metalloproteinases.

Metalloproteinases, such as collagenases and gelatinases, are the most important enzymes in neoplastic invasion. They digest the surrounding connective tissue, thus aiding invasion of the basement membrane.

Metastasis

Only a proportion of neoplastic cells within a malignant tumour can metastasize, having acquired genetic changes that facilitate invasion and spread. Metastatic deposits can become very high grade and aggressive, such that it is not possible to identify the primary lesion in some patients who present with extensive metastatic disease.

To metastasize through vessels, neoplastic cells undergo the following sequence of events:

- Detachment of tumour cells from neighbouring cells.
- Invasion of the tissue basement membrane and then surrounding connective tissue.
- Invasion into blood/lymphatic vessels.
- Evasion of the host's defence mechanisms, often by forming a tumour cell embolus with platelets or host lymphoid cells.
- Adherence to endothelium at a distant site.
- Infiltration of cells from vessel lumen into surrounding tissue.
- Growth in that tissue.

Following infiltration, the malignant cells proliferate and secrete more angiogenic growth factors for vascularization; hence a new tumour is formed. However, not all cancer cells will grow at all distant sites. This is the seed and soil effect: conditions must be appropriate for cell proliferation.

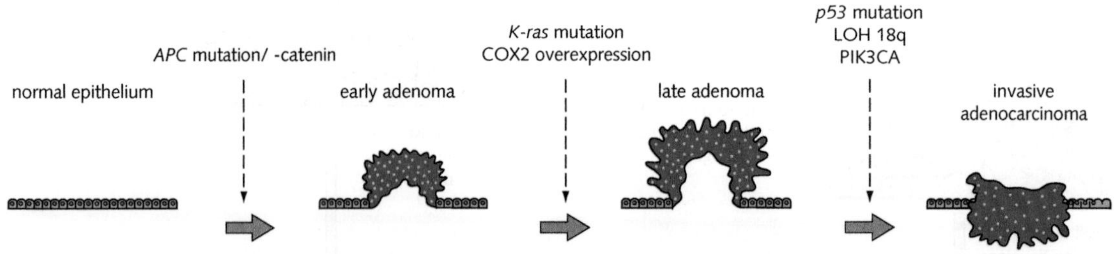

Fig. 4.7 Vogelgram. Multistep genetic model of colorectal tumorigenesis. The accumulation of key genetic mutations corresponds to the altered behaviour and a progressive increase in chromosomal instability leading to the development of cancer. *APC*, adenomatous polyposis coli; *LOH*, loss of heterozygosity; *PIK3CA*, phosphatidylinositol-4,5-bisphosphate 3-kinase catalytic subunit alpha. (Adapted from Underwood, 2009.)

> **CLINICAL NOTE**
>
> **SENTINEL LYMPH NODES (SLNS)**
>
> The SLN is the hypothetical first lymph node to which malignant cells will spread. These are selectively targeted and removed using radioactive tracers and coloured dyes at surgery. If the SLN is negative for tumour then metastasis to subsequent lymph nodes within the group is unlikely. This reduces the need for lymph node clearances and spares the patient unnecessary morbidity Fig. 4.8.

Main routes of metastasis

There are four main routes of metastasis:

1. Local invasion—most common pattern of spread of malignant tumours is by direct growth into adjacent tissues.
2. Lymphatic spread—forms secondary tumours in lymph nodes.
3. Haematogenous (blood-borne) spread—cells enter the bloodstream and form secondary tumours in organs perfused by blood that has drained from a tumour.
4. Transcoelomic spread (spread across a cavity)—in pleural, pericardial and peritoneal cavities.

CARCINOGENIC AGENTS

Carcinogens are substances known to cause an increased incidence of cancer.

Carcinogens can exert their effect either by genetic mechanisms causing DNA alteration (the majority of carcinogens) or epigenetic mechanisms by acting on the protein product of growth-regulating genes (see Chapter 6).

DNA repair mechanisms and their failure

DNA is sensitive to damage from both endogenous and exogenous agents, as well as inherent error within the polymerase (replication) enzymes. Fortunately, cells have multiple DNA repair mechanisms that deal with DNA damage. Repair occurs rapidly in the vast majority of cases, but damage is sometimes irreparable and major chromosomal and chromatid alterations occur. In these situations, the repair enzymes also play a role in inducing apoptosis.

A set of mismatch repair enzymes exists, which is concerned with correcting base to base mismatches and insertion and deletion errors (e.g., MLH1). This maintains the fidelity of the genetic code and integrity of the genome. An unchecked error can result in phenotypic alteration of a cell and subsequently become a permanent mutation in dividing cells. Defects within the mismatch repair genes increase the spontaneous mutation rate, predisposing the cell to neoplastic transformation.

Mutations within the mismatch repair genes can be hereditary e.g., Lynch syndrome (see Chapter 11) or sporadic, as is seen in 15% of colorectal cancers. Mismatch repair defects can lead to microsatellite instability. Microsatellites are short (<10) bases of non-coding repetitive DNA which are scattered throughout the genome and are prone to errors because of their repetitive nature.

> **CLINICAL NOTE**
>
> **LYNCH SYNDROME**
>
> An excellent example of failed DNA repair mechanisms is the autosomal dominant condition Lynch syndrome (discussed in Chapter 11). A DNA repair gene (e.g., *MSH2, MLH1*) is inactivated, resulting in failed mismatch repair and predisposition to multiple somatic mutations leading to various cancers.

Chemical carcinogens

Most chemical carcinogens are procarcinogens and require metabolic conversion into an active form (ultimate carcinogens), usually by the cytochrome P450 system, which shows significant variability in activity (gene polymorphisms) between individuals. Some people are therefore inherently more susceptible to producing ultimate carcinogens.

Some carcinogens act directly to induce cellular damage. Examples of chemical carcinogens are given in Table 4.5.

Stages of chemical carcinogenesis

The stages of chemical carcinogenesis (Fig. 4.9) are:

1. Initiation—induction of a genetic alteration in an oncogene or TSG.
2. Promotion—a stimulus for proliferation of the initiated cell; this may be an external agent or a further random mutational genetic abnormality.
3. Persistence—when proliferation of tumour cells becomes autonomous, i.e., it no longer requires the presence of initiators or promoters.

Radiation

Radiation can be:

- ionizing—natural radiation, therapeutic radiation and nuclear radiation
- nonionizing—ultraviolet (UV) radiation

Radiation can result in DNA damage in two ways:

1. directly—causing strand breaks, base alterations and cross-linking of DNA
2. indirectly—ionization of H_2O results in formation of reactive oxygen free radicals which damage DNA and cause structural cell damage

Table 4.5 Examples of chemical carcinogens

Chemical compound	Cancer type
Indirect carcinogens	
Polycyclic hydrocarbons	
Soot [benzo(a)pyrene; dibenzanthracene]	Skin, colon
Tobacco smoke	Lung, bladder, oral cavity, larynx, oesophagus
Aromatic amines	
Benzidine, 2-naphthylamine	Bladder
Nitrosamines	
Chemotherapeutic agents	Oesophagus, stomach
Cyclophosphamide, chlorambucil, thiotepa, busulphan	Leukaemias
Vinyl chloride	
	Liver (angiosarcoma)
Aflatoxins	
	Liver (HCC)
Unknown mechanisms	
Heavy metals	
Nickel, cadmium, chromium	Lung
Arsenic	Skin

HCC, Hepatocellular carcinoma.

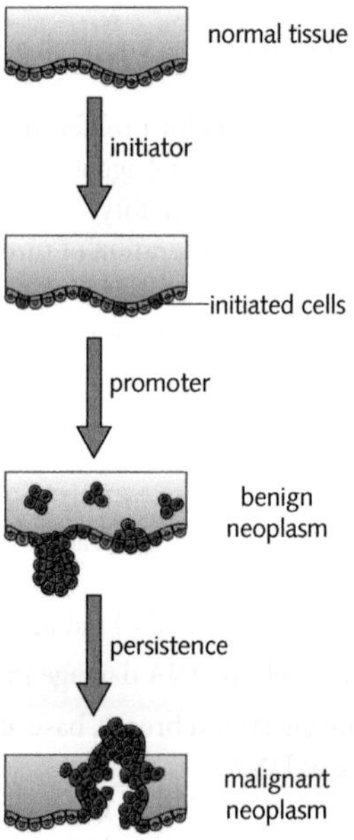

Fig. 4.9 Stages of chemical carcinogenesis.

Ionizing radiation

X-ray radiation

Radiotherapy can cause cancer as well as curing it! It is associated with radiation-induced malignant neoplasms, often sarcomas. These tumours may occur months or years after radiation therapy, in the lungs, breast, CNS, bones, kidneys and liver.

ETHICS

RADIOTHERAPY – CAUSE AND CURE OF CANCER

Although radiation therapy can be beneficial (e.g., treating cancer or providing palliative care), it may also induce cancer. Brachytherapy is used to target cancer and decrease exposure to radiation, and personalized radiotherapy is also being developed. Always discuss the potential risks and benefits of radiation therapy with patients, as it is a double-edged sword!

Using this therapy is potentially ethically challenging as, whilst it could effect a cure for the current cancer, it may also induce another cancer in the future. This is particularly relevant when considering treatment of children.

Radioisotopes

Radioactive iodine, which is used to treat hyperthyroidism, is associated with an increased risk of cancer development as much as 15–25 years after treatment.

Nuclear radiation

Survivors of the Hiroshima and Nagasaki atomic bombs, and of the accident at the Chernobyl nuclear power plant, have shown a greatly increased incidence of cancer, including leukaemia and carcinoma of the thyroid, breast and lung.

Nonionizing radiation

Ultraviolet radiation

UV radiation is associated with many different kinds of skin cancer, particularly:

- squamous cell carcinoma
- basal cell carcinoma
- melanoma.

Skin cancer is the most common type of cancer in the UK and the United States. It is more common in fair-skinned individuals.

UV light (especially UVB) is thought to cause DNA damage by inducing the formation of linkages between pyrimidine bases in the DNA molecule. The risk is greatly increased in patients with xeroderma pigmentosum, a rare autosomal recessive disease characterized by deficiency of DNA repair enzymes.

Bacteria

Some bacteria can cause neoplasia; the best known is *Helicobacter pylori* (group 1 carcinogen), which causes chronic gastritis and predisposes to development of gastric cancer (both gastric adenocarcinoma and mucosa-associated lymphoid tissue (MALT) lymphoma). Patients with gastritis are tested for *H. pylori* and treated with triple therapy (a proton-pump inhibitor and two antibiotics—usually amoxicillin and clarithromycin).

Viruses

Certain DNA viruses and retroviruses (Table 4.6) can cause neoplasia, as follows:

- DNA viruses insert viral DNA directly into the host genome.
- Retroviruses have reverse transcriptase enzyme to produce a DNA copy of viral RNA. The viral DNA copy is then inserted into the host genome.

Mechanism of viral carcinogenesis

Inserted viral genes may be viral oncogenes, expression of which may lead to uncontrolled proliferation, or they may be activators or repressors of important cell-cycle regulating genes.

The mechanism of viral carcinogenesis is understood best in one of the most studied tumour viruses, the human papilloma virus. This double-stranded DNA virus has a tropism for squamous epithelium, and subtypes 16 and 18 are implicated in cervical carcinoma. The viral genome incorporates into the host DNA and expresses the E6 oncoprotein, which inactivates the tumour suppressor protein p53. In addition, expression of the E7 oncoprotein inactivates the tumour suppressor protein RB1. These oncoproteins induce cervical intraepithelial neoplasia (CIN).

Table 4.6 Examples of oncogenic human viruses

Type	Virus	Tumour type
Retroviruses	Human T-cell lymphotropic virus (HTLV-1) HIV	T-cell leukaemia AIDS-related lymphomas
DNA viruses	Human papillomavirus	Skin papilloma (common wart) Cervical carcinoma
	Epstein–Barr virus	Carcinoma of the nasopharynx Burkitt lymphoma
	Hepatitis B virus	Hepatocellular carcinoma

CLINICAL NOTE

HUMAN PAPILLOMA VIRUS (HPV) SCREENING AND VACCINATION

Cervical screening aims to detect preinvasive atypical cells (cervical intraepithelial neoplasia (CIN)) by cytological examination of surface epithelial cells. In the UK, women between the ages of 25 and 49 years undergo cervical screening (Pap smears ± HPV testing) every 3 years, and every 5 years between the ages of 50 and 64 years. It is estimated that regular attendance at screening prevents up to 90% of cervical cancer. Management of CIN is by the local destruction of abnormal epithelium using cryotherapy, laser therapy or cone biopsy, following histological confirmation of its nature.

HPV vaccinations against serotypes 16 and 18 are now available. Cross-protection against other HPV serotypes (especially 31, 33 and 45) has been noted.

HOST DEFENCES AGAINST CANCER

Some tumours are known to stimulate both innate and adaptive immunological reactions in the host.

Innate immunity

Activation of macrophages and natural killer cells can prevent growth of some tumours. Other tumours can activate complement via the alternative pathway.

Adaptive immunity

Humoral

Antibodies may have a protective role through complement activation or opsonization of tumour cells for cell-mediated destruction. They are more likely to be effective against free cells (e.g., leukaemia or metastasizing tumours) than those in solid lumps.

Cell-mediated immunity

Cell-mediated immunity is involved in recognition and monitoring of cells progressing towards malignancy. Therefore, cells that become significantly different are recognized as 'foreign' and may be eliminated by the immune system. This is particularly true of those tumours with a suspected viral aetiology.

The importance of immune surveillance in the prevention of cancer is clearly illustrated in immunocompromised patients (Table 4.7). For example, lymphomas associated with Epstein–Barr virus can present 4–7 years after immunosuppressive therapy following organ transplant.

Cytotoxic T-cells are thought to play a role in tumour regression, particularly in virus-associated neoplasms. Infiltration of some tumours by lymphocytes and macrophages is associated with better prognosis. Immune therapies using biological agents like monoclonal antibodies (e.g., trastuzumab in breast cancer) are now regularly used in cancer treatment.

Although many immune mechanisms are known to be active against tumour cells, most tumours are not distinguishable from normal host cells and so are not easily detected by the immune system. Additionally, tumour cells develop mechanisms to evade the immune system. These are thought to include reducing the expression of the surface major histocompatibility complex (MHC), antigen masking and actually suppressing the host immune system through cytokine release or apoptosis stimulation.

EFFECTS OF CANCER ON THE HOST

Cancer is detrimental to the host as it elicits a number of pathological responses, which may themselves produce complications (Table 4.8). These include paraneoplastic disease, weight loss and cachexia, anaemia of chronic disease and obstruction (e.g. colonic, ureteric).

CLINICAL CANCER PATHOLOGY

Tumour markers are increasingly being used for prognostication and management decisions. These markers are products derived from the tumour that can be found in the blood and used for diagnosis, assessing response to treatment and detecting recurrence. Examples include the CA125 ovarian tumour marker, the prostate-specific antigen (PSA) marker in prostate carcinoma, CA19-9 in pancreatic carcinoma, and α-fetoprotein in hepatocellular carcinoma and testicular tumours.

Pathology reports of resected tumours contain macroscopic and microscopic descriptions that give information about the size and type of a cancer, local invasion, lymphovascular and perineural invasion, and lymph node metastasis. The appropriate stage and grade is also provided to inform management decisions.

ETHICS

PROSTATE-SPECIFIC ANTIGEN (PSA) AS A SCREENING MARKER

PSA is commonly used as a screening tool for detecting prostate carcinoma. Although it is a useful marker to provide a baseline score, there are many causes of a raised PSA (e.g., inflammation). It has a 51% sensitivity for detecting high-grade cancers and its specificity is 91%; this is lower for low-grade carcinomas. No UK prostate carcinoma screening programme exists as currently there are no screening markers (including PSA) that are sensitive or specific enough to indicate cancer. Screening with PSA would likely result in many unnecessary invasive procedures.

Table 4.8 Effects of cancer on the host

Feature	Effect
Anaemia of chronic disease	Fatigue, malaise, SOB, pallor
Bone metastases	Pathological fractures, pain
Constitutional symptoms	Weight loss, fever, night sweats
Hypercoagulability	Prothrombotic state → DVT/PE
Immunosuppression	Infection
Increased cell turnover	Cachexia
Paraneoplastic syndromes	Hypercalcaemia, SIADH, Lambert–Eaton syndrome, Cushing syndrome
Space-occupying lesions	Brain herniation, compression/obstruction of adjacent structures

DVT, deep vein thrombosis; PE, pulmonary thromboembolism; SIADH, syndrome of inappropriate antidiuretic hormone; SOB, shortness of breath.

Chapter Summary

- Tumours result from uncontrolled cell growth.
- Some benign tumours can metastasize, so not entirely accurate.
- Benign and malignant tumours have characteristic macroscopic and microscopic features.
- Malignant tumours are given a stage and a grade.
- The most common staging system is *T*umour *N*odes *M*etastasis (TNM) system.
- The most common cancers in the UK are prostate, breast, lung and colorectal.
- Screening programmes aim to detect cancer at an early stage to increase the success of treatment and improve survival.
- Proto-oncogenes promote growth. Mutations result in oncogene formation causing a gain of function.
- Tumour suppressor genes suppress growth by regulating the cell cycle. Mutations result in a loss of function.
- *p53* is a tumour suppressor gene and 'guardian of the genome' as it plays a key role in detecting DNA damage and preventing cell cycling.
- Tumorigenesis is a multistage process that results from the accumulation of mutations.
- Familial cancer syndromes occur because of an inherited mutation in a tumour suppressor gene or proto-oncogene, making the person at increased risk of developing malignancy.
- Microsatellite instability can lead to Lynch syndrome.
- There are three stages of carcinogenesis: initiation, promotion and persistence.
- Radiation, bacteria and viruses are all carcinogenic agents.
- Innate and adaptive immunity defend a host against cancer.
- Monoclonal antibodies are commonly used in cancer treatment.
- Tumour markers are used as screening tools, especially for cancer recurrence.

Infectious disease 5

GENERAL PRINCIPLES OF INFECTION

Infection and colonization

Globally, infectious diseases are a common cause of morbidity and mortality. The prevalence of infectious diseases varies considerably between developed and developing nations. The burden of specific diseases depends on the quality of the drinking water, sanitation, healthcare system and the prevailing social and climatic conditions.

Infection is the invasion and proliferation of microorganisms in the tissues of the body. This usually follows the successful breach of host barriers and immune defence mechanisms.

Transmission of infectious agents can be:

- human to human spread (horizontal and vertical transmission)
- animal to human (zoonoses)
- environment to human (airborne, water, fomites)
- healthcare-acquired (nosocomial).

Following invasion, infective organisms can spread to distant tissue sites by:

- local spread
- lymphatic spread
- haematogenous spread
- neural spread
- dissemination in tissue fluid.

Colonization is the inhabitation of external body surfaces—the skin, gastrointestinal (GI) tract, external genitalia and vagina—usually by harmless microorganisms. This generally occurs soon after birth.

Pathogens and commensals

Pathogens are microorganisms that are normally absent from the body, but which have mechanisms to invade and cause infection. Commensals are those microorganisms that constitute the normal flora of a healthy body. They do not normally cause disease and they are often advantageous to the host by the production of nutrients, such as vitamin B_{12}, and by the exclusion of harmful bacteria. For example, the normal commensal flora of the skin prevents colonization by pathogenic bacteria.

> **HINTS AND TIPS**
>
> **COMMENSALS VERSUS PATHOGENS**
>
> The distinction between commensals and pathogens is not absolute. Many commensals are potential pathogens, i.e., they are harmless only so long as they are kept at bay by the host's defence mechanisms.

Other characteristics of microorganisms

Pathogenicity

Pathogenicity is the capacity of a particular microorganism to cause disease.

> **COMMON PITFALLS**
>
> **ENDEMIC VERSUS EPIDEMIC**
>
> Endemic—the baseline level of a disease that is commonly found in a specific region.
>
> Outbreak—widespread increase in a level of a disease from baseline, within a limited region.
>
> Epidemic—the widespread (and usually rapid) increase in the level of a disease from baseline; it is not region-specific.

Virulence

Virulence is a measure of the pathogenicity of a microorganism. An organism is considered highly virulent if a small number of microorganisms can cause disease.

Opportunistic infection

Opportunistic infection is an infection by organisms of low pathogenicity when immune responses are impaired. Immunocompromised patients, such as those with a primary or secondary immunodeficiency, are most at risk. Examples include:

- Children with severe combined immunodeficiency (SCID): a rare group of inherited syndromes (often X-linked) that require bone marrow transplantation to prevent death in early infancy (see Chapter 17).

- Patients infected with HIV: destruction of $CD4^+$ T-cells (see HIV below).
- Transplant patients: using immunosuppressive drugs.

CLINICAL NOTE

PATTERNS OF INFECTION BASED ON DISEASE

Deficiency of specific immune defences predisposes individuals to characteristic patterns of infection. For example, in DiGeorge syndrome, T-cell deficiency results in chronic viral, fungal and intracellular bacterial infections (see Chapter 17).

CATEGORIES OF INFECTIOUS AGENT

There are numerous different categories of infectious agent. The classification of the major pathogens is shown in Table 5.1.

Viruses

Viruses are obligate intracellular parasites, i.e., they require a host cell to replicate. They show tropism towards specific cell types, e.g., hepatocytes, respiratory epithelium. The majority cause acute self-limiting infections; however, some can cause chronic infections and malignant transformation.

Classification

The Baltimore classification groups viruses based on the type of nucleic acid of their genome. They can also be subdivided based on other characteristics:

- Nucleic acid type, i.e., RNA or DNA (Baltimore classification).
- Capsid morphology, i.e., icosahedral, helical or complex.
- Presence of an envelope—phospholipid membrane from host cells.
- Size (nm).

Structure

Viruses are relatively simple organisms which share the same basic structure (Fig. 5.1):

- Nucleic acid core—DNA or RNA, linear or circular (Table 5.2).
- Capsid—protein coat formed from repeating identical protein units.
- Glycoproteins—binding sites for host cell receptors (tropism).
- Additional proteins—e.g., reverse transcriptase and RNA-dependent RNA polymerase.
- Envelope—acquired cytoplasmic membrane from budding of the host cell.

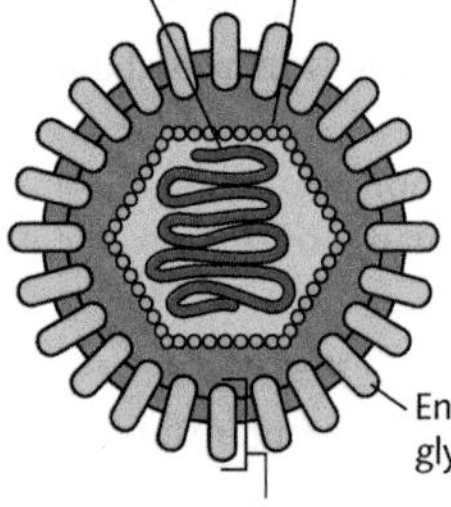

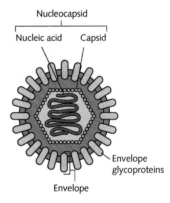

Fig. 5.1 Structure of a virus. Generalized structure of a virus showing the central nucleic acid (RNA or DNA) surrounded by a capsid formed of repeating protein units. Some viruses have an envelope which is derived from the host's cell membrane as a result of viral budding. Within the membrane, viral glycoproteins are inserted to form the viral envelope.

Table 5.1 Classification of major pathogens

	Viruses	Bacteria	Fungi	Protozoa	Helminths and ectoparasites
Size	20–300 nm	0.1–5 µm	2–10 µm	2-100 µm	0.5–35 cm
Prokaryote or eukaryote	Neither	Prokaryote	Eukaryote	Eukaryote	Eukaryote
Nucleic acid	DNA or RNA	DNA + RNA	DNA + RNA	DNA + RNA	DNA + RNA
Replication	Intracellular	Intracellular and/or extracellular	Intracellular and/or extracellular	Intracellular and/or extracellular	Extracellular
External cell wall	No	Yes (usually): peptidoglycan	Yes: rigid chitin	No	No
Reproduction	Assembly	Binary fission	Binary fission and sexual	Binary fission and sexual	Sexual

Table 5.2 Classification of viruses based on nucleic acid type

Nucleic acid	Mode of replication	Group	Example	Disease
dsDNA	Utilize host cell polymerases for mRNA synthesis. Can remain in infected cell and establish persistent infections (latent, immortalizing viruses)	Herpes viruses	HSV	Herpes skin lesions Oral genital lesions Encephalitis
			VZV	Chicken pox/shingles Chicken pox pneumonia
			CMV	In the fetus: ocular disease, death In the immunosuppressed: pneumonia, enteritis, retinitis
			EBV	Infectious mononucleosis Burkitt lymphoma Nasopharyngeal carcinoma
		Adenoviruses	Adenovirus	Respiratory tract infection Haemorrhagic cystitis Gastroenteritis
		Papoviruses	Papilloma virus	Warts Malignant tumours
		Hepadnaviruses	Hepatitis B virus	Hepatitis B
		Poxviruses	Variola virus	Smallpox
			Molluscum contagiosum virus	Molluscum contagiosum
ssDNA		Parvoviruses	Parvovirus	Erythema infectiosum Aplastic crisis
RNA	Encode their own replicative enzymes for formation of more mRNA (host enzymes cannot replicate RNA)	Picornaviruses	Coxsackie virus	Hand, foot and mouth disease
			Poliovirus	Poliomyelitis
			Hepatitis A virus	Hepatitis A
			Rhinovirus	Common cold
		Coronaviruses	Coronavirus	Common cold SARS
		Paramyxoviruses	Measles virus	Measles
			Mumps virus	Mumps
			Rubella	Rubella Congenital cataracts and deafness
			RSV	Bronchiolitis Bronchitis
		Orthomyxoviruses	Influenza virus	Influenza
		Rhabdoviruses	Rabies virus	Rabies
	Contain reverse transcriptase enzyme for production of viral mRNA. Viral DNA is inserted into host genome	Retroviruses	HIV	AIDS
			HTLV	Lymphoma

CMV, Cytomegalovirus; dsDNA, double-stranded DNA; EBV, Epstein–Barr virus; HSV, herpes simplex virus; HTLV, human T-lymphocyte virus; mRNA, messenger RNA; RSV, respiratory syncytial virus; SARS, severe acute respiratory syndrome; ssDNA, single-stranded DNA; VZV, varicella-zoster virus.

Viral replication

Viral genomes are relatively simple, containing very few genes coding for a limited repertoire of proteins, e.g., capsid proteins, glycoproteins and essential enzymes. These do not include synthetic enzymes, such that viruses are obligated to hijack the host cells' synthetic machinery to replicate. In essence, a host cell is turned into a virus-producing factory.

The rate of viral replication varies from virus to virus; however, the net result is always the same; the end virus titre is always greater than the initial one.

There are two basic types of replicative strategy depending on the nature of the nuclei acid, i.e., DNA or RNA.

The phases of viral replication are:

1. ***Adsorption and penetration***—the virus enters the host cell by binding to a receptor on the host's cell membrane.
2. ***Eclipse phase***—the virus particle is disassembled and the viral genome becomes free within the cytoplasm. The viral genome is replicated and translation of viral proteins occurs. This is achieved in different ways depending on whether the viral nucleic acid is DNA or RNA:
   - DNA → mRNA → protein
   - RNA antisense → RNA sense (mRNA) → protein
   - RNA sense (mRNA) → protein
   - RNA → dsDNA → host genome integration → mRNA → protein (retroviruses).
3. ***Assembly and release***—the viral proteins form the components of the new virus particles. These self-assemble into a capsid containing a copy of the viral genome at the core and are then released from the cell. Release occurs by cytolysis or budding (Fig. 5.2).
   - *Cytolysis*—non-enveloped viruses (e.g., adenoviruses) are released directly into the extracellular environment by lysis of the host cell; this results in the death of the cell.
   - *Budding*—enveloped viruses (e.g., HIV and herpes virus) are released by 'budding' from the host cell membrane:
     - Nucleocapsid proteins are inserted into the host cell membrane.
     - A modified area of host cell membrane extends out from the cell surface and is pinched off (i.e., budded) from the host cell, enclosing the new viral particle.

This mechanism does not cause the death of the cell, and so viral replication can continue.

Viral pathogenesis

The pathological effect of a virus depends on the cells it infects, e.g., hepatocytes versus B-cells versus neurones, and the scale and magnitude of the immune response. Tissue injury is produced in two ways:

- Direct cytopathic effect—cell lysis, e.g., respiratory epithelial cells infected with influenza virus.
- Indirect cytopathic effect—host immune response to viral proteins leading to cell destruction.

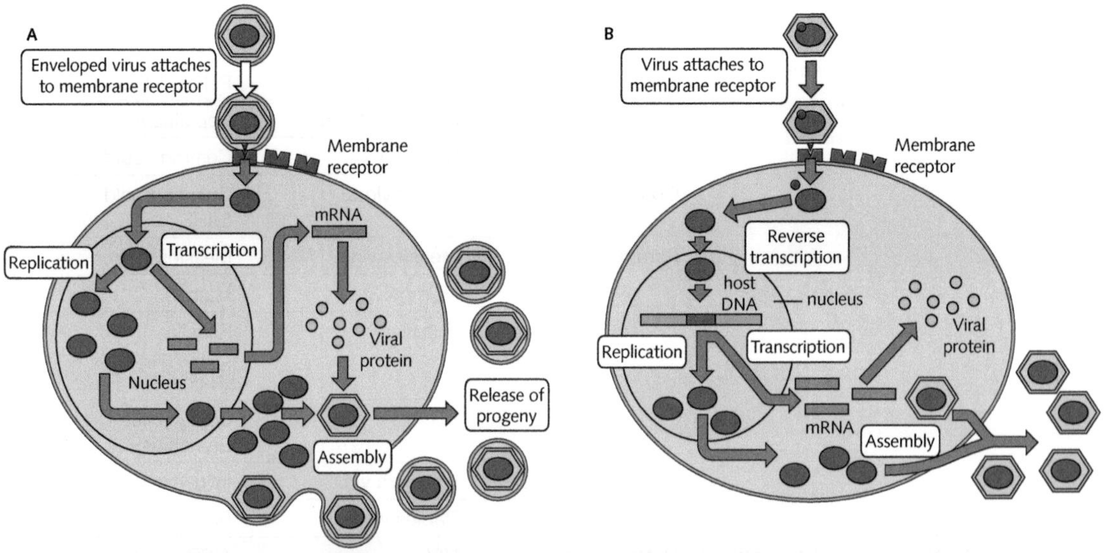

Fig. 5.2 Viral replication cycle. (A) DNA virus: viral DNA enters the host cell and utilizes the host's cellular machinery for transcription of the viral genome to messenger RNA *(mRNA)*. This is translated to viral proteins and glycoproteins and the viral DNA is replicated. New virus particles are assembled and released from the cell. RNA viruses can be translated to protein directly. (B) RNA retrovirus: viral RNA is converted to viral DNA using reverse transcriptase copackaged within the viral particle. Viral DNA is then inserted into the host genome and subsequently transcribed to mRNA. The viral mRNA is exported to the cytoplasm where it is translated to viral proteins. Together with viral RNA, these are assembled into new virions and released from the host cell.

Viruses can also produce morbidity with insertion of viral genes into the host genome causing:

- Persistent infections, e.g., hepatitis C and herpes simplex virus (HSV) with ongoing inflammation or recurrent infective episodes.
- Cellular transformation, e.g., Epstein–Barr virus (EBV), human papillomavirus (HPV) to produce cancers (see Chapter 4).

Therefore, the harmful effects of viral infections include cell death, acute and chronic tissue damage, immune response and transformation of cells to form tumours.

CLINICAL NOTE

VIRAL DETECTION

Viral infections can be detected by a variety of methods:

- Direct visualization by electron microscopy
- Observed specific cellular cytopathic effects
- Detection of viral proteins by immunofluorescence techniques
- Detection of antiviral antibodies produced by the host
- Detection of viral nucleic acid by polymerase chain reaction (PCR).

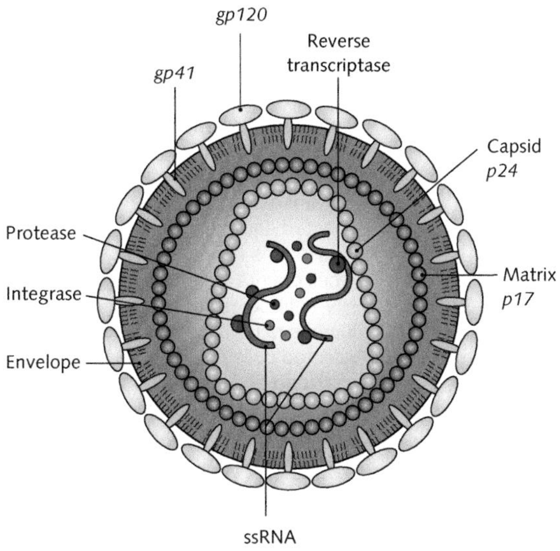

Fig. 5.3 Structure of HIV. The conical capsid of HIV is formed from the structural proteins *p24* and *p6* and contains two pieces of single-stranded RNA *(ssRNA)* and the enzymes reverse transcriptase, integrase and protease. The nucleocapsid is further surround by a matrix formed of *p17*. The membrane envelope is studded with the viral glycoprotein *gp41*, which anchors the nucleocapsid to the membrane, and *gp120*, which binds to CD4 on host cells.

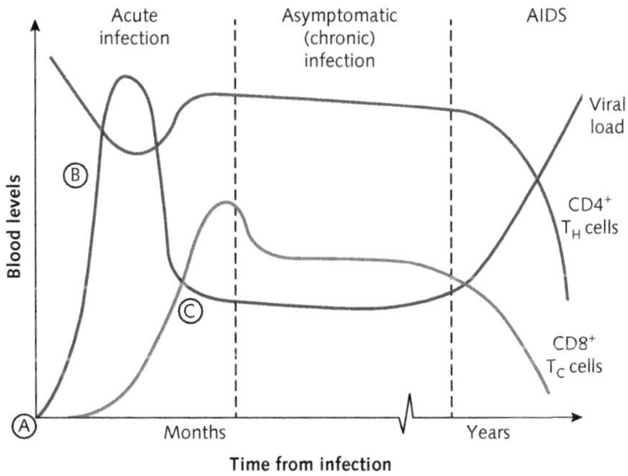

Fig. 5.4 CD4 count and viral load. Graph to show the time course of an untreated HIV infection. *(A)* Point of infection. *(B)* Dissemination of the virus. *(C)* Seroconversion. After the acute infection stage the virus is brought under control by the immune system and a steady state ensues. AIDS occurs when viral replication escapes immune control as seen by rising viral load and falling CD4 and CD8 T-cell counts, making the person susceptible to opportunistic infections. *T_C cells*, cytotoxic T-cells; *T_H cells*, T-helper cells.

HIV

HIV is a lentivirus of the retroviridae family from which two species infect humans: HIV-1 (the commonest worldwide) and HIV-2 (present mainly in West Africa). HIV has three main routes of transmission: sexual contact, blood-borne (transfusions or contaminated needles) and maternal (placental or via breast milk). HIV is a persistent infection and eventually progresses to cause acquired immune deficiency syndrome (AIDS).

Structure

HIV is an icosahedral enveloped RNA retrovirus (Fig. 5.3). It contains the following key genes which code for structural proteins:

- *gag*—inner structural proteins, e.g., *p24* forming the capsid, *p17* forming the matrix
- *pol*—reverse transcriptase, integrase and protease enzymes
- *env*—viral envelope proteins *gp120* and *gp41*.

Other genes include regulatory genes that aid the pathogenicity of HIV.

Pathogenesis of HIV infection

HIV infects cells by binding to the CD4 receptors on T-helper cells (T_H) and macrophages via the envelope glycoprotein spike *gp120*. Upon entry, the virus loses its capsid and utilizes the copackaged enzyme reverse transcriptase to make viral DNA. Integration into the host's genome occurs where viral DNA is transcribed to mRNA and subsequently translated to viral proteins which subvert the function of the cell (Fig. 5.4).

Clinically, there are three phases to HIV infection; these are outlined in Table 5.3 and relate to the natural history of

Table 5.3 Stages of HIV infection

Classification of HIV infection	
Stage I	Acute seroconversion: • widespread dissemination of the virus • plasma viraemia • proviral reservoir of persistently infected cells is created • viral load is initially high and $CD4^+$ T-cell counts are low • HIV antibodies are produced with increased $CD8^+$ T-cell killing of infected cells resulting in lowered viral load and increased CD4 counts • fever, lymphadenopathy, flu-like symptoms, rash occur in ~50% of infections.
Stage II	Chronic asymptomatic infection: • persists for years (>10 years) • viral load is stable and the immune response is effective • over time CD4 counts begin to decline. • No or limited symptoms, such as persistent lymphadenopathy, are seen at this time.
Stage III	AIDS: • Defined as CD4 count <200 cells/mm^3 or development of an opportunistic infection, e.g., *Pneumocystis jirovecii*, toxoplasmosis, *Cryptococcus.* • Development of secondary cancers e.g., Kaposi's sarcoma, non-Hodgkin's lymphoma, squamous carcinoma of the mouth or rectum • Symptoms are those of severe and recurrent infections • AIDS associated dementia/ encephalopathy and chronic diarrhoea.

the virus. The duration of each stage is highly variable; some patients pass directly from stage I to fully developed AIDS, whereas others remain in the earlier stages for months or years. Opportunistic infections tend to develop when the $CD4^+$ T-cell count drops below 200 cells/mm^3, which correlates with an increasing viral load. A small proportion of HIV-infected patients do not develop clinical AIDS.

Initially viral replication is repressed by intracellular factors and cell-mediated immunity by $CD8^+$ cytotoxic T-cells (T_C) so that the virus remains latent (i.e., dormant) for months or even years. Eventually $CD4^+$ T-cell numbers begin to decline, leading to B-cell dysfunction and severe impairment of cell-mediated immunity with a high risk of multiple opportunistic infections (usually viral or fungal).

HINTS AND TIPS

HIV COINFECTIONS

Patients infected with HIV will often be coinfected with other pathogens whose routes of transmission are similar to that of HIV. Examples include hepatitis C virus, hepatitis B virus and human herpes virus 8 (causative agent of Kaposi sarcoma), as well as other sexually transmitted infections.

CLINICAL NOTE

AIDS OPPORTUNISTIC INFECTIONS

Infections seen in AIDS include:

- Bacterial: Mycobacterium tuberculosis (tuberculosis), *Mycobacterium avium intracellulare.*
- Fungal: Toxoplasma, Cryptosporidium, Candida, Cryptococcus.
- Viral: cytomegalovirus (CMV), herpes simplex virus (HSV), *Pneumocystis jirovecii* (PCP).

Prognosis and treatment

The prognosis for HIV patients with access to highly active antiretroviral therapy (HAART) has improved dramatically, and there is a longer life expectancy. Treatment is combination antiretroviral therapy where two or more anti-HIV drugs are given to minimize the development of drug resistance. With no access to antiretroviral treatment, such as in the developing world, prognosis is poor, with mortality of >90%.

HINTS AND TIPS

CD4 COUNT AND VIRAL LOAD

CD4 cells are T-helper cells. As disease progresses, CD4 counts (i.e., the number of T-helper cells) decrease as they are destroyed, and viral load (i.e., the amount of detectable viral RNA) increases.

A low CD4 count puts the patient at high risk of acquiring opportunistic infections, which can be severe and life-threatening.

Bacteria

The number of bacteria in the body is estimated to be 3.8 × 10^{13}, which outnumbers human nucleated cells by 10:1. Bacterial infection can be localized or generalized and can be acquired directly (horizontal or vertical transmission) or indirectly through intermediate vectors such as food, water, fomites or soil.

Classification

The starting point of bacterial classification is the division of bacteria into Gram-positive and Gram-negative organisms based on the structure of the cell wall (Tables 5.4 and 5.5). Other characteristics are then assessed to aid further identification and classification, e.g., size, shape, type of respiration (aerobic, anaerobic, facultative or obligate) and nutrient requirements (growth on different culture media). It is also possible to assess different biochemical and immunological features, e.g., Gram-positive cocci can be catalase-positive (*Staphylococcus* species) or catalase-negative (*Streptococcus* species). Not all bacteria stain using the Gram method, e.g., *Mycobacterium tuberculosis,* as they lack a cell wall.

HINTS AND TIPS

GRAM STAINING

Gram staining involves using crystal violet and iodine to stain the bacterial cell wall. The crystal violet is trapped within the thick peptidoglycan wall of Gram-positive bacteria so that they stain purple. The crystal violet is lost from the wall of Gram-negative bacteria (lower peptidoglycan content) on washing with acetone such that they appear red/pink due to safranin counterstaining Fig. 5.5.

Table 5.4 Gram-negative bacteria

Cocci	Bacilli	Coccobacilli	Spiral	Spirochete	Comma
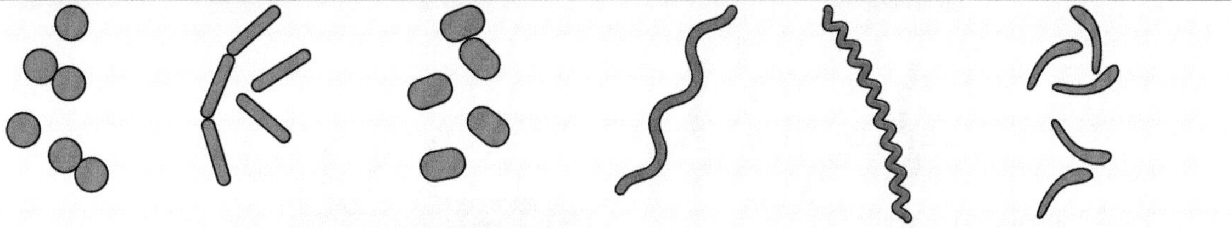					
Neisseria gonorrhoea (gonorrhoea), *N. meningitidis* (meningitis)	*Escherichia coli* (enterocolitis)	*Brucella abortus* (brucellosis)	*Helicobacter pylori* (gastritis, duodenal ulcers)	*Treponema pallidum* (syphilis)	*Campylobacter jejuni* (enterocolitis)
	Shigella (dysentery)	*Yersinia pestis* (plague), *Y. enterocolitica* (gastroenteritis)		Leptospira (Leptospirosis)	*Vibrio cholerae* (cholera)
	Salmonella typhi/paratyphi (enteric fever), *S. typhimurium* (food poisoning)	*Bartonella henselae* (cat scratch disease)		*Borrelia burgdorferi* (Lyme disease)	
	Klebsiella pneumoniae (pneumonia and HAI)	*Bordetella pertussis* (whooping cough)			
	Pseudomonas aeruginosa (respiratory and urinary tract infections)				

HAI, Healthcare-associated infection.

Table 5.5 Gram-positive bacteria[a]

Cocci	Bacilli
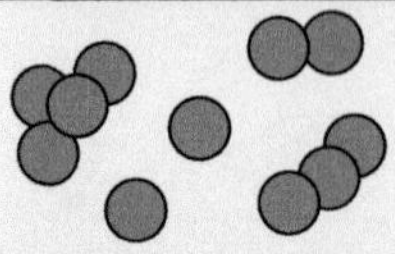	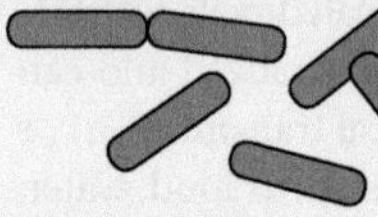
Staphylococcus aureus (soft-tissue infection, pneumonia, endocarditis)	*Bacillus anthracis* (anthrax) *B. cereus* (food poisoning)
Streptococcus pyogenes (sore throat, erysipelas, wound infection, septicaemia) *S. viridans* (dental caries, bacterial endocarditis) *S. pneumoniae* (pneumonia)	*Clostridium botulinum* (botulism) *C. tetani* (tetanus) *C. perfringens* (food poisoning, gas gangrene) *C. difficile* (pseudomembranous colitis)
Enterococcus faecalis (urinary tract, soft tissue and wound infections)	*Listeria monocytogenes* (meningitis, intrauterine death)
	Corynebacterium diphtheriae (diphtheria)

[a] *Bacteria, e.g., staphylococci and streptococci, can be further characterized by whether they form pairs (diplococci), clusters or chains.*

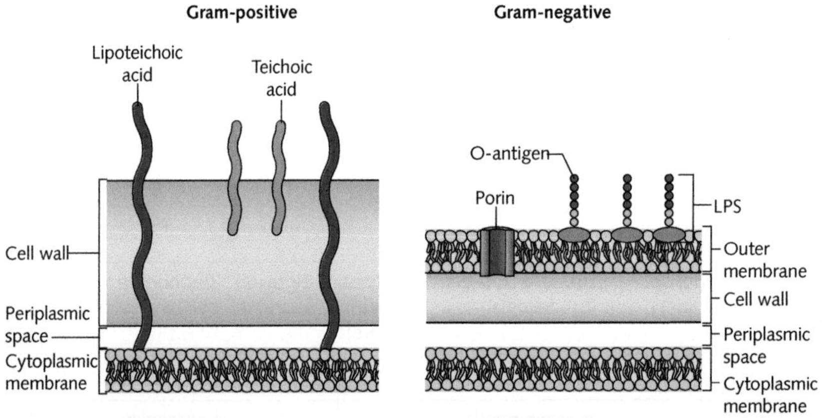

Fig. 5.5 Structure of the bacterial cell wall. Structure of GRAM-positive and Gram-negative bacterial cells walls. The outer membranes of Gram-negative walls contain the pore-forming protein perforin which allows transport of molecules across the cell wall. Lipopolysaccharide *(LPS)*, an endotoxin, is also present, with the lipid A component situated within the membrane and the O-antigen projecting from the surface membrane. The pericytoplasmic space contains enzymes involved in transport and antibiotic breakdown.

Structure

A generalized structure of a bacterium is shown in Fig. 5.6. Unlike other cells, bacteria do not have a nucleus or membrane-bound organelles and their genetic material lies free within the cytoplasm as a single circular piece of DNA. Additional extrachromosomal DNA may be present in the form of plasmids.

Bacterial pathogenesis

Bacteria are highly successful organisms as they have developed a number of virulence factors which allow them to overcome a host's defences, survive and propagate. The pathogenic effects of bacteria are the results of the release of endotoxins and exotoxins, which produce acute and chronic inflammation and tissue damage. Bacterial virulence factors include:

- adhesins
- lipopolysaccharide
- antigenic variation
- secreted enzymes
- exotoxins and endotoxins
- superantigens.

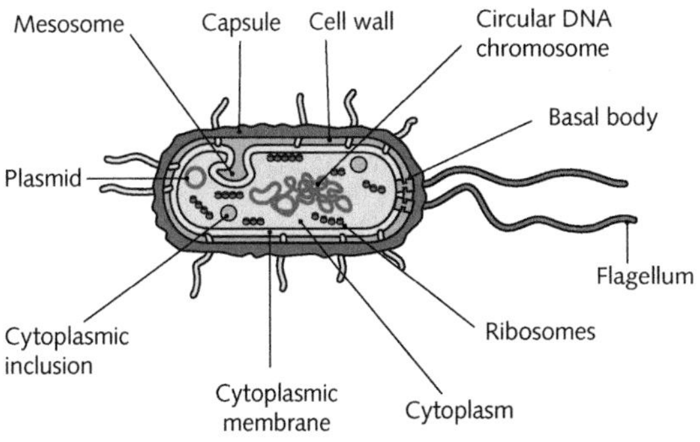

Fig. 5.6 Generalized structure of a bacterium. Bacteria are formed from a gelatinous cytoplasm in which the bacterial chromosome (nucleoid), ribosomes (30S + 50S), plasmids and cytoplasmic inclusions are located. Cytoplasmic inclusions are granules of various beneficial substances such as glycogen or fats. The bacterial envelope is comprised of the cytoplasmic membrane, cell wall and capsule. Within the cytoplasmic membrane, pili and flagella (present in some bacteria) are located and the membrane can focally in-fold to produce stacks of membrane (mesosomes). A peptidoglycan cell wall further surrounds the cytoplasmic membrane, the structure of which varies between GRAM-positive and Gram-negative bacteria. The capsule (glycocalyx) is the final layer which invests the bacterium.

CLINICAL NOTE

BACTERIAL DETECTION

Bacterial infections can be diagnosed from a number of different samples obtained from the patient. These include blood, faeces, urine, cerebral spinal fluid and swabs taken from infected wounds. Samples will generally be cultured to determine the species of bacteria and their sensitivity/resistance to different antibiotics.

Adherence

Certain bacteria are able to adhere specifically to epithelial cells or tissue matrix by means of pili (also called fimbriae), which are slender filamentous processes on the surfaces of some bacteria. Pili are coated in adhesins, which interact with specific molecules on surface epithelial cells to enable the bacterium to adhere to the host's cell membrane. Polymorphisms in host cell-surface glycoproteins may make an individual more susceptible to binding by certain types of bacterial adhesins. Pili are more common in Gram-negative bacteria.

Lipoteichoic acids (Gram-positive bacteria only) are surface-associated adhesion molecules that function in a similar manner to pili by binding to epithelial cells. It also induces immune responses in a similar manner to lipopolysaccharide (LPS).

Lipopolysaccharide

LPS is present on Gram-negative bacterial cell membranes and is composed of lipid A, a polysaccharide core and O-antigen. The O-antigen prevents the binding of the complement-formed membrane attack complex and therefore prevents cytolysis. Lipid A is an endotoxin.

Antigenic variation

Some bacteria can change the antigens that they present to the immune system by either shutting off expression of one gene in favour of another or rearranging DNA to change the composition of a surface antigen. Some bacteria can mimic host molecules to go undetected by the immune system.

Secreted enzymes

Bacteria secrete a variety of enzymes which aid infection and combat host defences. Examples include aggressins such as coagulase, streptokinase and collagenases, enzymes to cleave IgA, iron-binding proteins and defensins. They can also secrete β-lactamases, which confer resistance to penicillin.

Exotoxins and endotoxins

These toxins are produced by the bacteria and help survival, dissemination and transmission of the bacteria and are responsible for many of the local and distant effects of infection.

Exotoxins—Exotoxins are proteins secreted by bacteria which are highly toxic to the host, many of which are plasmid-encoded. Toxins are generally specific to a bacterial species. The modes of action of some exotoxins are considered below:

- Enzymatic lysis: α-toxin (phospholipase C) of *Clostridium perfringens* breaks down host cell membranes.
- Pore formation: a transmembranous pore is inserted into the host cell disrupting cellular function. Examples include α-toxin of *Staphylococcus aureus,* haemolysin of *E. coli*, and streptolysin O of *Streptococcus pyogenes.*
- Inhibition of protein synthesis, e.g., diphtheria toxin.
- Activation of adenylate cyclase: e.g., cholera toxin, *E. coli* toxin—this results in increased levels of cyclic adenosine monophosphate (cAMP), causing excess fluid and electrolyte secretion, leading to diarrhoea.
- Inhibition of neurotransmitter release, e.g., tetanus and botulinum toxins.

Treating exotoxin with formaldehyde or high temperatures can denature the toxin to form toxoids, which can be useful for vaccination.

Endotoxins—Endotoxins are LPSs, which form an integral part of the cell wall in Gram-negative bacteria. They are released when the bacterium dies. Endotoxins do not have enzymatic activity but can induce toxic effects by their potent activation of:

- The complement cascade, causing inflammatory damage.
- The coagulation cascade, potentially causing disseminated intravascular coagulation (DIC).
- Cytokines, notably tumour necrosis factor and interleukin-1 released from leucocytes, causing fever.

In overwhelming infections, the patient is said to suffer from 'endotoxic shock' with high fever, hypotension and DIC leading to multiorgan failure.

Superantigens

These are extremely potent bacterial toxins which directly stimulate T-cells, cross-linking the T-cell receptor and major histocompatibility complex (MHC) II directly outside of the peptide binding groove. T-cells are activated in an uncontrolled manner, resulting in a release of large quantities of proinflammatory cytokines that can lead to rash, fever, shock and death. Examples include:

- *S. aureus*: toxic shock syndrome toxin (TSST).
- *S. aureus*: staphylococcal enterotoxins, the cause of staphylococcal food poisoning.
- *S. pyogenes*: streptococcal pyrogenic exotoxin A causes the rash of scarlet fever and streptococcal toxic shock syndrome.

Avoiding death by phagocytosis

Successful microorganisms have evolved numerous ingenious antiphagocytic devices:

- Phagocyte killing, e.g., via exotoxin release.
- Prevention of opsonization—the microorganism produces protein that prevents interaction between opsonizing antibody and phagocyte.
- Preventing phagocyte contact—some bacteria have an external capsule of polysaccharide, which gives a slimy surface and provides protection against phagocytosis, e.g., *Streptococcus pneumoniae*.
- Protection against intracellular death—this allows the microorganism to survive within the phagocyte by, for example, inhibition of phagosome and lysosome fusion *(Mycobacterium tuberculosis)* or escaping from the phagolysosome into cytoplasm *(Listeria monocytogenes)*.

Antibiotic resistance and plasmids

Many bacteria are resistant to antibiotics. Resistance is conferred by genes that encode bacterial proteins which can ameliorate the effect of an antibiotic. Resistance can occur in two ways:

1. Genetic mutation conferring a survival advantage.
2. Transfer of resistance genes by mobile genetic elements (e.g., plasmids).

Transfer of genetic elements can occur by conjugation, transduction or recombination. Plasmids are circles of extrachromosomal DNA that are capable of self-replication and can be transferred between bacteria. Antibiotic-susceptible bacteria can acquire plasmids from resistant bacteria and so gain antibiotic resistance. These newly resistant forms are then positively selected under antibiotic treatment, with the nonresistant bacteria being deleted from the population.

Mechanisms of bacterial antibiotic resistance

There are various mechanisms which bacteria employ to overcome the effects of antibiotics. Usually multiple mechanisms exist such that there is resistance to several classes of antibiotic. The mechanisms include:

- *Inactivating enzymes:* production of enzymes which inactivate or degrade the antibiotic.
- *Modified target*: bacterial modification of the antibiotic target such that it is no longer recognized by the antibiotic.
- *Change in cell wall permeability*: a conformational change in the bacterial cell wall to render it less permeable, or the development of efflux pumps which actively remove the antibiotic from the bacterium.
- *Metabolic bypass*: bacterial development of an alternative synthetic/metabolic pathway to circumvent the effect of the antibiotic.

Multidrug resistance

Resistance to all classes of antibiotics has been increasing at a rapid rate, outstripping the rate of new antibiotic development. There is now a serious danger that in the near future common infections will no longer be curable. This has led to the development of antibiotic administration policies in an attempt to reduce the rate of resistance development. Examples of resistant organisms include:

- Methicillin-resistant *S. aureus* (MRSA)—contains a methicillin-hydrolysing β-lactamase, rendering penicillin class antibiotics obsolete.
- Vancomycin-resistant *S. aureus* (VRSA)—vancomycin is used to treat MRSA, which has led to the development of VRSA. The vancomycin resistance gene was acquired from enterococci.
- Vancomycin resistance enterococci (VRE)—vancomycin resistance is achieved by alteration in the bacterial cell wall which reduces affinity, and therefore efficacy, of vancomycin.
- Carbapenem resistance Enterobacteriaceae (CRE)—resistance to carbapenem class antibiotics owing to carbapenemase enzyme. They include bacteria such as *Klebsiella* and *E. coli*.

Fungi

Fungi are unicellular, multicellular or multinucleate organisms (Table 5.6). They are eukaryotes and contain ergosterol instead of cholesterol in their plasma membranes.

Fungi have a well-defined cell wall composed of polysaccharides and chitin; they can be moulds, yeasts or dimorphic.

Table 5.6 Classification of fungi

Yeast-like form	Hyphal form	Dimorphic form
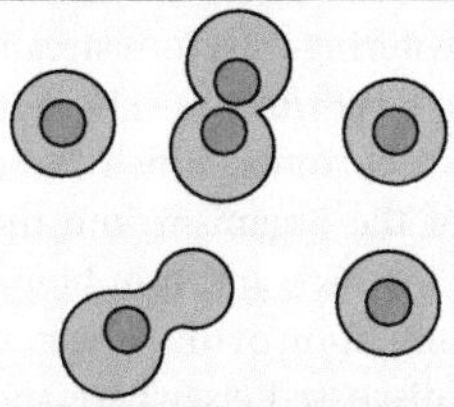	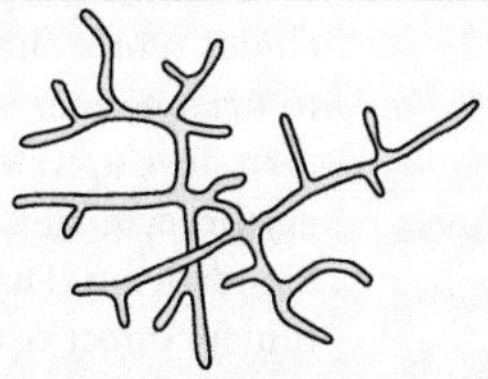	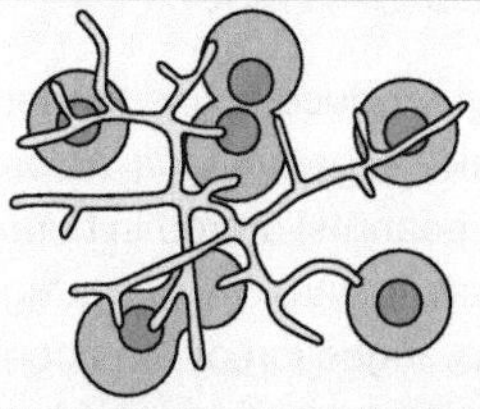
Single, rounded cells	Branching filaments interlaced to make mycelium or mould	Can assume either yeast or hyphal form depending on environment
Multiply by budding	Produce spores	
	Hyphae may be several hundred millimetres in length,	
e.g., *Candida albicans*, *Cryptococcus neoformans*	e.g., *Aspergillus fumigatus*, dermatophytes	e.g., *Histoplasma capsulatum*, *Blastomyces dermatitidis*

Fungal infections are either superficial (e.g., involving the skin, hair, nails and mucous membranes) or deep/systemic (e.g., involving the lungs, brain or heart); the latter are usually opportunistic, found only in the immunocompromised. Such opportunistic fungi include Candida, Aspergillus, Mucor, *Pneumocystis jirovecii* and Cryptococcus (Fig. 5.7).

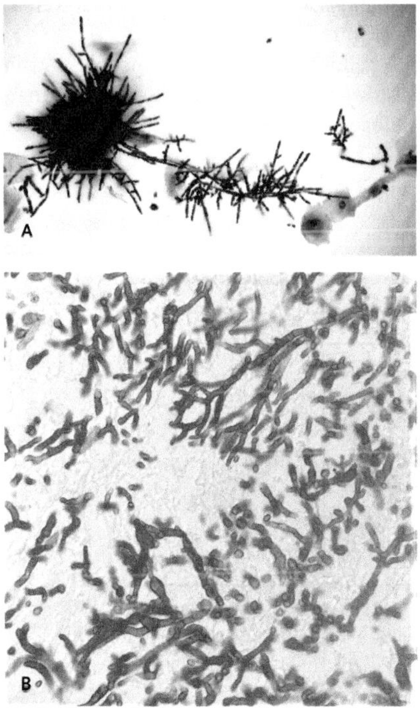

Fig. 5.7 Candida and Aspergillus. (A) Cytology of *Candida* spp. (B) Grocott stain showing *Aspergillus* hyphae.

- *Candida*—see Chapters 10 and 11.
- *Aspergillus*—a fungal infection of septate hyphae with branching at 45 degrees. Aspergillus infection is not uncommon in patients on immunosuppressive therapy (e.g., posttransplant). Infection may be noninvasive or invasive (extending into blood vessels) and can colonize lung abscesses/cavities or form fungal balls (aspergillomas). See Chapters 7 and 10 for further discussion.
- Mucor—this fungal infection with broad, non-septate hyphae branching at 90 degrees, may affect both the upper and lower respiratory tract. Angioinvasion is associated with haemorrhage and necrosis.
- *P. jirovecii* (PCP)—previously known as *P. carinii*, this opportunistic infection may be seen in any immunocompromised patient, but is also considered an AIDS-related illness. It infects the lungs and appears as cup-shaped cysts within alveolar casts (see Chapter 10).
- Cryptococcus—this encapsulated yeast may be inhaled from pigeon droppings. It causes meningitis and bronchopneumonia (see Chapter 7).

Deep mycoses are systemic diseases caused by fungal invasion (see Chapter 18). They include:

- Blastomycosis—found in decomposing plant matter. Spores are inhaled and may cause dermal plaques/ulcers or pneumonia.
- Histoplasmosis—spores are inhaled from bird or bat droppings; may cause granulomatous inflammation in the lungs or skin.
- Mycetoma—can be caused by bacterial or fungal (e.g., Aspergillus) infection; it is characterized by chronic granulomatous inflammation and sinus tract formation.

CLINICAL NOTE

ASPERGILLUS FLAVUS

Some fungi produce toxins termed mycotoxins. For example, *Aspergillus flavus* proliferates on food (e.g., peanuts) stored in humid conditions and produces aflatoxins, which are highly carcinogenic mycotoxins. Ingestion of food contaminated with aflatoxins causes an increased risk of hepatocellular carcinoma in humans, particularly where there is underlying hepatitis B infection (see Chapter 12).

- Sporotrichosis—also known as 'rose gardener's disease'; it is due to infection by *Sporothrix schenckii*. The classic presentation is of an ascending nodular skin infection following a cut from a rose bush. The infection tracks along lymphatic channels.

Protozoa

Protozoa are unicellular eukaryotes that may develop into cysts in harsh environmental conditions. The main divisions of protozoa are shown in Fig. 5.8. Protozoa species are capable of replicating intracellularly or extracellularly. The most important protozoal disease worldwide is malaria, which is caused by the *Plasmodium* species.

Identification of protozoa often occurs by microscopy of patient specimens. Specimens include faeces, blood and tissue. Culture methods are not routinely applied for identification purposes.

Malaria is carried by the female *Anopheles* mosquito; this tropical disease is due to infection by *Plasmodium* species (see Chapter 17). The highest mortality rate is from infection with *Plasmodium falciparum*, which can cause fatal haemorrhage and cerebral malaria. The life cycle includes sporozoites in hepatocytes entering the bloodstream to become merozoites which infect erythrocytes. These in turn develop into trophozoites and schizonts, which cause erythrocyte rupture and release of the organism into the bloodstream. Diagnosis is usually by thick and thin blood film for direct visualization and quantitation of the parasites.

Other protozoal infections are discussed elsewhere and include:

- Gastrointestinal tract (Chapter 11)—Giardia, Trypanosoma.
- Hepatopancreaticobiliary system (Chapter 12)—amoeba.
- Reproductive system (Chapter 15)—*Trichomonas vaginalis* (also genital and sexually transmitted infections below).
- Skin (Chapter 18)—Leishmania, cutaneous larva migrans, Onchocerca.

Helminths and ectoparasites

Helminths are a group of parasitic worms, as shown in Fig. 5.9. Ectoparasites (e.g., bed bugs, crab lice, fleas, etc.) are parasites that live on the outer surfaces of the host.

Microscopy of patient specimens (faeces, blood, tissue) allows the identification of most helminths and ectoparasites.

Taenia solium—a tapeworm found in undercooked pork; it becomes clinically significant when it infects the central nervous system, causing neurocysticercosis (cerebral cysts) which usually presents as seizures.

Other helminth infections include Strongyloides and Schistosomiasis (both discussed in Chapter 11), and Echinococcal infection (hydatid cyst, discussed in Chapter 12).

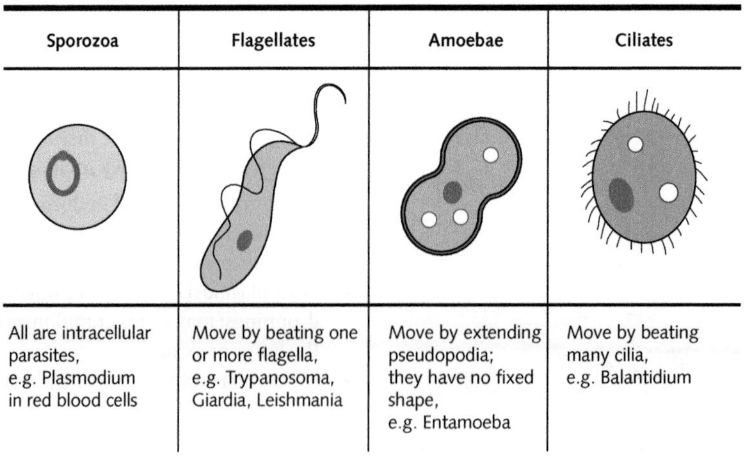

Sporozoa
Flagellates
Amoebae
Ciliates
All are intracellular parasites, e.g. Plasmodium in red blood cells
Move by beating one or more flagella, e.g. Trypanosoma, Giardia, Leishmania
Move by extending pseudopodia; they have no fixed shape, e.g. Entamoeba
Move by beating many cilia, e.g. Balantidium

Fig. 5.8 Main divisions of protozoa

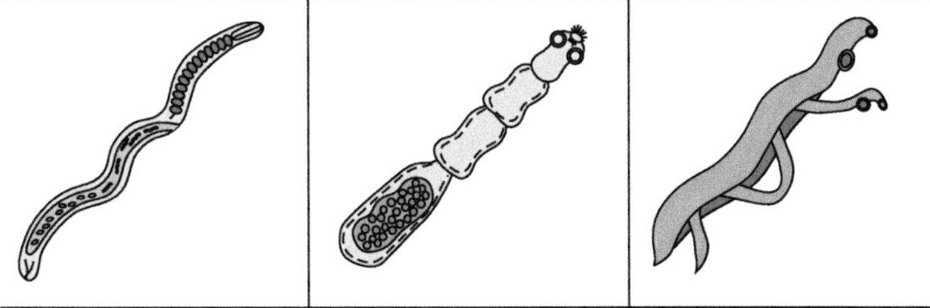

Nematodes (roundworms)	Cestodes (tapeworms)	Trematodes (flukes)
Resistant cuticle; longitudinal muscles; complete digestive system; separate sexed reproductive system, e.g., *Ascaris lumbricoides, Strongyloides stercoralis*	Cellular epithelium; no digestive system; all hermaphrodites, e.g., *Taenia solium, Echinococcus granulosus*	Cellular epithelium; circular and longitudinal muscles; incomplete digestive system; mostly hermaphrodites, e.g., *Schistosoma*

Fig. 5.9 Main groups of helminths.

Chlamydiae, Rickettsiae and Mycoplasma

Chlamydiae and *Rickettsiae* are obligate intracellular organisms. Chlamydia (a bacteria) replicates within vacuoles formed inside epithelial cells. *Chlamydia trachomatis* (see genital and sexually transmitted infections) is an important cause of female infertility (scarring of fallopian tubes) and preventable blindness (corneal scarring and opacification).

Rickettsiae are small Gram-negative bacteria transmitted by arthropod vectors (e.g., lice, ticks, mites), that replicate in the cytoplasm of epithelial cells. They cause a variety of diseases, including typhus and Rocky mountain spotted fever (*Rickettsia rickettsii*).

Mycoplasma lack cell walls and are the smallest free-living organisms known to man (typically 125–300 nm). They can be transmitted between people by aerosol to produce an atypical pneumonia (see Chapter 10).

Prions

Prions are proteinaceous infectious particles which are not microorganisms and do not contain nucleic acids. They are the responsible agent for transmissible spongiform encephalopathies (Table 5.7) (see Chapter 7). Prions are an abnormal isoform (PrP^{Sc}) of the normal 'prion protein' (PrP), which is abundant within the brain but whose function is unknown. PrP^{Sc} is able to induce conformational shape changes in the normal PrP, converting it to PrP^{Sc}. This can then convert more PrP to PrP^{Sc}, causing a self-propagating chain reaction. The newly formed PrP^{Sc} aggregates to form long amyloid fibres and can subsequently be deposited as protease-resistant amyloid plaques within the brain. Neuronal intracytoplasmic vacuoles and spongiform degeneration of the neuropil with neuronal loss, gliosis and atrophy occur by an unknown mechanism. These changes occur in the absence of inflammation. There is no cure for prion disease; it is fatal in 100% of cases.

Table 5.7 Diseases caused by prions

Human	Animal
CJD	Scrapie (sheep)
vCJD	BSE (cows)
Kuru	Wasting disease in deer and elk
Gerstmann–Sträussler–Scheinker syndrome	Transmissible mink encephalopathy
Fatal familial insomnia	

BSE, Bovine spongiform encephalopathy; CJD, Creutzfeldt–Jakob disease; vCJD, variant Creutzfeldt–Jakob disease.

PrP^{Sc} transmission is by direct inoculation with highly infectious tissues (brain, spinal cord, eye) into the skin or brain (such as in neurosurgery). PrP^{Sc} is highly resistant to standard decontamination methods so stringent disposal methods must be used, ideally with the incineration of ***all*** equipment used.

GENITAL AND SEXUALLY TRANSMITTED INFECTIONS

Viral infection

Viral infections of the genitalia are typically due to either HSV or HPV.

CLINICAL NOTE

TORCH INFECTIONS

These are the most common infections associated with congenital abnormalities.

***T**oxoplasmosis*
***O**ther (syphilis, varicella-zoster, parvovirus B19)*
***R**ubella*
***C**MV*
***H**erpes*

Herpes simplex virus

HSV is a DNA virus and member of the herpesvirus group. Two types of virus exist: HSV-1 and HSV-2. HSV-1 shows orofacial tropism and HSV-2 shows genital tropism; however, lesion location does not strictly correlate to viral type.

HSV-2 is considered a major sexually transmitted infection (STI) causing genital herpes of the vulva in women (herpes vulvitis) and glans penis in men. Infection with HSV-1, which usually causes oral infection, may also cause genital herpes. Transmission is by contact with infected genital epithelium or genital secretions and can occur in the absence of symptoms.

Eighty percent of infections are asymptomatic; however, initial infection may produce painless, herpetic vesicles on the genital mucosa which subsequently break down to produce shallow painful ulcers. This is accompanied by fever, aches and lymphadenopathy. Recurrent outbreaks are common and are usually preceded by a prodrome of genital pain or a tingling sensation.

The virus may remain latent in sensory neurones (e.g., trigeminal ganglia or sacral root ganglia) and cause recurrent herpes outbreaks (overt or covert) upon reactivation of the virus. This can be precipitated by a febrile illness, immune suppression, emotional stress or ultraviolet light.

Complications

- Bacterial superinfection (balanitis, candidal vulvovaginitis).
- Persistent severe ulcers in those who are HIV positive/immunosuppressed.
- Dissemination with impaired T-cell immunity affecting multiple organs, e.g., fulminant hepatitis.
- Rarely, aseptic meningitis (HSV-2) and HSV encephalitis (HSV-1).
- Neonatal HSV disease and congenital malformations.

Human papillomavirus

HPV is a double-stranded DNA (dsDNA) virus belonging to the papillomavirus family and comprises >40 types. It infects the basal cell layer of squamous stratified epithelium within the cervix, vulva, vagina, anus, penis and oropharynx. It is the most common STI, with the majority of infections being transient and subclinical. Ninety percent of infections are cleared within 2 years; however, some persist.

HPV is known to be the causative agent in benign and malignant neoplasms within the genital tract and, as such, is classified by its oncogenic potential:

- Low-risk HPV: causes warts (e.g., HPV types 6 and 11).
- High-risk HPV: causes dysplastic and malignant transformation (e.g., HPV types 16 and 18).

Within the high-risk group, viral proteins have been identified that inactive tumour suppressor genes: E6 inhibits *p53* and E7 inhibits *Rb*, which predisposes a cell to neoplastic transformation. A discussion of the premalignant and malignant lesions caused by HPV can be found in Chapters 4 and 15.

Condyloma acuminatum (genital warts)

These cauliflower-like warts are seen on the penis, vulva, vagina and around the perineum/perianal area. They are caused by sexual transmission of the human papillomavirus subtypes HPV6 and HPV11, which have very low neoplastic potential.

Bacterial and protozoal infections

Gardnerella vaginalis

This Gram-negative bacillus forms part of a polymicrobial infection causing bacterial vaginosis and is often associated with other sexually spread infections. The patient complains of a foul-smelling discharge, which is thin and greyish in appearance. *G. vaginalis* is also found as a commensal in a large proportion of women without evidence of bacterial vaginosis. Squamous cells with adherent bacteria (clue cells) are seen microscopically.

Chlamydia trachomatis

Chlamydia is a Gram-negative obligate, intracellular organism, of which 15 serotypes are responsible for a spectrum of diseases:

- Serotypes A–C: trachoma (chronic conjunctivitis associated with blindness, predominantly seen in Africa and Asia).
- Serotypes D–K: urogenital infections.
- Serotypes L1–L3: lymphogranuloma venereum (LGV).

Chlamydia is one of the most common STIs in the UK; 80% of women and 50% of men are asymptomatic, increasing the likelihood of silent transmission amongst the population. It is the leading cause of infertility in women and dual infection with *Neisseria gonorrhoeae* occurs in 30%–40% of cases. Diseases caused by Chlamydia include:

1. Women: pelvic inflammatory disease leading to increased risk of ectopic pregnancies, infertility, chronic pain and dyspareunia.
2. Men: orchitis, epididymitis, urethritis, LGV.
3. Neonates (vertical transmission): conjunctivitis, pneumonia.

Lymphogranuloma venereum

LGV is an STI which initally causes genital papules or ulcers followed 2–6 weeks later by painful inguinal lymphadenopathy. The third stage is characterized by proctitis, which is more common in women and in men who have sex with men. The incidence within the UK and Europe has been increasing. Chronic infections can lead to genital disfigurement, lymphatic obstruction (non-pitting oedema) and rectal strictures/fistulas. Real-time polymerase chain reaction (PCR) is the best diagnostic test as serology is not reliable.

Trichomonas vaginalis

This sexually transmitted flagellated protozoan is typically asymptomatic in men, but in women it often produces an intensely irritating vaginal discharge with inflammation of the vulva, vagina and cervix. The discharge is often frothy and offensive.

Treponema pallidum

Syphilis was thought to be a rare STI; however, its incidence is increasing. Primary syphilis presents with a painless chancre 3–6 weeks after initial infection. It is highly contagious as numerous organisms are present within the overlying ulcer exudate. The chancre spontaneously heals within 3 months with pronounced fibrosis. If left untreated, infection can progress to secondary or tertiary forms (see Chapter 7).

Histologically, the hallmarks of syphilis are endarteritis and a plasma cell–rich inflammatory infiltrate.

Haemophilus ducreyi

This Gram-negative coccobacillus is the commonest cause of genital ulceration worldwide (although uncommon in Europe and the UK) and is thought to be an important factor in HIV transmission.

It presents with a tender papule on the penis or vagina, which breaks down to form painful shallow ulcers. Unlike syphilis, ulcers may be multiple and inguinal lymphadenitis may be present. Involved lymph nodes may progress to buboes if the infection is left untreated.

Yeast and fungal infections

Candidiasis

Candida is a commensal yeast of the vagina whose growth is regulated by the normal commensal vaginal flora, e.g., Lactobacillus and Corynebacterium, which maintain an acidic environment. Loss of the normal bacterial flora can result in Candida overgrowth and candidiasis.

Candidiasis is a very common infection and presents with vulvovaginal itching, soreness, superficial dyspareunia and a white curd-like discharge. It is commonly known as 'thrush'. *Candida albicans* is the causative agent in 80–90% of cases, but other species include *Candida glabrata* and *Candida tropicalis*.

Conditions that predispose to candidal overgrowth are:

- oestrogenic states: pregnancy/oestrogen contraceptives
- immunosuppressed states: e.g., cytotoxic drugs, corticosteroids, HIV infection
- diabetes
- obesity
- broad spectrum antibiotic therapy: loss of the normal commensal bacteria.

Macroscopically, white plaques of fungal hyphae develop on inflamed vaginal mucosa. Most infections are mild; however, some can be severe. Candidiasis can be chronic or recurrent.

HEALTHCARE-ASSOCIATED INFECTION

Healthcare-associated infection (HAI), previously known as hospital-acquired infection and nosocomial infection, is infection acquired as a direct result of healthcare interventions, i.e., medical or surgical treatments, or from being in contact with a healthcare setting. Three hundred thousand patients per year acquire an HAI, with a prevalence of 6.4%; in 20–40% of cases the acquisition of an HAI is thought to have been preventable. The most common sites of infection are:

- respiratory tract
- urinary tract
- surgical site
- blood (bacteraemia).

A variety of pathogens are responsible for HAI, the most well known being MRSA and *Clostridium difficile*. Others include *S. aureus*, *E. coli*, *Klebsiella*, *Pseudomonas aeruginosa*, *Enterobacter* and *Salmonella*. Of particular concern are the multidrug-resistant infections that do not respond to traditional broad-spectrum antibiotics, i.e., MRSA and VRE. HAIs can delay recovery, increase complication rates and ultimately result in the death of a patient. They are also a significant economic burden to the NHS.

The highest rates of HAI are seen in patients on intensive treatment units (ITUs), as they are the most vulnerable and are often intubated, followed by those on surgical wards because of surgical wounds, drains and urinary catheters.

Public Health England monitors the rates of certain infections with routine surveillance programs, e.g., Gram-negative bacteraemia, MRSA, *C. difficile* and *E. coli*.

CLINICAL NOTE

MEASURES TO REDUCE HOSPITAL-ASSOCIATED INFECTION (HAI)

Important measures to reduce levels of HAI include:

- Handwashing/use of alcohol gels for staff and visitors.
- Isolating infected patients in side rooms and using barrier nursing techniques.
- Use of personal protective equipment.

- Appropriate use of antibiotics following local guidelines.
- Use of aseptic techniques when siting indwelling devices such as intravenous cannulas and urinary catheters.
- Minimizing the length of preoperative hospital stays.
- Regular cleaning of clinical areas.

HOST DEFENCES AND ROUTES OF ENTRY

The majority of infectious agents encountered by an individual are prevented from entering the body by a variety of biochemical and physical barriers. These include anatomical barriers such as the skin and mucous membranes or physiological factors such as pH, temperature and commensal flora, which provide an unfavourable physical environment for the growth of microorganisms (Table 5.8).

Commensal microflora

Commensal microflora form an important part of the innate immune system by providing a microenvironment which is unfavourable for pathogen growth.

Interest has been rapidly increasing in the human microbiome with the realization that these organisms provide a genetic contribution and play a role in health and disease states.

MOLECULAR

HUMAN MICROBIOME

The microbiome is the collective term for the genomes of all the microorganisms that live inside and on the human body. Microorganisms are required for digestion, vitamin synthesis, detoxification of carcinogens, drug metabolism and immune system support. It is becoming apparent that differences exist in the microbial populations in health and disease, and that disease states may in part arise from alterations in the microbiome, e.g., Crohn disease, bacterial vaginosis.

The human microbiome project arose as an extension of the human genome project to investigate the diversity and composition of microbial populations which exist at different sites within the body.

Innate immunity

Innate immunity consists of nonspecific mechanisms, cellular and serum, that contribute to resistance and recovery from infection. It preexists and acts within minutes to

Table 5.8 Host defences against infectious agents

Host defence	Features	Effects
Protein secretions	Lysozyme Complement Interferons	Lysozyme causes cell lysis of Gram-positive bacteria Complement has a range of antimicrobial functions
Skin	Dry, acidic, cool and salty Continual cell sloughing Sebaceous gland fatty acid secretion	Physical barrier to microbial invasion Unfavourable growth conditions Fatty acids retard growth Continual sloughing prevents prolonged adhesion
Mucous membranes	Mucin layer Gastric acid Bile salts Cilia Cell-to-cell tight junctions	Captures microorganisms and facilitates physical removal Acid kills ingested microorganisms. Tight junctions retard microbial invasion/penetration into host tissues
Microflora	Commensal organisms, especially in skin and gastrointestinal tract	Physical density prevents growth of pathogens Secretions that regulate and retard growth of pathogens Lower pH Lactoferrin and transferrin—iron limitation Toxic metabolites produced inhibiting growth of other microorganisms
Ciliary clearance	Lining of the respiratory tract, gastrointestinal tract	Move particulate matter out and prevent stasis
Washing of mucosal surfaces	Urine, tears, vaginal secretions, nasal secretions, saliva	Removes organisms and prevents stasis Often fluid contains lysozyme

prevent infection from becoming established. There is a restricted repertoire of responses as the genes are encoded within the germline and have evolved to recognize common pathogenic epitopes, e.g., LPS. Innate immunity has no memory, so the response is generic and will occur again and again.

Innate immunity includes:

- **Complement:** (see Chapter 3) which has many functions, including opsonization of pathogens, cell wall lysis, chemoattraction and to increase the immunogenicity of antigens. Complement receptors can also recognize LPS, which is important in the costimulation of B-cells.
- **Leucocytes with innate cellular immunity:**
  - Macrophages:
    - engulf microorganisms via Fc receptors (for antibodies) and C3b receptors
    - prevent dissemination of microorganisms
    - kill organisms via oxidative burst (free radical production) and other proteins which damage microbial membranes, e.g., cathepsin G, defensins and lysozyme with help from natural killer (NK) and T-helper cells (T_H1)
    - secrete cytokine (tumour necrosis factor (TNF) α, interleukin (IL) 1 and IL-12)
    - are involved in antigen processing and presentation for adaptive immune response (professional antigen-presenting cells).
  - Neutrophils:
    - engulf microorganisms
    - kill microorganisms (reactive oxygen species and nitric oxide)
    - secrete chemoattractants to recruit other immune cells
  - NK cells:
    - are cytotoxic lymphocytes
    - are important in viral infections, intracellular pathogens and tumour cells
    - can activate apoptotic pathways via Fas (see Chapter 3)
    - have antibody-dependent cell cytotoxicity and natural killing via specific receptors
    - secrete cytokines for T- and B-cell help.
- **Immunoglobulins:** produce nonselective IgA and IgM from B-cells, which recognize common bacterial antigens.

Adaptive immunity

Adaptive immunity is specific and includes cellular immunity (T- and B-cells) and humoral immunity (selective immunoglobulins). It is characterized by antigen specificity and clonal expansion of antigen-specific lymphocytes. The response generated is tailored towards the type of pathogen encountered, e.g., T_H versus T_C responses. The genes underlying the adaptive immunity are somatically rearranged and theoretically have infinite variability. Unlike innate immunity, adaptive immunity has immunological memory such that, on reexposure to an antigen, there is a heightened and specific immune response.

> **HINTS AND TIPS**
>
> **T_H CELLS VERSUS T_C CELLS**
>
> Each type of T cell is biased towards a particular microorganism or emergency situation due to its particular skill set and the way it becomes activated. Generally speaking, their roles are as follows:
>
> **T_H cells:**
>
> Provide help to other immune cells to enable them to do an efficient job e.g., to B-cells to produce better antibodies, to macrophages to activate them to become more efficient killers and to T_C cells to enhance killing. B-cells and macrophages are concerned with extracellular pathogens: in essence, antibodies immobilize the roaming pathogen and macrophages phagocytose (eat) the pathogen.
>
> **T_C cells:**
>
> Specialize in killing cells with intracellular pathogens e.g., viruses.

Immune reaction to virally infected cells

Cytotoxic T cells (Tc) kill virally infected cells as follows (Fig. 5.10):

- Virally infected cells express viral peptides bound to MHC class I on their cell surfaces.
- T_C cells recognize viral antigen via the T-cell receptor.
- T_C cells secrete cytolysins, which results in the lysis of the virally infected cells.

NK cells can do the same, but less effectively. The activity of these cells is enhanced by interferons produced by T_C and T_H cells. Interferons also prevent adjacent cells from becoming infected by intercellular viral transport.

Immune reaction to bacterial infections

Macrophages ingest bacteria/bacterial components and present bacterial peptides on MHC class II proteins on their cell surfaces (Fig. 5.11).

T_H cells recognize bacterial antigens via the T-cell receptor and secrete a variety of cytokines.

These cytokines act to help B-cells and T_C cells and to activate macrophages. B-cells produce antibodies, which enable opsonization for complement-mediated lysis or macrophage ingestion. Activated macrophages become more efficient at destroying engulfed material.

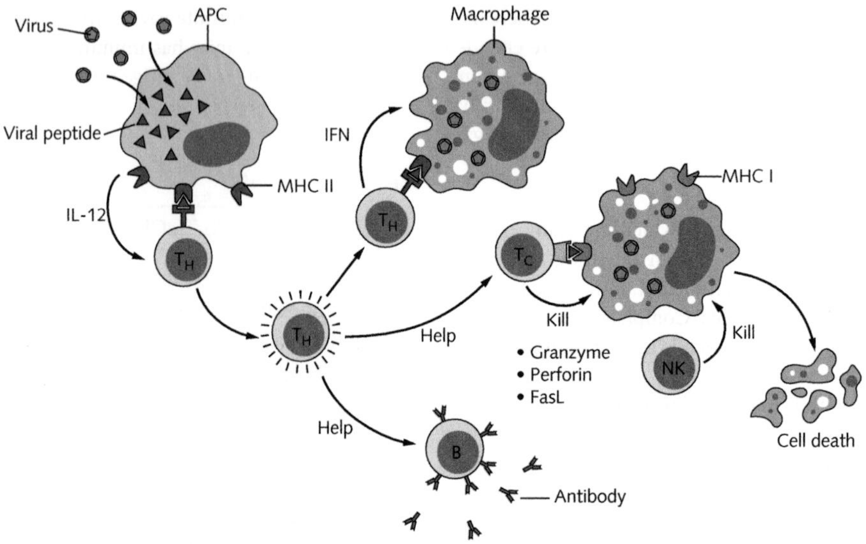

Fig. 5.10 Immune response to viral infection. Intracellular viral proteins are processed and presented as peptides on major histocompatibility complex class I *(MHC I)* molecules on the surface of an infected cell. CD8$^+$ cytotoxic T-cells *(T_C)* recognize the viral peptides and kill the infected cell. Professional antigen-presenting cells *(APC)* uptake viral debris from the interstitium and present viral peptides on MHC class II *(MHC II)* molecules. CD4$^+$ T-helper cells *(T_H)* become activated on recognition of the viral peptide and provide help to T_C and B-cells *(B)*. B-cells are then stimulated to produce antibodies which help to neutralize the virus. Viruses induce the downregulation of MHC I as part of immune evasion. Natural-killer *(NK)* cells recognize this downregulation and kill these cells. *IFNγ*, Interferon-γ; *IL-12*, interleukin 12.

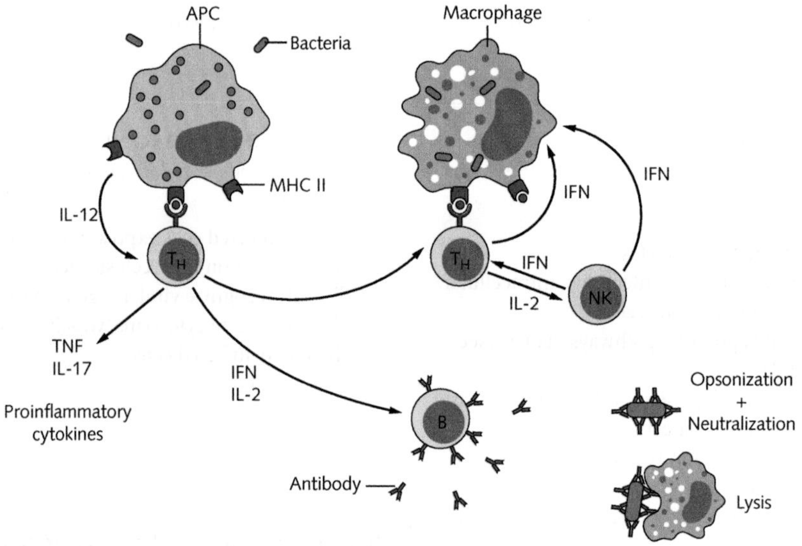

Fig. 5.11 Immune response to bacterial infection. Bacteria/bacterial antigens are ingested from the interstitium by professional antigen-presenting cells *(APC)* and processed and presented as bacterial peptides on major histocompatibility complex class II *(MHC II)* molecules. CD4$^+$ T-helper cells *(T_H)* become activated on recognition of the bacterial peptide and carry out several functions. They can activate infected macrophages, via interferon-γ *(IFNγ)* production, which enhances macrophage intracellular killing and activates natural-killer *(NK)* cells and B-cells *(B)* via interleukin *(IL)* 2. B-cells are stimulated to differentiate and produce antibodies, which opsonize the bacteria allowing efficient phagocytosis by macrophages, neutralization and complement-mediated lysis by formation of the membrane attack complex. T_H cells also release proinflammatory cytokines which facilitate the recruitment of leucocytes. *TNF*, Tumour necrosis factor.

SEPSIS

Sepsis is defined as the association of systemic inflammatory responses with evidence of a microbial origin. In the absence of infection, this is known as systemic inflammatory response syndrome (SIRS), in which there are abnormal clinical physiological variables, such as heart rate, respiratory rate, body temperature, and abnormal leucocyte count. The source of the infection may be organ-specific (e.g., lung in pneumonia), but often there is only bloodstream infection—bacteraemia. The diagnosis is often presumptive because blood and other microbiological cultures may be negative, partly from previous antibiotic administration.

A key concept in sepsis is the host response with production of cytokines (see Chapter 3). If organ dysfunction occurs, then severe sepsis has developed, and if hypotension occurs then septic shock has ensued and multiorgan failure is imminent.

NECROTIZING INFLAMMATION

Gangrene

Gangrene occurs when necrotic tissue is invaded by putrefactive organisms, notably Clostridia. Tissue appears green or black because of the breakdown of haemoglobin. The subtypes of gangrene include wet, dry and gas forms.

Necrotizing fasciitis

A deep-seated, rapidly spreading infection of subcutaneous fat, fascia and muscle. It is usually polymicrobial and commonly includes infection by *S. pyogenes*. It can occur in otherwise healthy subjects after minor trauma, but is not uncommon in diabetic patients. It may lead to toxaemia and multisystem organ failure.

The condition presents as ill-defined erythema, with pain out of proportion to the clinical appearance. Pain extends beyond the area of erythema as the infection tracks along deep fascial planes with infected tissues becoming rapidly necrotic. There is rapid progression of the erythema and necrosis, which has earned it the title of 'flesh-eating bacteria'. Diagnosis is clinical, and action must be taken immediately—'time is tissue!'

Necrotizing fasciitis can occur anywhere but is often seen on the legs or in the groin region (known as Fournier gangrene).

Management—emergency surgical debridement (removal of dead tissue) until viable tissue is identified—this can often be extensive and may lead to amputation; systemic antibiotics are essential. Even with rapid and aggressive management, morbidity and mortality are high.

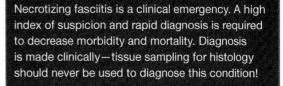

RED FLAG

NECROTIZING FASCIITIS

Necrotizing fasciitis is a clinical emergency. A high index of suspicion and rapid diagnosis is required to decrease morbidity and mortality. Diagnosis is made clinically—tissue sampling for histology should never be used to diagnose this condition!

Chapter Summary

- Infection is invasion and proliferation of microorganisms in the body; colonization is merely inhabitation of an external surface by organisms.
- Opportunistic infections occur in immunocompromised hosts.
- Viruses are obligate intracellular parasites and are classified according to their genomic material, e.g., RNA or DNA.
- HIV is an example of a retrovirus. It infects $CD4^+$ T-cells and, if unchecked, leads to AIDS.
- Bacteria are single cell prokaryotes and can be commensal or pathogenic.
- Bacteria are classified using Gram staining into Gram-positive and Gram-negative bacteria.
- Bacterial virulence factors are distributed via plasmids, e.g., antibiotic resistance genes.
- Bacteria cause disease via the action of exotoxins, endotoxins and superantigens.
- Tissue damage is caused in part by the direct effect of pathogens and in part by the action of the immune system.
- Fungal infections can be superficial or deep/systemic.
- Malaria is an important protozoal infection.
- Multidrug-resistant bacteria are a serious threat as the rate of resistance is outstripping the rate of new antibiotic development.
- Prions are proteinaceous infectious particles which are not microorganisms and do not contain nucleic acids. They are the cause of transmissible spongiform encephalopathies e.g., Creutzfeldt–Jakob disease.
- Healthcare-associated infections are attained as a direct result of healthcare interventions, i.e., medical or surgical treatments, or from being in contact with a healthcare setting. They are a significant source or morbidity/mortality and a burden on the NHS.
- Commensal microflora play a crucial role in the host's defence mechanisms against pathogens.
- Innate immunity consists of nonspecific cellular and humoral mechanisms that preexist and act within minutes to prevent infection.
- Adaptive immunity is specific and includes cellular immunity (T- and B-cells) and humoral immunity (selective immunoglobulins).
- Sepsis is systemic inflammatory response syndrome (SIRS), with evidence of microbial infection.
- Necrotizing fasciitis is a clinical emergency.

Molecular pathology 6

INTRODUCTION

The concept of molecular pathology and personalized medicine has been in existence for at least a decade; however, it is now becoming a more realistic and tangible goal. This is because of the rapid growth in the genomics/genetics arena, both in our molecular understanding of disease and technological abilities.

The traditional paradigm of one gene causing one disease has progressed as we now begin to appreciate the vastly complex web of interconnected pathways within a cell whose dysregulation results in disease. Our knowledge is still in its infancy, but the molecular potential is far-reaching in terms of understanding of both neoplastic and nonneoplastic disease processes, e.g., inflammatory and autoimmune diseases.

Basic terms

The nomenclature used within molecular pathology can be perplexing and seemingly impenetrable! Having a basic understanding of the terminology used goes a long way to demystifying it (Table 6.1).

UNDERSTANDING THE GENOME

Our understanding of the genome has gone beyond that of just genes coding for proteins. How it is constructed, packaged, regulated, maintained and the role of noncoding DNA sequences is vastly complex. These 'epigenetic' processes play a role in the aetiology of diseases such as immune disorders, neuropsychiatric conditions and cancers. Environment also directly interacts with the genome.

MOLECULAR

GENOME STATS

Length of genome: 3.2×10^9 nucleotide pairs
Protein coding genes: 21,000
Nonprotein coding genes: 9000

Table 6.1 Genetic nomenclature

Term	Definition
Chromothripsis	'Chromosomal shattering'. In some cancers a catastrophic event occurs, causing an extensive number of genomic rearrangements, generating carcinogenic mutations.
CpG islands	Are rare areas of noncoding DNA that are rich in C and G and are devoid of methylation. They are usually located near promoter regions.
DNA methylation	Covalent bonding of methyl groups to C molecules resulting in the silencing of gene expression.
Epigenetics	DNA modifications which do not alter the coding sequence of the DNA but influence its expression, e.g., histone configuration, methylation.
Exome	All of the exons within a genome, i.e., the coding portion of the DNA.
Mutator phenotype	Mutations that cause a cell to have an increased rate of mutation, e.g., mutations in DNA repair genes.
Noncoding RNAs	RNA sequences which do not code for a protein but have other functions, e.g., miRNA, siRNA, long ncRNA (see molecular box above).
Polymorphism	Normal individual variation in genetic code.
Promoter	A length of DNA (usually upstream from the gene) where transcription factors assemble before transcription occurs.
Proteome	All of the proteins that are expressed by a genome, cell or tissue.
SNP	'Single nucleotide polymorphism'—a substitution of a single nucleotide at a given position in the genome. Occurs in approximately 1/1000 nucleotide pairs.
Transcription factors	Proteins that bind to promoter regions to initiate the transcription of a gene.
Transcriptome	All of the RNA transcripts produced by an organism or by an individual cell/tissue.

C, cytosine; G, guanine; long ncRNA, long noncoding RNAs; miRNA, microRNAs; siRNA, small interfering RNAs.

Genes

Genes can be coding (when translated they ultimately form proteins) or non-coding. Genes are primarily formed from introns and exons which are then transcribed to mRNA. This undergoes posttranscriptional modification with removal (splicing) of introns and ligation of exons. Genes are also closely associated with portions of noncoding DNA such as promoters. It is important to note that it is not only mutations occurring within the genes themselves that can precipitate disease; various events can occur in the regions of noncoding DNA. For example, mutations far upstream of the gene can affect DNA packaging, causing aberrations in gene expression.

MOLECULAR

100,000 GENOMES PROJECT

The 100,000 Genomes Project commenced in the UK in 2012 with the aim to elicit a better understanding of the genes involved in cancer and rare (hereditary) diseases by sequencing and comparing '100K genomes'. Whole-genome sequencing is performed on both the patient's normal cells and cancer cells to identify genetic differences.

Epigenetics

Epigenetics is the study of potentially inheritable patterns of gene expression with no alteration of the DNA sequence, i.e., change of phenotype without a change in genotype. This can be achieved by controlling the activation or suppression of genes so that they are 'read' or 'not read'. Epigenetic phenomena occur in normal physiological and disease states. As the underlying genetic code is preserved, theoretically the epigenetic modifications are reversible and could potentially be targeted to halt and/or reverse disease processes. Examples of epigenetic modifications include:

- ***DNA methylation:*** covalent bonding of methyl groups to cytosine residues in the DNA strand results in the silencing of gene expression. In females, an entire X chromosome is silenced by methylation. When cells divide, daughter cells inherit the methylation patterns of the parent cell's DNA; thus liver cells remain liver cells.
- ***Histone modification:*** histones are the packing beads around which DNA is wrapped and organized. How loosely or tightly the DNA is packaged controls access to certain areas of the genome to allow transcription to occur. Genes can be silenced by being tightly packed.
- ***Noncoding RNA gene silencing:*** transcribed RNA sequences which do not code for a protein but themselves have other functions.

MOLECULAR

TYPE AND FUNCTIONS OF NONCODING RNAS

- *microRNAs (miRNA):* approximately 22 base pairs (bp) long. Help to regulate gene expression by binding with mRNA transcripts, reducing their stability and therefore translation.
- *long noncoding RNAs (long ncRNA):* longer version of miRNA (>220 bp).
- *small interfering RNAs (siRNA):* bind to and remove foreign RNA sequences, e.g., viral.

MOLECULAR TECHNIQUES

Molecular techniques are continuously evolving and, as our understanding of pathology and medicine moves to a molecular level, a basic knowledge of the technology is required.

Polymerase chain reaction

The polymerase chain reaction (PCR), put simply, is a technique used to amplify the amount of DNA present within a sample, creating sufficient quantities for further analysis. It incorporates thermal cycling and chemical reaction.

Method: a mix of sample DNA, labelled deoxynucleoside triphosphates (dNTPs), DNA polymerase, buffer and primers is made. dNTPs are the nucleoside base building blocks for the new strands of DNA that will be made (i.e., C, G, A and T) and are labelled (fluorescence/radioactivity) so they can be detected at the end of the reaction. DNA polymerase is the builder and the sample DNA is the template/plan; primers are the starting points.

The mix is heated to high temperatures, causing the DNA helix to separate (melt). The temperature is then reduced to allow the primers to stick (anneal/hybridize) at opposite ends. DNA polymerase binds to the primers and builds a complementary strand of DNA using the original sample DNA as a template (extension). At the end of a cycle the DNA has doubled. The cycle is repeated 20–40 times, resulting in exponential amplification (Fig. 6.1).

The technique of sequential addition of bases using a template and primers forms the basis of many sequencing reactions and the foundation of molecular genetics. It is therefore important to understand this fundamental process. RNA can also be amplified using this method by first converting it into copy DNA (cDNA) using reverse transcriptase. Real-time PCR (qPCR) is a variant of PCR that allows quantification of the DNA product as the reaction is monitored whilst it occurs.

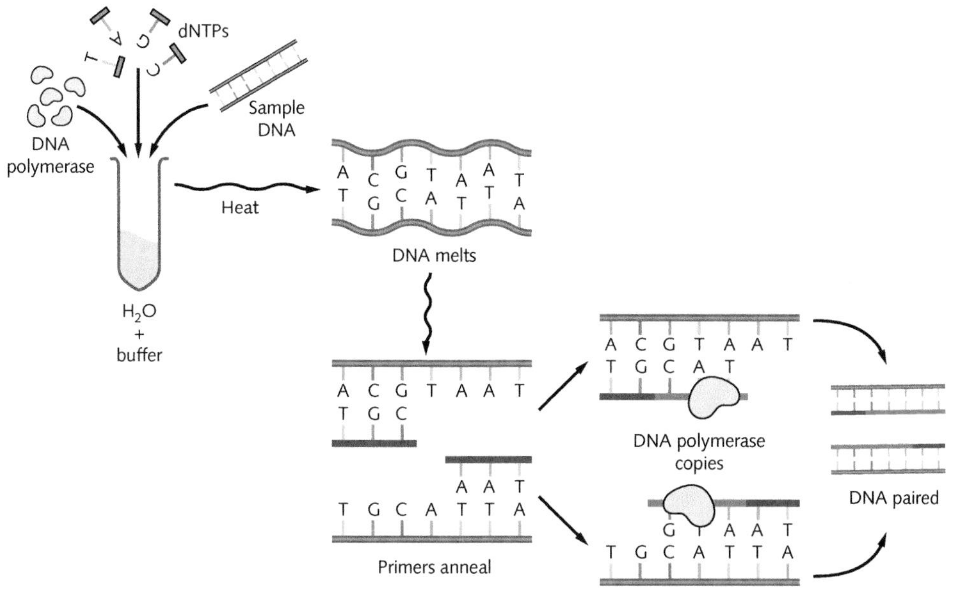

Fig. 6.1 Polymerase chain reaction. Primers flank a known region of interest in the DNA. They are carefully designed so that they do not stick to themselves and are unique for the part of the DNA you are interested in. Primers can also be designed to attach to mutant sequences and not wild type ones. *dNTPs*, Deoxynucleoside triphosphates.

DNA sequencing

DNA sequencing is the elucidation of the order (sequence) of DNA/RNA bases, e.g., AATCGGA. Sequencing offers a vast potential for diagnostics and therapeutics as it can be used to identify what is normal, what is mutant, and specific mutations. We are currently at the threshold of the third generation of sequencing techniques, with an astonishing gain in speed and efficiency, making sequencing more available, practical and cost effective as a day-to-day tool.

> **MOLECULAR**
>
> **HUMAN GENOME PROJECT**
>
> The first draft of the human genome was published in February 2001 in *Nature* (*Nature* 409:860–921). It was the result of 13 years of work by 20 international groups which began in 1990. This unprecedented momentous achievement has given birth to new DNA technologies, research and drugs. The sequence is open to all and can be found online.
>
> The majority of sequencing was performed using the laborious Sanger method. Now a whole genome can be sequenced in a matter of hours on the work bench.

First generation: Sanger sequencing

This was the first sequencing method and is considered the gold standard. It utilizes a modified PCR reaction.

Method: the reaction mix is the same as for PCR; however, four separate reactions are carried out using dideoxynucleoside triphosphates (ddNTPs), which are chain-terminating dNTPs for the A, T, G and C bases. These can be labelled with ethidium bromide or fluorescent probes. The reaction proceeds as with normal PCR; however, variable lengths of product are generated owing to incorporation of ddNTPs at variable points. The end products contain different lengths of DNA which have been terminated at each nucleotide position in the template molecule.

The products of the four reactions are then separated by size using electrophoresis to generate the DNA sequence. Large fragments move slowly and small fragments move quickly towards the end of the gel, creating a ladder effect. Originally electrophoresis was manually performed on a gel; this has been superseded by automated fluorescent capillary electrophoresis. The gel is read horizontally from bottom to top to determine the sequence, whereas the florescent trace is read like a sentence (Fig. 6.2).

Second generation: Next-generation sequencing

Next-generation sequencing (NGS) is ultimately massively parallel sequencing, i.e., 1000s of sequencing reactions occurring at the same time. This allows very high throughput, such that vast quantities of DNA can be sequenced in a short space of time, making whole genome sequencing a viable possibility.

Method: different manufacturers make different machines that harness different technologies/methods for sequencing (platforms), which have moved away from the

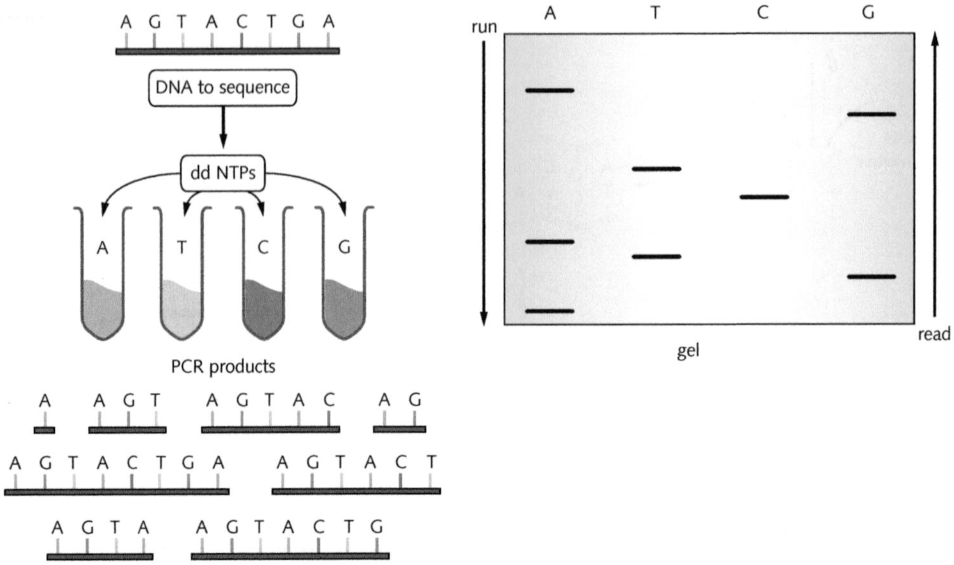

Fig. 6.2 Sanger sequencing. Dideoxynucleoside triphosphates *(ddNTPs)* lack the 3'-OH group of deoxynucleoside triphosphates that is essential for DNA polymerase–mediated chain elongation and therefore act as chain terminators. Gel separates fragments based on size and charge. DNA molecules carry a negative charge and migrate to the positive terminal. The bigger the molecule, the greater the charge, the slower it is; it is therefore seen at the top of the gel. The smaller fragments migrate more rapidly and are therefore seen towards the bottom. *PCR,* Polymerase chain reaction.

Sanger method. The process (workflow) of preparing the DNA/RNA sample for sequencing is largely the same across all platforms (Fig. 6.3). The material for sequencing can be whole-genome, whole-exome, RNA or disease-specific gene panels. The workflow is as follows:

(1) **Fragmentation of the sample:**
  (a) Fragmentation of the DNA into manageable bite-sized chunks to generate a library.
  (b) A library is a collection of DNA/cDNA fragments.

(2) **Library preparation:**
The library needs some organization before it can be sequenced, as currently all the DNA pieces are jumbled and ragged.
  (a) Blunt-ended fragment generation:
    (i) Any unpaired bases (sticky ends) are repaired into blunt ends, i.e., there are no unpaired bases.
  (b) Single adenosine (A) addition to 3' ends.
  (c) Adapter ligation:
    (i) Short adapter sequences are added (ligated) to the As at the ends of the fragments.
    (ii) These are 6–8-base pair (bp) oligonucleotides that allow the fragments to be stuck down to a solid surface during the sequencing reaction (a bit like Velcro).
    (iii) The adapters can also contain barcodes (short sequences), allowing different samples to be mixed together in one sequencing reaction for efficiency (multiplexing) and then unmixed using the barcodes at the end (demultiplexing). This is akin to painting ping pong balls and throwing them into a pot and then separating them later according to colour.

(3) **Target enrichment—hybrid capture:**
  (a) An optional step.
  (b) Allows sequencing of the desired areas of interest only, i.e., looking at books on sport rather than all the books in the library.
  (c) This can be done by adding a probe for the sequences of interest and having a mechanism for binding the probe and therefore the DNA whilst washing the unbound DNA away.
  (d) Alternatively, biotinylated baits or amplicon sequencing (primers to amplify areas of interest selectively) can be used.

(4) **Amplification of library:**
  (a) Creating a sufficient quantity of DNA within the sample to enable downstream reactions to work.
  (b) The fragments are attached (hybridized) to a solid surface (bead or flat surface) via physically tethered complimentary adapters (the other half of the Velcro).
  (c) Amplification is achieved by PCR, resulting in clusters of product.
  (d) The result is multiple copies of your books.

(5) **Evaluation of quality and quantity of DNA:**
  (a) A quality control step to assess what is present. Low-quality and -quantity DNA can result in low-quality data owing to read problems or reduced coverage because of insufficient amounts of DNA.

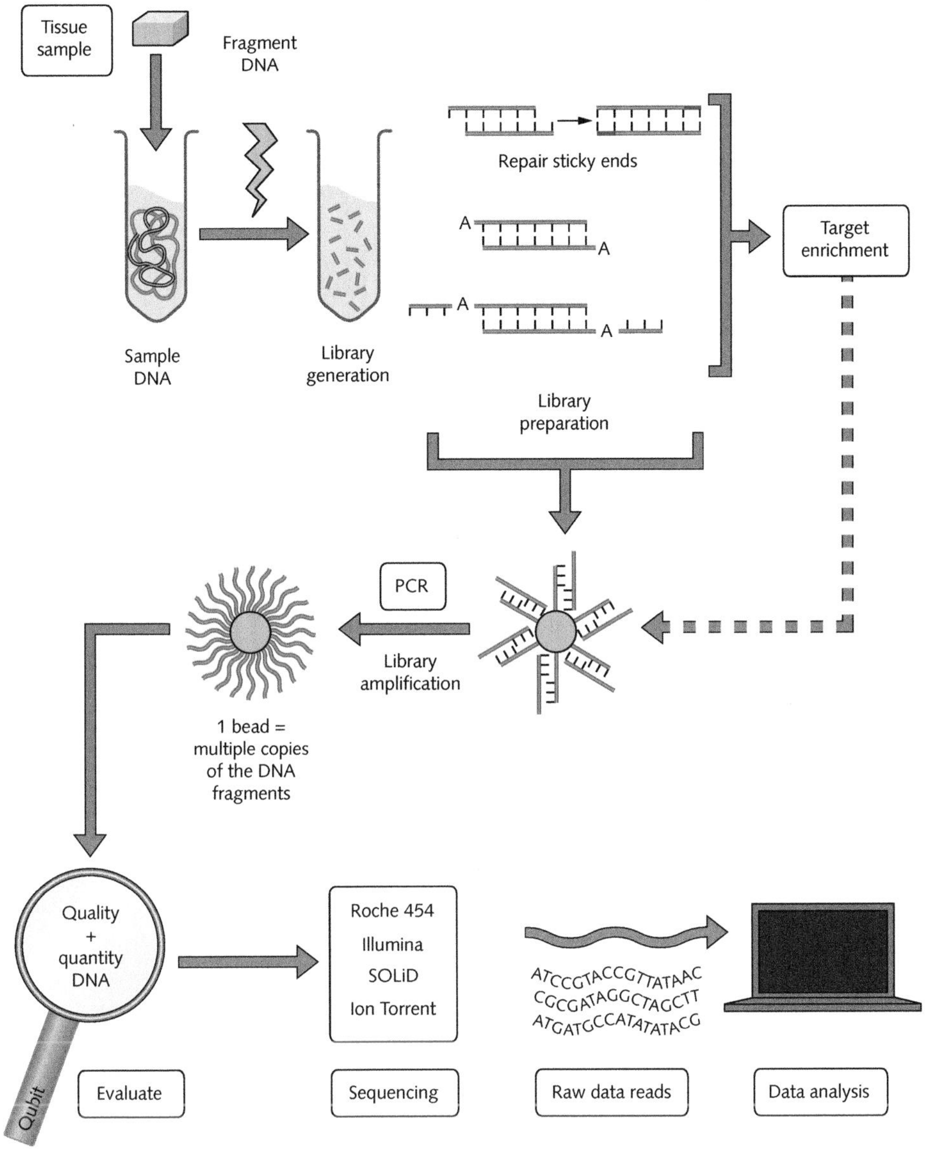

Fig. 6.3 Next-generation sequencing workflow. *PCR,* Polymerase chain reaction.

(b) This is akin to a stock check, i.e., are the books intact? Is the printing of good quality? Do you have enough?

(c) Quantity is checked using qPCR or a Qubit machine.

(d) Quality is assessed by looking at size distribution of fragments, and whether sizes selected in the preparation are present. This is performed by a Bioanalyser.

(6) **Sequencing:**

How this is achieved depends on the platform used:

(a) Sequencing by synthesis (reversible terminator technology):

(i) Illumina—DNA is hybridized to a flow cell with sequencing primers attached to both ends and amplified to form clusters of identical fragments of DNA. Fluorescently labelled dNTPs of different colours are introduced and compete to be sequentially added into the new complementary DNA strand being synthesized using the bound DNA fragment as a template. The fluorescent signals are read every time a dNTP is incorporated to generate the sequence.

(ii) Pyrosequencing: Roche (454) measures light emission caused by the release of inorganic pyrophosphate when a new base is incorporated into the DNA chain.

(b) Sequencing by ligation—DNA (SOLiD), synthesis is by DNA ligase rather than DNA polymerase and uses octamer primers which are fluorescently labelled and ligated to the sample DNA strand. The label is read and then cleaved off to allow the next octamer to be ligated to the preceding one. The reaction is repeated many times with offsetting of the bases to generate the sequence.

(c) Ion semiconductor (Ion Torrent)—every time a dNTP is incorporated into the DNA chain an H^+ ion is released and the pH changes. Different dNTPs are sequentially washed over the amplified DNA fragments attached to beads and pH is monitored as a marker for dNTP incorporation.

(7) **Data analysis:**

A vast amount of raw data is generated, which needs to be interpreted. Raw data consists of the bases as they are identified ('called'). If the samples were barcoded and mixed, they must first be separated (demultiplexed). Bioinformatics is essential and various computer programmes are required to support analysis, which requires several steps.

(a) Sequence alignment:

Required to arrange all the fragments generated into the correct order/sequence as currently they are jumbled. This can be done by:

(i) Alignment to a reference sequence, i.e., the human genome, which is now the most commonly used method.

(ii) De-novo alignment: when no reference sequence exists, fragments are aligned against themselves to build larger sequences called contigs. The idea is to build a single contig to encompass all of the genome (which was how the human genome was constructed).

(b) Variant calling:

(i) After alignment, variations in the sequence can be sought, either by known mutations or new single nucleotide polymorphisms (SNPs), etc.

(c) Visualization of data:

(i) Output can be seen visually and the data assessed manually if required.

HINTS AND TIPS

NEXT-GENERATION SEQUENCING DEPTH AND READ

Read—the raw sequence of a DNA fragment, e.g., ATTCTGGACAT.

Depth—the number of times a nucleotide is sequenced, i.e., average number of reads across a genomic location.

Coverage—the portion of the total intended sample (e.g., genome) that is represented in the data set, i.e., breadth of the sequence generated. Coverage improves with depth.

Greater depth and coverage are required to detect alleles of low frequencies.

A wide variety of mutations can be detected by NGS, including:

- Copy number variations
- Chromosomal inversions
- Translocations
- Insertions/deletions
- Large deletions
- Large amplifications
- Point mutations (SNPs)
- Splice variants.

MOLECULAR

PITFALLS OF NEXT-GENERATION SEQUENCING

- False-positive artifacts—DNA polymerase is 99% accurate. Therefore in 1/100 bases a mistake will be made. If error occurs early on in amplification it can appear as a true variant.
- Epigenetic variants are lost during amplification.
- NGS has shorter read lengths 100–200 bp versus 800 bp in Sanger sequencing.
- Preferential amplification—smaller fragments amplify better so there can be an overrepresentation of a fragment and fragment duplication.

Clinical applications of next-generation sequencing

The increasing speed, accuracy, availability and cost reduction of NGS is allowing it to become an everyday, standard diagnostic tool, with many clinical applications as outlined in Table 6.2.

Third-generation sequencing

This is cutting-edge technology that sequences DNA a single base at a time, allowing for long read length, speed and efficiency. Various techniques and kits are becoming available. Examples include:

- ***Nanopore technology***—the DNA chain is pulled through a nanopore sited on an electrically resistant

Table 6.2 Clinical applications of next-generation sequencing

Diagnostics	
To identify and type disease/cancer accurately	Gene panels for different cancers Whole-exome sequencing Whole-genome sequencing
Targeted therapies	
Molecular level specificity of treatment Reduce toxicity Cost-effective	Examples include: CML: BCR-ABL fusion protein—imatinib Breast cancer: HER2—trastuzumab (Herceptin)
Evaluation of clinical response Use of ctDNA	Quantify tumour load Assess effectiveness of treatment Track mutations in tumour genome to monitor for resistance Detect early recurrence Prenatal testing
Screening	
For inherited diseases For cancer	Common and rare inherited mutations Prenatal testing
Personalized therapies In the future...	Creating personalized vaccines against specific tumour epitopes, e.g., melanoma

CML, Chronic myeloid leukaemia; ctDNA, circulating tumour DNA.

polymer membrane. Translocation of different nucleotides/combinations of nucleotides through the pore give different characteristic changes in the flowing electrical current, allowing sequence determination.

- *SMRT*—'Single molecule sequencing in real time'. DNA is sequenced in real time as fluorescently labelled bases are sequentially added to the DNA strand using the sample DNA as a template. As each base is incorporated, its fluorescent colour is recorded and then the label is removed. The next base in the DNA chain is then added and recorded.

Fluorescent in-situ hybridization

Fluorescent in-situ hybridization (FISH) uses fluorescently labelled probes to identify a known target on a chromosome. The probes are short lengths of single-stranded DNA that can hybridize to their complementary sequence, making it visible (Fig. 6.4). There are various ways FISH can be utilized:

- ***Break-apart probes:*** to detect chromosomal translocations, e.g., EWSR1. The two signals e.g., red and green, flank the translocation break point. In an unmutated situation they appear together on the chromosome. If translocation occurs the red and green signals are seen to split ('break apart') from each other. This is good for diagnosis; however, it requires the gene of interest or break point to be known.

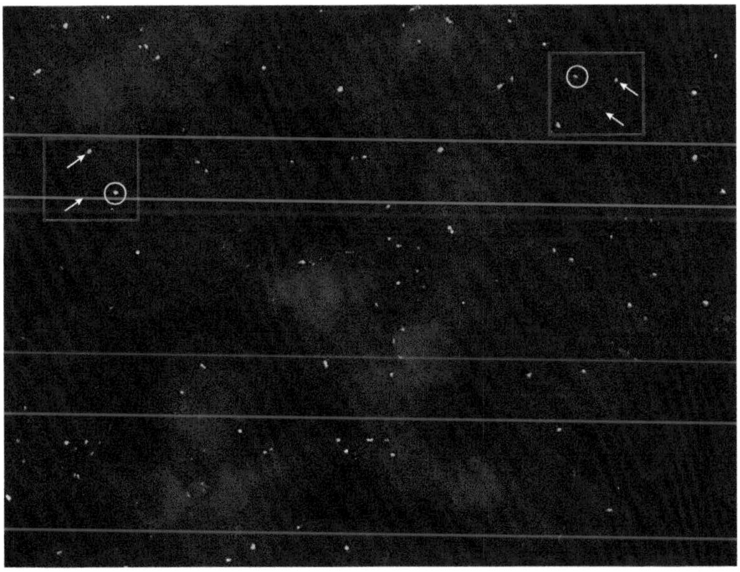

Fig. 6.4 Fluorescent in-situ hybridization (FISH) analysis. FISH image showing a break apart probe for the *MYC* gene. The blue fluorescence stains the nuclei of cells. The red and green probes are either sides of the break point on the *MYC* gene. The normal gene shows the red and the green signals together yellow circle. The rearranged gene shows the red and green probes apart (white arrows).

- ***Fusion probes:*** these work in the opposite way to break-apart probes. In unmutated chromosomes, the signals are separate. If translocation occurs, the signals are seen to associate, creating a 'fusion' signal with the colours now adjacent to each other on the same chromosome. This method is of limited use, as the translocation partner needs to be known, whereas in break-apart the partner does not.
- ***Copy number evaluation:*** increased numbers of genes/chromosomes or loss of a gene/chromosome can be detected by counting the ratio of probes present.

Chromosomal in-situ hybridization

Chromosomal in-situ hybridization (CISH) is the less glamorous sibling of FISH. Horseradish peroxidase-labelled DNA probes are hybridized onto paraffin tissue sections to detect specific genes, e.g., HER2 expression in breast cancer. The label is seen as a brown stain and creates a stable and permanent preparation, akin to immunohistochemistry (IHC).

Immunohistochemistry

IHC is the use of antibodies on paraffin/fixed tissue sections to identify specific protein epitopes within a population of cells, e.g., tumour cells. Positive staining can be further characterized by the intensity of the stain, location, distribution and pattern (Fig. 6.5). IHC can be used as a surrogate molecular marker as well, e.g., c-kit identification in gastrointestinal stromal tumours (GIST). It is currently cheaper and easier to perform than sequencing. Examples of IHC use include:

- Identification of cells, e.g., T- or B-cells in lymphoma.
- Subtyping a primary tumour.
- Confirming the origin of a metastasis from an unknown primary tumour.
- Characterization of spindle cell tumours, e.g., GIST, leiomyoma.
- Help to identify benign/malignant processes.
- The proliferation index, e.g., in lymphomas, neuroendocrine tumours.
- Identification of viruses/bacteria, e.g., Epstein–Barr virus infection.

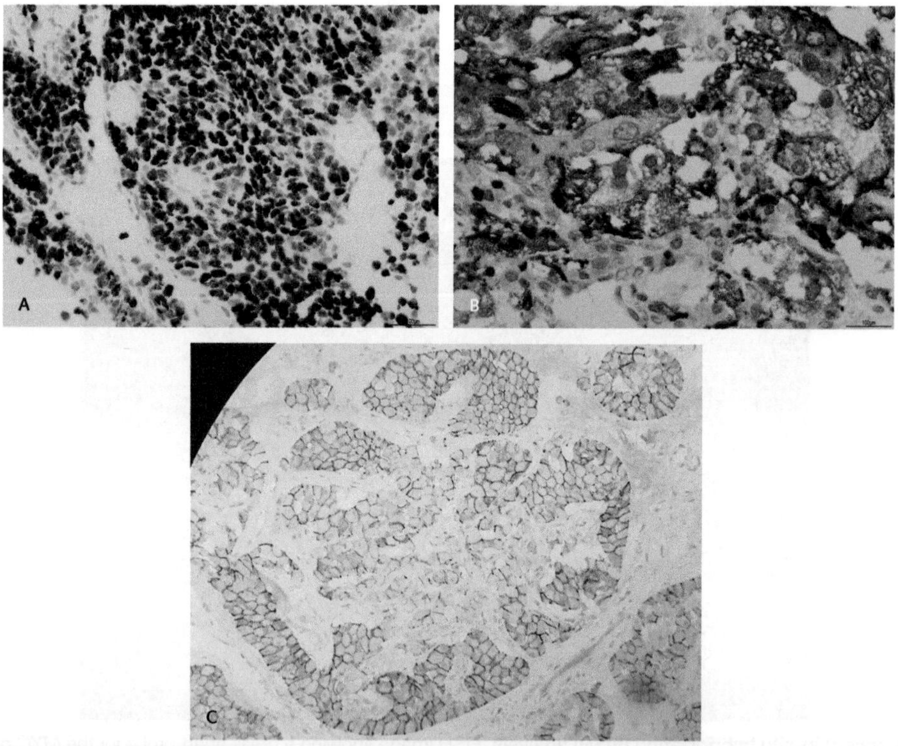

Fig. 6.5 Immunohistochemistry. Immunohistochemistry showing positive (brown) and negative (blue) cells. It is used to pick out a specific population of cells, e.g., myeloma cells within bone marrow. The location of the stain is also important. (A) Nuclear positive stain. (B) Cytoplasmic and membranous staining. (C) Membranous staining.

- Provide prognostic/therapeutic information, e.g., oestrogen and progesterone receptor positivity in breast cancer.
- Surrogate molecular markers, e.g., MLH-1, MSH-6 to assess microsatellite instability.

MOLECULAR BIOLOGY OF CANCER

Cell cycle

Cancer is fundamentally a genetic disease of uncontrolled growth, differentiation and failure of death (apoptosis) of a cell. It follows that the cell cycle and its drivers/suppressors play key roles in the development of cancer (Fig. 6.6).

Cell cycling and replication are tightly controlled events. Broadly speaking, different combinations of cyclins and their kinases (cyclin-dependent kinases (CDKs)) drive the cell cycle by concentration increases and decreases at different intervals (hence the name 'cyclin'). The net result is the transcription of the genes necessary for the completion of each stage and progression to the next.

Checkpoints (built-in fail-safes) exist within the cell cycle, and these must be overcome for the cell to progress. Here the balance of inhibitory versus stimulatory signals must be tipped in favour of the stimulatory signals. Tumour suppressor genes (TSGs) act at these checkpoints to prevent the cell cycling if it is damaged or if conditions are unfavourable for division and hence they maintain the integrity of the genome (see Chapter 4). It is therefore not surprising that many of the key genes within the cancer genotype are found at these checkpoints with mutations giving rise to uncontrolled division and genetic instability, which are the hallmarks of cancer.

G1-S restriction point: this is commonly deregulated in cancer. At this checkpoint the integrity of the cell's DNA is assessed. The cell either continues into S phase or exits the cycle to undergo DNA repair or apoptosis if DNA damage is irrevocable. The key proteins acting at this point include: RB-1, INK-4 and CDKs.

S-G2 restriction point: after DNA replication in S phase, DNA integrity is checked again. The key proteins acting at this point include: P53, MDM-2, P21 and ATR/ATM. They act directly to inhibit cyclins (therefore halting the cycle) and indirectly as transcription factors whose downstream genes include further TSGs, enzymes and proapoptotic molecules.

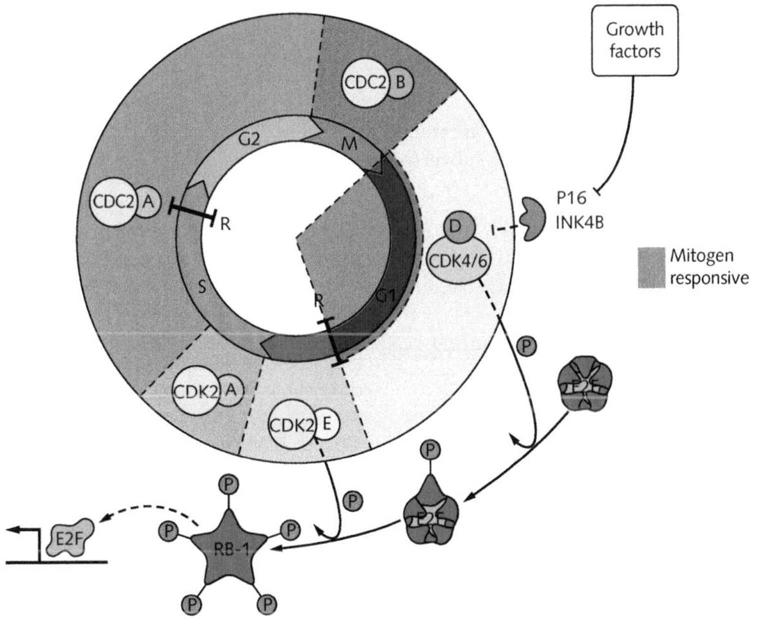

Fig. 6.6 The cell cycle. The cell cycle progresses through the different phases (M, G1, S and G2), driven by rising and falling concentrations of cyclins. Cyclin-dependent kinase *(CDK)* concentration remains static. The role of the tumour-suppressor gene (TSG) *RB-1* is illustrated here; however, many TSGs act at various points of the cycle. Through the majority of G1 phase, the cell cycle is under the influence of external growth factors (mitogens). The presence of mitogens inhibits P16/INK4B proteins, which are inhibitors of cyclin D/CDK4/6. Inhibition release of cyclin D/CDK4/6 results in activation and hypophosphorylation of *RB-1*. As the restriction point is passed, *RB-1* is subsequently hyperphosphorylated by cyclin E/CDK2, releasing the transcription factor *E2F*. Transcription and translation of genes needed for cell cycle progression can now occur. In carcinogenesis, a loss of *RB-1* means that E2F activity is uncontrolled, resulting in continual transcription of genes that drive the cell cycle, which ultimately predisposes to cancer. *CDC,* Cell division cycle protein; *P*, phosphate; *R*, restriction point A, B, C, D E, cyclin A, B, C, D, E.

COMMON PITFALLS

KINASES AND PHOSPHATASES

A common mechanism for controlling the activity of a protein is by the addition and removal of phosphate groups (e.g., on tyrosine or serine residues). Enzymes that add phosphate groups are called kinases (e.g., tyrosine kinases). Enzymes that remove phosphate groups are called phosphatases. Tyrosine kinase inhibitors are a class of drug that block the action of kinases and therefore block the activity of the kinase's target proteins.

Signalling cascades

A mind-boggling array of intracellular, interconnected signalling pathways exist within the cell; however, cancer mutations cluster on a few fundamental pathways. Unsurprisingly, these pathways are involved in the regulation of growth and apoptosis. The epidermal growth factor receptor (EGFR) is the prototypical example of this (Fig. 6.7).

Epidermal growth factor receptor

The mechanism of EGFR exemplifies how signals are transduced within the cell and how these can become subverted in cancer.

1. An extracellular signal is received for growth, e.g., binding of epidermal growth factor (EGF) to EGFR on the cell membrane. This causes receptor dimerization, resulting in receptor autophosphorylation.
2. Activated receptors recruit GRB2 and SOS, causing RAS to become phosphorylated via guanosine triphosphate and activated.
3. A mitogen-activated protein kinase (MAPK) signalling cascade then commences whereby RAS activates RAF, RAF activates mitogen-activated protein kinase kinase (MEK), and MEK activates MAPK.
4. Activated MAPK enters the nucleus and activates various transcription factors, resulting in gene expression.

Therapeutic targets

To offer patients the most effective, appropriate and specific treatments for their disease, genetic testing must be undertaken to identify the mutations present. The mutations that are screened for depend on current knowledge of the cancer in question, which are clinically relevant, and those for which a therapy exists.

The various stages of cancer development and signalling pathways are all legitimate therapeutic targets, e.g., membrane receptors and cytoplasmic signal transduction, amongst others.

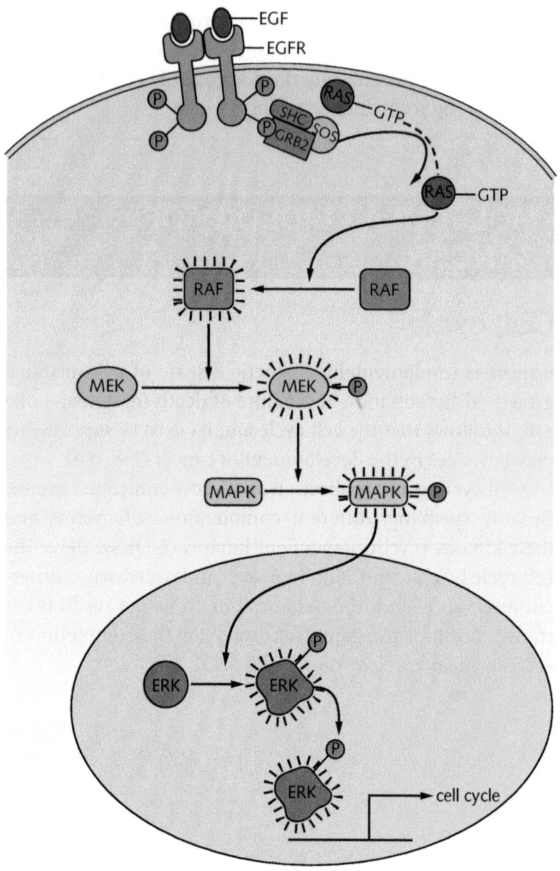

Fig. 6.7 EGFR signalling pathways. Binding of epidermal growth factors *(EGF)* to the epidermal growth factor receptor *(EGFR)* results in heterodimer formation and activation of the receptor by transphosphorylation of the cytoplasmic domains. This signal is conveyed to the nucleus (transduced) by the activation of RAS (a small GTPase), which in turn initiates a signalling cascade resulting in the activation transcription factors (e.g., *ERK* extracellular signal related kinase). The downstream genes that are transcribed are those required in the cell cycle GRB2/SHC/SOS are adapter proteins connecting the membrane receptor to the intracellular signaling cascade. *GTP*, Guanosine triphosphate; *MAPK*, mitogen-activated protein kinases; *MEK*, MAPK kinase; *P*, phosphate.

COMMON PITFALLS

NEGATIVE IS NOT NECESSARILY NEGATIVE

'Genetic testing' is not 100% accurate. A positive or negative result is highly dependent on the method that is used, mutations screened for and the quality and quantity of the DNA sample. A negative result is only negative for those mutations that have been sought; it is not to say that there is not a mutation in the gene somewhere else.

Membrane receptors

Mutations can cause membrane receptors to be permanently active, sending continuous signals for the cell to divide independent of growth factors/extracellular signals, e.g., HER2 in breast cancer and RET in thyroid carcinoma. These constitutively active receptors are potential drug targets in cancer, e.g., trastuzumab (Herceptin) in breast cancer.

It follows that, for a drug to work, the cancer must harbour that mutation. Both monoclonal antibodies and tyrosine kinase inhibitors are used therapeutically to target membrane growth factor receptors in a variety of cancers. Successful anti-EGFR therapy is dependent on the *RAS* gene status of the cancer. If *RAS* is mutated, EGFR signalling will have no influence over its activity, therefore drugs targeting EGFR will be ineffective (see Fig. 6.7).

Cytoplasmic signal transduction

Permanent activation of the intracellular signalling cascades can occur if a component of the cascades becomes mutated. The cell is positively driven to divide regardless of whether there is transduction of extracellular signals to do so. Examples include *RAS* mutations.

Currently there are no effective RAS inhibitors available; however, inhibitors to downstream effectors have been produced, e.g., sorafenib targeting RAF.

Other strategies

- Angiogenesis: another way to target cancers is to deprive them of their blood supply and to this end antiangiogenic drugs have been developed. These are not only proving useful in cancer but are used to treat other conditions such as macular degeneration, e.g., Avastin.
- P53 correction: to reestablish the cell's innate apoptotic mechanisms.
- Modulating the immune system to recognize cancer cells.
- Vaccines against oncogenic agents, e.g., human papilloma virus.
- Personalized antibodies: in the future it may be possible to design antibodies specific to a patient's cancer.

However, these strategies are currently only partially effective as mutations occur which allow cancer to circumvent the effects of treatment, becoming resistant and 'escaping'. It is important to appreciate that there is a large complex web of networks and pathways of interactions that we are only just beginning to understand. Targeting one point of the web is perhaps a drop in the ocean, and delusionally hopeful, but one must start somewhere.

HINTS AND TIPS

IT'S ALL IN THE NAME

The nature of a drug can be determined from the suffix of its generic name:

'-inib'—tyrosine kinase inhibitor e.g., erlotinib.
'-mab'—monoclonal antibody (common stem).
'-ximab'—chimeric monoclonal antibody e.g., infliximab.
'-zumab'—humanized monoclonal antibody e.g., trastuzumab.
'-umab'—human monoclonal antibody e.g., adalimumab.

The paradigm of cancer is shifting such that it is the overactivity or underactivity of a pathway that is important. This had led to so-called 'basket trials' for which a specific mutation qualifies for entry into a trial regardless of the type of cancer.

Apoptosis

The subversion of apoptotic pathways is another contributory mechanism by which cells become neoplastic. A more detailed discussion of apoptosis can be found in Chapter 3.

SYSTEMIC MOLECULAR PATHOLOGY

Currently there are a limited number of recognized mutations of clinical use and significance. These enable targeted drug therapies, define a cancer, provide prognostic information or are useful diagnostically. Table 6.4 outlines some of the current relevant mutations of the different organ systems.

NEW AGE OF GENETICS

Molecular taxonomy

The classification of cancer and some diseases is beginning to move away from pure morphology to a combination of genetic and morphological classification. Some cancers are defined solely on the basis of the mutations they contain, especially with regard to lymphomas. More cancers are now being considered in terms of their mutations rather than their primary site. This is important, as it changes the way in which we think about and treat disease.

Liquid biopsy

Fragments of circulating tumour DNA (ctDNA) can be found at low concentrations within the peripheral blood of cancer patients. They have also been detected in cerebral

Table 6.4 Clinically relevant mutations

System	Gene	Disease	Function/role	Clinical significance
Gastrointestinal	*RAS* (*N* and *K*)	Colorectal carcinoma	Signalling cascade	These can be mutated or wild type. If mutated, anti-EGFR drugs (e.g., cetuximab) will be ineffective
	Mismatch repair/ microsatellite instability (*MLH1, MSH6, MSH2, PMS2*)	Colorectal carcinoma	DNA mutation repair	If mutated, raises the possibility of Lynch syndrome (see Chapter 11)
	HER2	Gastric carcinoma	Growth factor receptor	A small subset of gastric carcinomas shows this mutation and may respond to treatment with trastuzumab
	C-KIT *PDGFRA*	Gastrointestinal stromal tumours (GIST)	Tyrosine kinases	Defines a GIST. Treatment is with TKIs
Breast	*ER/PR*	Breast carcinoma	Transcription factors	If positive, allows for treatment with ER and PR antagonists, e.g., tamoxifen
	HER2	Breast carcinoma	Growth factor receptor	If mutated, can be treated with Herceptin; mutation is an adverse prognostic indicator
	BRCA1 and 2	Hereditary breast carcinoma	Tumour suppressor gene involved in DNA repair	If present, at high risk of developing breast cancer; screening/prophylactic mastectomies required
Female genital tract	*TP53*	High-grade serous carcinoma of uterus and ovary	Tumour suppressor gene involved in regulation of cell cycle	Diagnostic identification of tumours
	PTEN *PIK3CA*	Endometrial carcinomas	Tumour suppressor genes	Often involved in endometrial cancer
	BRCA	Fallopian tube dysplasia/ovarian carcinoma	Tumour suppressor genes	May be a germline mutation so there is a risk of other cancers
Haematology	*C-MYC*	Burkitt lymphoma	Oncogene that drives cell cycle	Disease-defining
	BCR-ABL translocation	CML	Oncogene formed from chromosomal translocation (Philadelphia chromosome)	Disease-defining. Concentration can be monitored to assess response to treatment (imatinib)
	t14:18	Follicular lymphoma	Translocation of bcl-2	Disease-defining—present in 90% of cases
Lung	*EGFR*	Lung adenocarcinoma	Growth factor receptor	If mutated, patients can benefit from treatments with anti-EGFR
	ALK	Lung adenocarcinoma	Alk rearrangement	If ALK is rearranged, targeted therapies are available
	PD-L1	Lung adenocarcinoma and SCC	Prevents apoptosis when expressed	If overexpressed, targeted therapies are available
Soft tissue	*EWSR-FLI*	Ewing sarcoma	Oncogene acting as a transcription factor	Disease-defining

CML, Chronic myeloid leukaemia; EGFR, endothelial growth factor receptor; ER, oestrogen receptor; GIST, gastrointestinal stromal tumour; PDGFR, platelet-derived growth factor receptor; PR, progesterone receptor; SCC, squamous cell carcinoma; TKI, tyrosine kinase inhibitor.

spinal fluid, cyst fluid, faeces and urine. A great potential therefore exists to utilize this novel resource, especially as we now have the means to analyse the DNA meaningfully and interpret the result, i.e., rapid sequencing and expanding genomic knowledge, respectively.

Potential uses for ctDNA include:

- Tumour identification—it is not always easy or possible to obtain a biopsy of a lesion for tissue diagnosis. It can also be very distressing and cause significant morbidity for the patient.
- Treatment decisions—e.g., the use of appropriate biological therapies governed by mutations present.
- Monitoring for early recurrence—research has shown that tumour ctDNA appears up to 8 months before there are clinical signs of a recurrence.
- Assessing treatment efficacy—there is a link between ctDNA concentration and tumour burden/stage but this is not linear, neither is it currently properly understood.
- Tumour evolution—monitoring for escape mutations.

The use and validation of this novel approach is a work in progress as we try to gain a fuller understanding of the dynamics/aetiology of this process. Not all tumours release DNA equally and not all tumours have a characteristic defining mutation. However, it is feasible to develop a specific individualized biomarker for a patient's tumour and monitor for this.

The phenomenon of foreign ctDNA is also true in pregnancy, where fetal DNA can be identified in maternal blood. This has obvious implications for antenatal diagnostics.

Chapter Summary

- Cancer is essentially a genetic disease.
- Mutations in cancer cluster within a few fundamental pathways.
- Mutations can be within tumour suppressor genes or proto-oncogenes.
- There are various molecular techniques used to analyse genes.
- Next-generation sequencing is enabling genetic testing to become commonplace, efficient and cost-effective.
- Polymerase chain reaction (PCR) is a fundamental reaction which amplifies DNA.
- Sanger sequencing uses a modified PCR reaction.
- NGS is massively parallel sequencing.
- Circulating free tumour DNA is a novel way of gaining information about tumours.
- Taxonomy of some cancers is now based on their molecular genotype rather than morphological phenotype.

Pathology of the nervous system

7

DISORDERS OF THE CENTRAL NERVOUS SYSTEM

Common pathological features

Intracranial herniation

Intracranial herniation is the movement of part of the brain from one space to another, with resultant damage. It usually occurs following a critical increase in intracranial pressure caused by an expanding lesion, e.g., tumour or haematoma. However, it may be inadvertently precipitated by withdrawing cerebrospinal fluid (CSF) at lumbar puncture.

Fig. 7.1 shows a diagrammatical representation of the sites of intracranial herniation.

Cerebral oedema

This is abnormal accumulation of fluid in the cerebral parenchyma. It may be the result of disruption of the blood–brain barrier (vasogenic oedema), parenchymal cell membrane injury (cytotoxic oedema) or a combination of the two. Possible causes include:

- ischaemia, e.g., from infarction
- trauma, e.g., from head injury
- inflammation, e.g., encephalitis or meningitis
- cerebral tumours (primary or secondary)
- metabolic disturbances, e.g., hyponatraemia or hypoglycaemia.

The condition is associated with raised intracranial pressure and may result in herniation.

> **RED FLAG**
>
> **SYMPTOMS OF RAISED INTRACRANIAL PRESSURE**
>
> Always think of raised intracranial pressure in patients presenting with headaches, vomiting and blurred vision!

Hydrocephalus

Hydrocephalus is an increase in the volume of CSF within the brain resulting in the expansion of the cerebral ventricles and eventual increase in intracranial pressure. It can occur by one of three mechanisms:

1. Obstruction to flow of CSF (the most common form).
2. Impaired absorption of CSF at arachnoid villi (rare).
3. Overproduction of CSF by choroid plexus neoplasms (very rare).

Hydrocephalus can be classified as noncommunicating and communicating.

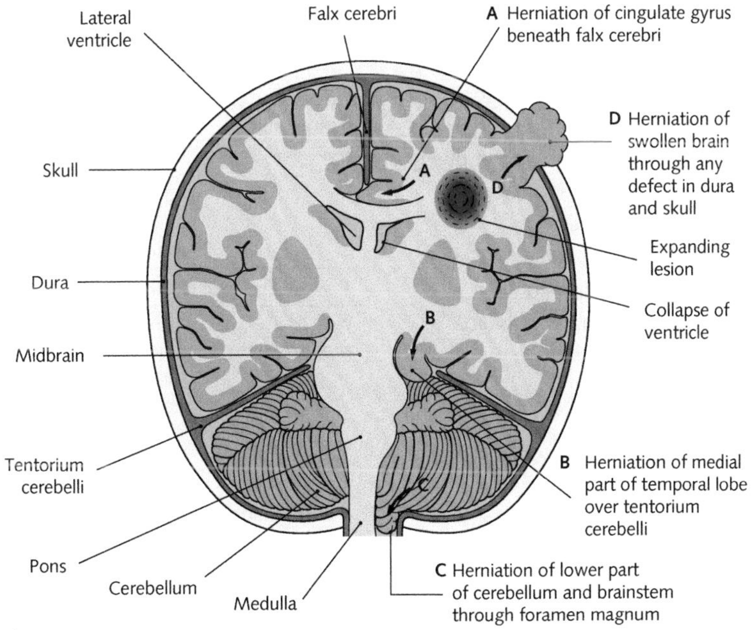

Fig. 7.1 Sites of intracranial herniation. *(A)* Subfalcine herniation. *(B)* Transtentorial herniation. *(C)* Tonsillar herniation. *(D)* Herniation of swollen brain through any defect in the dura and skull.

Noncommunicating (obstructive hydrocephalus)

This can be congenital or acquired. Congenital hydrocephalus occurs in 1 per 1000 births, owing to Arnold–Chiari and Dandy–Walker malformations (Table 7.1), arachnoid cysts and cerebral aqueduct stenosis. Acquired obstructive hydrocephalus can result from any lesion that obstructs the CSF within the ventricles, thus preventing flow into the subarachnoid space, such as:

- tumours—especially of the posterior fossa, as the fourth ventricle aqueducts are easily obstructed
- haemorrhage—intraventricular or in the posterior fossa.

Communicating hydrocephalus

This is caused by an impairment outside the ventricular system in the absence of any CSF flow obstruction, e.g., meningitis or subarachnoid haemorrhage. Normal pressure hydrocephalus is a particular form of communicating hydrocephalus. This is a rare condition of abnormal gait, urinary incontinence, and progressive (although potentially reversible) dementia associated with ventricular dilatation. Random sampling shows normal CSF pressure, but continuous monitoring may reveal intermittent increases.

Secondary or compensatory hydrocephalus

In this special type of hydrocephalus, an increase in CSF occurs as a compensatory measure following loss of brain tissue, e.g., due to infarction or atrophy. There is no associated increase in CSF pressure.

CLINICAL NOTE

CONGENITAL HYDROCEPHALUS

Congenital hydrocephalus may be diagnosed antenatally via ultrasound (if severe) or present as a considerably enlarged head at birth. In acquired hydrocephalus, skull expansion is prohibited owing to cranial suture fusion, resulting in increased intracranial pressure.

Treatment involves insertion of a ventricular shunt to drain cerebrospinal fluid into the peritoneum, attempting to prevent irreversible brain damage.

Malformations, developmental disease and perinatal injury

Neural tube defects and posterior fossa abnormalities

The aetiology of CNS malformations includes genetic factors, maternal infections, toxicity, metabolic factors (e.g., folic acid deficiency, diabetes) and in-utero irradiation.

Neural tube defects are the most common congenital abnormalities of the CNS and are caused by defective closure of midline structures over the neural tube. The most common forms in the newborn affect the spinal cord (e.g., spina bifida). Screening for neural tube defects is performed with ultrasound and measurement of α-fetoprotein in maternal serum or amniotic fluid (raised in 90% of cases).

Posterior fossa abnormalities are the second most common developmental abnormality of the CNS (e.g., Arnold–Chiari malformations). Table 7.1 summarizes the common types of congenital abnormalities.

Table 7.1 Types of congenital abnormalities

Condition	Features
Neural tube defects with cranial involvement	
Anencephaly	Absence of the cranial vault and failure in the development of the cerebral hemispheres from failure of the cranial portion of the neural tube to close
Encephalocele	Herniation of the brain and meninges through a defect in the centre of the skull, most commonly posterior (occiput), owing to failure of neural tube closure.
Neural tube defects with spinal involvement	
Spina bifida cystica	Abnormal development of the vertebral arches results in cystic outpouching through a defect in the vertebral column (90% lumbosacral): • Meningomyelocele: protrusion of spinal cord and meninges (90% of cases) • Meningocele: protrusion of only the dura and arachnoid matter (10% of cases)
Spina bifida occulta	Abnormal development of the vertebral arches but the spinal cord and meninges are normal. The defect is fully covered by skin, which may show an overlying herald mark, e.g., a hairy patch, haemangioma, pigmented lesion
Posterior fossa abnormalities	
Arnold–Chiari malformation	Abnormalities (types I–IV) of the hindbrain (pons, medulla oblongata, cerebellum). There is downward displacement of the brainstem/cerebellum through the foramen magnum into the spinal canal
Dandy–Walker malformation	Hypoplastic development and abnormal positioning of the cerebellar vermis with cystic dilatation of the fourth ventricle and enlargement of the posterior fossa. Associated with hydrocephalus owing to occlusion of the aqueduct of Sylvius and foramina of Luschka and Magendie.

Syringomyelia and hydromyelia

Syringomyelia is a rare condition in which a closed fusiform cyst (syrinx) develops within the spinal cord (Fig. 7.2). Progressive dilatation and dissection through ependymal cells occurs with CSF leaking into the spinal cord. It is most common in the cervical portion of the spinal cord. It is a primary condition in adults with type I Arnold–Chiari malformation, or can be acquired from trauma. Syringobulbia is the extension of the syrinx into the medulla.

Syringomyelia may produce a loss of pain and temperature sensation bilaterally at the level of the lesion (upper limbs if cervical) as it initially affects the decussating (crossing) spinothalamic tracts. Touch sensation is maintained as this is transmitted in the dorsal (posterior) columns (dissociated sensory loss). Symptoms progress as the syrinx expands to affect the ventral horn or descending motor tracts.

Hydromyelia is the dilatation of the central canal of the spinal cord (lined by ependymal cells) with connection to the fourth ventricle. It presents in infants/childhood with hydrocephalus or associated Arnold–Chiari malformation.

Perinatal brain injury

This term refers to any brain injury sustained in the period shortly before and after birth. It is an important cause of childhood disability.

Hypoxic–ischaemic injuries are major causes of severe perinatal brain damage. Perinatal hypoxia is usually due to asphyxiation associated with the trauma of birth, whereas perinatal ischaemia is commonly caused by intracranial haemorrhages.

Premature infants are highly susceptible to intraventricular haemorrhage owing to the fragility of the germinal matrix circulation which lines the lateral ventricles during development. In full-term infants, intracranial haemorrhages are uncommon and are related to instrumented deliveries or birth trauma. Subarachnoid haemorrhages are the most common type; intraventricular haemorrhages are rare owing to regression of the germinal matrix.

Overall mortality and morbidity is high, with survival conferring a spectrum of significant neurological sequelae, e.g., cerebral palsy, learning difficulties, and others.

Cerebral palsy

Cerebral palsy results from damage (nonprogressive) to the motor pathways of the brain. It is the leading cause of motor disability in children, affecting 2 per 1000 live births. Other impairments include postural problems, epilepsy, learning difficulties and visual and aural deficits. The different presentations of cerebral palsy are outlined in Table 7.2. Most cases are caused by antenatal developmental problems, with ~10% due to perinatal hypoxic–ischaemic injuries.

Table 7.2 Types of cerebral palsy and their associated characteristics

Type	Characteristics
Spastic cerebral palsy (70%)	Hypertonia, ankle clonus and extensor plantar reflexes. Three main types: • Hemiplegia: unilateral, arm and leg affected • Diplegic: all four limbs, but arms less affected than legs • Quadriplegic: all four limbs affected.
Dyskinetic cerebral palsy (10%)	Irregular, involuntary muscle movements of all four limbs: dystonia, athetosis or chorea.
Ataxic cerebral palsy (10%)	Trunk and limb hypotonia, uncoordinated movements and intention tremor
Mixed cerebral palsy (10%)	Combinations of the above characteristics.

COMMON PITFALLS

ISCHAEMIA AND HYPOXIA

Hypoxia and ischaemia are both related to inadequate oxygen supply, but are subtly different.

Hypoxia: oxygen deficiency owing to insufficient oxygen to meet demand either globally or focally.

Ischaemia: reduction in blood supply to tissues, resulting in reduction in oxygen and glucose, which are necessary for metabolism.

Hypoxaemia: low arterial concentration of oxygen.

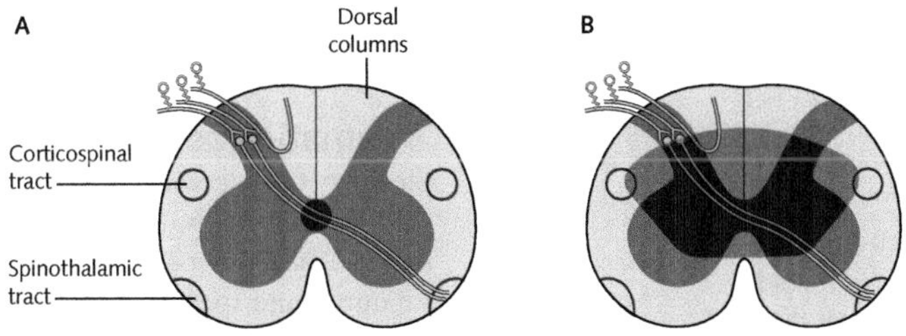

Fig. 7.2 Syringomyelia. (A) Early effects: damage to the decussating spinothalamic fibres (shaded area), with loss of pain and temperature in the upper limbs. (B) Late effects: progressive outward destruction of spinal cord to affect the dorsal columns and long tracts (shaded area) with loss of local reflexes, severe sensory loss and spastic paralysis.

Traumatic and ischaemic injuries to the central nervous system

The common types of CNS trauma are summarized in Table 7.3 and discussed in more detail below.

Skull fractures

Skull fractures occur in approximately 80% of fatal head injuries. Types of skull fractures are:

- linear—the commonest
- depressed—may be open (compound) or closed
- basilar—fracture of the base of skull; may present with clear CSF emanating from the nose or ears
- diastatic—fracture occurs along suture lines; most common in infants.

Sequelae include:

- cerebral oedema
- raised intracranial pressure
- laceration of cranial nerves
- infection (in cases of scalp laceration or tearing of the dura)
- parenchymal damage.

HINTS AND TIPS

FRACTURE OF THE PTERION

The pterion is the point at which the frontal, parietal, temporal and sphenoidal bones meet to form the temple, which is the thinnest part of the skull. The middle meningeal artery lies beneath the pterion, therefore fracture at this site is important as arterial laceration can result in extradural (epidural) haemorrhage.

Table 7.3 Examples of common central nervous system trauma

Level of injury	Pathology
Skull	Fracture
Parenchymal tissue	Concussion Contusions and lacerations Diffuse axonal injury
Vascular system	Extradural (epidural) haemorrhage Subdural haemorrhage Subarachnoid haemorrhage Intracerebral haemorrhage
Spinal cord	Complete Incomplete Penetrating

Parenchymal damage

Concussion

This is an abrupt, transient loss of consciousness owing to temporal neuronal dysfunction following a relatively slight impact. It is caused by an enormous, but short-lived, increase in pressure within the cranium at time of impact. Full recovery usually ensues, although amnesia for the event often persists.

Contusions and lacerations

A contusion is a bruise with extravasation of blood and is caused by blunt force injury. A laceration, however, is due to a tearing force. Within the skull, both are focal types of intracerebral damage occurring at the moment of injury, caused by the brain striking adjacent bone. Contusions are most common at the frontal and occipital poles of the cerebrum and mainly affect the crests of gyri. Both lesions are characteristically haemorrhagic.

Types of contusion:

- Fracture contusion—occurs at the site of fracture.
- Coup contusion—occurs at point of impact in absence of fracture.
- Contrecoup contusion—occurs diametrically opposite to the site of impact.
- Herniation contusion—e.g., when the cerebellar tonsils are impacted and bruised by the foramen magnum.
- Gliding contusion—caused by a shearing force after a rotational movement of the brain; it often accompanies diffuse axonal injury.

Diffuse axonal injury

This condition is produced as a result of rotational movements of the brain within the skull during angular acceleration or deceleration. It often occurs in the absence of any skull fracture or cerebral contusions. There are two main features:

1. *Macroscopic:* small haemorrhagic lesions in the corpus callosum and the dorsolateral quadrant of the brainstem.
2. *Microscopic:* widespread tearing of axons, usually at the nodes of Ranvier.

Diffuse axonal injuries are present in up to 50% of patients who develop coma shortly after trauma. It is associated with head injuries involving vehicular accidents.

Traumatic vascular injury

Bleeding from craniocerebral trauma is often associated with high mortality. It can occur in one or more of the potential spaces surrounding the brain, (e.g., extradural and subdural) and specific vessels are associated with different types of bleeds (Table 7.4).

Table 7.4 Cranial vessels and types of bleeds

Vessel	Vascular injury
Middle meningeal artery	Extradural haemorrhage
Bridging veins	Subdural haemorrhage
Predominantly anterior circulation (usually rupture of berry aneurysms)	Subarachnoid haemorrhage
Lenticulostriate vessels (branches of the middle cerebral artery)	Intracerebral haemorrhage

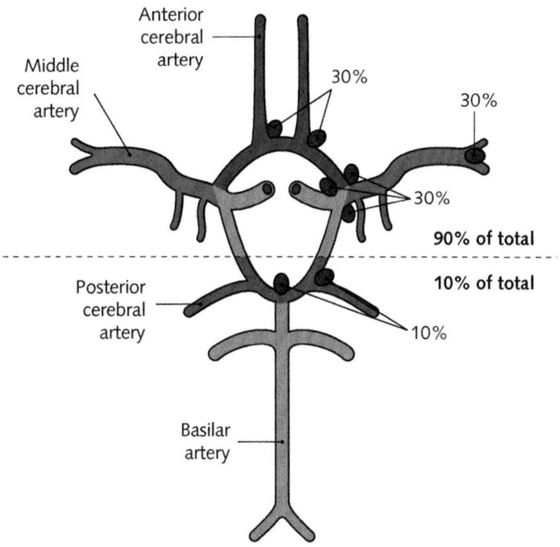

Fig. 7.3 Sites of berry aneurysms. The approximate frequency and distribution of berry aneurysms within the circle of Willis. The dotted line separates anterior from posterior circulation. (Redrawn with permission from Damjanov I and Linder J (eds) *Anderson's Pathology*, Mosby, 1995.)

Extradural (epidural) haemorrhage

This type occurs in 2% of all head injuries and in 15% of fatal cases. Haemorrhage occurs into the potential space between the skull and dura, gradually stripping dura from bone to form a large, saucer-shaped haematoma (as expansion of the haematoma is limited by dura-to-skull attachments at the suture lines).

This injury is almost always the result of skull fracture, usually of the temporal bone, with laceration of the middle meningeal artery that runs through it (a branch of the maxillary artery).

It is associated with a posttraumatic lucid interval of several hours followed by a rapid increase in intracranial pressure resulting in reduction of consciousness.

Subdural haemorrhage

Haemorrhage occurs into the potential space between the dura and the outer surface of the arachnoid membrane. It is usually caused by rupture of the small bridging veins or the venous sinuses within the subdural space. The resulting haematoma is often extensive because of the loose attachment of the dura and arachnoid membranes.

Subdural haemorrhage can be acute, following severe head injury or chronic, occurring over days to weeks. Chronic subdural haemorrhage is more common in:

- The elderly and chronic alcohol abusers—even with minimal trauma, because of brain atrophy and subsequent stretching of bridging veins.
- Infants—because the bridging veins have thin walls.

Subdural haemorrhage may present with focal signs relating to compression of a particular brain area. Personality change, memory loss and confusion are commonly seen.

Subarachnoid haemorrhage

Subarachnoid haemorrhages can occur at any age and are due to arterial rupture into the subarachnoid space. Small amounts of blood can be disposed of by arachnoid granulations. Larger haemorrhages cause arachnoid fibrosis, leading to meningeal irritation and raised intracranial pressure.

The majority of subarachnoid haemorrhages are caused by saccular (berry) aneurysms, which develop at proximal branch points in the major cerebral vessels of the circle of Willis (Fig. 7.3). These aneurysms occur in 1%–2% of the population. They are more common in the elderly and those with hypertension. Subarachnoid haemorrhage may also be caused by superficial contusions of the brain or rupture of arteriovenous malformations.

Intracerebral haemorrhage

This is caused by direct rupture of the intrinsic cerebral vessels (e.g., lenticulostriate vessels) at the time of injury. The majority of intracerebral haemorrhages are thought to arise from Charcot–Bouchard microaneurysms associated with hypertension and diabetic vascular disease. These haemorrhages occur most frequently in the basal ganglia. Other causes include trauma, rupture of an arteriovenous malformation or bleeding diathesis. The resulting haematoma acts as a space-occupying lesion, leading to increased intracranial pressure and herniation.

Cerebrovascular disease

Cerebrovascular disease is the third leading cause of death in the UK.

Stroke is a common outcome of cerebrovascular disease and is defined as a sudden event in which neurological deficit develops over minutes or hours and lasts for longer than 24 hours.

If CNS disturbance lasts for less than 24 hours the condition is termed a transient ischaemic attack (TIA).

> **RED FLAG**
>
> **FAST SYMPTOMS**
>
> The most important features of stroke can be remembered using the mnemonic FAST:
>
> *F*ace—look for unilateral drooping
> *A*rms—look for unilateral weakness
> *S*peech—listen for slurring
> *T*ime—call for help immediately

The incidence of stroke is highest in the elderly, affecting males more often than females. Causes are:

- cerebral infarction (80%)
- intracerebral haemorrhage (10%)
- subarachnoid haemorrhage (10%).

Pathological effects occur because of extensive hypoxic neuronal damage. The area of brain affected can be readily localized since the blood supply of the brain has a fairly constant anatomic distribution. Fig. 7.4 shows the territories of the major arteries.

Clinical features of stroke depend on localization and the nature of the causative lesion. Risk factors are atherosclerosis, ischaemic heart disease, hypertension and diabetes mellitus.

Hypoxia, ischaemia and infarction

Cerebral infarction (stroke) is the process whereby a focal area of necrosis is produced in the brain in response to a decreased supply of oxygen (and glucose) in the territory of a cerebral arterial branch. There are two main causes of infarction:

1. Hypoxia—the reduction of oxygen supply to tissues despite an adequate blood supply, e.g., following respiratory arrest.
2. Ischaemia—blood supply to tissues is absent, or severely reduced, usually as a result of constriction or obstruction of a blood vessel.

Ischaemia accounts for the majority of cases of cerebral infarction. Nontraumatic haemorrhage (including

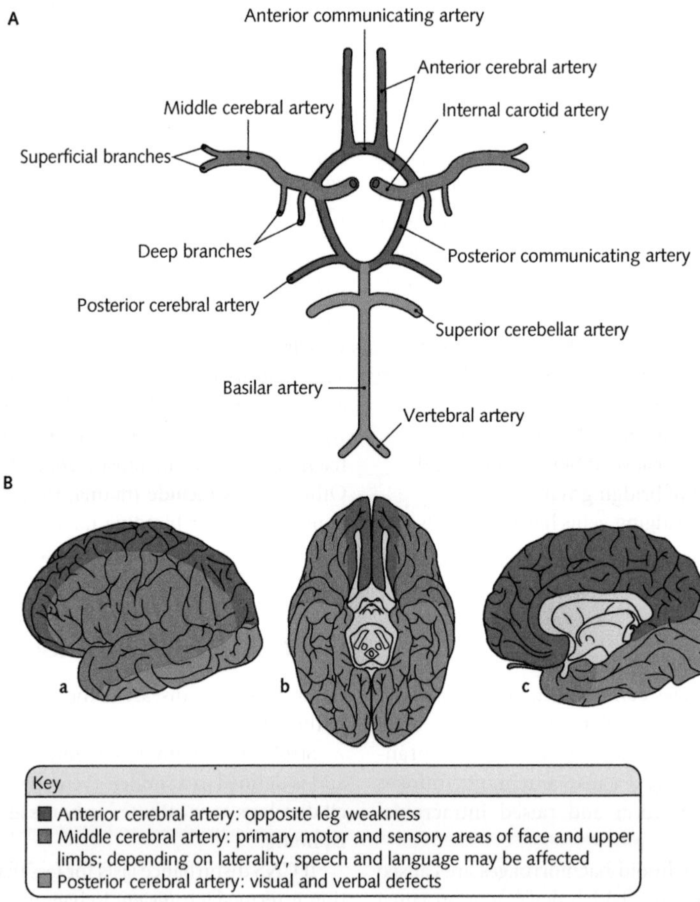

Fig. 7.4 Territories of major arteries. Territories of the major arteries and effects of cerebrovascular disease. (A) Main cerebral arteries forming circle of Willis. (B) Their territories: (a) lateral view; (b) inferior view; (c) medial view. (Reproduced with permission from Damjanov I and Linder J (eds) *Anderson's Pathology*, Mosby, 1995.)

intracerebral haemorrhage and subarachnoid haemorrhage) accounts for approximately 25% of strokes.

Mechanisms of ischaemia

Ischaemia may be caused by:

- Vascular disease, e.g., thrombosis, embolic occlusion or vasculitis.
- Cardiac disease, e.g., prolonged hypotension (producing global cerebral ischaemia) or cardiac embolism.
- Trauma—head injury leading to vascular occlusion, dissection or rupture.
- Infarcted tissue becomes swollen and soft with loss of definition between grey and white matter. It undergoes liquefactive necrosis and shows microglial macrophage infiltration. Eventually, the necrotic tissue is completely phagocytosed to leave a fluid-filled cystic cavity with a gliotic wall.

In global cerebral ischaemia, the peripheral cortex undergoes infarction, starting at the watershed areas where cerebral artery territories appose.

Table 7.5 shows the macroscopic and microscopic pathological features of cerebral infarction.

Sequelae:

- aspiration (secondary to dysfunctional swallowing)
- immobility, predisposing to urinary tract infections, pneumonia and pulmonary embolism
- depression
- recurrent strokes
- seizures
- incontinence (secondary to neurogenic bladder).

Hypertensive cerebrovascular disease

Systemic hypertension can affect the CNS, resulting in neurological dysfunction:

- Atheroma of the larger cerebral vessels leads to a loss of autoregulation of cerebral bloodflow. It may also allow small cavitary (lacunar) infarcts to develop, particularly in the lenticular nucleus and thalamus.
- Aneurysms—both saccular (berry) and microaneurysms—may cause spontaneous intracerebral haemorrhage.
- Encephalopathy—pathogenesis is uncertain but damage to the blood–brain barrier leads to forced cerebral hyperperfusion.

Chronic hypertension may lead to multiple small vessel infarcts, often producing vascular (multi-infarct) dementia (see later).

Table 7.5 Pathological features of cerebral infarction

Time	Macroscopic	Microscopic
Before 24 h	No naked eye abnormalities	Some neuronal damage
After 24 h	Softening and swelling (oedema) of affected tissue	Line of demarcation between normal and abnormal myelin in white matter
After a few days	Necrotic tissue	Infiltrating macrophages Proliferating astrocytes and capillaries
After weeks/ months	Fluid-filled cystic cavity with gliotic wall	Necrotic tissue removed Thickened capillary walls Only astrocytes remain

CLINICAL NOTE

SIGNS OF STROKE

Strokes caused by cerebral infarction clinically present with evolving signs and symptoms depending on the area of the brain affected. Intracerebral haemorrhage commonly gives rise to sudden headache, vomiting, and impairment of consciousness. Mortality is about 40%, increasing to 75% with brainstem involvement.

Subarachnoid haemorrhage presents with a sudden-onset intense headache accompanied by neck pain/stiffness and vomiting. Only 30%–40% survive the first few hours and their prognosis remains poor.

Spinal cord injuries

Most spinal injuries occur in males, usually less than 30 years or more than 70 years of age, with falls and road traffic accidents accounting for more than 70% of such injuries. Fracture or dislocation of the spinal column may cause compression of the cord by distortion of the spinal canal. The consequences depend mainly on the site and severity of the lesion. Cervical lesions may result in tetraplegia; lower thoracic lesions may result in paraplegia.

HINTS AND TIPS

EFFECT OF CENTRAL NERVOUS SYSTEM (CNS) LESIONS IS SITE DEPENDENT

Remember that, with limited CNS repair mechanisms, the site of trauma is more important than the size of lesion. For example, a small lesion of the frontal lobe may be clinically silent, but would cause tetraplegia if located in the cervical spinal cord, and death if in the brainstem.

Remember the rhyme: C3, 4 and 5 keeps the diaphragm alive!

Spinal cord injury can be subtyped as complete, incomplete or penetrating:

- Complete—there is complete loss of sensory and motor sensation below the level of the injury.
- Incomplete—there is partial loss of sensation below the level of injury, e.g., Brown-Séquard syndrome.
- Penetrating—these are a result of direct trauma to the spinal cord and nerve roots and may be associated with haemorrhage, infection or leakage of CSF.

Cauda equina syndrome

Compression of the distal nerve roots of the spinal cord (which have the appearance of a horse's tail, hence the name) causes characteristic symptoms of low back pain radiating down the leg, anaesthesia of the pubic and perineal region ('saddle anaesthesia'), in addition to bladder and bowel dysfunction.

INFECTIONS OF THE CENTRAL NERVOUS SYSTEM

Meningitis

Meningitis refers to inflammation of the meninges; specifically, the leptomeninges and CSF within the subarachnoid space.

- Pachymeningitis: inflammation centred on the dura.
- Meningoencephalitis: inflammation of the meninges and brain parenchyma.

RED FLAG

SYMPTOMS OF MENINGITIS

Vomiting
Fever
Headache
Limb pain
Cold hands and feet
Stiff neck
Nonblanching petechial rash (late sign)
Pale or mottled skin
Photophobia
Altered mental state/unconscious
Confusion/delirium
Seizures
Focal neurological deficits

Aseptic (viral) meningitis

Aseptic meningitis refers to an absence of recognizable bacterial pathogens on culture or Gram staining. It is usually caused by viral infection and is the most common cause of meningitis. Other causes include syphilis, Lyme disease, malignant infiltration, sarcoidosis, systemic lupus erythematosus (SLE), drugs, parasites, fungi, mycobacterium and partially treated bacterial meningitis.

Viral meningitis is a relatively benign, self-limiting illness and is usually less severe than bacterial meningitis.

Common causative organisms

The common causative organisms are:

- echovirus
- coxsackievirus
- poliovirus
- mumps virus
- measles
- herpes simplex virus 2 (HSV2)
- HIV
- adenovirus
- arbovirus.

Affected individuals present with headache, irritability and rapid development of meningeal irritation.

Acute bacterial meningitis

Organisms that typically cause this condition vary between age groups. Table 7.6 shows common macroscopic and microscopic features of bacterial meningitis. Table 7.7 highlights common causative organisms by age group.

The clinical features are signs of systemic infection (e.g., fever) and those of meningeal irritation (e.g., headache, photophobia, drowsiness and neck stiffness). The development of a petechial rash is a late sign.

Treatment is with vigorous intravenous antibiotic therapy.

Important complications include:

- brain abscess (see below)
- subdural empyema
- arterial and venous cerebral infarction
- obstructive or communicating hydrocephalus owing to subarachnoid adhesions blocking CSF flow
- epilepsy
- disseminated intravascular coagulation (DIC)
- adrenal haemorrhage (Waterhouse–Friderichsen syndrome).

Table 7.6 Macroscopic and microscopic features of bacterial meningitis

Macroscopic features	Microscopic features
• Diffuse cerebral swelling • Oedematous white matter • Congested meninges • Subarachnoid purulent exudate • Ventricular compression or dilatation • Purulent ventricular fluid • Possible haemorrhagic infarcts	• Parenchymal surface coated in inflammatory exudate - neutrophils and fibrin (pus) • Cortical perivascular spread of inflammatory exudate • Thrombosis of meningeal/cortical vessels with associated focal infarction

Table 7.7 Causes of meningitis by age group[a]

Neonates	Infants	Young adults	Elderly
Escherichia coli Group B streptococci *Staphylococcus aureus* *Listeria monocytogenes*	*Neisseria meningitidis* *Haemophilus influenzae B* *Streptococcus pneumoniae*	*Streptococcus pneumoniae* *Neisseria meningitidis* *Haemophilus influenzae B* Gram-negative bacilli (neurosurgery/head injury)	*Streptococcus pneumoniae* *Neisseria meningitidis* *Listeria monocytogenes*

[a] *Vaccination has changed the epidemiology of bacterial meningitis within the UK; however, in unvaccinated and immunosuppressed populations these are the common causes.*

Mortality varies by bacterial type, but may be as high as 60%, with *Streptococcus pneumoniae* particularly affecting the very young and the elderly.

Chronic meningoencephalitis

Tuberculous meningitis

This is meningitis due to infection by *Mycobacterium tuberculosis*. It is rare in the UK but a major problem in developing countries. The disorder is almost always secondary to tuberculosis elsewhere in the body, usually from haematogenous spread to the CNS.

Macroscopic appearance: the basal meninges of the brain are covered in a gelatinous, greenish-yellow exudate. Tuberculomas may be seen on the meninges or the lining of the ventricles, appearing as small white nodules.

Microscopic appearance: granulomatous inflammation affects the basal meninges, large arteries and cranial nerves. The meningeal exudate is composed of lymphocytes, macrophages, fibrin and necrotic debris. The superficial cortex may be gliotic and cortical tuberculomas may be present. Infarcts secondary to thrombosis from endarteritis are seen.

Clinical presentation is with slow-onset, subacute meningitis and may be accompanied by isolated cranial nerve palsies. Hydrocephalus may result from impaired reabsorption of CSF or obstruction of CSF outflow from arachnoid fibrosis.

CSF shows an initial increase in mononuclear cells and polymorphs (Table 7.8) with low glucose and raised protein. Outcome is variable based on age and stage of the disease at diagnosis. Untreated, the disease is usually fatal. Intensive treatment with antituberculous drugs lowers mortality to 15%–20%.

Table 7.8 Typical cerebrospinal fluid test results from lumbar puncture

	Bacterial	Tuberculosis	Viral–aseptic
Appearance	Turbid	Fibrin webs	Usually clear
Predominant cell	Neutrophils	Lymphocytes	Lymphocytes
Cell count/mm^3	90–1000+	10–1000	50–1000
Glucose (CSF:serum)	<0.5 plasma	<0.5 plasma	>0.5 plasma
Proteins (g/L)	>1.5	1–5	<1
Organisms	On Gram stain and culture	On Ziehl–Neelsen stain	Not seen

Redrawn with permission from Dr P. Xiu.

Neurosyphilis (tertiary syphilis)

This occurs in 30%–50% of patients with untreated syphilis owing to chronic inflammation following spirochaete infection with *Treponema pallidum*. It can occur months or years after initial infection (primary syphilis). Neurological manifestations of tertiary syphilis include:

- Syphilitic meningitis: 1–2 years post primary infection.
- Meningovascular syphilis: 7 years post primary infection. Thickening of meninges with hydrocephalus and syphilitic arteritis leading to parenchymal infarction.
- Chronic meningoencephalitis: 10–20 years post primary infection. Results in progressive neurological decline, general paresis and death.
- Tabes dorsalis: 15–20 years post primary infection. Loss of motor neurones in the dorsal root ganglia and posterior column degeneration.
- Gummatous inflammation: gummas (granuloma-like lesions) rarely involve the CNS to cause solitary space-occupying lesions. They are more commonly present in the liver.

See Chapters 5 and 18 for further discussion of syphilis.

Lyme disease (neuroborreliosis)

This disorder is caused by the tick-borne spirochaete *Borrelia burgdorferi*. It is a systemic illness characterized by skin lesions (erythema chronicum migrans) and neurological features (see Chapter 18). Neurological involvement includes lymphocytic meningitis, cranial nerve palsies, radiculopathies, encephalomyelitis and stroke.

Viral encephalitis

This is a virally induced diffuse inflammation of the brain parenchyma, which is usually concomitant with meningoencephalitis. It is a common complication of many viral illnesses. Common causative viruses are:

- arbovirus
- parainfluenza
- HSV1 and HSV2
- measles
- adenovirus
- cytomegalovirus
- polio
- enteroviruses (coxsackie and echovirus)
- rabies
- HIV.

Prognosis depends on immune status and viral virulence. Most cases are mild and self-limiting; however, in some cases fatality is 100% (e.g., varicella zoster in immunosuppressed patients and rabies).

Mortality for other types ranges up to 50%, with variable degrees of permanent morbidity, e.g., learning disabilities, seizures and motor deficits.

Brain abscess

A brain abscess is a severe focal infection of the brain and is typically 1–2 cm across. It starts as an area of cerebritis—inflammation of the brain parenchyma—and develops into a pus-filled cavity bounded by a capsule and surrounded by cerebral oedema. It often results in raised intracranial pressure.

The aetiology of brain abscesses is as follows:

Direct extension of infection:

- Middle ear infection (60%)—temporal lobe and cerebellar abscesses
- Frontal sinusitis (20%)—frontal lobe abscesses
- Dental root infection
- Secondary to meningitis.

Haematogenous spread:

This is usually mutlifocal, occurring at the junction of gray/white matter. Causes include:

- Children: congenital cardiac defects
- Adults: subacute endocarditis, bronchiectasis, lung abscess, septicaemia/bacteraemia.

Implantation:

- Penetrating skull trauma
- Neurosurgery.

Common causative organisms are *Streptococcus viridans, Streptococcus milleri, Staphylococcus* spp., but can also be caused by fungal infection.

Overall mortality is between 10% and 20%.

Subdural empyema

This is a collection of pus surrounded by granulation tissue in the subdural space, usually situated supratentorially. It is relatively uncommon. In adults, it usually results from frontal sinusitis/otitis media, whereas in infants it is usually secondary to meningitis.

Clinically, patients with subdural empyema are usually very ill. The pus spreads rapidly on the surface of a hemisphere, producing hemiparesis, raised intracranial pressure, fits and meningism.

Fungal infections

These are relatively rare and occur mainly in the immunosuppressed (e.g., associated with chemotherapy, lymphoma/leukaemia, diabetes mellitus, alcoholism, steroid use and AIDS), but a few organisms, e.g., *Coccidioides immitis,* can produce disease in the absence of immunosuppression. The clinical picture is that of meningitis or intraparenchymal abscesses/granulomas.

Nearly all infections are caused by spread from another site. Spread is mainly haematogenous (e.g., from the lungs), or by direct extension in a minority of cases (e.g., from the nose and paranasal sinuses).

The most common causative organism is *Cryptococcus neoformans.* Other common organisms include: *Aspergillus* spp., *Candida albicans* and mucormycosis.

Cryptococcosis

Most cases of cryptococcosis are from primary lung disease with haematogenous spread. CNS manifestations are meningitis ± parenchymal cysts or cryptococcal abscesses (cryptococcomas). Cryptococcomas may have a gelatinous texture and contain variable numbers of organisms, mononuclear cells and granulomas. Meningitis results in thickened, fibrotic meninges with a variable number of perivascular cysts within the grey matter.

Cryptococci are visualized with India ink or mucicarmine staining as budding yeasts with thick capsules. They may be identified within CSF.

Aspergillosis

Aspergillus is an angioinvasive hyphal fungus which can cause CNS disease from haematogenous spread from the lungs or by direct extension from the orbit, paranasal sinuses or middle ear (Fig. 7.5). Angioinvasion causes vascular occlusion and thrombosis resulting in haemorrhage and infarction which may develop into abscesses. Infection presents as multiple space-occupying lesions with focal symptoms.

Protozoal infection

Protozoan organisms that may cause infection of the CNS are:

- Toxoplasma
- *Plasmodium falciparum*
- Trypanosoma
- free-living amoebae.

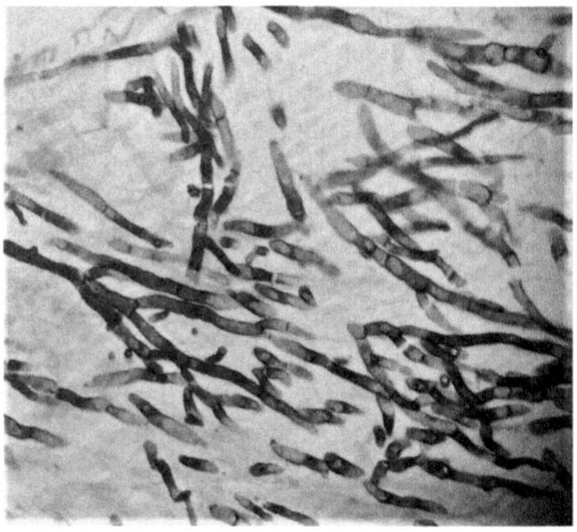

Fig. 7.5 Aspergillosis. Microscopic photograph of a Grocott preparation showing the branched fungus Aspergillus. This has the ability to invade blood vessel walls, causing infarction of the supplied tissue. It can also colonize cavities, such as in the lung, to form fungus balls (aspergillomas).

Toxoplasmosis

This is caused by infection with *Toxoplasma gondii.* It may be acquired by eating poorly-cooked infected meat (usually lamb or pork) or food contaminated with feline faeces. It has two forms: congenital and acquired.

In the congenital form, the organism is transmitted to the fetus through the placenta during maternal infection, potentially leading to:

- prematurity, abortion or stillbirth
- chorioretinitis
- hydrocephalus
- intracranial calcification (bilateral ring-enhancing lesions)
- moderate brain damage.

Acquired toxoplasmosis is usually subclinical; however, severe infection occurs in immunocompromised adults (e.g., AIDS) where it is the most common cause of brain abscess. It results in:

- necrotizing cerebritis
- chronic abscesses
- meningoencephalitis.

Multiple ring-enhancing lesions (abscesses) are seen on imaging, located in the basal ganglia and at the junction of the grey and white matter. The necrotic foci contain free tachyzoites with encysted bradyzoites at the periphery.

CLINICAL NOTE

HIV AND THE BRAIN

Sixty percent of patients with AIDS develop neuropathological-based sequelae, which include:

Opportunistic infections:
- Cytomegalovirus
- Toxoplasma
- Cryptococcus
- Varicella zoster virus
- Herpes simplex virus

Primary CNS lymphoma:
- High-grade non-Hodgkin lymphoma (Epstein–Barr virus–driven)

Cranial and peripheral neuropathies:
- Motor and sensory

Children:
- Microcephaly
- Mental retardation
- Intracranial calcification

Direct effect of HIV infection:
- Aseptic meningitis
- HIV encephalitis

Progressive multifocal leucoencephalopathy

Destruction and demyelination occurs with infection of oligodendrocytes by the JC polyoma virus in immunosuppressed individuals. Progressive multifocal leucoencephalopathy (PML)-associated immunodeficiency states include AIDS, lymphoproliferative disorders, carcinoma and SLE.

Patients present with progressive, multifocal neurological symptoms secondary to multiple patches of subcortical white matter destruction. Viral inclusions are present within oligodendrocytes and bizarre astrocytes are seen. The disease is progressive, and death usually occurs within a few months.

Subacute sclerosing panencephalopathy

Subacute sclerosing panencephalopathy (SSPE) is subacute chronic encephalitis occurring in children or teenagers years after measles infection. This is because of persistent infection by an altered measles virus. It presents with progressive neurological impairment, limb jerks, spasticity and eventually coma and death. Death can occur within months of onset, or progression can be intermittent with survival for more than 10 years. SSPE is now rare due to immunization with the MMR vaccine.

Pathologically, the white and grey matter are affected with severe gliosis and myelin degeneration. Lymphocytic infiltration is present within the leptomeninges and parenchyma. Viral inclusions are sparse and are seen within oligodendrocytes and neurones.

Transmissible spongiform encephalopathies

Creutzfeldt–Jakob disease (CJD) is the most common type of transmissible spongiform encephalopathy (TSE), and presents with rapidly progressive dementia, coordination loss, visual impairments and myoclonus; it is always fatal, usually within 6–12 months of the onset of symptoms. It is rare in the UK, affecting 1 per million people per year, with an average age of onset of 60 years. It may be sporadic (85% of cases), hereditary (5%–10% of cases) or iatrogenic (1%) from exposure to infected brain tissue or CSF.

The incubation period is estimated to be 11 years and the infectious agent is a prion protein (PrP^{Sc}). Prion proteins are abnormal isoforms of normal glycoproteins (see Chapter 5).

Other types of TSE include variant CJD (vCJD) and kuru (now extinct) and the rare hereditary forms: familial fatal insomnia and Gerstmann–Straussler–Scheinker disease. The animal forms of TSEs are bovine spongiform encephalopathy (BSE) in cows and scrapie in sheep.

Pathology: grey matter demonstrates spongiform changes caused by the formation of small intracellular vacuoles within neurones and the surrounding neuropil. Microvacuolation may be focal or widespread and classically distributed within the cerebral and occipital cortex. PrP^{Sc} deposition can be present, forming variable numbers of amyloid plaques. As the disease progresses there is neuronal loss, gliosis and atrophy.

Variant Creutzfeldt–Jakob disease

This disease was first recognized in 1995 in the UK and is thought to have been transmitted from cows infected with BSE. Sporadic CJD is not caused or linked to BSE. Variant CJD affects younger individuals (mean age of onset 28 years). Neurological decline appears slower, but progression is fatal at ~14 months. Presentation is with prominent psychiatric symptoms and ataxia. Pathologically, vCJD is similar to CJD; however, florid amyloid plaques within the occipital cortex and cerebellum are present and severe spongiform change is seen within the thalamus, cerebral cortex and cerebellum.

Demyelinating diseases

This group of diseases has a common factor of primary damage to myelin of nerves while the axons and nerve cells remain relatively intact.

Multiple sclerosis

Multiple sclerosis (MS) is the most common demyelinating disorder of the CNS, affecting up to 200 per 100,000 in the UK. Peak incidence is between 20 and 40 years, with a slight female predominance.

MS is usually characterized by relapsing and remitting episodes of immunologically mediated demyelination within the CNS. Recovery from each episode of demyelination is usually incomplete, leading to progressive deterioration. There is an association between the disease and certain human leucocyte antigens (HLA, e.g., A3, B7, DR2 and DQ1). The incidence also increases with distance from the equator, suggesting vitamin D deficiency as a possible environmental trigger. Other associations include smoking and viral infections, particularly Epstein–Barr virus (EBV).

Pathogenesis: activated T-lymphocytes cross the blood–brain barrier, reacting to self-antigens against myelin that are presented by microglia. A strong inflammatory reaction follows, enhanced by the release of proinflammatory cytokines. Acute demyelination occurs in the central white matter in discrete areas known as plaques.

Abnormalities are confined to the CNS; the peripheral nervous system (PNS) is usually spared. Common sites are the optic nerve, brainstem, cerebellum, periventricular regions and cervical spinal cord.

Table 7.9 lists the clinical manifestations of MS and their causes.

CLINICAL NOTE

MULTIPLE SCLEROSIS (MS)

MS diagnosis clinically involves multiple symptomatic episodes which are separated in time and space (region affected). Imaging may show abnormal areas in the brain and the cerebrospinal fluid may show increased lymphoid cells and oligoclonal bands of IgG. Most follow a relapsing–remitting course with variable disability, but a minority (5%) suffer rapidly progressive (fulminant) disease, which is fatal within 5 years.

Table 7.9 Clinical manifestations of multiple sclerosis and their causes

Manifestations	Causes
Early clinical symptoms	
Blurring of vision (diplopia)	Optic neuritis
Incoordination	Cerebellar peduncle disease
Abnormal sensation	Disease of long ascending sensory tracts
Late stages	
Blindness, paraplegia and incontinence	Spinal tract involvement
Dysarthria, ataxia, tremor (Charcot triad)	Spinal and cerebellar involvement
Intellectual dysfunction	Loss of hemispheric white matter

Degenerative disorders and dementia

These diseases primarily affect the grey matter, with progressive neuronal loss. A common feature of this group is the development of protein aggregates (cellular inclusions) that are resistant to degradation.

Dementia is defined as progressive memory loss and cognitive impairment, and occurs because of degeneration of the cerebral cortex.

Cortical

Alzheimer disease

This is the most common cause of dementia in developed countries. Alzheimer disease affects 7% of people over 65 years, and 15% of people over 80 years in the UK, with females affected more often than males. Also of significance is the subgroup of early-onset patients (40–60 years).

The aetiology and pathogenesis are unknown; some cases (5%) are familial, but most (95%) are sporadic. Genetic studies have shown that there is an increase in incidence of sporadic cases in individuals with apoE E4 genotype on chromosome 19. The amyloid precursor protein *(APP)* gene on chromosome 21 has been implicated in familial cases.

Macroscopically, there is marked cortical atrophy, especially of the frontal lobes; the brain is reduced in weight to 1000 g or less (normal average is 1400 g). There is a loss of cortical grey and white matter.

Histological hallmarks are as follows:

- Senile (neuritic) plaques—also known as β-amyloid plaques; composed of an extracellular core of amyloid protein (10–150 nm in diameter) surrounded by dystrophic neurites; occur most frequently in the hippocampus, cerebral cortex and deep grey matter. The main component of the core is β-amyloid, a readily aggregating peptide that is thought to be central in the pathogenesis of dementia.
- Neurofibrillary tangles—abnormal tangles of insoluble cytoskeletal-like proteins (tau proteins—paired helical filaments) that form within the cytoplasm of neurones.
- Neuropil threads—distorted dendritic processes and axons found around amyloid plaques.

Clinically, there is loss of memory and emotional lability. There tends to be progressive physical decline affecting nutrition and mobility. Death is commonly caused by the development of pneumonia.

CLINICAL NOTE

SALIVA TEST FOR ALZHEIMER DISEASE

A saliva test for Alzheimer disease is currently being developed.

Vascular dementia

This is the second most common cause of dementia and is usually seen in adults over 65 years. It is caused by small-vessel disease in the brain, and is usually multifocal (multiinfarct dementia). Hypertension is the underlying cause in over 50% of cases.

Frontotemporal dementia

This is a group of diseases characterized by atrophy of the frontal and/or temporal lobes. It results in personality and behavioural changes and alteration in speech, depending on the site of atrophy. One of the better-known subtypes is Pick disease, in which Pick bodies (neuronal inclusions) are found in the frontal and temporal lobes.

Basal ganglia

Parkinsonism

This term is used to refer to patients whose clinical presentation mimics Parkinson disease and typically consists of:

- akinetic rigidity
- stooped posture with slow voluntary movements (question mark posture)
- diminished facial expression (mask-like features)
- festinating gait (progressively shortened, accelerated steps)
- shuffling gait
- resting ('pill-rolling') tremor.

The main causes include neuroleptic drugs, cerebral anoxia, and Lewy body dementia.

Parkinson disease

This is characterized by resting tremor, bradykinesia, and cogwheel rigidity. It occurs in 1 per 500 adults, with increasing incidence over the age of 65 years. The aetiology is unknown.

Pathogenesis:

- The disorder shows degeneration of pigmented dopaminergic neurones of the substantia nigra, the locus coeruleus and several other brainstem nuclei.
- Degeneration of these cells causes disease by reducing the amount of dopamine in the corpus striatum.
- Surviving cells in the substantia nigra contain eosinophilic spherical inclusions (Lewy bodies), which contain cytoskeletal filaments.

The disease can be symptomatically treated with drugs, such as L-DOPA, that correct neurotransmitter imbalance. Eventually, there is failure of response to treatment and patients die from wasting and poor nutritional intake. Several genes have been implicated in the development of Parkinson disease, including those encoding the proteins α-synuclein and parkin.

COMMON PITFALLS

LEWY BODY DEMENTIA

Lewy bodies are abnormal clusters of α-synuclein protein found within diseased neurones. In Parkinson disease, Lewy bodies are seen; however, it is a different entity from Lewy body dementia, which is characterized by anterograde amnesia.

Motor neurones

Motor neurone disease (amyotrophic lateral sclerosis)

This progressive, neurodegenerative disease is characterized by the selective loss of both upper and lower motor neurones from the spinal cord, brainstem and motor cortex. Its prevalence is 2 per 100,000 of the population, with male incidence greater than female. The majority of cases are sporadic but 5% of cases are familial.

It eventually progresses to severe paralysis, with death from aspiration pneumonia and respiratory failure, occurring usually within 2–3 years of diagnosis.

Other degenerative disorders are considered in Table 7.10.

Metabolic disorders and toxins

Vitamin deficiencies

Vitamin B1 (thiamine) deficiency

This is common in chronic alcoholics, resulting in:

- Wernicke encephalopathy—memory impairment, ataxia, visual disturbances and peripheral neuropathy.
- Korsakoff psychosis—confused state, memory loss and confabulation.

Table 7.10 Additional types of degenerative disease

Degenerative disorder	Features
Pick disease	Progressive dementia with severe memory and speech loss. Cortical atrophy of the frontal and temporal lobes. Surviving neurones contain Pick bodies.
Huntington disease	Autosomal dominant trinucleotide repeat disorder (chromosome 4) characterized by chorea and progressive dementia. Cerebral atrophy in the caudate nucleus and putamen.
Friedreich ataxia	Autosomal recessive spinocerebellar disease. Degeneration of the posterior columns, corticospinal and spinocerebellar tracts.

If both occur, it is known as Wernicke–Korsakoff syndrome.

Vitamin B6 (pyridoxine) deficiency

This deficiency may cause microcytic anaemia, dermatitis and peripheral neuropathy as pyridoxine is a cofactor in pathways involving haemoglobin, sphingolipids and neurotransmitters (e.g., gamma-aminobutyric acid (GABA)). Pyridoxine is also involved in metabolism of tryptophan to niacin, therefore deficiency results in pellagra (niacin deficiency causing dermatitis, diarrhoea and dementia).

Vitamin B12 (cyanocobalamin) deficiency

This deficiency causes demyelination of nerve sheaths, particularly involving the posterior and lateral columns of the spinal cord. The result is subacute combined degeneration of the cord, producing weakness and paraesthesia in the lower limbs with loss of vibration and proprioception (Fig. 7.6).

Replacement therapy at an early stage reverses the degenerative process, but longstanding cases show irreversible axonal damage with reactive gliosis.

Folate deficiency

This deficiency is associated with anaemia and hyperhomocysteinaemia. Folate is a cofactor in the metabolism of homocysteine to methionine, therefore deficiency results in increased homocysteine levels, and consequently an increased risk of stroke. Folic acid is also important in pregnancy to reduce the risk of neural tube defects within the developing fetus.

Iodine deficiency

Severe iodine deficiency causes hypothyroidism; it is the most important endocrine disorder to affect the CNS in children. In the fetus, severe iodine deficiency causes cretinism characterized by dwarfism, mental defect and spastic diplegia.

Toxins

Carbon monoxide

Carbon monoxide (CO) binds with such a strong affinity to haemoglobin (forming carboxyhaemoglobin) that erythrocyte oxygen delivery is severely impaired. The resultant

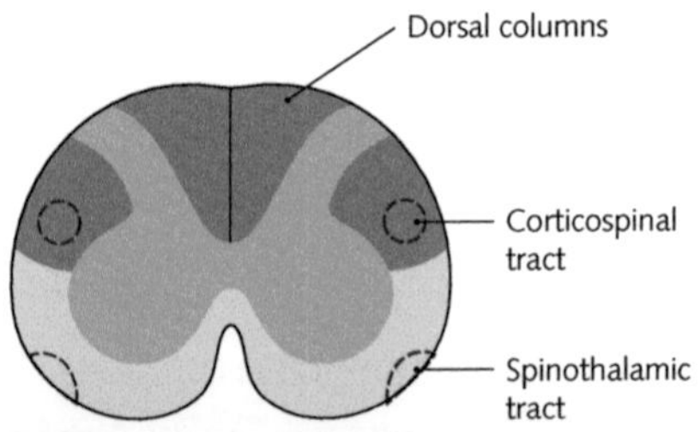

Fig. 7.6 Subacute combined degeneration of the cord. Degeneration of posterior columns leads to sensory loss (vibration and proprioception) causing ataxia. Degeneration of corticospinal tracts leads to upper motor neurone damage causing spastic paralysis.

hypoxia therefore causes cerebral ischaemia. Histologically, this is seen as neuronal necrosis with a predilection for the globus pallidus. Other selectively vulnerable regions are the hippocampus and the cerebral and cerebellar cortices.

CO levels of 3%–4% are considered normal, with levels up to 10% being normal in smokers.

Clinical symptoms correspond to the amount of carbon monoxide-bound haemoglobin as follows:

- 10%–20%—dyspnoea and slight headache
- 20%–40%—severe headache, fatigue and impaired judgement
- 60–70%—loss of consciousness
- >70%—rapidly fatal.

Methanol

Methanol is highly toxic to the CNS, particularly to the retina. It is lipid-soluble, so readily diffuses into the CSF and aqueous humour in concentrations higher than in plasma.

Methanol is metabolized into formic acid and formaldehyde. Formaldehyde is thought to mediate the toxic effects. Methanol poisoning can cause a spectrum of changes. These range from subacute and chronic toxicity causing blindness to sudden death. Blindness occurs through atrophy of the retinal ganglion cells, with secondary optic nerve degeneration, and sudden death by multiple haemorrhagic lesions in the cerebral hemispheres, especially the putamen.

Ethanol

The consequences of excessive ethanol intake on the CNS are manifold (Table 7.11).

Table 7.11 Consequences of excess ethanol intake on the central nervous system

Disease	Features	Mechanism
Fetal alcohol syndrome	Cognitive impairment Facial malformations Growth retardation	Direct toxicity
Acute intoxication	Cerebral oedema	Direct toxicity
Cerebral and cerebellar atrophy	Neuronal loss	Direct toxicity
Nutritional disorders	Wernicke encephalopathy Korsakoff syndrome	Deficiency of vitamin B1
Hepatocerebral syndromes	Hepatic encephalopathy Chronic hepatocerebral degeneration	Hepatic toxicity with secondary effects on CNS
Demyelinating disorders	Central pontine myelinolysis	Electrolyte disturbances

Neoplasms of the central nervous system

Primary CNS neoplasms account for 3% of all adult tumours, with secondary (metastatic) lesions outnumbering primary lesions by 3:1. Presentation is variable dependent on the tumour location, producing focal deficits, epilepsy or symptoms and signs associated with raised intracranial pressure. Neoplasms arise from a variety of cell types, the most important of which are glial cells.

> **HINTS AND TIPS**
>
> **CELLS OF THE CENTRAL NERVOUS SYSTEM**
>
> **Neurones**—sensory and motor
> **Neuroglia**—support cells of the CNS and peripheral nervous system (PNS)
> ***CNS neuroglia***
> - Astrocytes (largest population of cells in the CNS)
> - Oligodendrocytes (myelin-forming cells)
> - Ependymal cells (line the ventricular system of brain and spinal cord canal and help propel cerebrospinal fluid)
> - Microglia (chief CNS macrophages and antigen-presenting cells)
>
> ***PNS neuroglia***
> - Schwann cells (myelin-forming cells)
> - Satellite cells (support cells for neuronal cell bodies within the spinal ganglia)

Gliomas

Gliomas are tumours that arise from supportive neuroglial cells of brain. They are the most common primary brain tumours, accounting for up to 50% of all CNS tumours. Types include astrocytomas, oligodendromas and ependymomas.

Astrocytomas

These are a group of gliomas derived from astrocytes. They are the commonest primary CNS tumour in children and adults. Different subtypes of astrocytomas exist and occur on a spectrum graded I–IV (Table 7.12). The majority of astrocytomas are high-grade, infiltrative types (II–IV); grade I pilocytic astrocytomas are considered a separate entity to these as they are genetically different. Common types of astrocytomas include:

- *Pilocytic astrocytoma (WHO grade I)*: relatively benign tumour with minimal infiltration into the surrounding brain parenchyma. They have a favourable prognosis. Characteristically it appears on imaging as having a cystic component with a mural nodule. Microscopically, astrocytic cellularity is low with no

Table 7.12 Tumours of the central nervous system

Tumour	Location	Age	Features
Pilocytic astrocytoma	Cerebellum, optic chiasm/nerve	Child/young adult	Commonest primary brain tumour of childhood. Narrow/no infiltrative margin. Strong association with neurofibromatosis type 1. Rarely progresses.
Diffuse (fibrillary) astrocytoma	Cerebral hemispheres (adults) Brainstem (children)	Children: 6–12 years Adults: 26–46 years	Infiltrative tumour with indistinct borders. May involve entire cerebral hemisphere. Progresses to anaplastic and glioblastoma types. No mitoses or necrosis. Associated with Li-Fraumeni syndrome.
Anaplastic astrocytoma	Cerebral hemispheres	30–50 years	More cellular with increased nuclear pleomorphism. Mitoses but no necrosis.
Glioblastoma	Cerebral hemispheres	Adults over 40 years; peak 65–75 years	Can be primary or secondary. Pleomorphic with serpentine necrosis, mitoses, vascular proliferation. Multifocal in 20% of cases. Death <1 year.
Oligodendroglioma	Cerebral hemispheres—commonly temporal lobe	Tumour of adults 40–60 years	Most present with epilepsy. *IDH-1* mutated and 1p19q codeletion required for diagnosis.
Ependymoma	Intracranial—posterior fossa. Intraventricular—fourth ventricle Spinal—conus or filum terminale.	Children <4 years (intracranial) Adult 20–40 years (spinal and intraventricular)	CSF involvement. Spinal forms associated with neurofibromatosis type 2. Rosettes and pseudorosettes microscopically.
Medulloblastoma	Cerebellum, fourth ventricle	Children (majority)	Rapidly growing, infiltrative and aggressive. Four distinct, genetically defined subgroups exist. Second commonest childhood cranial neoplasm. Seeds the cerebrospinal fluid.
Meningioma	Parasagittal, sphenoid ridge and lateral sulcus	Adults—increasing frequency with age	Arise from meningoepithelial cells of arachnoid mater. Grow in pregnancy. Associated with cranial irradiation and neurofibromatosis type 2. Form whorls ± psammoma bodies.

mitoses or necrosis. Eosinophilic 'Rosenthal' fibres and hyalinized blood vessels are present. They are associated with *BRAF* mutations with wild type *TP53* and isocitrate dehydrogenase (*IDH-1*).

Fifteen percent of patients with neurofibromatosis type I develop astrocytomas.

- *Diffuse (fibrillary) astrocytoma (WHO grade II):* poorly defined, highly infiltrative tumour with indistinct borders that can invade the whole cerebral hemisphere. It commonly presents with epilepsy. Imaging shows an isodense/hypodense mass which can be macroscopically subtle, appearing as an area of abnormal texture or mild discoloration. These lesions can progress to anaplastic and glioblastoma types of tumour identified on imaging by acquisition of enhancing areas. Microscopically, a mild increase in cellularity with a fine felt-like network of astrocyte cell processes is seen. Cytological atypia is mild, and necrosis and mitoses are absent.

Diffuse astrocytomas are associated with Li–Fraumeni syndrome.

- *Anaplastic astrocytoma (WHO grade III):* features are between grade II astrocytomas and glioblastomas. Microscopically, more densely cellular areas are seen with increasing nuclear and cytological pleomorphism. Mitoses and vascular proliferation are variable, but necrosis is absent. Eighty percent of grade II and III astrocytomas have mutated *IDH-1*. Transformation to glioblastoma is heralded by rapidly worsening, progressive neurological symptoms.
- *Glioblastoma (WHO grade IV):* previously known as glioblastoma multiforme (Fig. 7.7); the most common and, unfortunately, malignant type of primary brain tumour in adults, accounting for up to 80% of adult gliomas. It is highly infiltrative and poorly demarcated with a propensity to spread along white matter tracts, e.g., corpus callosum, to involve contralateral hemispheres, hence the description 'butterfly tumour'. The majority

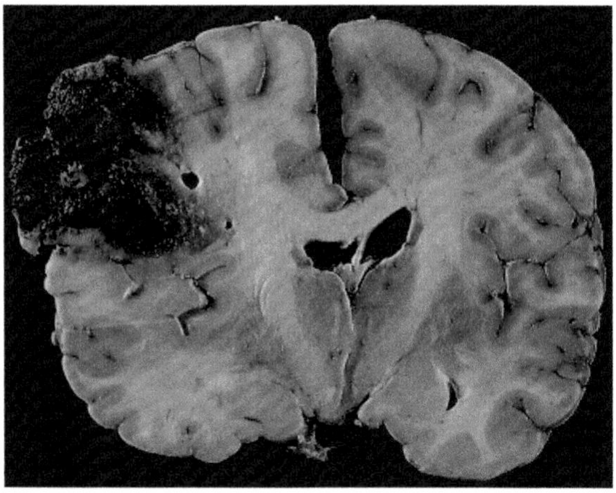

Fig. 7.7 Glioblastoma. A coronal section through the brain showing a left haemorrhagic glioblastoma with associated asymmetric swelling of the cerebrum. There is displacement of the midline structures to the right causing compression of the lateral ventricle, downwards displacement of the diencephalon, and part distortion of the left cingulate gyrus secondary to subfalcine herniation. (Reprinted with permission from Ellison D, Love S. *Neuropathology*, 3rd edn. Elsevier Mosby, 2013: pp. 697–704. © 2013 Elsevier.)

arise de novo (90%), whilst secondary forms occur from progression of preexisting lower grade diffuse astrocytomas (10%). These are associated with mutated *IDH-1* whereas primary forms are *IDH-1* wild type with epidermal growth factor receptor amplification.

Imaging reveals large, spherical masses with thick enhancing margins, central necrotic cavities, mass effect and surrounding oedema. Microscopically, glioblastomas are similar to anaplastic astrocytomas with additional areas of geographic necrosis, 'pseudopalisaded' tumour cells and vascular/endothelial cell proliferation and haemorrhage.

MOLECULAR

ISOCITRATE DEHYDROGENASE *(IDH-1)* MUTATIONS

IDH-1 is a key genetic marker in gliomas. Diffuse astrocytomas with mutated *IDH-1* have a better prognosis than those with wild-type *IDH-1*, which behave more aggressively. *IDH-1* mutation with 1p12q codeletion is also necessary for the diagnosis of an oligodendroglioma.

Oligodendrogliomas

These ill-defined, slow-growing tumours arise from oligodendrocytes in the white matter of the cerebral hemispheres, especially the temporal lobe. They account for 3% of all primary CNS neoplasms in adults and 2%–25% of gliomas. Imaging shows mixed density masses ± enhancement. Microscopically, they are characterized by uniform cells with so-called 'fried egg' appearance (spherical nuclei with perinuclear halos), which readily infiltrate grey matter and frequently invade the subarachnoid space. A fine anastomosing network of capillaries is also seen, and dystrophic calcification is common.

IDH-1 must be mutated with 1p19q codeletion for the diagnosis of an oligodendroglioma.

Ependymoma

These tumours arise from the ependymal cells lining the ventricles and central canal of the spinal cord. In children they account for 30% of primary CNS tumours and occur intracranially. In adults they occur within the spinal cord or ventricles, accounting for 2% of all primary CNS neoplasms. Microscopically, they are formed of uniform cells with indistinct cell borders and can demonstrate rosette and pseudorosette formations.

Spinal ependymomas are associated with neurofibromatosis type 2.

Other tumours

Medulloblastoma

This highly malignant tumour of primitive neuroepithelial cells arises in the cerebellum of children. It is the second commonest childhood CNS tumour. Clinically, the onset is rapid over a course of a few weeks owing to the rapid growth rate of these tumours. The tumours are variably infiltrative and tend to form a midline mass in the roof of the fourth ventricle ± extension over the pia mater with widespread underlying invasion. Microscopically, they are characterized by sheets of small round hyperchromatic cells with scant cytoplasm. The background is finely fibrillary with necrosis and mitosis. Homer Wright rosette formation may be seen (Fig. 7.8). Genetically they are subclassified into four groups.

CLINICAL NOTE

CENTRAL NERVOUS SYSTEM TUMOURS OF ADULTS AND CHILDREN

The commonest intracranial tumours in descending order of frequency:

Children

1. Astrocytomas (75% pilocytic)
2. Medulloblastoma
3. Ependymomas

Adults

1. Gliomas (80% glioblastomas)
2. Meningiomas
3. Pituitary tumours

The tumour is highly radiosensitive, but without treatment it is rapidly fatal.

Meningiomas

These account for approximately 21% of adult intracranial tumours and are the second most common primary intracranial neoplasms; incidence increases with age. They arise from the arachnoid cells of the leptomeninges. They are usually benign (although they may be locally aggressive) and external to the brain, occurring anywhere within the CNS, preferentially parasagittal, sphenoid ridge and lateral sulcus locations. They are often dural based and well-defined, with a shape related to their location.

Microscopically, appearance is variable as they show both epithelial and mesenchymal differentiation. Characteristically, a whorled appearance is seen with a variable presence of psammoma bodies.

The risk of recurrence is related to coexisting underlying parenchymal invasion. They are associated with previous cranial irradiation and neurofibromatosis type 2 when found in young patients. They are oestrogen- and progesterone-sensitive, so may enlarge during pregnancy. Fig. 7.9

Metastatic tumours

Metastatic tumours are more common than any primary intracranial neoplasms and are the most common mass lesions in the brain. Any part of the brain can be affected (cerebrum, cerebellum and brainstem) as well as other intracranial structures, especially meninges (malignant meningitis). Metastases often occur at the boundary between grey and white matter or vascular watershed areas. Appearance is variable on imaging; however, they are usually well demarcated and surrounded by a zone of peritumoral oedema. They may be solitary or multiple.

The most common metastatic CNS neoplasms are:

- lung carcinomas
- melanoma
- breast carcinomas
- renal carcinomas
- colonic carcinomas.

DISORDERS OF THE PERIPHERAL NERVOUS SYSTEM

Disorders of peripheral nerves are termed neuropathies. They can be predominantly sensory, motor or mixed, depending on which nerves are affected. Examples can be found in Table 7.13.

Terminology:

Mononeuropathy = disorders affecting one nerve

- Distal asymmetric weakness
- ± Sensory changes
- Can be symmetrical if affects more than one nerve.

Mononeuritis multiplex = disorders affecting multiple individual nerves

- Asymmetrical (can be symmetrical depending on nerves involved).

Polyneuropathies = disorders affecting multiple peripheral nerves

- Distal symmetrical weakness
- ± Sensory changes
- Usually lower limbs then upper limbs affected.

Radiculopathies = disorders affecting the nerve roots

- Proximal or distal asymmetric weakness
- Dermatomal sensory loss
- Pain

Table 7.13 Examples of mononeuropathies and polyneuropathies

Mononeuropathy	Polyneuropathy
• Median nerve palsy (carpal tunnel syndrome) • Ulnar nerve palsy • Radial nerve palsy • Peroneal nerve palsy • Sciatic nerve (sciatica)	• Hereditary motor and sensory neuropathies • Guillain–Barré syndrome • Diabetic neuropathy • Renal (uraemic) neuropathy • Alcohol • B12 and thiamine deficiency • Drugs (e.g., cisplatin, isoniazid, vincristine)

Hereditary motor and sensory neuropathies

Peroneal muscular atrophy (hereditary motor and sensory neuropathies I and II; Charcot–Marie–Tooth disease)

This disorder is characterized by pronounced atrophy of the calf muscles with associated sensory deficits as a result of slowly progressive symmetrical neuropathy. It is the commonest of the hereditary neuropathies, and is usually autosomal dominant. It impedes ambulation and causes foot deformities (pes cavus), but it does not shorten the lifespan (Table 7.14).

Mononeuropathies

These are usually caused by nerve compression (see Traumatic neuropathies). A common example is carpal tunnel syndrome. Each mononeuropathy will have a pattern of sensory loss and muscle weakness dependent on the innervation of that nerve.

Carpal tunnel syndrome

This is a disorder in which the size of the carpal tunnel is significantly reduced, causing compression of the median nerve, resulting in:

- Weakness: thenar muscles of the hand and atrophy of pollicis brevis.
- Sensory loss: palm and lateral 3.5 fingers (inclusive of thumb).

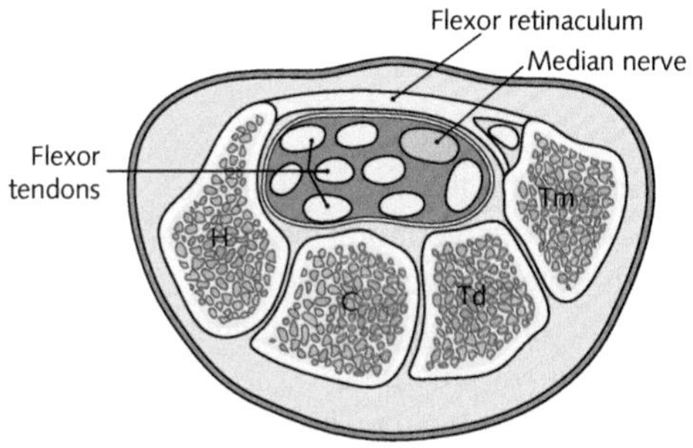

Fig. 7.10 The carpal tunnel. The carpal tunnel showing the anatomical limitation of size and how any decrease in aperture of the tunnel will lead to compression of the structures within, i.e., median nerve. *C*, Capitate; *H*, hamate; *Td*, trapezoid; *Tm*, trapezium.

Causes include inflammation of the flexor retinaculum, hypothyroidism, diabetes mellitus, pregnancy, obesity, acromegaly and arthritic changes (Fig. 7.10).

Polyneuropathies

There are lots of types and causes of polyneuropathies, including diabetes and alcohol. The key is to remember that they are generalized disorders so the underlying causes tend to be ones that have global (systemic) rather than focal (localized) effects. As such, the distribution is usually bilateral and symmetrical. The longest nerves are affected first, as they are the most vulnerable, meaning that deficits begin distally, usually in the lower limbs, and spread proximally as shorter nerves are progressively involved. The pattern of deficit usually has a 'glove and stocking' distribution. Examples of polyneuropathies are discussed below.

Inflammatory neuropathies

Guillain–Barré syndrome (acute inflammatory demyelinating polyradiculoneuropathy)

This is the most common form of acute neuropathy and is caused by immune-mediated demyelination of peripheral nerves, usually occurring 2–4 weeks after an infection, most commonly respiratory (e.g., cytomegalovirus) or gastrointestinal (e.g., *Campylobacter jejuni*). It is thought that the infectious agent causes production of cross-reactive antibodies, which recognize glycolipids present in the myelin sheaths surrounding nerves triggering a T-cell–mediated response.

Affected patients develop a progressive ascending motor neuropathy ('ascending paralysis') of the peripheral limbs because of widespread demyelination of the peripheral nerves. Initial presentation is with proximal lower limb weakness. Lesser sensory changes (usually toes and finger tips) also occur but these do not ascend. Mechanical ventilation is required in approximately one-third of patients. Recovery (i.e., remyelination) occurs over 3–4 months and in the majority is complete; however, the condition is associated with long-term morbidity. Death can occur owing to the sequelae of long-term immobility, e.g., thromboembolic disease, pneumonia, arrhythmias.

Infectious neuropathies

Leprosy (Hansen disease)

A chronic granulomatous disease caused by *Mycobacterium leprae*. It is the most common cause of peripheral neuritis worldwide. The clinicopathological features of leprosy are discussed in detail in Chapter 18. Nerve involvement is outlined in Table 7.15.

Varicella zoster virus (shingles)

A neuropathy of cutaneous sensory nerves discussed in detail in Chapter 18.

Metabolic neuropathies

Peripheral neuropathy of diabetes mellitus

This occurs in both type 1 and 2 diabetes mellitus, with a prevalence of 10%–60% clinically, but up to 100% when evaluated by nerve conduction studies. There is increased prevalence with increased duration of the disease (see Chapter 14).

Uraemic neuropathy in renal failure

Approximately 60% of patients with chronic renal failure have symptoms of uraemic neuropathy at the onset of dialysis. It is typically a distal, symmetrical, sensorimotor polyneuropathy producing pain and paraesthesia preferentially

Table 7.15 Peripheral nerve damage in leprosy

	Lepromatous	Tuberculoid
Distribution in nerves	Widely disseminated diffuse nerve involvement	One or a few sites (asymmetrical)
Nerve enlargement and damage	Intense infiltration of nerves by vacuolated macrophages	Hallmark of nerve involvement is discrete, well-formed granulomas
Peripheral nerves	Nerves palpable but degree not as severe as tuberculoid form. Remain functional early on in disease so sensation is maintained	Palpable thickened nerves supply the lesion and may be painful
Neurological deficit	Sensory and motor involvement, patchy loss of sensation	Sensory, motor and autonomic involvement. Peripheral nerve palsies. Anaesthetic areas prone to injury and secondary infection

within the lower extremities. Motor symptoms of weakness and atrophy follow sensory symptoms. Dialysis usually improves symptoms.

Toxic neuropathies

Many toxins cause damage to peripheral nerves. The most common toxins are:

- Drugs: e.g., amiodarone, lithium, phenytoin, isoniazids, sulphonamides, vinca alkaloids, dapsone and chloroquine.
- Alcohol: in cases of chronic abuse.
- Industrial toxins: e.g., acrylamide, carbon disulfide, hexane, organophosphates, lead, arsenic, mercury.

Most toxins produce a 'dying back' pattern of axonal damage resulting in a distal symmetric pattern of sensorimotor involvement. There is a 'stocking-glove' distribution at onset but continued exposure to the toxin extends the deficit to the lower calves and forearms.

Neuropathies associated with malignancy

Cancer patients frequently have neuropathies that can be caused by direct infiltration of individual nerves or plexuses, e.g., brachial plexopathy due to apical lung cancer, as a result of treatment (surgery, chemotherapy/radiotherapy) or, rarely, as a paraneoplastic syndrome.

Traumatic neuropathies

Peripheral nerves arise from the roots of the spinal cord and consist of motor and sensory components that supply specific muscle groups and dermatomes. They may be injured anywhere along their course, especially in vulnerable areas, e.g., superficial under the skin or traversing a bony prominence. The resultant symptoms are dependent on the nerve/spinal cord root that is involved and whether damage occurs to the sensory/motor components or both.

Mechanisms of injury

There are various ways in which nerves can become injured:

- *Crush injuries:* usually result from acute, traumatic compression from blunt force trauma. Different degrees of damage are sustained.
- *Compression injuries:* can be acute, e.g., from sleeping with an arm over a chair (Saturday night palsy—radial nerve neuropathy) or chronic, e.g., nerves which pass through narrow anatomical locations. Compressed nerves undergo segmental demyelination, causing decreased nerve conduction velocity. Axons are preserved; however, if compression is prolonged or severe, axonal degeneration may occur.

Symptoms of nerve compression are paraesthesia, anaesthesia and muscle weakness.

CLINICAL NOTE

COMMON SITES OF NERVE COMPRESSION

- Nerve roots in the intervertebral foramina by prolapsed intervertebral discs or osteophytes due to spinal osteoarthritis
- Median nerve in the carpal tunnel at the wrist—carpal tunnel syndrome
- Ulnar nerve at the medial epicondyle of humerus—cubital tunnel syndrome
- Common peroneal nerve at the neck of the fibula—foot drop

- *Transection/laceration injuries:* complete or partial division of axons and epineural (connective) tissue resulting in discontinuity of the nerve. These injuries occur from sharp force trauma, e.g., knife wounds or bone shards at fracture sites.
- *Stretch/traction injuries:* nerves can be stretched beyond their elastic limits, ranging in severity from myelin degeneration to rupture depending on the degree of force applied. These commonly affect the brachial plexus, e.g., when head is forced in the opposite direction to the shoulder, such as in a motor cycle accident or poorly-executed rugby tackle.

Types of injury

Injuries may be mild or severe and, depending on the type of damage, have a different potential for healing and restoration of normal function. Damage to peripheral nerves results in demyelination, axonal degeneration or both. Types of damage include:

- *Avulsion:* the nerve is removed from the spinal cord. It may be complete or partial.
- *Neuropraxia:* focal demyelination with axons and connective tissue remaining intact resulting in a temporary loss of conduction. Results from mild compression or traction.
- *Axonotmesis:* axons are divided with focal demyelination occurring whilst nerve continuity is maintained as the covering nerve sheath remains intact. This occurs commonly with traction or crush injuries. Loss of function is variable, depending on the degree of injury.
- *Neurotmesis:* partial or complete transection of the axons and nerve sheath, with loss of nerve continuity. Depending on the nature of the injury surgical repair may be possible.

Healing

After an axon has become crushed or cut a reparative process is attempted. The axon is now divided into distal and proximal segments. The distal segment undergoes Wallerian degeneration where axon and myelin sheath degenerate at the site of injury with absorption of axonal debris by Schwann cells and recruited macrophages. The proximal nerve ending develops neuritic sprouts (collateral branches) with growth cones which grow towards the distal portion in an attempt to locate the distal Schwann cells of the severed axons. The Schwann cells and surrounding nerve sheath act as guide for the slow regrowth of the axons (1 mm/day). Outcome is variable and functional recovery may not be complete.

If continuity of a nerve is completely interrupted (i.e., endoneurium, perineurium and epineurium are dissected) there are no longer continuous tubes to guide regeneration of Schwann cells and neuritic sprouts so the potential for recovery is limited.

Neoplasms of peripheral nerves

The common neoplasms of peripheral nerves are outlined in Table 7.16. It is important to note that 'neuromas' are non-neoplastic proliferations of Schwann cells and fibroblasts around peripheral nerves in response to trauma and are usually associated with pain. Common examples include:

- *Traumatic neuroma*: a tangled mass of axons, Schwann cells and fibroblasts of an injured proximal nerve segment which has attempted regeneration but failed to locate the distal nerve segment.
- *Morton neuroma*: occurs specifically on the plantar interdigital nerve of the foot, usually within the third metatarsal space, in response to repeated trauma. It is a fusiform mass of perineural and intraneural fibrosis ± nerve degeneration.

Neurofibromatosis

Also known as Von Recklinghausen disease, this is a genetic condition principally characterized by neurofibroma formation. It affects the skin, soft tissues, bone and nervous system and is subclassified into two distinct types, the features of which are outlined in Table 7.17.

Tuberous sclerosis complex

This is an autosomal-dominant inherited disease characterized by multiple hamartomatous lesions and benign tumours. It can affect any organ system but predominantly neurological and cutaneous features are seen. Mutations in the *TSC1* (hamartin protein) and *TSC2* (tuberin protein) genes are responsible.

Cutaneous features: ash leaf patches, shagreen patches (roughened) and angiofibromas in a butterfly distribution on face.

Neurological features: epilepsy, intellectual impairment, infantile spasms and cortical, subependymal calcified nodules/tubers.

Table 7.16 Common neoplasms of peripheral nerves

Tumour	Location	Macroscopic features	Microscopic features	Other
Benign				
Schwannoma[a]	Commonly cutaneous on head and flexor surfaces of upper/lower limbs and trunk. May be intracranial	Well-circumscribed mass, encapsulated. Attached/associated to a peripheral nerve	Diffuse spindle cells. Areas of different cellular densities: Antoni A (dense), Antoni B (less dense with fibrillary collagen). Verocay bodies (parallel columns of nuclei). Axons excluded from tumour	NF-2, known as acoustic neuroma when occurs at cerebropontine angle attached to VIII cranial nerve (see Chapter 8)
Neurofibroma	Solitary or multiple. Cutaneous: head, neck, trunk, proximal limbs. Within a peripheral nerve	Localized nodules within the dermis or infiltrative masses within nerves. Unencapsulated	Spindle cells. Collagenous/myxoid stroma. No Verocay bodies. Mast cells. Axons within the tumour. Plexiform type within a nerve bundle	NF-1 associated if plexiform or multiple lesions
Malignant				
MPNST	Medium to large peripheral nerves anywhere in the body. Common sites: nerve roots, extremities, pelvis, sciatic nerve	Not circumscribed. Locally invasive within nerves and adjacent soft tissue	High-grade tumours. Spindle cells forming fascicles. Mitoses. Necrosis. Nuclear anaplasia	Fifty percent of cases associated with NF-1. Rapid growth. Commonly metastasizes to lung

[a] *Schwannomas are also known as neurilemmomas.*
MPNST, Malignant peripheral nerve sheath tumour; NF, neurofibromatosis 1 and 2.

Table 7.17 Neurofibromatosis type 1 and type 2

	Neurofibromatosis type 1[a]	Neurofibromatosis type 2
Inheritance	Autosomal dominant	Autosomal dominant
Incidence	1/3000	1/50,000
Gene (protein)	*NF1* (neurofibromin)	*NF2* (merlin)
Age of onset	Childhood—adolescence	Late adolescence—early adulthood
Characteristic tumours	Neurofibromas ++ Optic nerve glioma Small bowel GIST Phaeochromocytomas	Schwannomas (especially spinal cord) Bilateral acoustic neuromas Meningiomas Neurofibromas Gliomas (ependymomas)—spinal cord
Other clinical features	Café-au-lait spots Axillary/inguinal freckling Lisch nodules in iris Short stature Scoliosis Learning difficulties/ADHD Hypertension	Cataracts
Morbidity	MPNST risk 10% Cosmetic issues	Bilateral deafness Enlargement of brain or spinal cord lesions can cause significant neurological deficits and pain, and may be life-threatening

[a] *Neurofibromatosis type 1 has greater cutaneous involvement than neural involvement, whereas neurofibromatosis type 2 has greater central and peripheral nervous system involvement by tumours and few cutaneous lesions.*
ADHD, Attention deficit hyperactivity disorder; GIST, gastrointestinal stromal tumour; MPNST, malignant peripheral nerve sheath tumour.

Tubers are haphazardly arranged neurones which display a mixed phenotype between neurones and glial cells. Macroscopically they resemble potato tubers.

DISORDERS OF THE AUTONOMIC NERVOUS SYSTEM

Disorders of the sympathetic nervous system

Horner syndrome

An uncommon condition caused by loss of sympathetic innervation to the eye. It is characterized by:

- Pupillary constriction (miosis) owing to unopposed action of the pupillary constrictor.
- Partial ptosis (drooping) of the upper eyelid owing to paralysis of smooth muscle fibres contained in the levator muscle of the upper eyelid.
- Enophthalmos (eye sunken into socket).
- Anhidrosis (loss of sweating) on affected side of the face.

HINTS AND TIPS

HORNER SYNDROME

Lesions affecting any part of the sympathetic pathway may produce Horner syndrome:

- Brainstem—tumours, vascular lesions or syringobulbia
- Cervical cord—tumours or syringomyelia
- Cervical sympathetic chain—Pancoast tumours (apical tumours of the lung) frequently invade adjacent sites, including the sympathetic chain.

Trauma/surgical section of the sympathetic trunk

Surgical sympathectomies are sometimes performed for the relief of such conditions as:

- Raynaud phenomenon—pallor, pain and numbness of the fingers caused by vasospastic constriction of the digital arteries; sympathectomy is occasionally performed to improve limb perfusion (Fig. 7.11).
- Causalgia—severe burning pain that occurs following injury to the major peripheral nerves of the limbs (e.g., median, ulnar, sciatic) presumed to be because of disturbances of sympathetic reflexes.
- Hyperhidrosis—excessive sweating.

The consequences of either traumatic or surgical section of the sympathetic chain depend on the level of the section, but may cause:

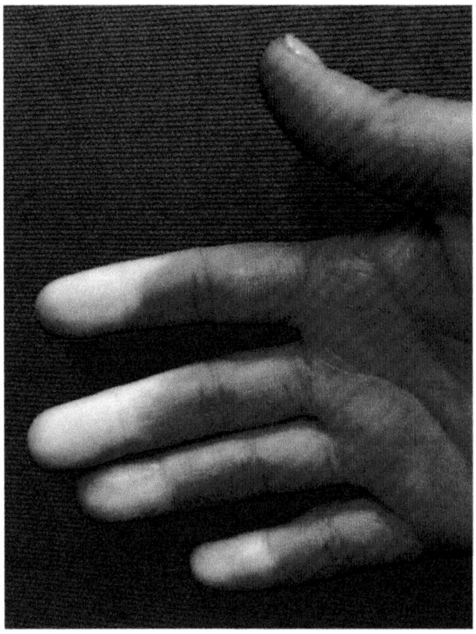

Fig. 7.11 Raynaud disease. Photograph of fingers showing the changes seen in Raynaud disease. Arteriole vasospasm leads to complete blood loss of the finger(s), rendering them white (dead) in appearance. On restoration of bloodflow, the fingers turn blue then bright red, which is associated with burning pain.

- impairment of sweating → hyperpyrexia
- impairment of bladder and bowel functions
- interruption of pathway to erectile tissue → impotence.

Diseases of the parasympathetic nervous system

Effects of ablation of parasympathetic innervation

Parasympathetic nerve ablation is uncommon, but may be performed in cases of refractory atrial fibrillation. Catheter ablation of atrial parasympathetic nerves is performed.

CLINICAL NOTE

MORBIDITY OF TRANSURETHRAL RESECTION OF THE PROSTATE (TURP) AND AXILLARY NODAL CLEARANCE (ANC)

Iatrogenic autonomic dysfunction is a known side-effect of some common surgical procedures. Impotence owing to thermal injury of periprostatic nerves may occur in TURP. Anhidrosis may occur after ANC in patients undergoing mastectomy and axillary lymph node clearance.

Chapter Summary

- Hydrocephalus can be congenital or acquired, communicating or non-communicating.
- Neural tube defects are the most common central nervous system (CNS) abnormality, e.g., spina bifida.
- Hypoxic ischaemic injuries are major causes of severe perinatal brain damage.
- Cerebral palsy is caused by damage to the motor pathways in the brain and is nonprogressive.
- Extradural haemorrhage is associated with a lucid interval and is usually due to rupture of the middle meningeal artery.
- Subdural haemorrhage is usually due to rupture of the bridging veins.
- Berry aneurysms and trauma are the commonest causes of subarachnoid haemorrhage.
- Rupture of Charcot–Bouchard microaneurysms in hypertensive patients is associated with intracerebral haemorrhage.
- Meningitis is inflammation of the meninges and can be caused by infectious agents, e.g., bacteria, viruses, fungi and protozoa or by other conditions such as metastatic disease.
- Creutzfeldt–Jakob disease is a transmissible spongiform encephalopathy caused by prions.
- Degenerative diseases not only include multiple sclerosis and Parkinson disease, but also many forms of dementia.
- Multiple sclerosis is characterized by oligoclonal bands of IgM in the cerebrospinal fluid.
- Parkinson disease is characterized by loss of the substantia nigra.
- Alzheimer disease is characterized by senile plaques (β-amyloid protein) and neurofibrillary tangles (tau protein).
- CNS tumours include gliomas (astrocytomas, oligodendrogliomas and ependymomas), medulloblastomas, meningiomas and metastatic tumours.
- The most common CNS tumours are gliomas.

- Damage and disorders of the peripheral nerves are termed neuropathies. They can be sensory, motor or mixed and involve one or many nerves.
- The pattern of sensory loss and muscle weakness in peripheral neuropathy is dependent on the sensory area/muscle groups that the nerve innervates.
- Neuropathies can be traumatic, infectious, inflammatory or toxic.
- Mechanisms of nerve injury include crush, compression, stretch and laceration.
- The potential for a peripheral nerve to regenerate depends on the type of injury and degree of residual nerve connective tissue continuity.
- Peripheral nerve neoplasms include schwannoma, neurofibroma and malignant peripheral nerve sheath tumours.
- Horner syndrome is caused by compression of the sympathetic cervical chain and is characterized by miosis, ptosis, anhidrosis and enophthalmos.

Pathology of the head and neck 8

INTRODUCTION

Although composed of part of both the respiratory and gastrointestinal tract, the ear, nose and throat form their own subspecialty. Lesions specific to the head and neck may be found in this region and thus they are classed together.

DISORDERS OF THE UPPER RESPIRATORY TRACT

The nose and nasopharynx

Rhinitis

Rhinitis, inflammation of the nasal mucosa, is the most common nasal disorder seen in general practice. The condition may be either acute or chronic.

Acute rhinitis

Aetiology of acute rhinitis is either:

- Infective
- Allergic
- Iatrogenic.

Infectious rhinitis is usually of viral origin, e.g., the common cold (rhinoviruses, adenoviruses). Virally induced inflammation of surface epithelial cells is followed by exudation of fluid and mucus from the damaged surface ('runny nose'). Later, submucosal oedema produces swelling, which may lead to partial blockage of the nasal airways.

Allergic rhinitis ('hay fever') is a type I (immunoglobulin (Ig) E-mediated) hypersensitivity reaction to inhaled materials such as pollens, producing a mixed serous/mucous exudate and submucosal oedema leading to nasal blockage. Eosinophils are prominent in the inflammatory infiltrate.

Iatrogenic rhinitis can occur secondary to frequent use of nasal sprays.

Chronic rhinitis

Chronic rhinitis can be caused by repeated attacks of acute rhinitis, which often develop a secondary bacterial infection. It may result in the development of nasal polyps.

- Macroscopically, nasal polyps are typically smooth-surfaced, creamy, semitranslucent, ovoid masses.
- Microscopically, they have oedematous tissue with a scattered infiltrate of chronic inflammatory cells. Eosinophils are often very numerous in allergic polyps.

Sinusitis

Sinusitis is inflammation of the paranasal sinuses (maxillary, ethmoidal, frontal, sphenoidal), usually secondary to acute or chronic rhinitis. Sinusitis usually results in inflammation of the sinus linings, engorging the mucosa around the draining foramen of the maxillary sinus in the nasal cavity. This may cause stasis of maxillary sinus secretions. Stasis predisposes to secondary bacterial infection with alteration of the static maxillary fluid from seromucous to purulent.

In severe cases, the infection may spread into the ethmoid and frontal sinuses, with a risk of spread to the meninges. Orbital cellulitis may also complicate acute sinusitis.

Chronic sinusitis is characterized by chronically thickened and inflamed mucosa of the sinuses and by persistent fluid accumulation.

RED FLAG

ORBITAL CELLULITIS

Orbital cellulitis is inflammation and infection of the posterior orbital septum and is characterized by pain, swelling, chemosis and sudden loss of vision. It is a clinical emergency.

Kartagener syndrome

This is a primary ciliary dyskinesia causing a syndrome of bronchiectasis, sinusitis and situs inversus (transposition of viscera) resulting in a failure to clear mucus and bacteria.

Necrotizing lesions

Granulomatosis polyangiitis

Formerly called Wegener granulomatosis, this autoimmune granulomatous vasculitis frequently presents with nasal lesions (see Chapter 10).

Lethal midline granuloma (NK/T-cell lymphoma)

This is a condition presenting with progressive granulomatous inflammation, ulceration and necrotizing destruction of the structures in the upper respiratory tract, i.e., the nose, nasopharynx, palate and sinuses. It is thought to be a form of lymphoma affecting natural killer (NK) cells, and may occur alongside lymphomatous disease elsewhere in the body.

Untreated, death occurs from systemic disease caused by erosion of blood vessels, local infection or the development of pneumonia.

Neoplastic disease

Benign

Nasal papilloma—This benign tumour composed of respiratory-type mucosa can arise in the lateral wall or the nasal septum. Treatment is via excision.

Nasopharyngeal angiofibroma—This rare benign tumour, composed of blood vessels and fibrous tissue, occurs almost exclusively in males between 10 and 25 years old. The lesions are typically located in the posterolateral wall of the nose and may mimic a malignant tumour, owing to their rapid growth and tendency to erode bone. Ulceration and bleeding are common.

Malignant

Nasopharyngeal carcinoma—This is a carcinoma of the nasopharynx with a characteristic abundant lymphoid stroma.

Most subtypes are strongly associated with Epstein–Barr virus infection, the virus being demonstrable in tumour cells in most cases. The carcinoma is most commonly found in North Africa and South-East Asia, and is rare elsewhere in the world.

The tumours often remain small and undetected until metastasis to the lymph nodes in the neck has occurred.

The prognosis is good with radiation therapy and immunotherapy.

Olfactory neuroblastoma—This tumour, located in the upper part of the nasal cavity, develops from neuronal cells found in the olfactory mucosa. It often presents as a haemorrhagic mass with evidence of bone destruction. Microscopically, Homer Wright rosettes may be seen.

The larynx

Acute laryngitis

Acute inflammation of the larynx is most commonly due to viral infection but may also be caused by bacteria, irritants (cigarette smoke), endotracheal intubation or overuse of the voice, e.g., shouting. It causes a hoarse voice due to oedema of the vocal cords impeding their ability to vibrate and produce phonation. It is usually self-limiting of less than 3weeks' duration.

Chronic laryngitis

Inflammation of the larynx persisting for >3 weeks. It is caused by repeated exposure of the laryngeal mucosa to irritants such as environmental pollutants, acid from gastro-oesophageal reflux, chronic sinusitis, allergens, smoking and excessive alcohol use. Long-term voice strain, e.g., in singers, is also common.

The laryngeal epithelium comprises a mix of nonkeratinized squamous epithelium (true vocal cords) and ciliated respiratory epithelium (false vocal cords). Metaplasia of the laryngeal mucosa from respiratory epithelium to keratinized squamous epithelium can occur in response to repeated irritation, e.g., smoking. This can progress to keratotic thickening with dysplastic changes predisposing to the development of squamous carcinoma of the larynx.

Acute laryngotracheobronchitis (croup)

Croup is a potentially life-threatening acute inflammation, causing swelling and obstruction of the upper respiratory tract involving the larynx, trachea, bronchi and subglottis. It usually affects young children aged 6 months to 3 years and is typically caused by parainfluenza virus infection. Coryzal symptoms precede characteristic hoarseness, inspiratory stridor, wheeze and barking cough. Severity is gauged by clinical signs and the degree of hypoxaemia.

Reactive nodules/polyps

These common benign lesions are usually unilateral and commonly involve the free edge of the vocal fold mucosa. They are thought to arise from phonotrauma or single episodes of haemorrhage. Presentation is with hoarseness that will not resolve until the polyp is removed.

Singer's nodules

These are small (1–3 mm), benign bilateral fibrous nodules covered by squamous epithelium located at the nodal point (junction between the anterior third and posterior two-thirds of the vocal cords), which corresponds to the area of maximal trauma on high-pitched phonation. Nodules are especially common in singers and professional voice users, and they can alter the character of the voice.

> **HINTS AND TIPS**
>
> **SINGER'S NODULES VERSUS POLYPS**
>
> Remember that polyps are unilateral lesions and are treated by excision, whereas singer's nodules are bilateral and are treated with voice rest. Reactive nodules of the larynx affect men more often than women.

Papilloma and papillomatosis

Papilloma

These lesions are usually solitary in adults and confined to the true vocal cords. Histologically they are formed of squamous epithelium covering finger-like fibrovascular cores. Recurrent papillomas can occur due to infection by human papillomavirus (HPV 11 and 16).

Juvenile laryngeal papillomatosis

These multiple, soft, pink papillomas on the vocal cords are largely confined to children. Lesions often extend into other parts of the larynx, sometimes even along the trachea, and they have the histological features of florid viral warts. Spontaneous regression often occurs at puberty, although the lesions are typically difficult to eradicate if this does not happen.

Squamous cell carcinoma of the larynx

The larynx is the most common site of head and neck cancer, followed by the tonsils, with squamous cell carcinoma (SCC) accounting for 95% of all laryngeal cancers. It typically presents after 45 years of age, affecting males more often than females (but the incidence is rising in females) and accounts for 3% of all cancers in the UK. The risk factors are smoking, alcohol, head and neck irradiation, and HPV infection. There is a linear association between the degree of smoking and alcohol consumption and the risk of SCC.

Laryngeal cancer is classified as:

- Glottic (60%)—arises from true vocal cords. The best prognosis follows early detection because this area is alymphatic, which restricts the routes for metastasis. The earliest symptom is hoarseness, which should always be investigated if persisting for more than 4 weeks.
- Supraglottic (30%)—involves the lower epiglottis, false cords, ventricles and arytenoids. It has a worse prognosis, as presentation is late owing to occult growth and rich lymphatic drainage.
- Subglottic region (10%)—arising below the true vocal cords and above the first tracheal ring; poor prognosis as presentation is late and there is rich lymphatic drainage. Extension to involve the trachea and thyroid is possible, with presentation often as respiratory distress rather than dysphonia.

RED FLAG

CANCER OF THE HEAD AND NECK

- The location of the cancer will determine the symptoms experienced.
- Persistent hoarse voice >3 weeks' duration.
- Unexplained lump in the neck.
- Unexplained weight loss.
- Dyspnoea.
- Dysphonia.
- Progressive dysphagia.
- Otalgia with normal otoscopy.
- Trismus (late sign).

Macroscopically, cancers appear as ulcerated, diffuse, grey solid or papillary lesions. Microscopically, the majority are well-differentiated, keratinizing SCCs with several recognized histological variants, e.g., verrucous, acantholytic. Dysplasia and carcinoma in-situ are well-recognized precursor lesions.

Spread:

- Local—to adjacent laryngeal structures but often confined by laryngeal cartilages for a considerable time.
- Lymphatic—to regional lymph nodes. The presence of a palpable neck lump usually indicates metastatic disease in adults.
- Haematogenous—occurs late if at all; lungs are the most common site.

Prognosis:

The prognosis depends on location, stage (local invasion) and the presence of lymph node metastasis. Sixty percent of patients present with advanced disease. The respective overall 5-year survival for stage I–IV disease is:

- supraglottic tumours: 59%–34%
- glottic tumours: 90%–44%
- subglottic tumours: 65%–32%.

THE MOUTH AND OROPHARYNX

Oral cavity

Cleft palate and cleft (hare) lip

These are the most common major congenital malformations of the mouth. They frequently occur together as a result of the same process, namely a failure of fusion during the embryonic period.

Aetiology:

A few cases are associated with a chromosomal abnormality (e.g., trisomy 13), but the majority have no identified cause. Retinoic acid (vitamin A) has recently been proposed as having teratogenic activity in the developing palate.

Morphology:

- Cleft lip—may be unilateral or bilateral, involving the lip only or extending upwards and backwards to include the floor of the nose and the alveolar ridge (Fig. 8.1).
- Cleft palate—considerable variation, from a small defect in the soft palate (bifid uvula) that causes little disability, to a complete separation of the hard palate combined with a cleft lip (Fig. 8.2).

The effects are an abnormal facial appearance, defective speech and feeding difficulty with extensive lesions (the child is unable to suck).

Leucoplakia

This premalignant epithelial dysplasia may precede the development of carcinoma. The condition is characterized by a white patch or plaque (hyperkeratosis) of the oral cavity that cannot be scraped away. The condition usually affects the tongue. All lesions are considered precancerous unless proven otherwise by histological evaluation.

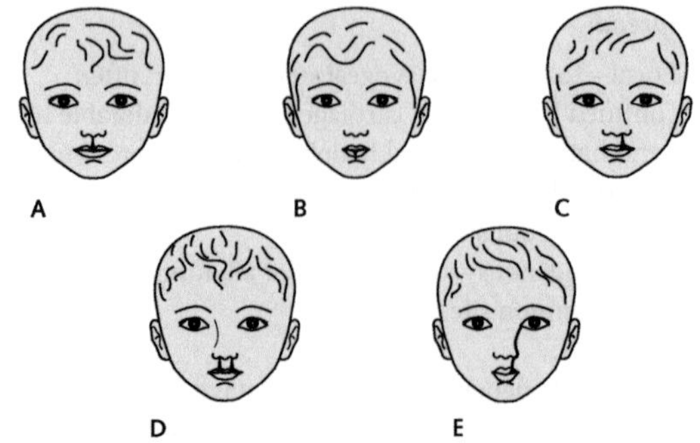

Fig. 8.1 Different types of cleft lip. (A) Median cleft upper lip. (B) Median cleft lower lip. (C) Unilateral cleft lip. (D) Bilateral cleft lip. (E) Oblique facial cleft.

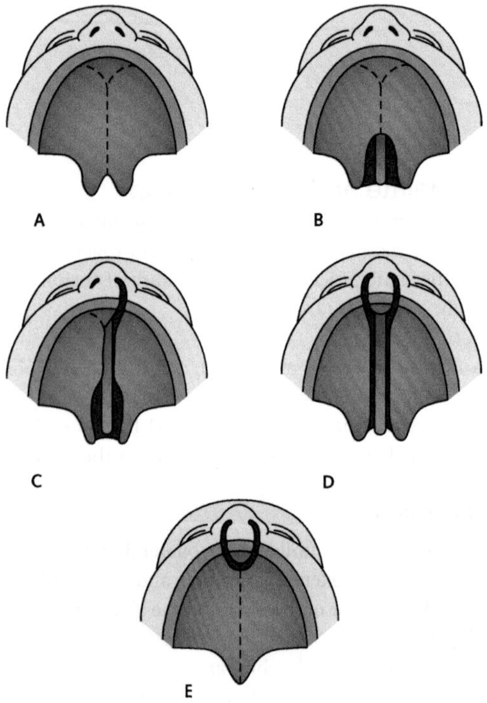

Fig. 8.2 Different types of cleft palate. (A) Cleft uvula. (B) Cleft soft and hard palate. (C) Total unilateral cleft palate and cleft lip. (D) Total bilateral cleft palate and cleft lip. (E) Bilateral cleft lip and jaw.

Erythroplakia

Less common than leucoplakia, this is characterized by the presence of red velvety patches of epithelial atrophy and dysplasia. It is seen mainly in elderly males on the buccal mucosa or the palate.

Malignant transformation is far more common than with leucoplakia. The development of erythroplakia is associated with heavy tobacco use.

Malignant neoplastic disease of the oral cavity

Squamous cell carcinoma

This is the most common tumour of the mouth, and it is derived from lining squamous epithelium. It may arise from preexisting dysplasia such as described above. Carcinoma occurs more often in men than women by a factor of about 2:1. The risk factors are:

- Smoking—there is a direct relationship between number of cigarettes smoked per day and the risk of developing oral cancer.
- Alcohol—moderate intake = decreased risk; excessive intake = increased risk.
- Nutritional deficiencies.
- Viral infections, particularly some forms of HPV.

Macroscopically, there are raised nodular lesions and central ulceration with hard raised edges.

Microscopically, the tumour is typically well-differentiated and keratinizing.

The sites are:

- Lips—usually recognized early and amenable to surgery.
- Tongue—typically occurring on the lateral border of the anterior two-thirds.
- Floor of the mouth—generally asymptomatic, resulting in extensive local invasion making surgical removal difficult.

Prognosis—may infiltrate locally and metastasize to regional lymph nodes in the neck. Five-year survival is about 50%.

HINTS AND TIPS

Remember that 95% of all cancers arising in the head and neck are squamous cell carcinomas, most commonly occurring in the oral cavity. These cancers are classically seen in men who are heavy tobacco smokers and alcohol drinkers.

Tonsils

The palatine tonsils are paired organs located between the faucial pillars of the oropharynx. They are formed of organized lymphoid tissue covered by squamous epithelium. As the tonsils are lymphoid organs they are subject to those pathologies affecting other lymphoid organs (see Chapter 17).

Tonsillitis

Inflammation of the tonsils can be viral, bacterial or fungal and is more common in children than adults. Viral aetiology accounts for 50% of cases, with causative organisms including rhinoviruses, adenoviruses and respiratory syncytial virus. Bacterial tonsillitis is caused by a variety of pathogens, most commonly β-haemolytic streptococci. Other important specific infections include diphtheria, mononucleosis (glandular fever), tuberculosis and syphilis.

Complications: these are now rare with the use of antibiotics but include:

- Peritonsillar abscess (quinsy)—usually unilateral, the patient has a severe sore throat and is unable to swallow saliva.
- Cervical adenitis with abscess.
- Ludwig angina—cellulitis of the neck with pus accumulation within the floor of the mouth causing upward displacement of the tongue and brawny induration.
- Additional group A β-haemolytic streptococcal infections, e.g., rheumatic fever, acute glomerulonephritis and scarlet fever.
- Acute otitis media—from adjacent spread of infection.

COMMON PITFALLS

AMPICILLIN AND EPSTEIN–BARR VIRUS

Do not give ampicillin to treat 'tonsillitis' as it characteristically causes a maculopapular rash in those with Epstein–Barr virus infection (glandular fever). The erroneous assumption could be made that the patient is allergic to ampicillin and they could thus be excluded from an entire class of antibiotics (penicillins) unnecessarily.

Squamous cell carcinoma

Fifty percent of all oropharyngeal SCCs arise within the tonsils, most commonly in elderly men. Two-thirds of cases present with advanced disease, e.g., regional lymph node metastasis, as the early stages are asymptomatic. Risk factors include smoking, alcohol and HPV infection.

Lymphoma

The tonsils are the commonest site of extranodal lymphoma, which presents as smooth unilateral tonsillar enlargement. The lymphoma is usually a non-Hodgkin high-grade B-cell lymphoma.

THE EAR

The ear is a complex organ in a complex location and is intricately associated with cranial and peripheral nerves. A plethora of conditions affect the ear, and these are beyond the scope of this book; however, there are a few pathologies that are peculiar to this region which will be discussed below.

Nonneoplastic conditions

Chondrodermatitis nodularis helicis

This is a benign inflammatory condition affecting the cartilaginous portion of the ear. It presents as a tender nodule (<2 cm), classically on the helix of the ear, which is extremely painful to lie on. It typically affects men over 40 years of age.

Clinically it can mimic an SCC as it may be ulcerated and crusted with discharge. Histologically, the features are of a benign ulcer with granulation tissue involving the underlying cartilage.

Cholesteatoma

This is an epidermal cyst of the middle ear, usually affecting men of 20–30 years. It is a nonneoplastic condition with no malignant potential; however, it can cause extensive morbidity owing to local destruction of the surrounding bone and the ossicles.

Cholesteatomas are formed of cysts of keratinizing squamous epithelium which may arise congenitally as embryological inclusions or as a result of trauma. Histologically they demonstrate keratinizing squamous epithelium with keratotic debris and granulation tissue.

Neoplastic disease

Acoustic neuroma

This is a schwannoma of the vestibulocochlear cranial nerve (VIII) that can arise in the internal auditory canal and cerebellar pontine angle. It is a rare benign tumour; however, it causes significant morbidity with hearing loss, tinnitus and balance problems. Continued growth can cause compressive symptoms, e.g., facial numbness owing to trigeminal nerve compression, brainstem compression, otalgia and ataxia.

Acoustic neuromas can be sporadic or familial, occurring as part of a syndrome, i.e., neurofibromatosis type II, where occurrence is bilateral in nearly all patients.

THE SALIVARY GLANDS

Inflammatory conditions

Several inflammatory conditions may arise within the salivary glands. They are usually infective or autoimmune in nature.

Sialolithiasis

Stone formation within the salivary gland is termed sialolithiasis and may occur secondary to infection, inflammation or dehydration. Stones usually form in the Wharton (submandibular) duct and can cause obstruction and further inflammation (termed sialadenitis). Presentation is with pain and swelling.

Küttner tumour

Küttner tumour is an inflammatory lesion formed when chronic sclerosing sialadenitis occurs in the submandibular gland. It is not neoplastic and is usually associated with IgG4 disease.

Mumps

This condition, caused by an RNA paramyxovirus, causes bilateral swelling of the parotid gland. Deafness, and infertility owing to testicular involvement (rarely ovarian) may also occur.

Sjogren syndrome

Please see Chapter 17 for discussion.

Benign neoplasms

Many neoplasms can arise in the major and minor salivary glands, and benign tumours account for most of these. The commonest entities are described below.

Pleomorphic adenoma

This is the commonest tumour of salivary glands, with 90% arising within the parotid gland. It presents as a painless mass, characterized histologically by epithelial cells, myoepithelial cells and myxofibrillary stroma. Treatment is by surgical excision, although multinodular recurrences may occur with incomplete excision.

Warthin tumour

This is the second commonest tumour of salivary glands and predominantly arises within the parotid gland. This tumour is commonly seen in middle-aged men with a strong history of smoking and may present bilaterally. It is characterized by cysts lined by papillary epithelium and lymphocytes (hence the alternative name papillary cystadenoma lymphomatosum). Treatment is by surgical excision.

Basal cell adenoma

This neoplasm presents as a solid, well-circumscribed, slow-growing tumour and is usually asymptomatic. Histologically, it is characterized by bland basaloid cells and must be differentiated from malignant basaloid tumours—basal cell adenocarcinoma and adenoid cystic carcinoma. Treatment is by excision, and recurrence rates are low.

Malignant neoplasms

Malignant primary salivary gland neoplasms are even more numerous than their benign counterparts. However, metastatic disease (especially SCC and melanoma) must always be considered.

Mucoepidermoid carcinoma

This is the commonest malignant salivary gland neoplasm and is also the commonest in children. It arises as a slow-growing, painless mass and may often arise in the minor salivary glands. Histologically, these tumours comprise mucous, squamoid and intermediate cells. It is associated with a t(11;19) *MECT1/MAML2* fusion gene.

Carcinoma ex pleomorphic adenoma

This tumour occurs when one or more components of a pleomorphic adenoma undergoes malignant transformation. It usually presents as a slow-growing mass (the benign component) with sudden rapid increase in size. Prognosis is dependent on degree of invasion; therefore wide surgical excisions are performed.

Acinic cell carcinoma

This tumour usually arises in the parotid gland and presents as a solid, well-circumscribed, slow-growing mass. It is characterized by acinic cells with basophilic cytoplasm and periodic acid schiff (PAS)-positive zymogen granules. Well-differentiated forms may closely resemble normal tissue. They are usually considered low-grade tumours; however, metastasis to lymph nodes, lung and bone can occur.

Adenoid cystic carcinoma

This tumour presents as a slow-growing but aggressive lesion, usually in the minor salivary glands. It is characterized by basaloid cells surrounding hyalinized cores. Perineural invasion is common. Recurrence rates after excision are high. The 5-year survival rate is 40–60%.

NECK

When faced with pathology arising in the neck, it is helpful to broadly divide the area into two anatomically-based triangles—anterior and posterior (Fig. 8.3). Each triangle contains different structures/organs and is therefore helpful in formulating a differential diagnosis.

Anterior triangle

Pharyngeal pouch/Zenker diverticulum

This is a pulsion diverticulum formed through the Killian dehiscence between the thyropharyngeus and cricopharyngeus muscles of the upper oesophagus. They occur most commonly in elderly men, with symptoms including a gurgling in the neck on palpation, chronic cough, regurgitation and halitosis. They can be complicated by aspiration pneumonia.

Carotid body tumour

These are parasympathetic paragangliomas arising from the carotid bodies located at the carotid artery bifurcation

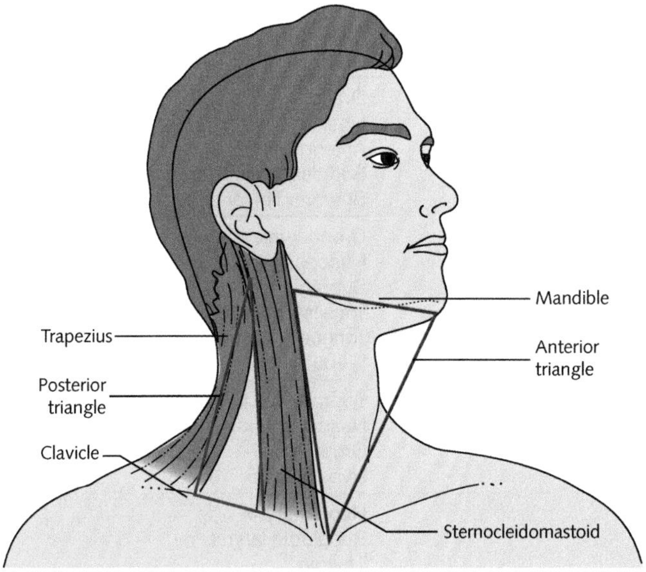

Fig. 8.3 Triangles of the neck. The anterior triangle is defined by: the midline anteriorly, the inferior border of the mandible superiorly and the medial border of the sternocleidomastoid (SCM) muscle laterally. The posterior triangle is defined by the posterior border of the SCM muscle anteriorly, the anterior border of the trapezius muscle posteriorly and the superior border of the clavicle inferiorly. (Redrawn with permission from Dhilon R.S. and East C.A., Ear, Nose and Throat: and Head and Neck Surgery, 3rd edn. Churchill Livingstone Elsevier, 2006.)

within the neck. These are rare tumours presenting in midlife as a painless, slow-growing lump near the angle of the mandible. The majority are benign (90%) and they can be unilateral or bilateral (5–10%).

Paragangliomas range in size from 2–6 cm and are composed of neuroendocrine cells arranged in a nested 'Zellballen' pattern surrounded by supportive sustentacular cells and slender fibrovascular septa.

Most are sporadic, but they can be familial as part of a syndrome, e.g., multiple endocrine neoplasia type II, neurofibromatosis type I and the Carney triad.

Thyroid

The pathology of the thyroid gland is covered in detail in Chapter 14. Lesions arising from the thyroid will occur in the midline of the neck and move with swallowing.

Thyroglossal duct cyst

Developmentally, the thyroid gland migrates from the base of the tongue down to its position in the anterior neck. The developmental tract it follows may fail to close completely and remnants can produce cysts. Classically these are in the midline and move upwards on protrusion of the tongue. As well as cysts, aberrant thyroid tissue can be found in various places along this tract, e.g., base of the tongue. For further discussion see Chapter 14.

Branchial cyst

This is an epithelial cyst caused by a remnant of the second branchial cleft. It typically presents as a mass along the sternocleidomastoid muscle in young adults (20–40-year-olds). Branchial cysts are lined by stratified squamous or ciliated columnar epithelium overlying lymphoid tissue and may connect to the skin surface (branchial fistula) and discharge following infection.

Clinically they can mimic cancer, becoming fixed hard masses secondary to postinfective inflammatory fibrosis. Cytologically they are a great mimic of SCC, such that a definitive diagnosis may necessitate excision.

> **HINTS AND TIPS**
>
> As a rule of thumb consider neck lumps to be:
> Adult: 80% malignant, 20% benign
> Children: 20% malignant, 80% benign

Posterior triangle

Cervical rib

A supernumerary cervical rib is present within 0.5% of the population and is associated with the last cervical vertebra (C7). This can be unilateral or bilateral, free-floating or connected to the first rib. It is significant as it can manifest as a mass or impinge on adjacent structures, e.g., brachial plexus or subclavian vessels, to cause thoracic outlet syndrome.

Cystic hygroma

This is a congenital lymphatic malformation (also known as lymphangioma) which can occur anywhere anatomically but is most prevalent on the left side of the neck and axilla. It is formed from cystically dilated, blind-ending lymphatic channels that have limited or no connection to the venous system. Over 50% of cystic hygromas are identified at birth, with the remainder becoming apparent by 2 years of age.

Presentation may be a rapid increase in size owing to secondary infection or haemorrhage. Depending on size and location, they can cause impingement (e.g., on neurovascular structures) and cosmetic issues.

Lymph nodes

Lymph nodes occur in both the anterior and posterior triangles and are subject to the pathologies of all lymph nodes (see Chapter 17).

Cervical lymph nodes are grouped into levels, with each level draining a specific region and its associated structures (Fig. 8.4). It is therefore important to specify which level or group of lymph nodes cervical lymphadenopathy affects as this will help to indicate the site of the primary pathology (Table 8.1). They are also important in the staging of some cancers.

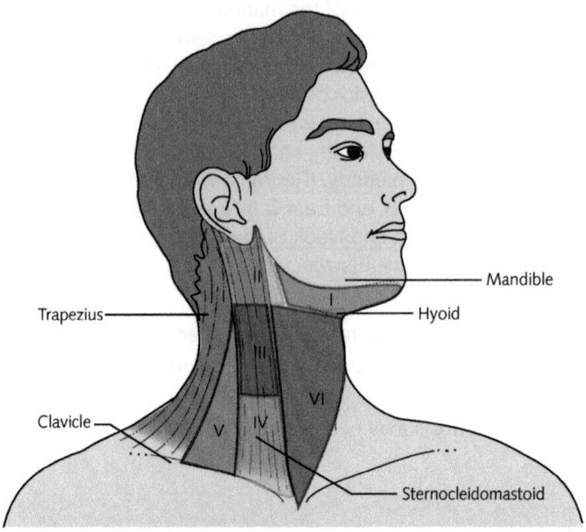

Fig. 8.4 Cervical lymph node levels. Level I: submental and submandibular; level II: internal jugular nodes; level III: middle jugular nodes; level IV: low jugular nodes; level V: posterior triangle nodes; level VI: anterior compartment nodes.

Table 8.1 Cervical lymph node drainage

Level	Structures and sites drained
I	Oral cavity Lips Anterior tongue Soft tissue mid face Submandibular gland
II	Oropharynx Nasopharynx Supraglottic larynx Tonsils Tongue Parotid
III	Supraglottic larynx Nasopharynx Oropharynx Hypopharynx
IV	Hypopharynx Subglottic larynx Thyroid Trachea Cervical oesophagus
V	Nasopharynx Thyroid Paranasal sinuses Posterior scalp skin Infraclavicular sites, e.g., stomach, breast, lung
VI	Thyroid Glottic and subglottic larynx Cervical oesophagus Lung

Chapter Summary

- Acute infective rhinitis is usually of viral aetiology.
- Orbital cellulitis may complicate sinusitis and is a clinical emergency.
- Many malignant tumours can arise in the nasal cavity. Nasopharyngeal carcinomas and olfactory neuroblastomas are two specific malignancies at this site.
- The commonest malignancy of the oral cavity is a squamous cell carcinoma (SCC). Metastases are usually to cervical lymph nodes.
- Pleomorphic adenoma is the commonest salivary gland tumour, usually arising in the parotid gland.
- Warthin tumours are the second commonest salivary gland tumour. They are often seen in smokers.
- Mucoepidermoid carcinomas are the commonest malignant salivary gland tumour and commonest paediatric salivary gland tumour.
- Ninety-five percent of head and neck cancers are SCCs.
- The larynx is the most common site of SCC in the head and neck.
- The commonest malignancies of tonsils are SCCs and lymphomas.
- Smoking and alcohol are the biggest risk factors for SCC of the head and neck.
- Thyroid lesions occur within the midline.
- Specific pathologies of the ear include chondrodermatitis nodularis helicis, cholesteatoma and acoustic neuroma.
- The neck can be anatomically divided into anterior and posterior triangles, and this is helpful in the formulation of a differential diagnosis list.
- Cervical lymph nodes are grouped according to levels which aid the location of the primary site of pathology in both benign and malignant disease.

Pathology of the cardiovascular system 9

CONGENITAL ABNORMALITIES OF THE HEART

Epidemiology

Congenital heart abnormalities are relatively common, affecting nearly 1% of live births. The incidence is higher in premature babies.

Causes

Sporadic

These are the majority of cases and no teratogenic factors can be identified.

Maternal factors

There is an increased incidence associated with certain maternal factors, including:

- maternal infection, especially with rubella
- maternal alcohol abuse (causes fetal alcohol syndrome)
- intrauterine radiation
- maternal use of teratogenic drugs, e.g., phenytoin, thalidomide.
- maternal medical conditions e.g., systemic lupus erythematosus (SLE), diabetes.

These factors are of greatest importance between the fourth and ninth week after conception.

Genetic or chromosomal abnormalities

These are associated with an increased incidence of congenital heart malformations (e.g., Down syndrome, Turner syndrome).

Clinical features

Most cardiac abnormalities are diagnosed antenatally at the 20-week scan or become apparent at or shortly after birth, usually by a manifestation of heart failure such as cyanosis, breathlessness, feeding difficulties or a failure to thrive. However, it is possible for some conditions to be undetected until adulthood.

Classification

Congenital heart defects may be divided into two main groups depending on whether the lesions cause:

1. Abnormal shunting of blood between the two sides of the heart. A shunt is defined as an abnormal passage of blood through an anomalous opening between the heart chambers or blood vessels. In congenital heart disease there may be either left-to-right (more common) or right-to-left shunts.
2. Obstruction to blood outflow by narrowing of the chambers, valves or blood vessels.

Fetal circulation

As the fetus does not breathe in utero, bloodflow and oxygenation are maintained by three unique mechanisms (Fig. 9.1):

- **Foramen ovale**—oxygenated blood returns from the placenta to the right atrium via the umbilical vein and inferior vena cava (IVC). From here the majority of the oxygenated blood passes through the foramen ovale (an opening in the atrial septum) to enter the left atrium and subsequent left ventricle before exiting through the aorta.
- **Aortic isthmus**—this is constriction in the fetal aorta after the origin of the head and neck arteries and limits bloodflow such that ~90% of the more oxygenated blood (originating from the left ventricle) is directed to supply the crucial arteries of the head and neck. Blood supply to the immature organ systems is mainly delivered via the ductus arteriosus.
- **Ductus arteriosus**—the blood within the right ventricle is generally less oxygenated than that in the left ventricle, having entered the right atrium from the superior vena cava avoiding diversion through the foramen ovale. The ductus arteriosus is a low-resistance connection between the pulmonary artery and aorta that allows blood from the right ventricle to be directed to the body rather than the lungs. The high resistance of the immature lungs promotes flow through this low-resistance pathway.

After birth, pulmonary vascular resistance drops, resulting in reduced pressure in the right atrium and increased return to the left atrium. The foramen ovale and the ductus arteriosus close at birth or shortly after and the aortic isthmus expands.

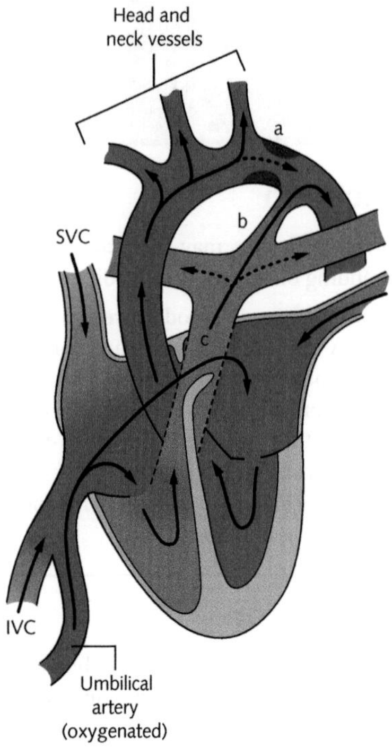

Fig. 9.1 Fetal circulation. Schematic representation of the fetal circulation. Note the role of the foramen ovale (c) and ductus arteriosus (b) in diverting blood away from the immature lungs. The aortic isthmus (a) ensures that highly oxygenated blood is delivered to the crucial head and neck structures, with less oxygenated blood supplying the immature organ systems. *IVC*, inferior vena cava; *SVC*, superior vena cava.

CLINICAL NOTES

CYANOTIC VERSUS ACYANOTIC HEART DISEASE

Acyanotic

- Left-to-right shunts
- Ventricular septal defect (VSD)
- Patent ductus arteriosus (PDA)
- Atrial septal defect (ASD)
- Outflow obstruction
- Pulmonary stenosis
- Aortic stenosis
- Coarctation of the aorta

Cyanotic

Result from right-to-left shunts, therefore reduced pulmonary bloodflow or mixing of systemic and pulmonary blood.

- Tetralogy of Fallot
- Transposition of the great arteries
- Complete atrioventricular septal defect (AVSD)

Left-to-right shunts

These are the most common group of congenital heart abnormalities and are malformations that result in the flow ('shunting') of blood from the left side of the heart to the right. The degree of shunting is determined by the site and size of the defect and occurs owing to the higher pressures in the left side of the heart. These abnormalities clinically are acyanotic as the blood does not bypass the lungs. Closure may be spontaneous or require surgical intervention to prevent shunt reversal.

Table 9.1 lists the prevalence of left-to-right shunts.

Ventricular septal defect

Defects of the interventricular septum are the most common cardiac abnormalities, accounting for 25%–30% of all cases of congenital heart disease (Fig. 9.2). The interventricular septum can be divided into a membranous/fibrous portion (below the valve cusp) and a muscular portion which abuts it. Defects can occur anywhere along the length of the septum but most are perimembranous, i.e., occurring at the junction of the membranous and muscular portions (80%).

They can be small or large:

- Small defects—often confined to the tiny membranous area, many of which spontaneously close.
- Larger defects—also involve the muscular wall of the septum.

Defects may present as cardiac failure in infants, or as a murmur in older children or adults.

CLINICAL NOTE

PRESENTATION OF VENTRICULAR SEPTAL DEFECTS

The clinical presentation of a ventricular septal defect includes:

- Pansystolic murmur, caused by flow from the high-pressure left ventricle to the low-pressure right ventricle during systole. The smallest defects generally produce the loudest murmurs
- Tachypnoea
- Indrawing of the lower ribs on inspiration.

Small defects need no treatment; larger ones require surgical repair to prevent cardiac failure.

Table 9.1 Prevalence of left-to-right shunts

Type	Percentage of all CHD abnormalities
Ventricular septal defect	25–30
Atrial septal defect	10–15
Patent ductus arteriosus	10
Atrioventricular septal defect	5

CHD, Congenital heart disease.

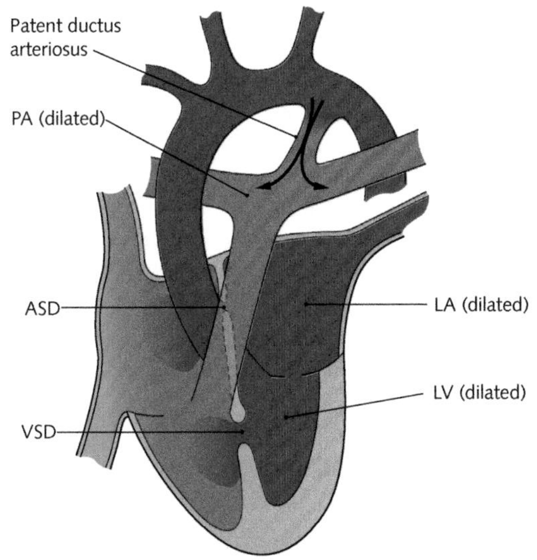

Fig. 9.2 Congenital heart defects. Ventricular septal defect *(VSD)*: larger defects involve septal muscle but smaller defects may be confined to a tiny membranous region (Maladie de Roger). Atrial septal defect *(ASD)*: the defect is usually located at the level of the fossa ovalis. Patent ductus arteriosus: persistence of the duct is more common in females, and is associated with maternal rubella. *LA*, Left atrium; *LV*, left ventricle; *PA*, pulmonary artery.

Atrial septal defect

This is a common congenital heart defect, affecting more females than males by a factor of 2:1. Blood flows from the left to the right atrium owing to higher left atrial pressures and the high compliance of the right ventricle. The defect may be of two types:

1. Ostium primum (20%)—incomplete flap closure of the fossa ovale with a defect at the level of the atrioventricular septum; it is associated with an abnormal mitral valve (split/cleft in the anterior leaflet).
2. Ostium secundum (80%)—the foramen ovale fails to close remaining patent as the fossa ovalis. This is the most common form of atrial septal defect.

Most children are asymptomatic; however, some children present with fatigue, exertional dyspnoea, chest infections, cardiac failure or arrhythmias (e.g., atrial fibrillation). The malformation may therefore not be detected until late childhood or adulthood.

The characteristic physical signs are a systolic flow murmur over the pulmonary valve and fixed wide splitting of the second heart sound.

Atrial septal defects should be closed surgically to prevent shunt reversal (see below). If performed before shunt reversal occurs, the prognosis is excellent.

COMMON PITFALLS

PARADOXICAL EMBOLI

These are emboli which arise within the venous system, usually deep veins of the legs, and enter the arterial circulation through an intracardiac defect, e.g., patent foramen ovale. This may result in a stroke.

Complete atrioventricular septal defect

This is a congenital defect involving both the atrial and ventricular septa, usually resulting in a single valve leaflet separating the atria and ventricles. Diagnosis is antenatal and clinically it results in cyanosis at birth or heart failure within the first few weeks. It is most commonly seen in Down syndrome.

Patent (persistent) ductus arteriosus

This persistence of the embryological connection between the aorta and the pulmonary artery beyond a month post term is shown in Fig. 9.2. Patent (open) ductus arteriosus occurs in about 10% of all cases of congenital heart disease, affecting females more often than males. There is a recognized association with maternal rubella.

A continuous 'machinery-like' murmur is classically detected, as high volumes of oxygenated blood are shunted from the high-pressure aorta back into the pulmonary artery and then the lungs. This can dramatically increase the work of the heart in a large defect, leading to eventual cardiac failure without early surgical correction.

Eisenmenger syndrome

All the left-to-right shunts described above have the potential to result in pulmonary hypertension owing to increased pulmonary bloodflow and the associated remodelling of the pulmonary microvasculature in response to this. Eventually, pulmonary vascular resistance can be so great that reversal to a right-to-left shunt occurs, producing marked progressive cyanosis as deoxygenated blood is pumped around the body (Eisenmenger syndrome). The condition is irreversible.

Right-to-left shunts

These are less common than left-to-right shunts. Right-to-left shunts cause deoxygenated blood to bypass the lungs and enter the systemic circulation. Cyanosis may, therefore, develop in the early neonatal period with any of these conditions.

> **HINTS AND TIPS**
>
> **EMBRYONIC HEART DEVELOPMENT**
>
> Understanding the embryonic development of the heart assists in the understanding of congenital abnormalities; for example, the involvement of the embryonic foramen ovale in the development of atrial septal defects and the congenital abnormality created by a persistent ductus arteriosus.

Tetralogy of Fallot

This is the most common cause of cyanotic congenital heart disease, occurring in about 3–6 in 10,000 live births. It is associated with prenatal factors such as maternal alcohol intake (fetal alcohol syndrome), maternal rubella and maternal age of more than 40 years. It is also seen in Down syndrome and Noonan syndrome.

There are four components (Fig. 9.3):

1. Ventricular septal defect.
2. Overriding aorta sitting astride the ventricular septal defect.
3. Pulmonary stenosis (causing systolic murmur).
4. Right ventricular hypertrophy.

Pulmonary stenosis leads to inadequate perfusion of the lungs and increased afterload for the right ventricle, resulting in ventricular hypertrophy. The overriding aorta straddles both left and right ventricles owing to the ventricular septal defect, such that it receives blood from both ventricles. The net result is that the systemic circulation contains deoxygenated blood, causing cyanosis in affected individuals.

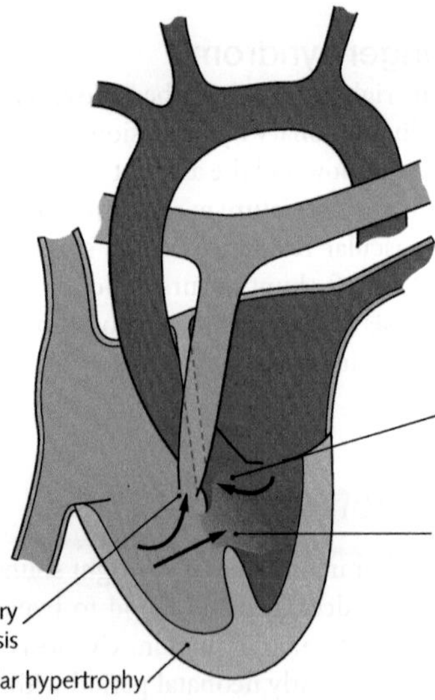

Fig. 9.3 Tetralogy of Fallot.

Clinical features are:

- Cyanosis—especially after a crying attack. This is termed a 'Fallot spell', as adrenergic stimulation exacerbates the right ventricular outflow obstruction, so increasing the amount of blood shunted. Squatting after exertion can relieve these symptoms by increasing the afterload of the left heart.
- Loud ejection systolic murmur—either from the ventricular septal defect or pulmonary stenosis.

Most cases are now surgically corrected, with a good prognosis if performed in early childhood. Complications include endocarditis and consequent cerebral infarction or brain abscess.

Transposition of the great arteries

The great arteries, aorta and pulmonary artery, are switched such that the aorta emanates from the right ventricle and the pulmonary artery arises from the left (Fig. 9.4). This results in two separate circulations. Survival after birth is therefore only possible if one or more shunts exist:

- Atrial septal defect.
- Ventricular septal defect.
- Patent ductus arteriosus.

Surgical correction is required.

Persistent truncus arteriosus

Both the aorta and pulmonary artery develop from a single tube: the truncus arteriosus. Persistence of the truncus results in a single great artery that receives blood from both ventricles. A ventricular septal defect is also present. Cyanosis occurs because of the mixing of blood from the right and left ventricles.

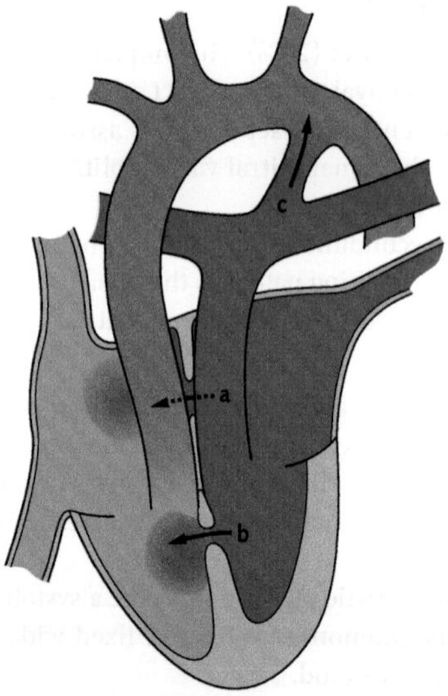

Fig. 9.4 Transposition of the great vessels. Survival is possible only if shunts are present at either the atrial *(a)*, ventricular *(b)* or ductus *(c)* level.

Obstructive congenital defects

Coarctation of the aorta

This is a stenotic narrowing of the aorta, usually located in the region where the ductus arteriosus joins the aorta (fetal aortic isthmus) (Fig. 9.5). This defect accounts for up to 5% of all forms of congenital heart disease, and it affects 1 in 4000 live births, incidence in males being greater than in females by a factor of 2:1.

Clinical features:

The stricture produces:

- Hypertension proximal to the stenosis, leading to symptoms such as headache and dizziness.
- Hypotension distal to the stenosis, leading to generalized weakness and poor peripheral circulation.
- Blood pressure is raised in the upper body but is normal or low in the legs.
- Absent or weak femoral pulses.
- Radio-femoral pulse delay.

Pathological complications—in untreated severe cases death may occur in several ways:

- Left ventricular failure—secondary to hypertension.
- Aortic dissection—particularly in patients with bicuspid aortic valves (50% have bicuspid valves).
- Bacterial endocarditis—usually at the site of aortic constriction.
- Cerebral haemorrhage—berry aneurysms of the cerebral circulation are more common in these individuals.

Pulmonary artery stenosis

This can arise in conjunction with other congenital cardiac malformations or in isolation. The pulmonary artery is stenosed either by partial commissural fusion of the valve leaflets, a dysplastic valve which is thickened and hypomobile or subvalvular stenosis.

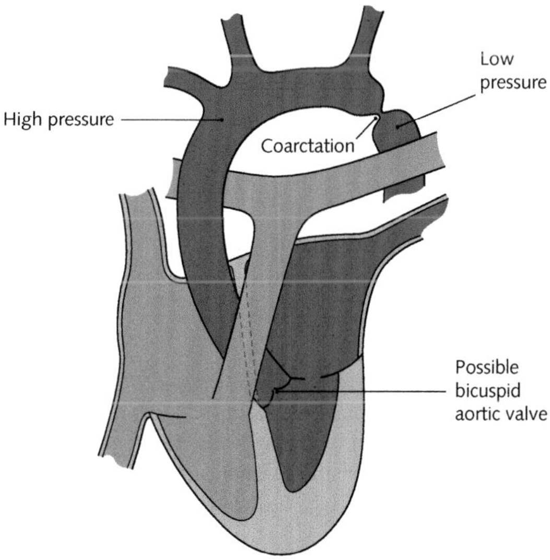

Fig. 9.5 Coarctation of the aorta. Signs and symptoms depend largely on the size of the narrowing.

Table 9.2 Congenital cardiac malformations

	Proportion of congenital cardiac malformations
Left-to-right shunts	
Ventricular septal defect	25%–30%
Atrial septal defect	10%–15%
Patent ductus arteriosus	10%
Atrioventricular septal defects	5%
Right-to-left shunts	
Tetralogy of Fallot	5%
Transposition of the great arteries	5%
Persistent truncus arteriosus	1%–2%
Total anomalous venous connection	1%
Obstructive congenital defects	
Pulmonary artery stenosis/atresia	10%
Coarctation of the aorta	5%
Aortic stenosis/atresia	5%

Aortic stenosis and atresia

Aortic stenosis can be mild to severe, and results in mild to severe left ventricular outflow tract obstruction (LVOTO). The valve is commonly bicuspid with a variable degree of commissural fusion and an eccentrically located orifice. LVOTO results in left ventricular hyperplasia or, if stenosis is severe in utero, a hypoplastic left ventricle can develop. Those with critical valvular stenosis present within the first week of life with symptoms of congestive cardiac failure, whereas those with little LVOTO may present as adults secondary to calcification of the bicuspid valve.

Table 9.2 gives a summary of congenital cardiac malformations.

ATHEROSCLEROSIS, HYPERTENSION AND THROMBOSIS: DEFINITIONS AND CONCEPTS

The structure of an artery is outlined in Fig. 9.6.

Arteriosclerosis

This is an imprecise term meaning thickening and loss of elasticity of the arteries caused by any condition (Fig. 9.6). Three patterns of arteriosclerosis exist:

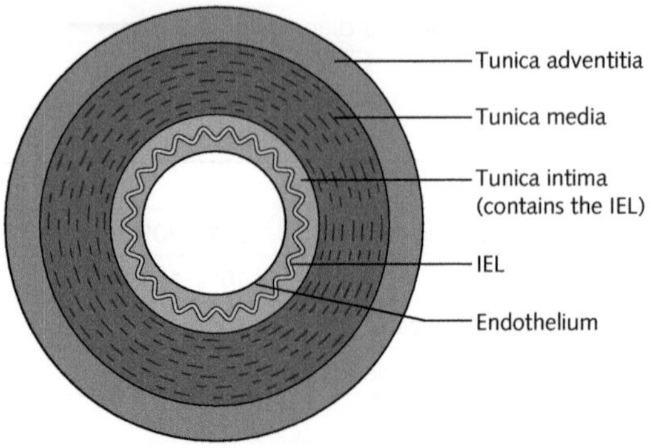

Fig. 9.6 Structure of an artery. Note: in a normal artery, the tunica media is thicker than in a vein. *IEL*, Internal elastic lamina.

1. Atherosclerosis—the most common form. A degenerative disease involving the intima of large- and medium-sized arteries. Atherosclerotic lesions are termed atheromas. This is discussed in greater detail below.
2. Mönckeberg medial calcific sclerosis—this degenerative disease of older individuals involves the deposition of calcium in the tunica media of medium-sized muscular arteries. These deposits do not reduce the size of the vessel lumen.
3. Arteriolosclerosis—the thickening of small artery and arteriole vessel walls, with subsequent reduction in lumen size. This is associated with systemic hypertension and diabetes mellitus, and particularly affects vessels in the kidney, pancreas, gallbladder, small intestine, adrenals and retina.

COMMON PITFALLS

ATHEROSCLEROSIS VERSUS ARTERIOSCLEROSIS

The terms 'arteriosclerosis' and 'atherosclerosis' are often confused. They are not synonymous and they should not be used interchangeably. Arteriosclerosis is hardening or loss of elasticity of the arteries from any cause, whereas atherosclerosis implies hardening or loss of elasticity due to atheroma.

Consequences of arteriosclerosis

The consequences of arteriosclerosis (and particularly of atherosclerosis) are:

- vessel thickening → narrowing of lumen → poor tissue perfusion
- inelasticity of vessels → predisposition to vessel rupture and haemorrhage
- alterations in vascular endothelium → increased predisposition to thrombosis.

Arteriosclerosis contributes to the high frequency of cardiac (myocardial infarction (MI), angina pectoris), cerebral (stroke, transient ischaemic attack), colonic (malabsorption, ischaemic colitis) and peripheral (intermittent claudication, rest pain) diseases in the elderly population.

Certain diseases are known to accelerate and aggravate arteriosclerosis, e.g., hypertension and diabetes.

Atherosclerosis

Atherosclerosis is a degenerative, progressive and inflammatory disease of large and medium-sized arteries (but not veins), characterized by the focal accumulation of lipid-rich material in the intima of arteries and associated cellular reaction. Although essentially a disease of the vessel intima, atherosclerosis also has an impact on the structure and function of the underlying media.

Atherosclerotic lesions are found to some extent in virtually every adult over the age of 40 years, as well as in many younger individuals. The consequences of atherosclerosis account for significant numbers of deaths in the developed world.

Commonly affected arteries are:

- aorta (especially the abdominal aorta)
- coronary arteries
- cerebral arteries
- common iliac/femoral arteries.

Atherosclerosis is rare in the arteries of the upper limb and in the pulmonary arteries.

Epidemiological studies have identified risk factors associated with atheroma development (Table 9.3). These can be broadly classified into:

- Nonmodifiable (fixed) risk factors, i.e., inherent to an individual.
- Modifiable risk factors, i.e., those that may be controlled.

Modifiable risk factors lead to increased severity of atherosclerosis. Such factors are multiplicative rather than additive.

Pathogenesis

Atherosclerotic plaques are hypothesized to be a chronic inflammatory response to arterial endothelial injury. Atherosclerosis begins early in life; the first signs of the disorder are termed fatty streaks, and usually occur in areas of altered arterial stress (e.g., bifurcations and sites of endothelial injury).

Low-grade endothelial injury may be induced by:

- Cigarette smoking.

Table 9.3 Risk factors for development of atherosclerosis

	Risk factors	Comments
Nonmodifiable	Age	Atherosclerotic lesions increase in number with increasing age
	Gender	Females have half the incidence of males up to the age of 55, owing to the protective effect of oestrogens; over 55 years, the male to female ratio is equal
	Familial traits	Familial increase in predisposition is often associated with familial hyperlipidaemia
	Race	Wide interracial variations exist in the incidence of atheroma, but this may be due to dietary differences. The condition is relatively uncommon in China, Japan and Africa
Modifiable	Hypertension	Increased blood pressure, both systolic and diastolic levels
	Diabetes mellitus	Probably because it is secondary to hypercholesterolaemia
	Cigarette smoking	There is a strong link between smoking and deaths from coronary artery disease; the mechanism is unclear
	Sedentary lifestyle	Exercise decreases the incidence of sudden death from ischaemic heart disease, but it is not clear whether it directly reduces atherosclerosis formation
	Obesity	Particularly central or truncal obesity, probably a reflection of poor diet and resultant hyperlipidaemia
	Hypercholesterolaemia (increased serum levels of cholesterol or low-density lipoprotein)	Usually dependent on diet, but may also be familial

- Altered haemodynamics—the damaging effect of turbulent bloodflow (e.g., at major arterial bifurcations) may be further worsened by hypertension.
- Homocysteine—this amino acid may directly damage the arterial wall. Individuals with the rare genetic disorder homocystinuria, which results in raised blood homocysteine levels, develop premature vascular disease.
- Hyperlipidaemia—possibly causing direct endothelial damage and promotion of platelet attachment.
- Others—viruses, other infectious agents and inflammatory cytokines have all been suggested as potential inducers of endothelial injury.

Stages of development in atherosclerosis

The key stages in the development of atherosclerotic plaques (atheromas) are as follows:

1. Chronic endothelial injury results in permeability of the vessel wall and the expression of receptors for leucocyte adhesion.
2. Plasma lipoproteins (especially low-density lipoprotein (LDL)) travel into the arterial intima and are prone to free radical oxidation.
3. Monocytes migrate into the intima, differentiating into macrophages. Macrophages phagocytose oxidized LDL and become foam cells, which can rupture and release their contents, causing more monocytes to migrate into the intima and creating a cycle.
4. Adhesion of platelets to the disrupted endothelium.
5. Release of cytokines and growth factors (e.g., platelet-derived growth factor) by platelets and activated macrophages results in the migration of smooth muscle cells from the media to the intima (myointimal cells). These muscle cells change from a contractile to secretory phenotype, producing collagen in an attempt to repair and stabilize the growing plaque.

Fig. 9.7 outlines the formation of a stable atherosclerotic plaque (which can remain asymptomatic for many years, slowly growing to the point where it may significantly obstruct bloodflow).

The maintenance of a stable atherosclerotic plaque depends on the balance between inflammation (macrophage-mediated) and repair (smooth muscle–mediated). If activated, macrophages start producing additional cytokines (e.g., interleukin-1, matrix metalloproteinases). The muscle cells forming the protective fibrous cap may become senescent, resulting in an unstable plaque. Thinning of the cap follows, with potential for erosion, ulceration or rupture (releasing prothrombotic material).

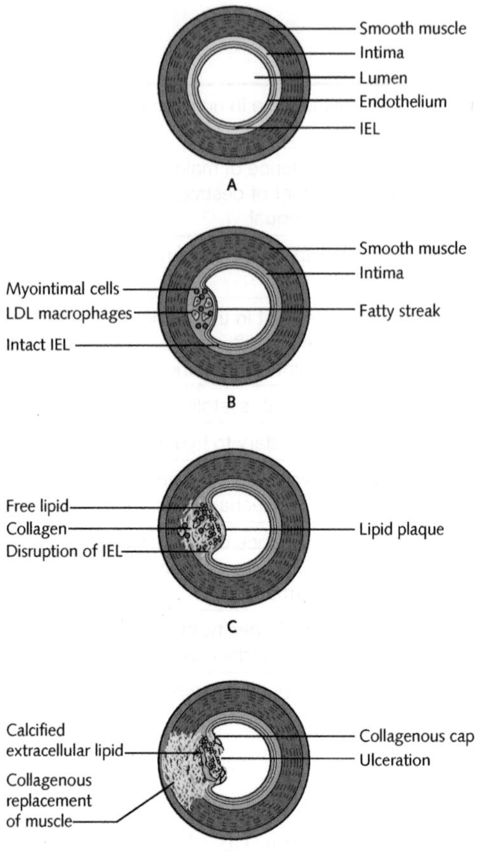

Fig. 9.7 Formation of atheroma. Formation of an atheroma. (A) Endothelial injury: allows entry of cholesterol-rich, low-density lipoproteins *(LDLs)* into the intima. (B) 'Fatty streaks': barely visible pale bulges form as a result of phagocytosis and accumulation of lipid by intimal macrophages. (C) Stable plaques: raised, yellow lesions within the intima consisting of free lipid released by macrophages and collagen deposited by myointimal cells (repair phenotype). (D) Unstable plaque with ulceration: allowing platelet aggregation and thrombosis with the potential for embolism to a distant site. Note that pressure atrophy of the underlying media and elastic lamina results in weakening of the arterial wall. *IEL*, Internal elastic lamina.

Arterial remodelling

The migration of smooth muscle cells away from the arterial media produces remodelling. Two types have been proposed:

1. Negative remodelling—some arterial segments affected by atherosclerosis constrict, increasing the likelihood of occluding the lumen.
2. Positive remodelling—affected arterial segments dilate, potentially compensating for the plaque and maintaining the size of the lumen.

However, thinning of the muscular arterial media predisposes an artery to aneurysm (Table 9.4).

Table 9.4 Complications of atherosclerosis

Complications of atherosclerosis
Ulceration
Plaque rupture
Stenosis/calcification/luminal occlusion
Aneurysm
Thrombosis

Lipids

Several plasma lipoproteins are found in the bloodstream and are important for cell structure but are also involved in atheroma formation. Chylomicrons, very low-density lipoproteins (VLDL) and intermediate-density lipoproteins (IDL) transport triglycerides, whereas low-density lipoproteins (LDL) transport triglycerides and cholesterol to fat cells. Increasing levels result in hyperlipidaemia. High-density lipoproteins (HDL) transport fat molecules (like triglycerides and chylomicrons) from fat cells to the liver; therefore it is often called the 'good' lipoprotein. Hyperlipidaemia may be familial or acquired. Family variants are subtyped by the Frederick classification (Table 9.5).

Hypertension

Elevated blood pressure is an important and treatable cause of cardiovascular disease. It is a major risk factor for atherosclerosis and cerebral haemorrhage. Any increase in blood pressure is associated with an increased risk of disease.

Functional or operational definition

Hypertension is increasingly being defined by the level at which intervention (e.g., antihypertensive medication) is of proven benefit. Sustained systemic blood pressure above 140 mmHg systolic and/or above 90 mmHg diastolic should be treated to reduce cardiovascular events. Target levels for those with diabetes and renal disease are lower.

Aetiological classification

Hypertension can be classified into two main types according to its aetiology (Table 9.6):

1. Primary (essential/idiopathic) hypertension—a complex, multifactorial disease in which blood pressure is elevated with age, but with no apparent cause. This accounts for 90% of all cases and probably has a strong genetic determinant.
2. Secondary hypertension—elevated blood pressure with an identifiable cause. It accounts for less than 10% of all cases of hypertension. Examples include renal hypertension, endocrine causes and coarctation of the aorta.

Table 9.6 Causes of hypertension

Primary hypertension: unknown aetiology but probably multifactorial involving:	
Genetic predisposition	Strong familial association
Socioeconomic factors	Related to social deprivation
Dietary factors	Obesity, high salt intake, high alcohol and caffeine intake
Hormonal factors	Abnormalities in renin–angiotensin–aldosterone system
Neurological factors	Excessive sympathetic nervous system activity
Secondary hypertension: secondary to:	
Renal disease	Parenchymal disease, e.g., chronic pyelonephritis, glomerulonephritis, polycystic kidneys, amyloidosis
	Vascular disease, e.g., renal artery stenosis
Adrenal disorders	Phaeochromocytoma, Cushing syndrome, Conn syndrome (primary hyperaldosteronism), congenital adrenal hyperplasia
Other endocrine disorders	Thyrotoxicosis, hypothyroidism, acromegaly, hyperparathyroidism, diabetes with renal involvement
Cardiovascular disorders	Coarctation of the aorta, arteriovenous fistulae and shunts
Drugs	e.g., Oral contraceptives, anabolic steroids, corticosteroids, adrenaline (epinephrine) and related sympathomimetic drugs
Pregnancy	Preeclampsia

Pathological classification

Hypertension can also be classified according to the clinical course of disease (Table 9.7):

- 'Benign' hypertension—stable elevation of blood pressure over many years.
- Malignant and accelerated hypertension—rare conditions characterized by a dramatic elevation of blood pressure over a short period of time.

Benign hypertension

Here, vessel changes develop gradually in response to a persistent elevated blood pressure; males are affected more often than females. Histologically, it is characterized by:

- hypertrophy and thickening of muscular media
- thickening of the internal elastic lamina
- fibroelastic thickening of intima
- hyaline deposition in arteriole walls (hyaline arteriolosclerosis).

Table 9.7 Features of benign and malignant hypertension

	Benign	Malignant
Incidence	Very common (at least 5% of UK population)	Rare
Age	Begins at <45 years but extends into the sixth and seventh decades	Young adults (25–35 years)
Sex	Females < males	Females = males
Aetiology	Majority of cases due to primary hypertension	Majority of cases secondary to renal disease (few cases arise out of benign essential hypertension)
Disease progression	Very slow (many years)	Rapid (months to 1–2 years)
Blood pressure	Very slow rise	Rapid rise
	Diastolic = 90–120 mmHg	Diastolic ≥120 mmHg
Arterial changes	Potentiates atheroma → accelerated arteriosclerosis	Intimal fibrous thickening → accelerated arteriosclerosis
Arteriole changes	Hyaline thickening with narrowed lumen	Fibrinoid necrosis of vessel wall
		Lumen occluded by thrombus
		Affects mainly kidney and abdominal viscera

The effects are:

- reduced size of vessel lumen leading to tissue ischaemia
- increased rigidity leading to limited capacity for expansion and constriction
- increased fragility of vessels leading to an increased risk of haemorrhage (especially cerebral).

After many years of benign progression, 1%–5% of such patients enter an accelerated or malignant phase.

Malignant hypertension

Acute, destructive changes occur in the walls of small arteries when there is a sudden marked rise in blood pressure, causing fibrinoid necrosis of the vessel wall.

The destructive changes lead to cessation of bloodflow through small vessels, with multiple foci of tissue necrosis, often with intravascular thrombosis. This results in end-organ damage and is referred to as accelerated hypertension. Areas typically affected include the retina (high-grade retinopathy) and the kidneys (glomerular disease). When papilloedema is also present, this is known as malignant hypertension.

Complications and effects of hypertension

Vascular effects

Hypertension accelerates atherosclerosis, which causes thickening of the media of muscular arteries, particularly the smaller arteries and arterioles. Structural changes perpetuate further rises in blood pressure, causing a progressively worsening clinical picture.

The normal flow of protein into the vessel wall is increased, resulting in intramural protein deposition, termed hyaline in benign hypertension and fibrinoid in malignant hypertension:

- Hyaline deposition—a common feature of aging small arteries (<1 mm diameter); refers to the homogeneous appearance of vessel walls due to infiltration by plasma proteins.
- Fibrinoid deposition—a combination of fibrin infiltration with necrosis of the vessel wall.

Heart

The left ventricle undergoes hypertrophy resulting from increased workload, causing increased susceptibility to spontaneous arrhythmias. Ischaemic heart disease owing to accelerated atherosclerosis is a common complication of hypertension.

Brain

Intracerebral haemorrhage is a frequent cause of death in hypertension. Small-vessel damage within the cerebral hemispheres may result in the development of microinfarcts, which form hypertensive lacunae, i.e., small areas of destroyed brain filled with fluid. Consequently, vascular dementia may occur (see Chapter 7).

Kidneys

Arteriolosclerosis leads to progressive ischaemia of the nephrons and chronic renal failure. This is termed benign hypertensive nephrosclerosis, and it is a common cause of chronic renal failure in the middle-aged and elderly population.

Retina

Hypertension may produce retinal ischaemia and infarction, visible on fundoscopic examination.

Table 9.8 outlines the complications and effects of hypertension.

Table 9.8 Complications and effects of hypertension

	Benign	Malignant
Vessels	Hyaline deposition due to infiltration by plasma proteins	Fibrinoid deposition due to combination of fibrin deposition and necrosis of vessel wall
Heart	Hypertrophy of left ventricle → ↑susceptibility to spontaneous arrhythmias	Hypertrophy of left ventricle → ↑susceptibility to spontaneous arrhythmias
	Heart failure in 60% of cases	Focal myocardial necrosis
	Ischaemic heart disease	Acute heart failure
		Ischaemic heart disease
Brain	Cerebral haemorrhage	Encephalopathy (fits and loss of consciousness) due to cerebral oedema
		Cerebral haemorrhage
Kidney	Nephrosclerosis, but not usually serious	Severe renal damage; death from uraemia
Retina	Ischaemia and infarction ('cotton wool' exudates)	Ischaemia and infarction ('cotton wool' exudates)
	Association with central retinal vein thrombosis	Association with central retinal vein thrombosis
Other organs	No significant damage	Focal necrosis, e.g., perforation of intestines

Pulmonary hypertension

Definition and causes

Pulmonary hypertension is defined as pulmonary arterial pressure in excess of 30 mmHg (see Chapter 10 for causes and effects of pulmonary hypertension).

Thrombosis

Thrombosis is the formation of a solid mass of blood constituents—thrombus—within the vasculature during life. It is not to be confused with a clot, which is coagulated blood outside of the vasculature (e.g., haematoma) or within the vascular system after death. Clots are not attached to the vessel walls, do not involve platelets and are gelatinous. In contrast, a thrombus is firm, attached to the vessel wall and contains platelets.

Thrombosis occurs when there is a change in any of the components of Virchow triad (see below) and can affect both arteries and veins. The structure and appearance of a thrombus depends on the site of formation and rate of bloodflow.

Arterial thrombosis

Arterial thrombi are compact, laminated masses characterized both microscopically and macroscopically by the lines of Zahn, which are alternating bands of pale fibrin and platelets with darker bands of erythrocytes.

They are commonly superimposed on atheromatous plaques as these have disrupted endothelial cells and cause turbulent flow. The plaque contents are extremely thrombogenic if rupture occurs. Thrombi, termed mural thrombi, can also develop over a dyskinetic portion of the myocardium, e.g., post-MI or in atrial fibrillation.

Arterial thrombi have retrograde growth (i.e., away from the heart) and can result in occlusion and/or embolization, both of which can result in ischaemia and infarction. The most commonly affected arteries are the coronary arteries, followed by the cerebral arteries and then the femoral arteries.

Venous thrombosis

Venous thrombi are less compact than their arterial counterparts and contain more red cells as they occur in areas of sluggish venous bloodflow. The thrombus propagates in the direction of bloodflow, i.e., towards the heart, and resembles a comet with long, friable tails that are prone to embolization. Occlusion also occurs as the thrombus molds itself to the shape of the vein.

The majority of venous thrombi occur within the legs as deep vein thrombosis (DVT), with many beginning at damaged valves that produce turbulence. Blood stasis during surgery or due to immobilization is a strong risk factor for the formation of DVTs. However, some thrombi form with no known predisposing factors.

Affected sites

The most commonly affected sites are:

- deep leg veins (90% of cases), particularly the lower leg
- upper arm veins
- pelvic veins
- skull and dural sinuses—venous sinus thrombosis
- portal and hepatic veins.

Complications

- Pulmonary embolism (PE)—the most serious acute complication is embolism of the thrombus to the pulmonary arteries and lungs. This is discussed in detail in Chapter 10.
- Chronic venous insufficiency—spectrum of varicose veins, venous hypertension, venous eczema and ulceration (see below).
- Thrombophlebitis.

RED FLAG

DEEP VEIN THROMBOSIS (DVT)

- Painful unilateral swollen calf
- Warm to touch
- History of a risk factor, e.g., recent operation, recent period of immobilization (e.g., long-haul flight), pregnancy, obesity, cancer, previous DVT.

DVT is a key clinical topic, as a resultant pulmonary embolus may be life-threatening. High-risk patients should be identified and offered prophylaxis.

The fate of thrombi

Outcomes of thrombosis include:

- Vascular stenosis and occlusion.
- Lysis—dissolution of the thrombus by activated fibrinolytic system.
- Propagation—spread of the thrombus proximally in the veins.
- Organization— thrombus undergoes an inflammatory reparative process with migration of fibroblasts, amalgamation into the vessel wall and reendothelialization. The result is a stenosed lumen.
- Recanalization—small new vascular channels occur within the organized thrombus with an incomplete reestablishment of bloodflow.
- Resolution—the thrombus is removed by the fibrinolytic system.
- Fibrosis—organization can result in fibrosis, such that the vessel is obliterated entirely.
- Embolism—thrombi (whole or fragments) migrate to a distant site.
- Infection—from transient bacteraemia or from adjacent tissue infection.

COMMON PITFALLS

WARFARIN DOES NOT DISSOLVE THROMBI

Warfarin and heparin are both used in the treatment and prevention of thrombosis. However, it is important to realize that they only prevent the propagation and growth of the thrombus—they do not dissolve it. Thrombus removal (thrombolysis) can be medically achieved using 'clot busters' such as streptokinase and alteplase.

Virchow triad

Factors that predispose any blood vessel to thrombosis can be classified into three main groups, collectively known as Virchow triad (Fig. 9.8). Changes in any one of the components of the triad is sufficient for thrombosis to occur:

1. Changes in the constituents of blood—causing a hypercoagulable state.
2. Changes in the blood vessel wall/endothelial injury.
3. Changes in the pattern of bloodflow—stasis or turbulence.

Hypercoagulability

Primary (hereditary)

Hereditary defects of hypercoagulability lead to a lifelong prothrombotic tendency (thrombophilia). Thrombosis usually affects the venous system:

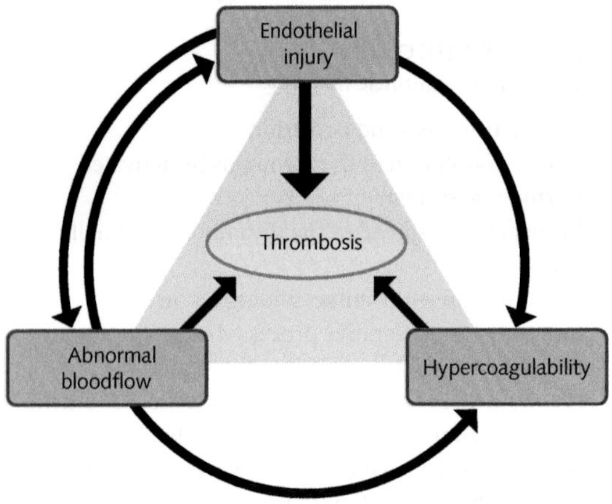

Fig. 9.8 Virchow triad. Virchow triad in thrombosis. Endothelial integrity is the single most important factor: injury can affect local bloodflow and/or coagulability. Abnormal bloodflow (turbulence or stasis) can, in turn, cause endothelial injury. The elements of the triad may act independently or combine to cause thrombus formation. (Redrawn with permission from Kumar V, Abbas A, Fausto N. Robbins & Cotran Pathologic Basis of Disease, 7th edn. Elsevier Saunders, 2005.)

- ***Factor V Leiden***—point mutation in the factor V gene causing resistance of factor V to degradation by protein C. This is very common, affecting up to 5% of whites.
- ***Prothrombin G20210A***—this prothrombin gene polymorphism occurs in 2% of the population and is associated with increased levels of prothrombin and venous thromboembolism.
- ***Protein C deficiency***—autosomal dominant condition resulting in failure of factor V and VIII inactivation owing to loss of protein C.
- ***Protein S deficiency***—protein S is a cofactor for protein C (therefore, protein S deficiencies produce a similar pathology).
- ***Antithrombin III deficiency***—autosomal dominant condition characterized by recurrent venous thromboses usually starting in early adult life. Primary defect is a deficiency of antithrombin III, which usually neutralizes thrombin and other activated clotting factors.

Secondary (acquired)

Acquired conditions associated with a procoagulant state are as follows:

- ***Malignancy***—patients with carcinoma of the breast, lung, prostate, pancreas or bowel have an increased risk of venous thrombosis.
- ***Tissue damage***—e.g., postoperative, trauma.
- ***Blood disorders***—e.g., increased viscosity (especially polycythaemia rubra vera and thrombocytosis) leads to an increased risk of venous thrombosis.
- ***Oestrogens***—associated with raised plasma levels of various clotting factors leading to an increased risk of venous thrombosis. This includes use of the oral contraceptive pill.
- ***Antiphospholipid syndrome***—leads to the interaction of autoantibodies (lupus anticoagulant and anticardiolipin antibodies) with phospholipid-bound proteins involved in coagulation. This causes prolongation of clotting times in vitro, with a paradoxical increased risk of venous and arterial thrombosis.
- ***Cholesterol***—partly genetic, partly acquired (diet/lifestyle), leads to an increased risk of arterial thrombosis.
- ***Smoking***—has been implicated as a predisposing risk factor for thrombosis, possibly by causing a hypercoagulable state and endothelial damage.

Endothelial injury

Endothelial cells are important in the balance of a prothrombotic/antithrombotic state, therefore direct injury to endothelial cells or endothelial dysfunction can result in a procoagulant state.

Direct injury to the endothelium is seen in trauma (including intravenous cannulation), inflammation (vasculitis), ulcerated atheromatous plaques and after MI. Endothelial dysfunction can result from toxins, e.g., bacterial, smoking-related, metabolic abnormalities or haemodynamic factors such as turbulent bloodflow and hypertension.

Alterations to bloodflow

Normal bloodflow is smooth and laminar such that cellular blood components are drawn into the centre of the stream where flow is maximal, and acellular serum is peripheral where flow is minimal. This discourages unwanted platelet-endothelial binding and ensures the dilution/removal of clotting factors in proximity to the endothelial cells.

Stasis and turbulence cause disruption of laminar flow, allowing platelets to come into contact with the endothelium and impaired removal and delivery of procoagulant and anticoagulant factors. Causes of altered bloodflow are summarized in Table 9.9.

Table 9.9 Causes of altered bloodflow

Venous	Arterial/cardiac chambers
Right-sided heart failure	Atherosclerotic stenosis
Immobilization	Aneurysm
Venous compression	Infarcted myocardium—akinetic wall segment
Varicose veins	Abnormal cardiac rhythm – e.g., atrial fibrillation
Increased blood viscosity, e.g., dehydration, sickle cell anaemia	
Immobilization	

Alterations in venous bloodflow are usually due to stasis whereas alterations to bloodflow in arterial/cardiac chambers are usually due to turbulence or occlusion.

ISCHAEMIC HEART DISEASE AND HEART FAILURE

Ischaemic heart disease (IHD) is a condition caused by a reduction or cessation of the blood supply to the myocardium (myocardial ischaemia). This is usually as a result of atherosclerosis, although in rare cases it may be caused by coronary artery embolism, arteritis or ostial obstruction. The left ventricle is more prone to ischaemia because of its greater bulk, work requirement and its higher oxygen demand.

IHD is the most common type of cardiac disease and a leading cause of death in the developed world. Risk factors for the development of IHD are the same as those for the development of atherosclerosis.

Classification

IHD results in four main syndromes:

1. Stable angina (chronic manifestation) or unstable angina (acute manifestation).
2. MI (acute manifestation).
3. Sudden cardiac death (acute manifestation).
4. Congestive cardiac failure (chronic manifestation).

The acute manifestations of cardiac ischaemia form a continuous spectrum of disease termed the acute coronary syndromes.

Angina pectoris

Angina pectoris is episodic chest pain caused by ischaemia of the myocardium following exercise (increased oxygen demand). Ischaemia is usually the result of stenosis of one or more of the coronary arteries, resulting in reduced bloodflow to the myocardium. Stenosis of the coronary arteries is typically the result of atherosclerosis.

Atheromatous plaques may be:

1. Eccentric—fibrolipid plaques affecting only one side of the wall of a coronary artery. Improvement of flow at the site of such plaques may be achieved by the use of vasodilator drugs. These drugs, such as glyceryl trinitrate, produce relaxation of the unaffected part of the vessel wall.
2. Concentric—collagenous plaques affecting the whole circumference of the arterial wall. As the whole wall is abnormal, drug therapy cannot improve flow over a narrowed segment. Stents may be inserted to improve lumen diameter.

Cardiac referred pain

Pain of angina (and MI) commonly radiates from the substernal and left pectoral regions to the left shoulder and the medial aspect of the left arm; this is known as referred cardiac pain.

Afferent fibres of the heart, and sensory fibres of affected cutaneous zones, enter the same spinal cord segments (T1–T4 on the left side) and ascend in the spinal cord along a common pathway. The brain is unable to discern the origin of the pain, hence the phenomenon of referred pain.

Less commonly, pain radiates to the jaw or right shoulder and arm, with or without concomitant pain on the left side.

Types of angina

Stable angina

This is a predictable angina that occurs at a fixed level of exercise, as a result of an increased demand in myocardial work, usually in the presence of impaired perfusion by blood. It is caused by a fixed obstruction of one or more of the coronary arteries, therefore limiting any increase in coronary bloodflow. Pain can usually be relieved by 1 or 2 minutes of rest. A stenosis of at least 70% of the lumen of the arteries is required to produce angina on exercise.

Unstable angina

Unstable anginal pain is unpredictable and not related to exercise. It reflects reversible ischaemia owing to variable luminal stenosis of some segments of the coronary arteries: so-called dynamic obstruction.

The condition is usually the result of active fissuring and/or rupture of plaques with intimal surface thrombus deposition, microembolization and occlusion. Unstable angina is an acute event, often preceding the development of acute MI. It is a medical emergency.

Prinzmetal angina (vasospastic angina)

This is angina at rest caused by an increase in the coronary vasomotor tone (rather than luminal occlusion). The mechanism for coronary spasm is unknown. Prinzmetal angina is particularly common in the early morning. Attacks are usually self-limiting and, although pain may be severe, they rarely progress to MI.

> **HINTS AND TIPS**
>
> **ANGINA**
>
> - Stable angina is predictable (i.e., it occurs at a fixed level of exercise) and it is caused by a fixed arterial obstruction
> - Unstable angina is unpredictable (i.e., it is unrelated to exercise) and it is caused by variable luminal stenosis of the coronary arteries
> - Prinzmetal angina is also unpredictable and this is caused by coronary artery spasm.

Myocardial infarction

MI is necrosis of the myocardium as a result of severe ischaemia. MI is extremely common, accounting for 10%–15% of all deaths and about 60% of sudden unexpected deaths. It typically affects middle-aged individuals, between the ages of 50 and 60 years, but can occur in younger patients. MI affects males more often than premenopausal females (by 5:1), but there is an increasing incidence in postmenopausal women.

Clinical features are central crushing chest pain accompanied by breathlessness, vomiting and collapse or syncope. Pain occurs in the same sites as angina, but it is usually more severe and lasts for longer.

Regional infarcts

Infarcts occur in the territory supplied by one of the major coronary arteries, involving a segment of the ventricular wall. The cause of infarction is often thrombus formation on a ruptured or eroded atheromatous plaque. Patterns of regional MI and sites of MI are shown in Figs 9.9 and 9.10.

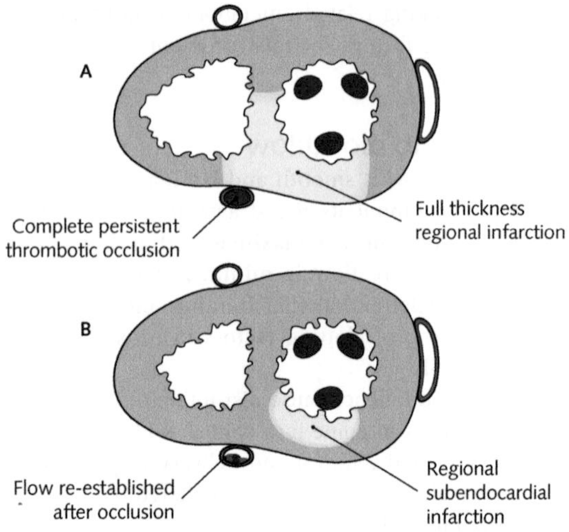

Fig. 9.9 Patterns of regional myocardial infarction. (A) Transmural or full-thickness infarct. (B) Regional subendocardial infarct.

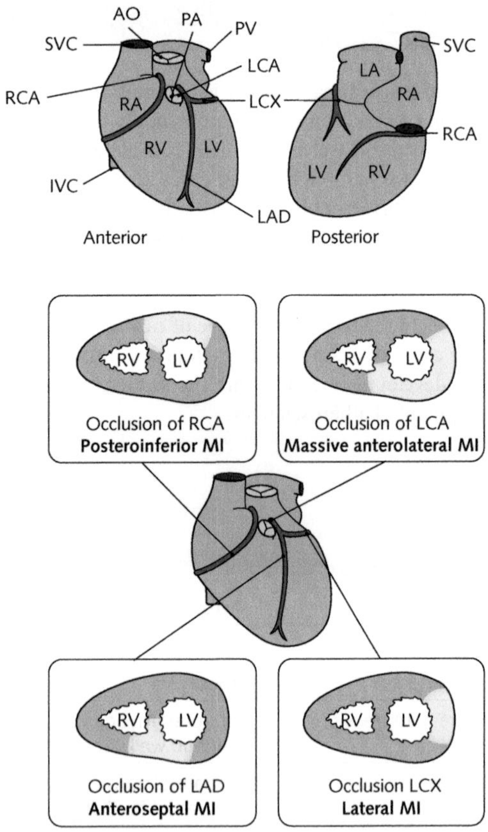

Fig. 9.10 Sites of myocardial infarction *(MI)* and vessel involvement. *AO*, Aorta; *IVC*, inferior vena cava; *LA*, left atrium; *LAD*, left anterior descending; *LCA*, left coronary artery; *LCX*, left circumflex; *LV*, left ventricle; *MI*, myocardial infarction; *PA*, pulmonary artery; *PV*, pulmonary vein; *RA*, right atrium; *RCA*, right coronary artery; *RV*, right ventricle; *SVC*, superior vena cava.

ST-segment elevation myocardial infaction and non–ST-segment elevation myocardial infaction

An acute MI should be classified as an ST-segment elevation myocardial infaction (STEMI) when there is:

- ST elevation (2 mm in two or more chest leads, or 1 mm in two or more limb leads).
- Chronic MI with Q wave formation.
- Imaging evidence of transmural involvement rather than MI limited to the subendocardium.

Other MIs that do not meet these criteria should be classified as a non-STEMI (NSTEMI). The main difference between the two classifications are their emergency management protocols. STEMI patients will have primary percutaneous intervention (PCI).

Histological changes following myocardial infarction

MI comprises coagulative necrosis and acute inflammation, which gradually progresses to chronic inflammation and then replacement by a collagenous scar. The entire process from coagulative necrosis to scar formation takes 6–8 weeks, with the macroscopic and microscopic appearances of the infarct changing with time (Fig. 9.11).

The extensive necrosis of cardiac muscle is associated with the release of cardiac enzymes and proteins that can be used as clinical markers for a cardiac event. Examples include troponin I and T, creatinine kinase (CK-MB cardiac isoform) and lactate dehydrogenase (Fig. 9.12).

Time	Macroscopic appearance	Microscopic appearance
0–12 hours	Not visible 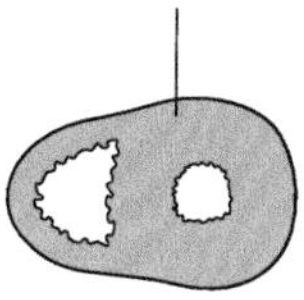	Subtle wavy change of fibroblasts
12–24 hours	Pale with mottled appearance 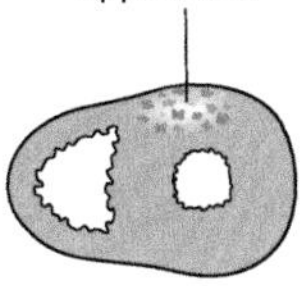	Infarcted muscle is brightly eosinophilic with intercellular oedema
24–72 hours	Infarcted area appears soft and pale with a slight yellow colour 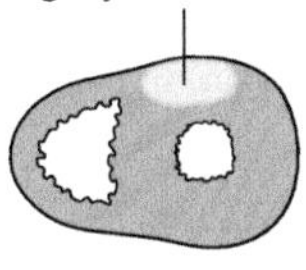	• Infarcted area excites an acute inflammatory response • Neutrophils infiltrate between cardiac muscle fibres
3–10 days	Hyperaemic border develops around the yellow dead muscle 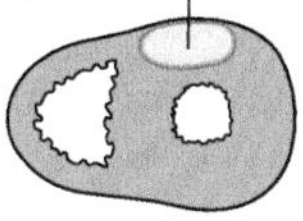	• Organization of infarcted area • Replacement with vascular granulation tissue
Weeks to months	White scar 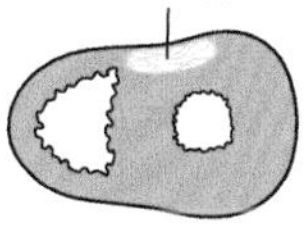	• Progressive collagen deposition • Infarct is replaced by a collagenous scar

Fig. 9.11 Morphological changes occurring following myocardial infarction.

> **CLINICAL NOTE**
>
> **TROPONIN I AND T**
>
> The troponins (I and T) are markers which become elevated during myocardial ischaemic events and are used to monitor development of a myocardial infarction. It should be noted that, although fairly sensitive, they are not specific—especially troponin I, which may be elevated with pulmonary embolism, heart failure and chronic renal failure.

Sequelae of myocardial infarction

The effects and sequelae of MI are variable, and can be classified into:

- Immediate effects—sudden cardiac death (described below).
- Short-term complications—occurring in the first 2 weeks following MI.
- Long-term complications—occurring over 2 weeks following MI (Table 9.10).

Sudden cardiac death is the most important immediate consequence of myocardial ischaemia. It is usually due to ventricular fibrillation. This may be the result of:

- Previous ischaemic heart disease, e.g., angina or previous infarction; cardiac arrhythmias can arise from muscle adjacent to an area of old scarring.
- Acute myocardial ischaemia, which, due to a new thrombotic event, may precipitate arrhythmia.

Other causes of sudden death include ruptured or dissecting aneurysms of the aorta and pulmonary emboli.

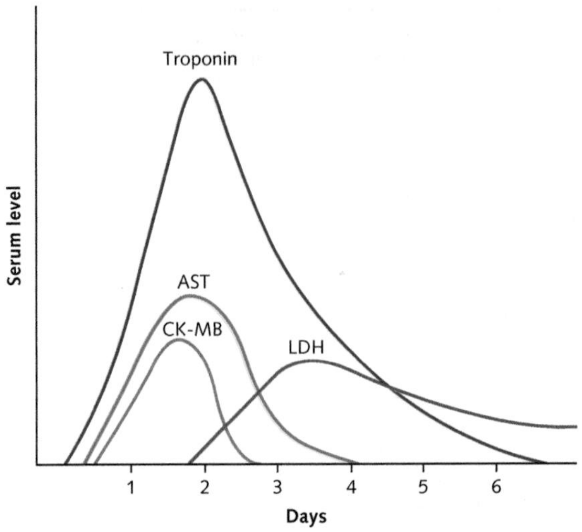

Fig. 9.12 Cardiac enzyme concentrations over time. *AST*, Aspartate aminotransferase; *CK-MB*, creatinine kinase found in myocardium (isoezyme variants CK-M and CK-B); *LDH*, lactate dehydrogenase.

Heart failure

Heart failure can result from many different types of heart disease. It develops when the heart is no longer able to maintain adequate cardiac output or can only do so by increasing the filling pressure. The prognosis of heart failure is worse than many cancers; half of those with severe left-ventricular impairment die within 2 years.

Heart failure may develop acutely (e.g., following MI) or chronically (e.g., gradually progressing from ischaemic heart disease) (Table 9.11).

Table 9.11 Causes of heart failure

Causes of left-sided heart failure	Ischaemic heart disease
	Hypertension
	Valve stenosis
Causes of right-sided heart failure	Left-sided heart failure
	Cor pulmonale
	Pulmonary emboli
	Pulmonary valve stenosis

Table 9.10 Short- and long-term complications of myocardial infarction

Short term complications of MI	**Arrhythmias**—owing to the involvement of conduction tissue, leading to ventricular fibrillation, atrial fibrillation, heart block and sinus bradycardia. Nearly all MI patients have some form of arrhythmia, usually resolving spontaneously.
	Left ventricular failure—this is common with large areas of infarction; the necrotic wall softens in organization, leading to cardiac dilatation. Ventricular remodelling is the process of thinning and stretching of the infarcted segment, with progressive dilatation and hypertrophy of the remaining ventricle.
	Rupture, which can be: I. External (majority)—blood bursts through the external wall into the pericardial cavity (haemopericardium); the sudden rise in intrapericardial cavity pressure prevents cardiac filling (cardiac tamponade), leading to rapid death II. Internal (rarely)—intracardiac rupture through the septum leads to an acquired septal defect, causing a left-to-right shunt and the development of left ventricular failure.
	Papillary muscle dysfunction—when one or more valve leaflets are unable to close during systole there is mitral valve incompetence.
	Mural thrombosis—on the inflamed endocardium over the area of infarction; there is a high risk of embolization producing infarction of various organs, e.g., brain, kidney, spleen, mesentery and lower limbs.
	Acute pericarditis—caused by inflammation over the infarct surface.
Long-term complications of MI	**Chronic intractable left-heart failure**—the long-term effects of ventricular remodelling result in inadequate left ventricular pumping action; common when the infarct is extensive and full thickness.
	Ventricular aneurysm (in 10% of long-term survivors)—gradual distension of the weakened fibrotic part of the left ventricular wall with thrombus formation, embolism or severe functional deficit.
	Recurrent MI—risk of developing a further episode owing to underlying coronary artery insufficiency.
	Dressler syndrome—a form of autoimmune-mediated pericarditis associated with a high erythrocyte sedimentation rate, pleuritis and persistent fever; develops in a very small number of cases after infarction.

MI, Myocardial infarction.

Classification

Left-sided heart failure

This occurs owing to either reduced output from the left ventricle or increased volume/preload from the left atrium. Common causes include:

- Ischaemic heart disease—including the effects of ventricular remodelling after infarction.
- Hypertension—pressure overload produces initial ventricular hypertrophy, but this compensatory change cannot be maintained indefinitely and the ventricle eventually dilates.
- Valve disease—either aortic or mitral.

Eventually, the increased pressure in the left atrium works back through the vasculature, resulting in pulmonary hypertension. Pulmonary oedema (also termed pulmonary congestion) and eventual right-sided heart failure may follow, resulting in symptoms of dyspnoea (breathlessness), orthopnoea (breathlessness on lying flat) and paroxysmal nocturnal dyspnoea (attacks of extreme breathlessness, usually at night).

Right-sided heart failure

The most common cause is progression of left-sided failure, so-called biventricular heart failure. In these cases, the right ventricle has to pump against increased resistance in the pulmonary circulation.

Rarely, isolated right heart failure may develop because of:

- chronic lung disease (cor pulmonale)
- pulmonary emboli (usually multiple)
- pulmonary valve stenosis.

This may result in peripheral oedema, congestive hepatomegaly and congestive splenomegaly.

DISORDERS OF THE HEART VALVES

Types of valvular disorder

Valvular disorders can be:

- stenosis—narrowing or abnormal rigidity of a valve
- regurgitation (or incompetence)—failure of a valve to close fully.

Both types may coexist in one valve, but one type is usually dominant.

Factors that may cause heart valve damage include:

- congenital abnormality
- postinflammatory scarring, e.g., after rheumatic heart disease
- degeneration with aging
- dilatation of the valve ring, e.g., in dilated cardiomyopathy (DCM)
- degeneration of collagenous support tissue of the valve
- acute destruction by necrotizing inflammation.

Commonly affected valves

The mitral and aortic valves are the most frequently affected; the tricuspid and pulmonary valves only infrequently.

Table 9.12 outlines the major causes and basic features of acquired valve disease.

Abnormalities of flow and their effects

Diseased valves often cause regurgitant jets of blood, with concomitant development of endocardial lesions opposite the jet's origin. These lesions (jet lesions) are typically seen on the septum opposite the aortic valve.

Degenerative valve disease

Calcific aortic stenosis

There are two types:

1. Degenerative calcific aortic valve stenosis—calcification of the aortic valve associated with increasing age; typically affects the elderly.
2. Bicuspid calcific aortic valve stenosis—calcification of a congenital bicuspid aortic valve (present in 1% of the population); quite common, usually manifesting by 40–50 years of age.

In both types, the valves become thick and fibrotic with fusion of the commissures. Large subendothelial nodular masses of calcium may be found within the sinuses of Valsalva, restricting opening of the aortic cusps.

Effects

There are two effects:

1. Aortic stenosis: thickening and fusion of valves → decreased valve lumen → reduced systolic flow.
2. Aortic regurgitation: increased rigidity of valves → failure to close properly → backflow into the left ventricle during diastole.

Stenosis and regurgitation result in left-ventricular hypertrophy, coronary insufficiency (often angina) and syncope or sudden death owing to acute left-sided heart failure or arrhythmias.

Mitral annular calcification

This is 'wear and tear' calcification of the mitral valve leaflets. Massive calcification can immobilize the valve and predispose to the development of either thrombosis (owing to change in bloodflow) or bacterial endocarditis.

Mitral valve prolapse ('floppy valve syndrome')

The changes here are due to myxomatous degeneration. The leaflets are thickened and redundant, containing large amounts of mucopolysaccharides and abnormal collagen. It most commonly involves the posterior mitral

Table 9.12 Major causes and basic features of acquired valve disease

Valve lesion	Causes	Effects	Physical findings
Mitral stenosis	Rheumatic fever Senile calcific degeneration	Left-sided cardiac failure with predisposition to atrial thrombosis. Left atrial hypertrophy and dilation leads to: • pulmonary vascular congestion • pulmonary hypertension • right ventricular hypertrophy • 'nutmeg liver' and congested kidneys	Loud S_1 Opening snap Diastolic rumble
Mitral regurgitation	Acute: • papillary muscle dysfunction • cusp damage by endocarditis Chronic: • postinflammatory scarring, commonly rheumatic • left ventricular dilation • floppy mitral valve syndrome (prolapse)	Acute: • pulmonary oedema Chronic: • left ventricular hypertrophy and dilation • giant left atrium • progressive left-sided cardiac failure develops with time	Pansystolic murmur Widely split S_2
Aortic stenosis	Calcification of congenital bicuspid aortic valve Rheumatic fever Senile calcific degeneration	Early: • asymptomatic but with slowly progressive left ventricular hypertrophy Late: • left ventricular failure • low cardiac output → breathlessness • coronary artery insufficiency → angina • cerebrovascular insufficiency → syncope, sudden death	Systolic ejection murmur reaching peak intensity in mid or late systole Narrow pulse pressure Slow-rising carotid pulse
Aortic regurgitation	Rheumatic fever Endocarditis Senile calcification Aortic root dilation	Left ventricular hypertrophy Progressive left-ventricular failure	Diastolic murmur Wide pulse pressure Collapsing pulse

leaflet, which is soft and bulges upwards into the atrium during systole. The net result is mild valvular incompetence and an increased risk of rupture of one of the chordae tendineae, which may lead to sudden, severe valvular incompetence.

Mitral valve prolapse can also be a feature of connective tissue disorders such as Marfan syndrome.

Rheumatic heart disease

Rheumatic fever is an autoimmune disorder that can occur 2–3 weeks after a streptococcal infection, usually tonsillitis or pharyngitis, and can result in development of rheumatic heart disease.

Epidemiology

This disease occurs mainly in children aged 5–15 years. It was once prevalent in Europe, including the UK, and in the USA. Its incidence has now decreased in the developed world due to antibiotics, and it is now most frequently seen in parts of central Africa, the Middle East and India.

Pathogenesis

Susceptible individuals develop antibodies to antigens produced by specific strains of group A streptococci; these antibodies then cross-react with host antigens, causing inflammation and fibrosis. The disease is a systemic disorder affecting the heart, joints, skin and arteries.

The most important target organ is the heart. Repeated attacks of rheumatic fever lead to progressive fibrosis of the endocardium and valves, which is the main cause of chronic scarring of the valves.

Diagnosis is via the Jones criteria (see online Table 9.13).

Aschoff bodies

These pathognomonic heart lesions consist of multinucleate giant cells surrounded by activated macrophages and lymphoid cells (predominantly T-cells). Caterpillar-shaped Anitschkow cells may also be seen.

Acute rheumatic heart disease

In the acute phase, rheumatic fever causes a pancarditis, the components of which are:

- Rheumatic pericarditis—acute inflammation of the pericardium.
- Rheumatic myocarditis—mild inflammation of the heart muscle with occasional muscle fibre necrosis.
- Rheumatic endocarditis—inflammation of the valves; mitral valves are most prone to the development of severe lesions.

Chronic rheumatic heart disease

Long-term morbidity from rheumatic fever occurs as a result of immune damage causing chronic scarring of valves, which develop fish-mouth deformities. Chronic valvular heart disease develops in about 50% of those affected by rheumatic fever with carditis. In developed countries, lesions may develop after 10–20 years, but much earlier in developing countries.

Pathogenesis

Endocardial valvular damage from the acute phase heals by progressive fibrosis. Valve leaflets and chordae tendineae become thickened, fibrotic and shrunken, often with fusion to their partners; there is frequent marked secondary deposition of calcium.

Once damage has developed, the altered haemodynamic stresses extend the damage even in the absence of continued autoimmune processes.

Infective endocarditis

This is an acute or subacute disease resulting from infection of a focal area of the endocardium, which usually has preexisting damage. It can affect almost any age group, but it is increasing in incidence in the elderly population and is more common in males than females (3:1). Predisposing factors in susceptible individuals include genitourinary infection, diabetes, tooth extraction, pressure ulcers and surgical procedures.

Morphological features

The characteristic lesions of endocarditis are termed vegetations. These are formed from deposits of platelets, fibrin and bacteria. The mechanism of formation is outlined in Fig. 9.13. Vegetations may form in areas of high-pressure gradients, e.g., at an incompetent valve.

Almost all vegetations occur on valve leaflets or chordae tendineae. The size varies from a small nodule to a large mass that may occlude the valve orifice. The mitral valve, followed by the aortic valve, is most commonly affected.

Causative organisms

Bacteria

Pathogens such as *Staphylococcus aureus*, α-haemolytic streptococci, pneumococci, meningococci and *Escherichia coli* are commonly responsible.

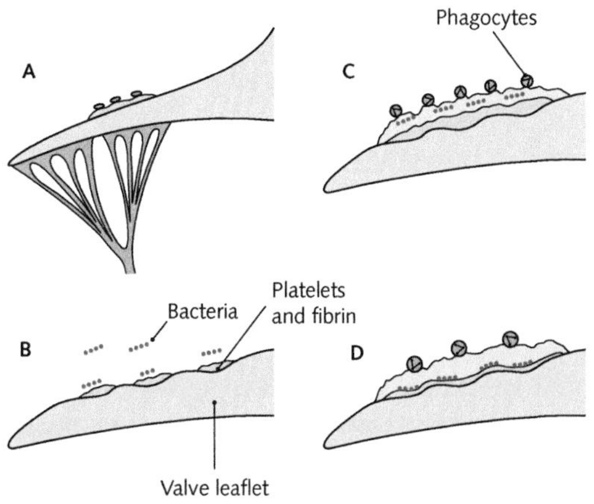

Fig. 9.13 Pathogenesis of vegetation formation. (A) An abnormality on the endocardium of the valve leaflet is coated with small deposits of platelets and fibrin (thrombus). (B) Circulating bacteria or fungi colonize the platelet thrombus. (C, D) Further layers of platelets and fibrin are deposited, and the microorganisms proliferate in the superficial layer of the vegetation. They are separated from blood by a thin layer of fibrinous material, which protects against immune destruction but allows diffusion of nutrients. (Adapted from Underwood, 2009.)

Fungi

Fungi such as *Candida* and *Aspergillus* can occasionally cause endocarditis, particularly in intravenous drug users, the immunosuppressed or those with valve prostheses.

The type of causative organism responsible depends on whether the affected valve is structurally normal or abnormal.

Infection of structurally normal valves

Infective organisms are pathogenic and directly invade the valve, causing rapid destruction. This is commonly seen in intravenous drug users (often affecting the tricuspid valve), after open heart surgery and following septicaemia from other causes. Highly virulent forms of *S. aureus* are often responsible for such infections.

Infection of structurally abnormal heart valves

Infective organisms are of low pathogenicity and are derived from normal commensal organisms of the skin, mouth, urinary tract and gut. Following trivial episodes of bacteraemia, organisms become enmeshed in platelet aggregates on the surface of the abnormal endocardium, growing to cause persistent infection. The main underlying abnormalities in this group are:

- congenital bicuspid aortic valves
- postinflammatory scarring
- mitral valve prolapse syndrome
- prosthetic valves.

The incidence has increased in developed countries in recent years, mainly as a result of patients surviving with structurally abnormal hearts and heart valves.

Types of infective endocarditis

Acute

The cause is usually a virulent organism, such as *S. aureus.* It can affect either normal or abnormal heart valves.

The bacteria proliferate in the valve, causing necrosis and the generation of thrombotic vegetations. Consequently, there is destruction of valve leaflets with perforation and acute disturbance of valve function leading to acute heart failure.

Prognosis—disease is rapidly progressive and often fatal owing to the incidence of embolic events, renal failure and acute heart failure.

Subacute

The typical cause here is when less virulent organisms, such as *Streptococcus viridans*, are involved.

The bacteria proliferate slowly in the thrombotic vegetation on damaged valve surfaces. Gradual valve destruction occurs, stimulating further thrombus formation with the potential for systemic embolization.

CLINICAL NOTE

INFECTIVE ENDOCARDITIS

Key clinical features of endocarditis are:

- Systemic symptoms—fever, weight loss and malaise due to cytokines (low-grade infection)
- Skin petechiae and microhaemorrhages in the retina and skin, particularly around the fingernails (splinter haemorrhages), caused by the deposition of immune complexes in small vessels—they also cause glomerulonephritis
- Finger clubbing (cause unknown), occasionally with characteristic Janeway lesions and/or Osler nodes
- Splenomegaly and anaemia owing to persistent bacteraemia

Sequelae

The sequelae are as follows:

- Valvular regurgitation owing to gradual destruction of valves leading to cardiac failure.
- Perivalvular abscesses following extension of the infection into the valve ring and myocardium, producing sinuses, fistulae, septal defects and abnormalities of conduction.
- Mycotic aneurysms—infection of the muscular wall of a medium-sized artery caused by emboli to the vasa vasorum.
- Multiorgan infarction—small emboli of infected thrombotic material enter the systemic circulation, producing infarction of many organs, especially the brain, spleen and kidneys. Infarcted organs may in turn become infected by organisms within the occluding thrombus.

Complications of infective endocarditis are summarized in Fig. 9.14.

Nonbacterial (marantic) endocarditis

Nonbacterial thrombotic endocarditis is inflammation of the valves with the formation of sterile thrombotic vegetations (marantic vegetations) on the closure lines of the valve cusps. It occurs in severely debilitated patients with serious systemic disease, particularly malignancy.

Endocarditis of systemic lupus erythematosus (Libman–Sacks disease)

Thrombotic vegetations complicate SLE in 50% or more of fatal cases. The vegetations are small, meaning that valvular changes rarely give rise to any appreciable functional deficiency (and therefore symptoms), but thrombotic material can fragment and cause distant embolic infarction.

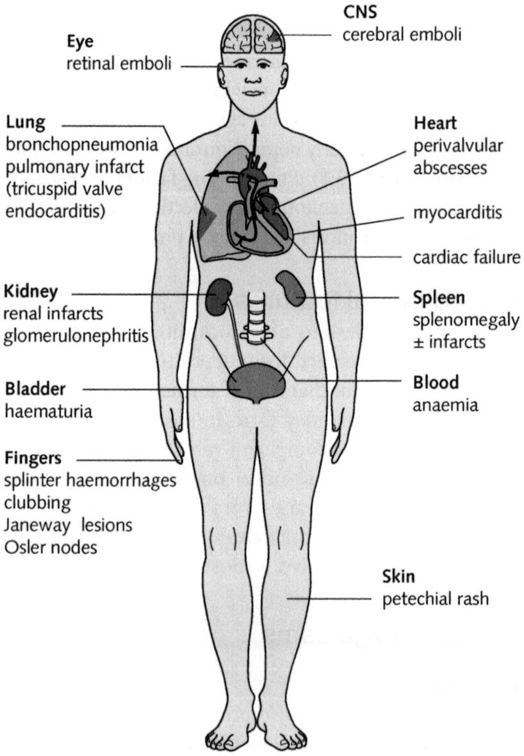

Fig. 9.14 Complications of infective endocarditis.

Carcinoid heart disease

Carcinoid syndrome is caused by excess serotonin secretion by a carcinoid (neuroendocrine) tumour. Serotonin secreted by the tumour (most commonly arising in the small intestine and metastasizing to the liver) acts on 5-hydroxytryptamine receptors and can result in endocardial fibrosis of the tricuspid and pulmonary valves, in turn resulting in stenosis or incompetence.

Complications of artificial heart valves

Prosthetic valve diseases

The prosthetic valve diseases include:

- Thrombosis leading to valve obstruction or embolism.
- Valve failure owing to breakage of a mechanical prosthesis, or tissue calcification and cusp rupture of a bioprosthesis.
- Infective endocarditis from turbulence and prosthetic material; its incidence is 1%–2% per year.
- Obstructive gradients—the valve may be too small or there may be tissue ingrowth of the pannus onto the valve ring.
- Haemolysis of red blood cells passing through a mechanical valve, occasionally leading to jaundice.

DISEASES OF THE MYOCARDIUM

Cardiomyopathy

This is a group of diseases cause by an abnormal myocardium. It should only be considered if all other potential causes of myocardial impairment have been excluded.

Effects of cardiomyopathy

Cardiomyopathies usually cause progressive development of cardiac failure. The timescale varies from weeks to years depending on the specific pathology. In some instances, sudden cardiac death is the first manifestation of disease owing to electrical dysfunction of the myocardium.

Classification

Cardiomyopathies are now classified into five groups:

1. Hypertrophic cardiomyopathy (HCM)—'too thick'
2. Dilated cardiomyopathy (DCM)—'too thin'
3. Arrhythmogenic right-ventricular cardiomyopathy (ARVC)—'too unstable'
4. Restrictive cardiomyopathy—'too stiff'
5. Unclassified.

The cause of each can be familial or nonfamilial. Nonfamilial causes include idiopathic (unknown) or acquired - i.e., the ventricular dysfunction is the complication of the acquired disease rather than an intrinsic feature of the disease.

Hypertrophic cardiomyopathy

This is the presence of increased ventricular wall thickness in the absence of loading conditions, e.g., hypertension and valvular disease sufficient to cause the abnormality. This condition may present in young adults and juveniles with sudden unexplained death on exertion or, less dramatically, with angina and breathlessness on exertion, syncope/presyncope and palpitations.

HCM is a complex disease of the contractile apparatus (sarcomere) of the myocardium with a highly variable clinical course and a high degree of heterogeneity. It is estimated to occur at a frequency of 1/500, with a death rate of 1%–2.5%.

Macroscopically: Eccentric hypertrophy (15–35 mm or more) involving the intraventricular septum is the most commonly seen form; however, any pattern of hypertrophy may occur. A quarter of cases are associated with subaortic obstruction and mitral valve regurgitation. Concentric thickening is more in keeping with metabolic disorders, e.g., glycogen storage diseases.

Microscopically:

- Bizarre myocytes—hypertrophied with Y-shaped forms and irregular side-to-side branch connections.
- Myocardial disarray—architectural distortion with haphazard arrangement of myocyte bundles.
- Myocardial fibrosis—from microvascular ischaemia.
- Small-vessel disease—hypertrophy of the tunica media causing stenosis of coronary arteries and capillaries.

These changes contribute to the haemodynamic and electrical instability of the myocardium, resulting in systolic dysfunction from marked reduction in systolic volume and difficulty in diastolic filling.

Genetics: Mutations can be inherited or sporadic and, to date, over100 mutations have been identified that are associated with HCM. These all code for a component of the sarcomere; the most common affecting the β-myosin heavy chain and cardiac myosin-binding protein C genes. Inheritance is mostly autosomal dominant with incomplete penetrance. Mutations confer different levels of risk for disease-related death. The *ARG 403 GLN* and *ARG 719 TRP* mutations are high risk for disease-related death.

Dilated cardiomyopathy

This is defined as a dilated left ventricle with poor systolic function in the absence of coronary (ischaemic) heart disease, or any conditions that may cause systolic impairment from abnormal loading, e.g., hypertension or valve disease. DCMs are not a single entity but a group of conditions which are characterized by:

- dilatation of the ventricles—usually left more often than right
- thin, stretched chamber walls
- hypocontractile myocardial muscle.

Aetiology is often unidentifiable but can be inherited in an autosomal dominant or X-linked pattern. More than 30 genes have been identified, many of which are concerned with the sarcomere. The most commonly mutated is the *TTN* gene that codes for the titin protein involved with the structural stability of the sarcomere.

DCM can represent end-stage myocardial damage from known causes, including viral myocarditis, alcohol (dilated alcoholic cardiomyopathy) and other forms of secondary cardiomyopathies.

Arrhythmogenic right-ventricular cardiomyopathy

ARVC is a progressive disease of the right ventricle with gradual patchy replacement of the myocardium by fibroadipose tissue. This acts as a substrate for electrical instability and subsequent ventricular arrhythmias causing sudden death.

It is an uncommon disease, with a prevalence of 1/5000. It is more common in people of Italian and Greek descent but is significant as it accounts for 11% of sudden cardiac deaths. Diagnosis is usually at 20–50 years and presentation includes palpitations, chest pain, dyspnoea, syncope on exertion and sudden death. However, a large proportion is asymptomatic.

The disease is largely familial, with an autosomal dominant pattern of inheritance with incomplete penetrance. There is large genetic heterogeneity with mutations in at least eight genes identified which involve desmosomes. The most common mutations are in the *PKP2* gene, which codes for plakophilin 2.

CLINICAL NOTE

SUDDEN CARDIAC DEATH

Sudden arrhythmic death syndrome (SADS) is an umbrella term for a group of genetic heart conditions that often present with death in teenagers/young adults who are otherwise healthy. It accounts for approximately 450 deaths per year in the UK and is caused by conduction disorders of the heart, such as Wolff–Parkinson–White syndrome, Brugada syndrome, long and short QT syndrome, catecholaminergic polymorphic ventricular tachycardia (CPVT) as well as hypertrophic cardiomyopathy (HCM) and arrhythmogenic right-ventricular cardiomyopathy (ARVC). Warning symptoms include syncope/seizures during exercise, excitement, startle or arousal from sleep, consistent or unusual chest pain ± abnormal shortness of breath during exercise and family history of sudden unexpected death in relatives <40 years of age.

Restrictive cardiomyopathy

Abnormal stiffness of the myocardium results in impaired ventricular filling during diastole. This leads to reduced diastolic volumes and normal or reduced systolic volumes, with normal ventricular wall thickness. The stiffness is caused by infiltration of the myocardium by disease processes, for example:

- Amyloidosis
- Scleroderma
- Sarcoidosis
- Carcinoid heart disease
- Endomyocardial fibrosis (fibrosis of thrombotic material deposited on the endocardial surfaces).

The condition causes high atrial pressures resulting in atrial hypertrophy → atrial dilatation → atrial fibrillation with pulmonary and systemic congestion as both sides of the heart are affected. It is not known to have a genetic cause.

Unclassified

This group includes Takotsubo cardiomyopathy, also known as acute stress-induced cardiomyopathy. This is a transient cardiomyopathy presenting with the symptoms of MI, with sudden and acute heart failure. Imaging shows ballooning of the left-ventricular apex associated with hypokinesis, dyskinesis or akinesis of the left mid ventricle ± apex. Coronary artery disease is absent.

It is usually preceded by stress (emotional or physiological) and is seen most commonly in postmenopausal women.

Myocarditis

This is an inflammatory disease of the myocardium with the presence of inflammatory cells in the myocardium. The clinical picture is highly variable, from an asymptomatic disorder with minor ECG changes to rapidly progressing heart failure.

Aetiology

The vast majority of cases of myocarditis are either infectious or immune-mediated. The infectious causes are:

- Viruses—viral infection is the commonest cause of myocarditis in the UK. Coxsackie virus is the commonest. Other agents include influenza, echovirus, HIV, cytomegalovirus, poliomyelitis or mumps virus.
- Bacteria and spirochetes, e.g., *Corynebacterium diphtheriae* (diphtheria), *Borrelia* (Lyme disease), *Chlamydiae*, *Rickettsiae* and syphilis.
- Fungi, e.g., Candida
- Protozoa, e.g., toxoplasmosis, Chagas' disease (*Trypanosoma cruzi)*, leishmaniasis.
- Helminths, e.g., trichinosis, schistosomiasis, filariasis.

The immune-mediated causes are:

- poststreptococcal, e.g., acute rheumatic fever
- postviral
- SLE
- drug hypersensitivity, e.g., sulfonamides, doxorubicin, cyclophosphamide.

Other less common causes include sarcoidosis (see Chapter 10) and giant cell myocarditis, an acute fulminating form of fatal myocarditis.

Neoplasms of the heart

Tumours of the heart are extremely rare. Examples include:

- Myxoma—a benign tumour of stellate myxoma cells, typically arising from the endocardium. Ninety percent are found in the atria (usually the left atrium).
- Connective tissue tumours, such as papillary fibroelastomas and lipomas.
- Rhabdomyomas—the most common primary cardiac tumour of infancy.
- Metastatic or locally invasive tumours—these are more common than primary tumours and include lung, breast and lymphoma.

DISEASES OF THE PERICARDIUM

Accumulation of fluid in the pericardial sac

Usually the pericardial sac is a potential space which contains minimal/no fluid.

Pericardial effusion

This is the accumulation of fluid within the pericardial sac. Effusions may be:

- Serous—transudate has a low protein content and usually contains only scanty mesothelial cells. Caused by heart failure, hypoalbuminaemia or myxoedema.
- Serosanguinous—exudate with high protein content. Occurring with infection, uraemia, neoplasia or connective tissue disorders.
- Chylous—accumulation of lymphatic fluid occurring in the presence of lymphatic obstruction of pericardial drainage, most commonly due to neoplasms and tuberculosis.

The aetiology is of two types: inflammatory (e.g., acute pericarditis) and noninflammatory. In noninflammatory causes at least one of the following must have occurred:

- ↑ capillary permeability, e.g., severe hypothyroidism
- ↑ capillary hydrostatic pressure, e.g., congestive heart failure
- ↓ plasma oncotic pressure, e.g., cirrhosis or nephrotic syndrome.

Clinical effects depend on the increase in pressure within the pericardium which, in turn, depends on:

- Volume of effusion—the greater the volume, the greater the pressure, the greater the interference with cardiac function.
- Rate of fluid accumulation—sudden increase → marked elevation of pressure → severe cardiac chamber compression. Slow effusion (over weeks to months) → pericardium stretches → no elevation of pressure.
- Compliance characteristics of the pericardium—even small effusions may cause marked elevation of pressure if there is stiffness of the pericardium, e.g., chronic constrictive pericarditis.

The condition is often asymptomatic, but it may present with a dull constant ache in the left side of the chest. Unlike ischaemic cardiac pain, it is accentuated by inspiration, movement and by lying flat.

Haemopericardium

This is the accumulation of blood in the pericardial sac. The causes of haemopericardium are outlined in Table 9.14. In most cases, death occurs rapidly owing to the sudden rise in intrapericardial pressure, which prevents cardiac filling (cardiac tamponade): as little as 200–300 mL usually being sufficient to cause death.

Cardiac tamponade

Fluid (of any kind) rapidly accumulates under high pressure, compressing the cardiac chambers to such an extent that filling of the heart is severely limited, resulting in acute heart failure. The condition is often associated with myocardial rupture following MI and malignant disease.

Diagnosis

The physical signs are:

- Sinus tachycardia.
- Increased jugular venous pulse (often with a further rise on inspiration—Kussmaul sign).
- Decreased systemic blood pressure (producing shock in severe cases).
- Cyclical decrease in systolic blood pressure during each inspiration—pulsus paradoxus.

The management of cardiac tamponade depends on the extent of haemodynamic compromise.

Table 9.14 Aetiology of haemopericardium

Causes	Example
Rupture of heart	Traumatic, e.g., stab wound Spontaneous, e.g., myocardial infarct
Rupture of intrapericardial portion of aorta	Dissecting aneurysm Syphilitic aneurysm Traumatic
Haemorrhagic tendencies	Purpura Scurvy Hypoprothrombinaemia Anticoagulant therapy

Pericarditis

Pericarditis, i.e., inflammation of the pericardium, is the main disorder of the pericardium. The condition is often complicated by the development of an effusion.

Acute pericarditis

In acute pericarditis both pericardial surfaces (visceral and parietal layers) are coated with a fibrin-rich acute inflammatory exudate. The loss of smoothness can be heard clinically as a friction rub. The causes of acute pericarditis are listed in Table 9.15.

Variants can be:

- Serous, nonbacterial inflammation—the exudate is a clear, straw-coloured and protein-rich fluid.
- Serofibrinous or fibrinous—occurs with MI. The exudate contains plasma protein, including fibrinogen. This is the most common form of acute pericarditis and macroscopically has a 'bread and butter' appearance.
- Suppurative (or purulent) pericarditis—associated with pyogenic bacterial infection; serosal surfaces are erythematous and coated with thick, creamy pus.
- Haemorrhagic—blood is mixed with inflammatory exudate.
- Caseous—fibrinous exudate with granulation tissue and areas of caseation caused by tuberculosis infection.

Clinical features

The clinical features of acute pericarditis are:

- pleuritic chest pain—typically retrosternal pain radiating to the shoulders and neck, relieved by leaning forward
- fever
- pericardial friction rub
- ECG abnormalities.

HINTS AND TIPS

THE 'FIVE IS' OF ACUTE PERICARDITIS'

Remember the 'Five Is' for possible causes of acute pericarditis:

Infarctive
Infective
Injury
Invasive
Immunological

Chronic pericarditis

Adhesive pericarditis

Although fibrinous pericarditis may resolve completely, it occasionally results in fibrinous adhesions or even in complete obliteration of the pericardial sac.

Constrictive pericarditis

Progressive fibrosis and calcification of the pericardium causes restriction of ventricular filling and interference with ventricular systole. The heart is effectively encased in a solid shell and filling is impaired. Calcification may also extend into the myocardium, producing impaired myocardial contraction.

This condition often follows tuberculous pericarditis, but it can also complicate haemopericardium, viral pericarditis, rheumatoid arthritis and purulent pericarditis.

Clinical features

In chronic pericarditis, the fibrous tissue impairs venous return, resulting in symptoms and signs of systemic venous congestion, namely raised jugular venous pressure, enlarged liver and ascites. Atrial fibrillation is also common.

Table 9.15 Aetiology of acute pericarditis

Infarction	Myocardial infarction: local pericarditis over an infarct is the commonest cause of pericarditis
Infective	Most often due to viral infections (second most common cause), usually clinically mild, rarely requiring hospital treatment Pyogenic: e.g., staphylococci, streptococci, haemophilus septicaemia or pneumonia Tuberculosis: spread to pericardium from tuberculous lymph nodes in mediastinum; now rare
Injury	Postoperative: following open heart surgery Pericarditis is diffuse, involving entire pericardial surface Heals by fibrosis → obliteration of pericardial cavity
Invasive	Malignant pericarditis: usually due to infiltration of the pericardium by local spread from a primary bronchial tumour; less commonly the cause is a bloodborne metastasis from a distant site, e.g., malignant melanoma
Immunological	Immune pericarditis: associated with rheumatic fever or may present in patients with systemic autoimmune disease, e.g., systemic lupus erythematosus, rheumatoid disease

Rheumatic disease of the pericardium

Rheumatic disease of the pericardium is an acute form of pericarditis occurring with generalized pancarditis following streptococcal infection.

ANEURYSMS

Definitions and concepts

Aneurysm

An aneurysm is an abnormal localized, permanent, dilatation of an artery. The term can also be applied to the wall of the heart. Types of aneurysm are shown in Fig. 9.15:

- True aneurysms—the wall is formed by one or more layers of the affected vessel.
- False aneurysms (pseudoaneurysms)—the vascular wall is breached (usually following trauma or infection), allowing communication with an extravascular space that is limited by surrounding tissue (usually an organized haematoma). There is no epithelial lining and the haematoma is expanding and pulsatile.

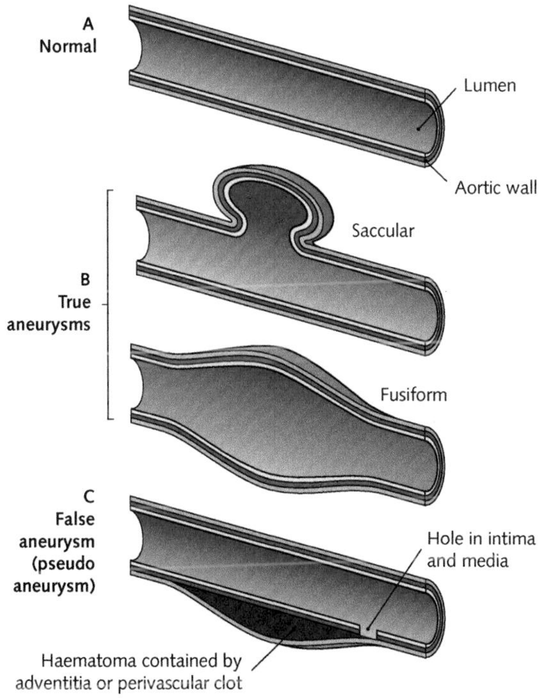

Fig. 9.15 Aneurysm morphology. (A) Normal. (B) True aneurysms—saccular aneurysms take the form of globular sacs, whereas fusiform aneurysms are spindle-shaped owing to long segments of the vessel wall being affected around the whole circumference. (C) False aneurysm (pseudoaneurysm).

Main causes of aneurysms

Any abnormality that weakens the tunica media may produce an aneurysm.

Congenital causes:

Localized weakness

- Cystic medial degeneration—focal degeneration of media with the formation of small cyst-like spaces filled with mucopolysaccharide. Aetiology may be idiopathic or associated with connective tissue diseases, e.g., Marfan syndrome and Ehlers–Danlos syndrome.

Acquired causes:

- Atherosclerosis—the most common cause, typically affecting the abdominal aorta, causing thinning and fibrous replacement of tunica media
- Trauma
- Infection
- Bacterial aortitis
  - mycotic aneurysms (small saccular dilatations with destruction of the wall caused by bacteria in an infected thrombus)
  - tertiary syphilis (typically affecting the ascending and transverse portions of the aortic arch, causing inflammatory destruction of the media with fibrous replacement)
- Vasculitic syndromes (see below)—inflammation of the vessels caused by immune-complex deposition or cell-mediated immune reactions of the arterial wall, leading to weakening of the vessel wall then aneurysmal dilatation.

Pathogenesis

The majority of aneurysms occur because of a weakening of the arterial wall with loss of elasticity and contractility. Stretching of the weakened wall is progressive owing to haemodynamic pressure forces producing an increased thinning of the wall. Wall tension increases with radius according to Laplace law (T=RP, where T=tension, R=arterial radius and P=pressure) until eventual rupture occurs. High blood pressure is the most important factor in increasing the rate of growth.

The build-up of layers of thrombus within the lumen of the aneurysmal sac is protective, but not usually sufficient to repair the defect and reconstitute a normal lumen to the artery.

HINTS AND TIPS

ANEURYSM AND ATHEROMA

The most frequent cause of an aneurysm is an atheroma. However, any abnormality that weakens the tunica media may predispose a patient to aneurysm formation. The commonest vessels involved are abdominal aorta, femoral and popliteal arteries.

Complications

- Rupture—increased risk of rupture with increasing size. Rupture may extend into the surrounding cavity, e.g., as a retroperitoneal haemorrhage or as a slow leak into the vessel wall.
- Thrombosis—can cause occlusion (usually popliteal) or embolize (typically to the feet or intestine).
- Pressure effects—can cause erosion of adjacent structures (e.g., vertebrae), displacement of structures (e.g., sciatic nerve) or occlusion by extrinsic pressure (e.g., femoral vein).
- Fistula formation—aortoduodenal (massive gastrointestinal bleeding) and aortocaval (raised jugulovenous pressure, plethora, lower body oedema).

Abdominal aortic aneurysms

Abdominal aortic aneurysms (AAAs) are more common in males, especially over 60 years of age.

Aetiology: atherosclerosis is the most common cause; however, they may also arise as a result of inflammation (vasculitis) or infection (mycotic aneurysms).

Site: 80% of AAAs are situated below the origin of the renal arteries and are thus amenable to repair.

Morphology: atherosclerotic aneurysms produce a fusiform dilatation of the wall.

Symptoms and signs: the majority of AAAs are asymptomatic. Symptoms may occur because of compression of neighbouring structures by the expanding aneurysm, e.g., back pain from vertebral compression, or vomiting following duodenal obstruction.

Consequences: rupture is the most devastating consequence and is often fatal, with an overall mortality of 85%.

Prognostic factors

Prognosis depends on the anterior–posterior diameter of the aneurysm:

- <5.5 cm: 1% rupture per year
- 5.5–6.5 cm: 5% rupture per year
- >6.5 cm: >25% rupture per year.

Fifty percent of all abdominal aortic aneurysms that are >6 cm in transverse diameter rupture within 2 years if not surgically resected. Aneurysms <6 cm across may also rupture, albeit less frequently.

Surgical mortality

Elective surgical repair carries a mortality rate of <5% and, therefore, is considered when the risk from operative death is lower than risk of aneurysmal rupture. For AAAs this is when the diameter is >5.5 cm in diameter or those that are rapidly progressing or symptomatic. Elective surgical repair has a much lower mortality than emergency surgery for rupture, which has a perioperative mortality of 50% (in the 30% of ruptures that survive to surgery).

Mortality for surgical repair of abdominal aneurysms is also lower than that of thoracic aneurysms.

Aortic dissection

An aortic dissection is a tear in the tunica intima of the aorta, allowing entry of blood into the tunica media, with dissection of a 'flap' of intima from the rest of the aortic wall. A false lumen is created, usually between the inner two-thirds and outer third of the tunica media, giving the appearance of a double-barrelled aorta ('tennis ball sign' on imaging). The false lumen inevitably ruptures, either:

- Extraluminally—external rupture leads to massive fatal bleed into the thoracic cavity or, less commonly, the pericardial sac (cardiac tamponade), mediastinum or abdomen.
- Intraluminally—rarely, blood tracks back and ruptures into the true lumen through the inner media and intima, forming a double-channelled aorta.

Types of aortic dissection

Aortic dissection is classified using the Stanford-DeBakey classification system (Fig. 9.16):

1. Stanford type A/DeBakey types I + II (67% of dissecting aneurysms)—arise in the ascending aorta with or without extension into the descending aorta. These can also involve the heart, causing cardiac tamponade.
2. Stanford Type B/DeBakey type III (33% of dissecting aneurysms)—are confined to the descending aorta, distal to the origin of the left subclavian artery.

Epidemiology—there are approximately 600 cases per year of aortic dissection in the UK, occurring most commonly in people between 50 and 70 years old, and affecting males more often than females by a factor of 2:1.

Predisposing factors are:

- hypertension
- aortic atherosclerosis
- aortic aneurysm
- connective tissue disorders (e.g., Marfan syndrome)
- pregnancy
- congenital abnormalities of the aortic valve
- trauma, e.g., cardiac catheterization, road traffic accident
- vasculitis, e.g., Takayasu arteritis, giant cell arteritis
- cocaine use.

RED FLAG

SYMPTOMS AND SIGNS OF AORTIC DISSECTION

The symptoms and signs of aortic dissection are:

- sudden-onset severe chest pain, radiating through to the back between the shoulder blades
- tearing pain
- usually hypertension
- asymmetry of brachial, carotid or femoral pulses

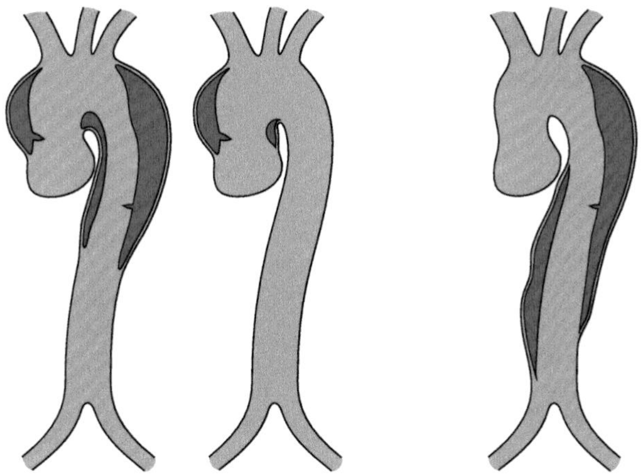

Fig. 9.16 Diagram of aortic dissection, Stanford and DeBakey classification. Stanford A: all dissections of ascending aorta; Stanford B: all dissections not involving ascending aorta. DeBakey I: originates in the ascending aorta and propagates to at least the aortic arch—60% of all dissections. DeBakey II: originates in the ascending aorta and is confined to the ascending aorta—10%–15% of all dissections. DeBakey III: originates in the descending aorta (distal to the left subclavian artery) and extends distally (occasionally proximally)—25%–30% of all dissections. The classification system is used to identify those that need surgical repair (type A) and those that require medical management.

- mediastinal broadening and aortic 'knuckle' distortion on chest radiography
- symptoms/signs of occlusion of aorta branches, e.g., MI—coronary artery, haematuria—renal artery, abdominal pain—mesenteric artery
- left-sided pleural effusion

Prognosis—the mortality rate without treatment is 20% before reaching hospital, 30% within 1 week, 80% at 2 weeks and 90% at 1 year. Overall, there is a 60% survival at 5 years for those who have surgery. Proximal dissections carry a higher mortality rate than distal.

PERIPHERAL VASCULAR DISEASE

This is vascular disease affecting the peripheral vasculature and is caused by similar pathologies to those of central arteries. It almost exclusively involves the legs and is divided into:

- **Intermittent claudication**—gripping cramp-like pain (usually the calf) that occurs on exercise and resolves on cessation. Oxygen delivery (vascular supply) to the tissues is insufficient to meet the increased oxygen demand of the exercising muscle.
- **Critical limb ischaemia**—this manifests as progressive, unremitting rest pain day and night, preventing the patient from sleeping. The vascular supply is insufficient for the basal metabolic needs of the tissues. Gangrene and ulceration may occur.
- **Acute limb ischaemia**—abrupt onset of severe limb pain owing to sudden interruption of the vascular supply to the leg, resulting in ischaemia. Causes include embolus and rupture of a thrombotic plaque.

HINTS AND TIPS

ACUTE LIMB ISCHAEMIA

Remember the six Ps for features of acute limb ischaemia:

- **P**ain (severe)
- **P**allor
- **P**ulselessness
- **P**araesthesia
- **P**erishing cold
- **P**aralysis

Clinically

An ischaemic limb will initially appear white, then blue, then blotchy and marbled. The muscles harden over time. If there is complete occlusion of an artery, then the limb is viable for ~6 hours; this is therefore a surgical emergency, with successful restoration of blood flow inversely proportional to the time elapsed since the onset of ischaemia. Neurosensory deficit is an ominous sign, and if skin staining becomes fixed, the limb is no longer viable.

INFLAMMATORY AND NEOPLASTIC VASCULAR DISEASE

Vasculitides

This is a group of disorders characterized by inflammation of the blood vessel walls (vasculitis) leading to occlusion. Vasculitis can affect capillaries, venules, arterioles, arteries and, occasionally, large veins.

Effects:

- Mild cases—transient damage to the vessel wall, which produces leakage of red blood cells.
- Severe cases—irreversible vessel wall destruction resulting in ischaemia and organ damage with associated systemic disturbances, commonly fevers, myalgias, arthralgias and malaise.

Classification:
Vasculitis can be classified either according to the size of the vessel affected—small, medium or large or according to the pathogenesis of the inflammation (Table 9.16).

Pathogenesis:

- Idiopathic vasculitis—the aetiology is unknown.
- Immune-mediated vasculitis—pathogenesis is caused by immune complex formation between antigens and antibodies, which become trapped in vessel walls and stimulate an acute inflammatory response with neutrophil chemotaxis. Neutrophils release enzymes that destroy the vessel wall. There are two main types:
  1. Hypersensitivity (neutrophilic) vasculitis—the most common pattern affecting capillaries and venules; usually manifests as a skin rash, often as a result of an allergy to a drug or occasionally arising as an allergic rash in viraemia or bacteraemia. It also occurs in Henoch–Schönlein purpura, serum sickness and cryoglobulinaemia.
  2. Multiorgan autoimmune diseases, e.g., SLE and rheumatoid disease (mainly affects the aorta).
- Infectious vasculitis—inflammatory destruction of the tunica media with fibrous replacement. The infection can be primary, e.g., tertiary syphilis, *Aspergillus* or via infected thrombi.

Table 9.16 Classification of vasculitis

Size of vessel	Disorders	Pathogenesis
Large and medium	Syphilitic aortitis	Infectious
	Takayasu disease	Idiopathic
	Giant cell arteritis	Idiopathic
	Rheumatoid disease	Immune-mediated
Medium and small	Polyarteritis nodosa	Immune-mediated
	Kawasaki disease	Idiopathic
	Buerger disease	Idiopathic
	Systemic lupus erythematosus	Immune-mediated
Small	Henoch–Schönlein purpura	Immune-mediated
	Granulomatosis with polyangiitis	Immune-mediated
	Microscopic polyangiitis	Immune-mediated
	Churg–Strauss syndrome	Immune-mediated

Large vessel vasculitides

Giant cell (temporal) arteritis

Giant cell arteritis is a systemic disease of large- and medium-sized arteries that has a predilection for arteries of the head and neck, particularly the temporal arteries. Vertebral, ophthalmic, occipital and carotid arteries are commonly involved.

Epidemiology: it is the commonest vasculitis, affecting 1–2 per 10,000 per year in the UK. Incidence increases with age, and it is rare in people under 50 years; it affects females more often than males by a factor of 3:1.

Aetiology: it is thought to be an immune-mediated T-cell response against an unknown antigen. Smoking increases the risk.

Pathology:

- patchy segmental disease
- transmural granulomatous inflammation with multinucleate giant cells
- concentric intimal proliferation and fibrosis
- fragmentation of the elastic lamina
- luminal narrowing
- thrombosis.

Clinical features: patients have ill-defined symptoms of:

- loss of appetite
- fatigue
- severe headaches/facial pain
- scalp tenderness
- visual disturbances, e.g., blurred vision, diplopia, amaurosis fugax from involvement of the ophthalmic arteries. This is an ophthalmic emergency requiring prompt treatment with high-dose corticosteroids to prevent blindness
- jaw claudication.

There is an association with polymyalgia rheumatica, a musculoskeletal condition causing muscle pain and stiffness classically in the upper body.

Investigations characteristically reveal high erythrocyte sedimentation rate and/or C-reactive protein. Diagnosis is made by histology on a temporal artery biopsy. Management is with high-dose corticosteroid therapy to control the disease. Uncontrolled, it can lead to blindness, stroke and MI.

Takayasu (pulseless) disease

This is a rare granulomatous inflammatory disorder of the aorta and its major proximal branches, typically affecting young or middle-aged females most commonly from Japan, China and the Far East. The condition is characterized by severe necrotizing granulomatous inflammation of all the layers of the arterial wall. There is successive occlusion of the aorta and its branches due to fibrosis, intimal proliferation and luminal narrowing. Clinically, pulses are delayed or absent in the upper arm, with ischaemic symptoms such as arm claudication, visual disturbances and stroke. Hypertension is also present secondary to renal artery stenosis.

Medium vessel vasculitides

Kawasaki disease

This is a self-limiting febrile disease of infants (6 months to 5 years), primarily in Japan and China, but seen worldwide. Presentation is with fever, bilateral conjunctivitis, fissuring/crusting of the lips, strawberry tongue, cervical lymphadenopathy, global erythema and desquamation of the palms and soles. It affects medium-sized vessels, particularly the coronary arteries, which can lead to coronary artery aneurysm formation and other myocardial sequelae such as infarction.

Polyarteritis nodosa

This systemic disease is characterized by inflammatory necrosis of the walls of small and medium-sized muscular arteries. Although the disease is systemic, it causes patchy and focal inflammation, with only parts of some arteries being involved.

Epidemiology: a rare disease (about 5–10 per million per year in most populations), typically affecting young adults but can occur in all age groups; males more often than females by a factor of 2:1.

Aetiology: the cause is unknown but there is an association with chronic hepatitis B infection.

Pathogenesis: transmural necrotizing inflammation of the vessel wall with necrosis of muscle cells and destruction of the elastic lamina resulting in microaneurysm formation. Fibrinoid necrosis of part of the vessel's circumference is seen. Healing occurs with fibrous replacement of the muscular media. Extensive damage to the intima predisposes to thrombosis, which is often followed by vessel occlusion and downstream infarction.

Clinical features depend on the vascular bed involved, with vessel occlusion producing small areas of ischaemia and infarction. Systemic features of inflammation (fever, weight loss, myalgia and muscle wasting) are also seen. Antineutrophil cytoplasmic antibodies (ANCA) tests are negative. The tissues most seriously affected are the kidneys, heart, liver and gastrointestinal tract.

Buerger disease (thromboangiitis obliterans)

This is a rare disease affecting the small- and medium-sized arteries of the lower legs and arms. It characteristically presents in young males (under 35 years old) and is seen almost exclusively in heavy smokers. Pathologically, sharply demarcated segments of vasculitis are seen accompanied by thrombosis containing microabscesses. This can extend to affect adjacent veins and nerves, resulting in fibrosis. Clinically, claudication in the peripheries and Raynaud phenomenon are early symptoms, later evolving to peripheral gangrene of the fingers and toes; the disease is progressive and amputations are often required.

Small vessel vasculitides

Microscopic polyangiitis

Also known as leucocytoclastic vasculitis, this is a multisystemic necrotizing vasculitis of small blood vessels, e.g., capillaries and venules. It is relatively rare, affecting 2 per 100,000 in the UK, with a slight male bias. The age of onset is around 50 years. It predominantly causes severe crescentic glomerulonephritis, but can also involve the skin, lung, brain and gastrointestinal tract. Necrotizing but not granulomatous inflammation of small vessels is seen and is described as pauci-immune, as little immunoglobin can be detected within the lesions.

Churg-Strauss (eosinophilic granulomatosis with polyangiitis)

See Chapter 10 for a full discussion.

Granulomatosis with polyangiitis (Wegener disease)

See Chapter 10 for a full discussion.

Henoch-Schönlein purpura

See Chapters 13 and 17 for a full discussion.
Table 9.17 compares small-vessel vasculitides.

Neoplastic vascular disease

Benign

Haemangiomas

Haemangiomas are benign tumours of blood vessels and can occur anywhere within the body but are most commonly appreciated on the skin. They are composed of dilated vascular spaces, varying from small to large to cavernous (which are derived from blood vessels). There are numerous histological variants; three of the commoner ones include:

1. Capillary haemangiomas (strawberry naevi), which are composed of small, capillary-like vessels. They have a tendency to grow and then spontaneously regress.

Table 9.17 Small-vessel vasculitides[a]

Systemic involvement/ ANCA status	GPA (Wegener granulomatosis)	EGPA (Churg-Strauss syndrome)	Microscopic polyangiitis
ENT	+++	+	–
Lung	++ (granulomas)	++ (asthma)	–
Kidney	++	+/–	+++
Nerves	+	++	++
GIT	++	++	–
ANCA	cANCA+ >90%	c+p ANCA+ ~40%	pANCA+ >90%

[a] *Table comparing the distribution of the small vessel vasculitides and ANCA associations as an aid to diagnosis.*
cANCA, cytoplasmic antineutrophil cytoplasmic antibodies; EGPA, eosinophilic granulomatosis with polyangiitis; ENT, ear, nose and throat; GIT, gastrointestinal tract; GPA, granulomatosis with polyangiitis; pANCA, perinuclear antineutrophil cytoplasmic antibodies.

2. Cavernous haemangiomas, which are composed of cavernous, endothelial-lined spaces (vein-like vessels). These can involve deep structures and do not regress.
3. Sclerosing haemangiomas, which are fibrous nodules containing iron pigment produced as a result of fibrosis or sclerosis of a capillary haemangioma.

Telangiectasias

These are dilatations of preexisting capillaries. They are often seen in the elderly, those with irradiated skin or liver failure (spider naevi). They can occur as part of a hereditary syndrome, e.g., hereditary haemorrhagic telangiectasia, and are nonneoplastic.

Malignant

Kaposi sarcoma

This is associated with human herpes virus 8 (HHV8) and immunosuppressed states, e.g., HIV, iatrogenic. It is primarily a vascular tumour of the skin with a variable course ranging from indolent to disseminated with organ involvement. It has three stages: patch, plaque and nodule, with lesions being solitary or multiple. Clinically, it manifests as red–purple plaques or nodules, most commonly on the lower legs. Histologically, spindle cells with extravasated red blood cells, slit-like vascular channels and mononuclear inflammation are seen.

Angiosarcoma

A malignant tumour of blood vessel endothelium. This most commonly occurs as a raised bluish-red patch on the head and neck of elderly people, and is often confused with a benign haemangioma. Other common sites include the breast and liver. Risk factors for development include radiation, polyvinyl chloride, thorotrast, arsenic exposure and lymphoedema.

Angiosarcomas are aggressive cancers which invade locally and easily metastasize. The prognosis is poor; the 5-year survival rate is approximately 20%–30%.

DISEASES OF THE VEINS AND LYMPHATICS

Chronic venous insufficiency

This is a condition caused by ineffective venous return in the lower extremities resulting in blood pooling within the legs. It is initiated by venous valvular incompetence either from inherited valvular dysfunction or valve destruction post thrombosis. This manifests clinically as varicose veins.

Symptoms include aching or heavy legs, especially after long periods of standing, itching and improvement of symptoms when legs are elevated.

Sequelae:

- Oedema (of lower limbs) owing to increased hydrostatic pressure.
- Stasis dermatitis—erythematous, crusted, cracked skin with pigmentation due to haemosiderin deposition.
- Lipodermatosclerosis—a type of panniculitis (inflammation of adipose tissue) resulting in skin induration and hardening, redness, hyperpigmentation and small white scarred areas (atrophie blanche).
- Venous ulcers—nonpainful, shallow ulcers with irregular sloping edges occurring on the medial gaiter area, especially around the medial malleoli. The base contains yellow slough or pink granulation tissue and can be very pungent. They are usually colonized, but not infected by microorganisms (no lymphadenopathy) and are slow to heal. The surrounding skin may show changes associated with venous insufficiency.

COMMON PITFALLS

STASIS DERMATITIS VERSUS BILATERAL CELLULITIS

Skin changes associated with stasis dermatitis and lipodermatosclerosis can be mistaken by the unaware as 'bilateral cellulitis'. Be suspicious of a diagnosis of bilateral cellulitis as, whilst it is possible, cellulitis is usually unilateral and of acute onset.

Varicose veins

Varicose veins are persistently dilated superficial veins in the lower limbs (long and short saphenous veins). They result from incompetent valves that allow the veins to become engorged with blood under the influence of gravity.

Epidemiology: the condition affects 10%–20% of the general population. There is an increasing incidence with age, and it is most common above 50 years. It affects females more often than males by a factor of 4:1.

Table 9.18 lists the predisposing factors of varicose veins.

Pathogenesis: blood returns into the superficial veins → deep veins via the perforating veins of the deep fascia with aid from the muscle pump (Fig. 9.17). Valves aid the return by preventing regurgitation and stasis of blood. If a valve in the perforating veins fails, there is a transmission of high venous pressure from the deep system into the low-pressure superficial venous system. The increased venous pressure of the superficial veins causes them to dilate and become tortuous, resulting in sequential valve failure as the leaflets are unable to achieve apposition. Variceal veins are the result.

Table 9.18 Predisposing factors of varicose veins

Defective support of vessel wall
Familial tendency: in approximately 40% of all cases
Sex: significantly increased incidence in females
Obesity: adipose tissue = poor venous support muscle = good venous support
Age: degenerative changes in surrounding tissues and decreased activity of muscles → loss of venous support
Increased venous pressure
Standing occupations: increased incidence in occupations involving prolonged standing (venous pressure is greater on standing)
Pregnancy
Intravascular thrombosis
Tumour masses pressing on veins (e.g., uterine fibroids and ovarian tumours)
Garters and other constrictions

Sequelae of varicose veins

The sequelae are those of chronic venous insufficiency with:

- Deep vein thrombosis (very rare; tends to affect deep veins)
- Haemorrhage
- Phlebitis.

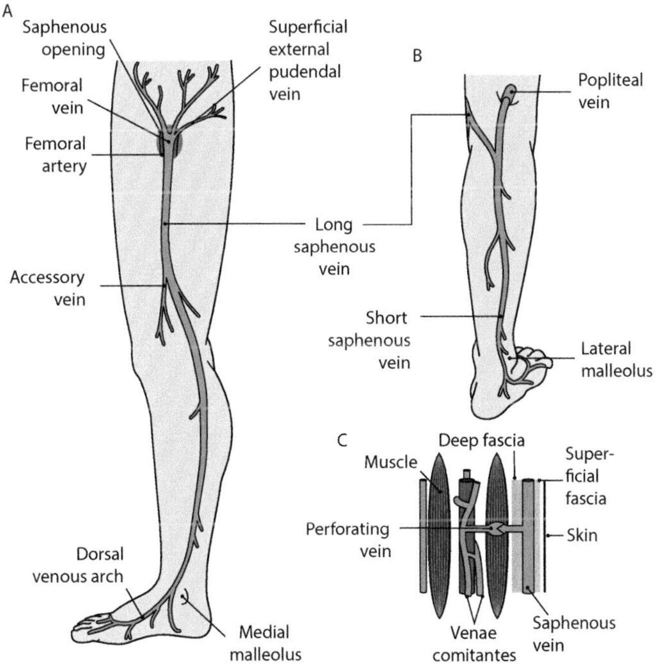

Fig. 9.17 Superficial veins of the right lower limb. (A) Long saphenous vein. (B) Short saphenous vein. (C) 'Venous pump' showing valved perforating veins, which link deep and superficial veins.

Lymphangitis and lymphoedema

Lymphangitis

Lymphangitis is inflammation of lymphatic channels draining any focus of infection. The channels are dilated and contain inflammatory cells and pathogenic organisms. This manifests as erythematous tracts on the skin, migrating proximally. The condition may result in the spread of the infection in some cases, e.g., in tuberculosis.

Lymphoedema

Lymphoedema is oedema of the tissues caused by obstruction of the lymphatics.

Causes

The causes of lymphoedema are:

- Primary
  - Congenital—simple congenital lymphoedema
  - Milroy disease—lymphatic agenesis or hypoplasia
- Secondary
  - Postinflammatory thrombosis and scarring, e.g., lymphogranuloma venereum.
  - Filariasis (elephantiasis)—nematode infection of lymph nodes (most common organism is *Wuchereria bancrofti);* transmitted by the bite of an infected mosquito.
  - Post-irradiation fibrosis.
  - Surgical removal of lymph nodes (e.g., axillary node clearance in breast carcinoma).
  - Metastatic spread of tumours causing mechanical blockage.

Effects

The effects of lymphoedema are:

- Gross oedema.
- Increased predisposition to attacks of lymphangitis and ulceration.
- Severe cases result in thickening of skin and overgrowth of dermal connective tissues leading to elephantiasis.

Chapter Summary

- Congenital heart disease can affect any structure within the heart, e.g., myocardium, valves, conducting system. It is divided broadly into cyanotic and acyanotic disease and can be described further by the direction of blood shunting, i.e., left to right or right to left.
- The commonest congenital heart defect is a ventricular septal defect.
- Atherosclerosis is associated with significant numbers of deaths in developed countries, therefore a thorough understanding of its pathogenesis is required.
- In 90% of patients, hypertension is idiopathic; hypertension arises from secondary causes in only 10% of patients.
- A thrombus occurs during life and may be arterial or venous.
- A pulmonary embolism is a feared complication of a deep vein thrombosis.
- Virchow triad is a change in the endothelium, a change in the flow of blood and a change in the constituents of blood (hypercoagulable state).
- A thrombus develops if any component of Virchow triad is altered.
- Ischaemic heart disease causes four syndromes: stable angina, unstable angina, myocardial infarction (MI) and sudden cardiac death.
- The site of an MI corresponds directly to the coronary artery that supplies a specific region of the heart.
- Hypertension and ischaemic heart disease are the commonest cause of left-sided heart failure.
- Left-sided heart failure is the commonest cause of right-sided heart failure.
- Rheumatic heart disease is diagnosed via the Jones criteria.
- Infective endocarditis is associated with classic clinical signs. Causative organisms differ depending on whether a heart valve is normal or abnormal.
- Cardiomyopathies are intrinsic disease of the myocardium and can be divided into hypertrophic, restrictive, dilated, arrhythmogenic right-ventricular cardiomyopathy and unclassified.
- Cardiac tumours are rare; examples include (atrial) myxoma and rhabdomyoma.
- Rapid accumulation of fluid in the pericardium results in cardiac tamponade.
- The main subtypes of acute pericarditis are fibrinous and suppurative; the main subtype of chronic pericarditis is constrictive.

- An aneurysm is a permanent dilatation of a blood vessel wall. The risk of rupture increases with increasing size.
- Aortic dissection is the entrance of blood into the wall of a blood vessel and tracking ('dissecting') between the layers.
- Vasculitis can be classified by vessel size (large, medium and small) and produces symptoms according to the affected vascular bed.
- Antineutrophil cytoplasmic antibodies (ANCA) are useful in the diagnosis of small-vessel vasculitis.
- Giant cell arteritis is the most common vasculitis.
- Chronic venous insufficiency results from venular valve incompetence causing pooling of blood within the lower limbs.
- Lymphoedema is oedema of the tissues caused by obstruction of lymphatics and may be congenital or acquired.

Pathology of the respiratory system 10

CONGENITAL AND DEVELOPMENTAL LUNG DISORDERS

Bronchogenic cysts

These are unilocular cysts arising most commonly in the anterior mediastinum or along the trachea and main bronchi, with which they can communicate. They arise from abnormal buds of the primitive foregut and do not form connections with alveolar tissue, unlike congenital pulmonary airway malformations (CPAMs) (see below).

The cyst walls contain a variable amount of cartilage and submucosal glands, and are lined by ciliated columnar epithelial cells.

Sequestration

Sequestrations are pieces of lung tissue which do not communicate with the tracheobronchial tree and derive their blood supply from systemic rather than local pulmonary supply, i.e., akin to an 'accessory lobe'. They can be extralobular (outside the visceral pleura) or intralobular (within the parenchyma). Microscopically they resemble normal lung; however, intralobular sequestra are prone to recurrent infection and show chronic inflammatory changes.

Congenital pulmonary airway malformations

Previously known as congenital cystic adenomatoid malformations, these are masses of maldeveloped tissue of the lower respiratory tract that are usually cystic and have abnormal bronchial proliferation. Typically, they are unilateral and affect a single lobe.

There are five subcategories based on histological appearance and size, reflecting the normal bronchial tree anatomy, e.g., proximal (bronchi) to distal (alveoli) (Table 10.1). They are usually identified antenatally by ultrasound or neonatally with respiratory distress. However, if small, they may not become apparent until adulthood where presentation is with repeated chest infections.

DISORDERS OF THE LUNGS

Numerous lung diseases and conditions exist, and categorization of them may be confusing. Fig. 10.1 is an aid in the subclassification of lung pathology.

Table 10.1 Congenital pulmonary airway malformation classification

CPAM type	Features
Type 0	Acinar dysplasia—global arrest of lung development with only dilated branching airways and no alveoli present. This represents a proximal bronchial anomaly and is incompatible with life.
Type 1[a]	Larger unilocular or multilocular cystic spaces 2–10 cm in diameter, may be lined by ciliated or mucinous epithelium and have cartilage within the walls.
Type 2[a]	Smaller cystic spaces <2 cm diameter, surrounded by alveolar tissue. Can be associated with pulmonary sequestration and renal agenesis.
Type 3	Solid lesion usually involving an entire lobe or lung. Appears like pulmonary hyperplasia. Rare.
Type 4	Large peripheral cyst, may be lined by flattened alveolar epithelium. Some cases represent low-grade cystic pleuropulmonary blastoma.

[a] *Types 1 and 2 are the most common, accounting for 70% and 20% of lesions, respectively. CPAM, Congenital pulmonary airway malformation.*

Atelectasis

This is defective expansion and collapse of the lung. It may occur as a result of:

- obstruction
- compression
- scarring
- surfactant loss

Obstructive causes

Obstruction of the larger bronchi leads to resorption of air from the distal lung, causing collapse. Causes of obstruction can be within the lung (e.g., mucus plugs in bronchiectasis, asthma, inhaled foreign bodies) or outside the lung (enlarged lymph nodes, as in tuberculosis (TB) or lung cancer).

Patchy atelectasis describes the pattern of atelectasis associated with chronic obstructive airway diseases.

Compressive causes

Compressive atelectasis is the compression of the lung caused by the accumulation of fluid or air in the pleural cavity, e.g., following a pneumothorax.

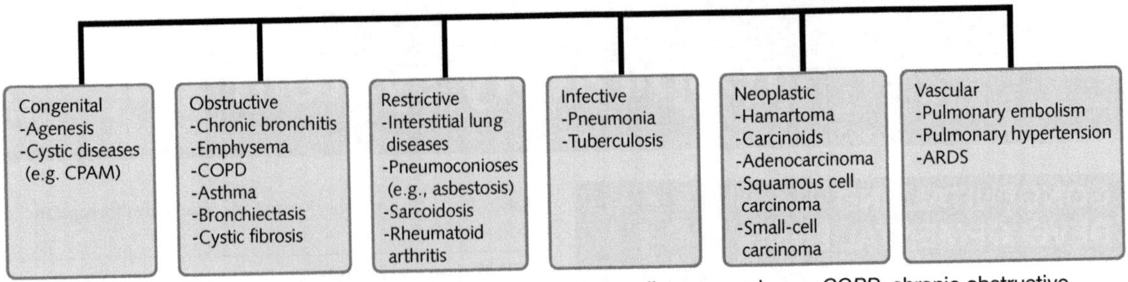

Fig. 10.1 Classification of lung pathology. *ARDS*, Acute respiratory distress syndrome; *COPD*, chronic obstructive airway disease; *CPAM*, congenital pulmonary airway malformation.

Scarring

Scarring of the lung may cause contraction of the parenchyma and lung collapse.

Surfactant loss

Surfactant is produced by type 2 pneumocytes (alveolar cells) reducing the surface tension of the alveoli and giving the lung sufficient compliance to expand without collapse. Surfactant loss can be either developmental or acquired and leads to a generalized failure of lung expansion, termed microatelectasis.

Lack of surfactant causes respiratory distress in premature infants; steroids may be administered to the mother to aid fetal lung development (and surfactant production) if premature labour is inevitable.

Consequences of atelectasis

The collapse of a lung has important clinical consequences as respiratory function will be disturbed and there is a predisposition to infection.

CLASSIFICATION OF DIFFUSE LUNG DISEASE

Diffuse lung disease can be classified as obstructive or restrictive based on the characteristics of pulmonary function tests (Fig. 10.2 and Table 10.2). They can both cause significant respiratory impairment.

Table 10.2 Patterns of lung function

	Obstructive lung diseases	Restrictive lung diseases
VC	↓ or normal	↓↓
FEV_1	↓↓	↓
FEV_1/VC ratio	↓	Normal or ↑
PEFR	↓	Normal

FEV1, Forced expiratory volume in 1 second; PEFR, peak expiratory flow rate; VC, vital capacity.

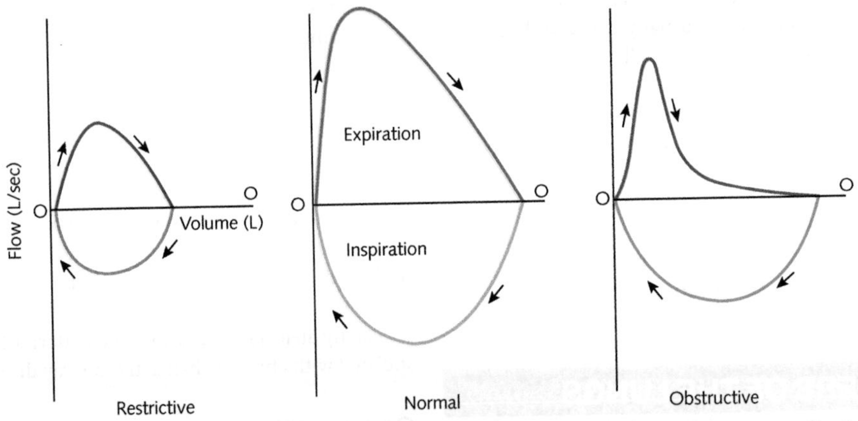

Fig. 10.2 Characteristic patterns of obstructive and restrictive lung diseases. Flow–volume loops illustrating normal, obstructive (chronic obstructive pulmonary disease) and restrictive deficits. Restrictive deficit shows a decrease in total lung volume with maintained flow as the airways are normal. Obstructive deficit shows a collapse (concave shape) in the expiration loop as flow rate reduces dramatically owing to partial obstruction of the small airways, impeding air expulsion.

Obstructive lung diseases

Obstructive lung diseases are those in which there is obstruction to the airflow within the lungs, although the lungs themselves may be hyperinflated. Disorders include emphysema, chronic bronchitis, bronchiectasis and asthma.

Chronic obstructive pulmonary disease

Chronic obstructive pulmonary disease (COPD) is a chronic, slowly progressive disease of airflow limitation caused by an abnormal inflammatory response of the lungs to noxious substances (usually from long-term cigarette smoking). COPD is used clinically where emphysema and chronic bronchitis occur together.

Pathological changes

COPD classically involves three overlapping pathological processes:

1. Chronic bronchitis—this causes hyperplasia of the bronchial submucosal glands, leading to an increased Reid index.
2. Emphysema—abnormal dilatation of air spaces with destruction of alveolar walls.
3. Bronchiolitis—this describes inflammation of the small airways (bronchioles).

Chronic bronchitis and emphysema are considered in more detail in separate sections below.

Diagnosis

Common symptoms of COPD are persistent cough, sputum production and breathlessness. If combined with a strong history of tobacco or pollutant exposure, lung function tests are performed (see Fig. 10.2 and Table 10.2). These are suggestive of COPD if:

- Forced expired volume in 1 second (FEV_1) is less than 80% predicted.
- FEV_1/forced vital capacity ratio is less than 70% predicted.
- The limitation is incompletely reversible with bronchodilators (e.g., inhaled salbutamol). This distinguishes the result from asthma, which is fully reversible.

A chest X-ray may show hyperinflation, flat hemidiaphragms, reduced peripheral vascular markings and bullae.

Complications

The frequency of complications increases with progression of the disease:

- Infection—this produces acute exacerbations of symptoms requiring hospital admission.
- Pneumothorax—bullae are thin-walled airspaces created by alveolar collapse. Rupture of subpleural bullae may produce a pneumothorax (Fig. 10.3).
- Respiratory failure—with hypoxia and hypercapnia (type 2 failure).
- Cor pulmonale—right-sided heart failure (see Chapter 9).

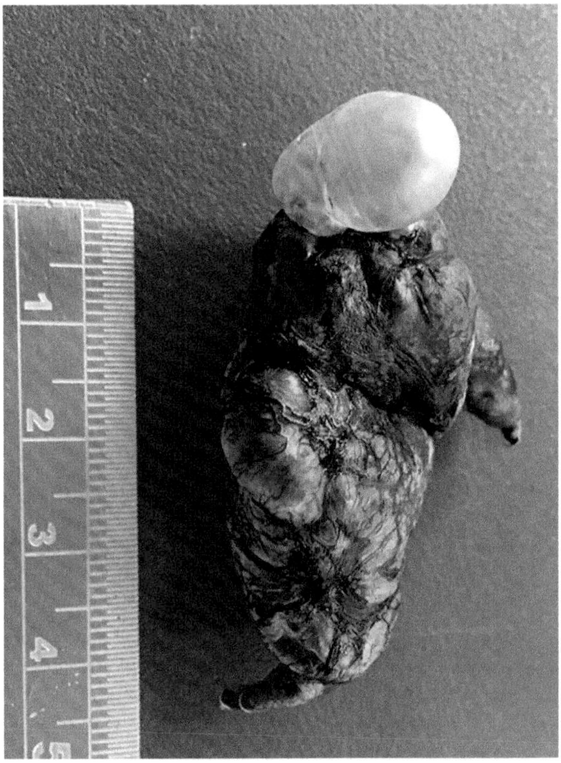

Fig. 10.3 Subpleural bulla. An apical wedge resection of lung showing subpleural bullae/blebs. It is easy to see how this could spontaneously burst and result in a pneumothorax.

Emphysema

Emphysema is a permanent dilatation of any part of the air spaces distal to the terminal bronchiole, occurring with tissue destruction but without fibrosis. It is a common condition, which usually forms part of COPD, but may occasionally present alone.

The aetiology is unclear, but risk factors are the same as for COPD, including cigarette smoking, occupational dusts or chemicals and atmospheric pollution. The inherited disorder α_1-antitrypsin deficiency (see Chapter 12) predisposes to early emphysema.

Pathogenesis

In normal individuals, extracellular elastases secreted into the lung by inflammatory cells are inhibited by protease inhibitors (particularly α_1-antitrypsin). In emphysema, these inhibitors are either inactivated (e.g., by cigarette smoke) or absent (inherited disorder), resulting in continued activity of the elastases with destruction of lung parenchyma. Destruction of respiratory tissue leads to a loss of elastic recoil in the lungs and a decreased area available for gaseous exchange. About one-third of lung capacity must be destroyed before clinical symptoms of emphysema appear.

Types of emphysema

There are several forms of emphysema, defined by the location of damage in the respiratory acinus (Fig. 10.4):

- Centrilobular—dilatation of the respiratory bronchioles at the centre of the acinus. It is most common in males and is closely associated with cigarette smoking. Lesions are usually found in the upper lobes.
- Panacinar—dilatation of the terminal acinus, which later affects the respiratory bronchioles, thereby affecting the whole acinus. This typically affects the lower lobes. This pattern is typically seen in inherited α_1-antitrypsin deficiency (caused by variants of the *pi* gene with the homozygous *piZZ* state resulting in hepatic cirrhosis as well).
- Paraseptal—involves air spaces at the periphery of lobules, typically subpleural. Usually affects the upper lobes adjacent to areas of scarring or atelectasis.
- Irregular—irregular involvement of the respiratory acinus and almost always associated with scarring. It is thought to be caused by the trapping of air following lung fibrosis and it is, therefore, commonly present around old healed tuberculous scars at the lung apices.

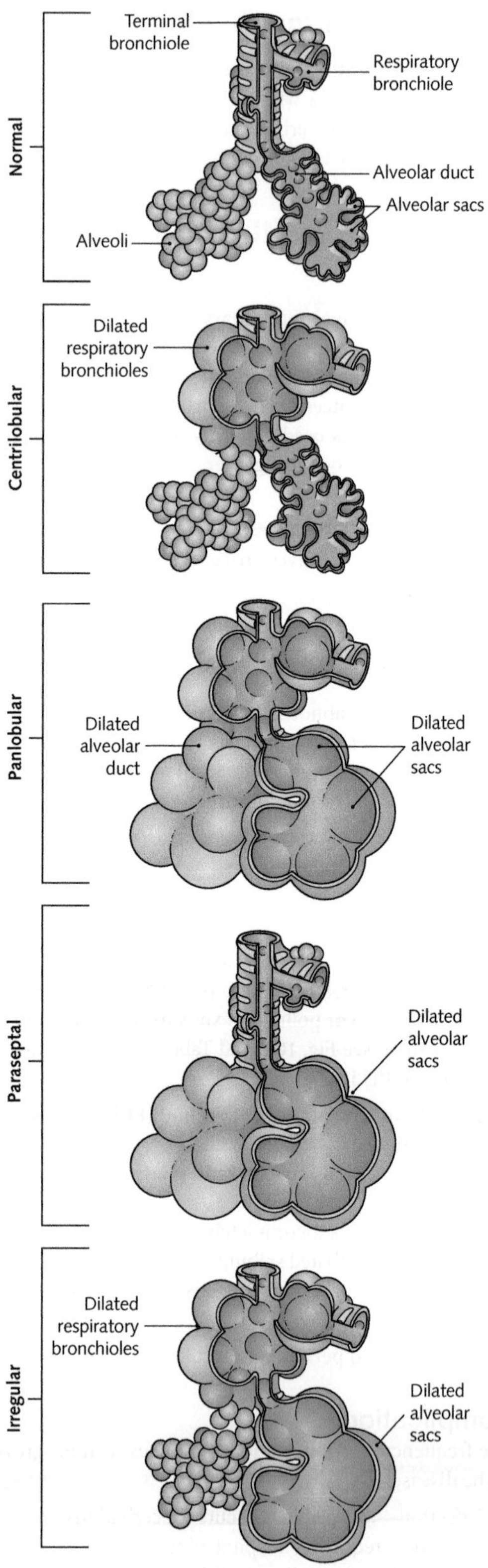

Fig. 10.4 Types of emphysema.

Clinical features

In the early stages of emphysema, a rapid respiratory rate enables individuals to maintain blood oxygenation, such that partial pressure of carbon dioxide ($PaCO_2$) and partial pressure of oxygen (PaO_2) are near normal. Patients are breathless but not cyanosed (so-called *'pink puffers'*). However, on the slightest exertion patients become increasingly breathless and ultimately hypoxic (type 1 respiratory failure). Complications are the same as described for COPD.

The lungs are hyperinflated, and the accessory muscles may be hypertrophied. Associated chronic bronchitis may produce cough and sputum. Breath sounds are quiet, especially over bullae, often with crepitations or wheezes.

Chronic bronchitis

Chronic bronchitis is defined as a cough productive of sputum on most days for 3 months of the year for at least 2 successive years. It typically affects middle-aged men and normally forms part of COPD; most cases are due to cigarette smoking.

Pathogenesis

Constant irritation by cigarette smoke causes chronic inflammation of the respiratory bronchioles (bronchiolitis) and increased mucus secretion.

Hypersecretion of mucus is associated with hyperplasia of the submucosal mucus-secreting glands. Proteases stimulate this hypersecretion following their release by neutrophils recruited as part of the inflammatory response. The Reid index gives the ratio of gland to wall thickness in the bronchus, and it is significantly increased in cases of chronic bronchitis.

Clinical features

Bronchiolar obstruction must be extensive and widespread to give clinical symptoms. Eventually, extensive mucus plugging leads to the clinical obstructive features of the disease with typical cough and sputum production.

In later stages of the disease, progressive obstruction may result in patients with hypercapnia, hypoxaemia and cyanosis (so-called '*blue bloaters*'). Other complications include:

- Recurrent low-grade bronchial infections caused by bacteria such as *Haemophilus influenzae* and *Streptococcus pneumoniae*, or viruses such as respiratory syncytial virus and adenovirus.
- Squamous metaplasia—loss of ciliated cells as a result of squamous metaplasia can further exacerbate the problem.
- Malignancy—persistent injury by smoking may invoke dysplastic changes in metaplastic squamous epithelium, which may ultimately become malignant (squamous cell carcinoma of the bronchus).

Asthma

Asthma is an increased irritability of the bronchial tree with paroxysmal narrowing of the airways, which may reverse either spontaneously or after treatment with bronchodilators.

This is a common disorder, affecting around 15% of children and 7% of adults. Its incidence is thought to be rising, possibly owing to environmental atmospheric pollution.

Classification

Asthma can be classified into two categories, depending on whether there is an allergic basis to the disease:

1. Extrinsic asthma (atopic)—this is the most common type of asthma. It is early-onset asthma triggered by environmental allergens. Individuals often have a family history of allergic disorders. IgE levels are raised and an immediate type 1 hypersensitivity to the allergen is produced on skin challenge.
2. Intrinsic asthma (nonatopic)—adult-onset asthma often associated with chronic bronchitis, as well as other asthma triggers such as cold or exercise. IgE levels are normal, there is no family history of allergic disorders and skin testing is negative.

However, there is often much overlap between the two types and many patients do not fit neatly into any one type.

Pathogenesis

There are three key features in both types of asthma:

1. Airflow limitation—obstruction is caused by a combination of bronchospasm, oedema and mucus plugging. This may be spontaneously reversible, or reversible with bronchodilator treatment.
2. Airway hyperresponsiveness to bronchoconstrictor trigger factors, e.g., cold air.
3. Airway inflammation—it appears that the allergic inflammatory process of extrinsic asthma is driven by type 2 helper T-cells (Th2). With time, airway remodelling occurs so that the smooth muscle of the bronchial wall becomes hypertrophied, increasing airflow limitation.

HINTS AND TIPS

DIFFERENTIATING ASTHMA FROM CHRONIC OBSTRUCTIVE PULMONARY DISEASE

Remember that both asthma and chronic obstructive pulmonary disease (COPD) are obstructive lung diseases, but there are key differences between them:

- Asthma is due to a sensitizing agent; COPD is due to a noxious agent.
- Asthmatic airway inflammation is predominated by CD4+ T-cells and eosinophils; COPD occurs with predominantly CD8+ T-cells, macrophages and neutrophils.
- Asthma airflow limitation is completely reversible with bronchodilator medication; COPD is only partially reversible.

The three phases of extrinsic asthma

- Early (15–20 minutes)—a rapid onset of bronchoconstriction caused by histamine release from mast cells. The allergen binds to IgE antibodies on the surface of mast cells, causing cross-linking and degranulation (Fig. 10.5).
- Late (4–6 hours)—following recovery from the early phase, inflammatory mediators released by mast cells cause activation of macrophages and chemotaxis of polymorphs and eosinophils into the bronchial

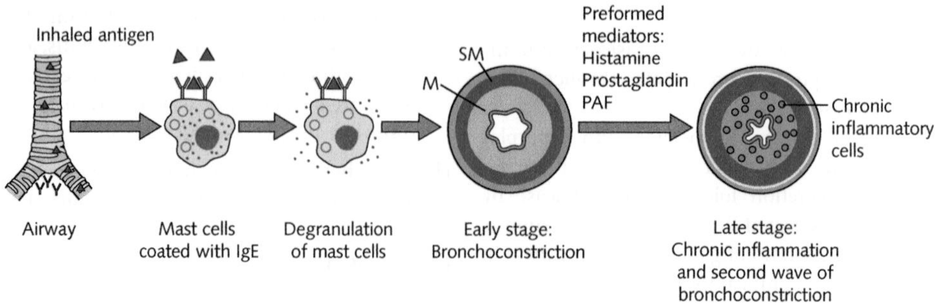

Fig. 10.5 Pathogenesis of asthma. Pathogenesis of the early and late stages of asthma. ▲, antigen; *M*, mucosa; *PAF*, platelet-activating factor; *SM*, smooth muscle; *Y*, IgE.)

mucosa. These cells release inflammatory mediators, causing a secondary wave of bronchoconstriction unrelated to exposure to the original antigen.

- Prolonged hyperreactivity (over days)—an exaggerated response of the airway on further reexposure to the allergen or other bronchoconstrictor trigger factors over ensuing days. Persistence of inflammatory cells within the bronchial wall leads to damage and loss of epithelial cells.

Structural changes

The main structural changes that take place in asthmatic airways are listed below and illustrated in Fig. 10.6:

- Immune cell infiltration—the bronchial mucosa is infiltrated by eosinophils, mast cells, lymphoid cells and macrophages.
- Mucosal oedema—extravasation of plasma into submucosal tissues produces a narrowing of the airways.
- Mucus hypersecretion leads to plugging of airways.
- Hypertrophy of bronchial smooth muscle owing to recurrent bronchoconstriction.
- Focal necrosis of the airway epithelium, caused by prolonged inflammation.
- Deposition of collagen beneath the bronchial epithelium in longstanding cases.
- Sputum contains Charcot–Leyden crystals (derived from eosinophil granules) and Curschmann spirals (composed of mucus plugs from small airways) (Fig. 10.7).

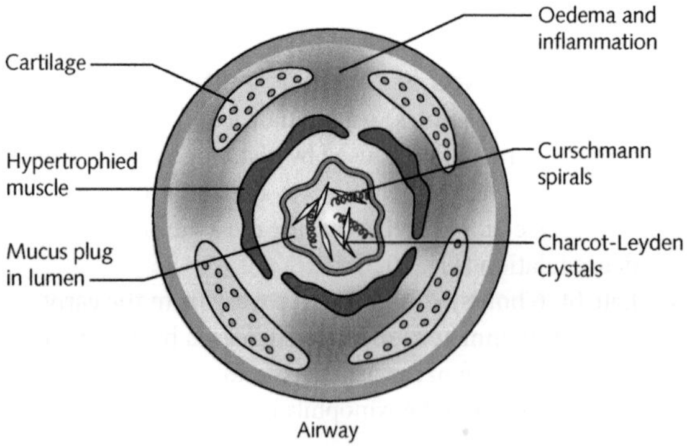

Fig. 10.6 Morphological airway changes in asthma.

Clinical features

Clinical features are as follows:

- Mild disease (majority of cases)—acute, intermittent episodes of bronchospasm (high-pitched wheezing, dyspnoea or coughing) are triggered by well-recognized causes.
- Moderate to severe disease (small percentage)—increasingly severe and irreversible asthma in middle or old age (chronic asthma); patients may present with signs of respiratory distress and may develop a barrel chest.
- Acute severe asthma (status asthmaticus)—severe, acute disease usually presenting with tachypnoea/respiratory distress, tachycardia and pulsus paradoxus. Death may result from acute respiratory insufficiency.

RED FLAG

STATUS ASTHMATICUS

In status asthmaticus, the silent chest is an ominous sign as air entry is so inadequate that the patient is unable to generate any wheeze! It is a life-threatening medical emergency.

Prognosis

- Remission—approximately 50% of cases of childhood asthma resolve spontaneously but may recur later in life; remission in adult-onset asthma is less likely.
- Mortality—death occurs in approximately 0.2% of asthmatics. Mortality is usually (but not always) preceded by an acute attack and about 50% are more than 65 years old.

Bronchiectasis

This is an irreversible dilatation of the bronchi or their branches. Its causes are:

- Congenital—cystic fibrosis (CF), primary ciliary dyskinesia and Kartagener syndrome (bronchiectasis, situs inversus and sinusitis).

- Acquired—infection (especially whooping cough, necrotizing pneumonia or measles in childhood) and obstruction (either by an inhaled foreign body or by tumour).
- Widened bronchi are more prone to infections, *Haemophilus influenzae* and *Pseudomonas aeruginosa* being the most common pathogens. Patients often cough up purulent sputum, which may contain blood.

Cystic fibrosis

CF is a hereditary multisystem disease characterized by the production of abnormally thick mucus, and primarily affects the lung and the pancreas. It is the most common autosomal recessive disorder, affecting 1 in 2000 newborns, with approximately 1 in 25 whites heterozygous carriers of the *CF* gene.

Pathogenesis

The mutated gene is found on chromosome 7 and encodes for a protein termed the cystic fibrosis transmembrane regulator (CFTR). The most common mutation is deletion of the phenylalanine residue at position 508 (ΔF508), which is found in 70% of cases. This protein normally enables the transport of chloride ions across cell membranes. In CF, defective CFTR results in impaired chloride transport, which prevents the release of sodium and water to liquefy mucus. The net result is the production of extremely thick and viscid mucus by the exocrine glands.

CLINICAL NOTE

CHLORIDE SWEAT TEST

The chloride sweat test is used in the diagnosis of cystic fibrosis; sweat is collected over 30 minutes and the concentrations of sodium and chloride are measured—these are elevated in cystic fibrosis.

Table 10.3 shows the organ systems affected by the epithelial dysfunction in CF.

In the respiratory tract, the bronchi and bronchioles become obstructed by abnormally viscid mucus, which leads to four main problems:

1. Infections—obstruction and stagnation of secretions leads to repeated bouts of infection, particularly with *Staphylococcus aureus* and *Pseudomonas aeruginosa*. *Burkholderia cepacia* infection is often intrinsically resistant to multiple antibiotics and some forms are transmissible between patients. This has resulted in the segregation of CF patients in hospitals and the community.
2. Bronchiectasis—a frequent complication (see section on 'Bronchiectasis' above).

Table 10.3 Organs affected in cystic fibrosis

Organ	Key features
Lungs	Abnormally viscid mucus cannot be cleared from the lungs, resulting in repeat infection and lung destruction
Intestine	Thick secretions cause meconium ileus in newborn babies and distal intestinal obstruction syndrome later in life
Pancreas	Causing deficiency of the pancreatic enzymes, resulting in malabsorption and failure to thrive
Liver	Thickened bile may cause biliary cholangitis and hepatic cirrhosis
Vas deferens	Failure of the vas deferens to develop leads to male infertility (though not sterility)
Cervix	Thickened cervical mucus can affect female fertility

3. Hyperinflation—due to air trapping behind mucus plugs; increased risk of developing spontaneous pneumothorax.
4. Hypoxia—scarring and destruction of the pulmonary vascular bed leads to pulmonary hypertension and cor pulmonale.

Prognosis

The previous median age of survival is just over 30 years, but nowadays CF sufferers are expected to live beyond 40 years. New drugs appear to reduce the rate of decline, as does lung transplant.

Restrictive lung diseases

Restrictive lung diseases are those in which there is dysfunctional lung expansion (e.g., due to fibrosis or oedema). In these diseases, although the lungs are often underinflated, the rate of airflow is unaffected.

Diffuse interstitial diseases

Interstitial lung diseases are a broad group of noninfectious, nonmalignant disorders in which there are varying degrees of inflammation and fibrosis of the lung parenchyma with characteristic patterns. This large group of diseases occurs with a mainly restrictive pattern. Disorders can be classified into broad groups, as shown in Table 10.4. There are thought to be over 200 distinct diffuse interstitial conditions and, confusingly, some of them have different histological names. The most important of these are discussed below.

Idiopathic pulmonary fibrosis

This disease, of unknown aetiology, is rare but increasing in incidence. It mainly affects the elderly and affects males

Table 10.4 Interstitial lung diseases

Groups	Clinical name	Histological pattern
Fibrosis	Idiopathic pulmonary fibrosis	Usual interstitial pneumonia
	Acute respiratory distress syndrome (ARDS)	Diffuse alveolar damage
	Cryptogenic organizing pneumonia	Organizing pneumonia
	Pneumoconiosis	Pneumoconiosis (several subtypes)
Smoking-related	Desquamative interstitial pneumonia	Desquamative interstitial pneumonia
	Respiratory bronchiolitis	Respiratory bronchiolitis
Granulomatous	Sarcoidosis	Sarcoidosis
	Hypersensitivity pneumonitis	Hypersensitivity pneumonitis
Eosinophilic	Pulmonary eosinophilia	Pulmonary eosinophilia (several subtypes)

more often than females. Clinical features of early-stage disease are a slowly increasing respiratory insufficiency owing to reduced lung capacity and residual volume, reduced compliance and reduced diffusion capacity. The characteristic signs are dyspnoea, cough and finger clubbing. There is a restrictive pattern of lung function tests.

Macroscopically, the lung is converted into a mass of cystic airspaces separated by areas of dense collagenous scarring. Microscopically, fibrosis occurs in a subpleural and paraseptal location. Characteristic 'honeycombing' (which may also be seen macroscopically or using high-resolution CT scanning) is seen, as are fibroblastic foci. Histologically this entity is known as usual interstitial pneumonia.

Median survival is 4 years, although the response to traditional end-stage drug regimens is very variable.

The pneumoconioses

This is a group of interstitial lung diseases resulting from chronic exposure to inorganic dust. The three most common types of pneumoconioses are coal-worker's pneumoconiosis (CWP), silicosis and asbestosis. If pneumoconiosis is associated with rheumatoid arthritis, this is known as Caplan syndrome.

In the normal lung, inhaled dust is coughed out or ingested by macrophages. However, if the dust is toxic to macrophages there is local inflammation, secretion of cytokines and stimulation of fibrosis. The result is a restrictive pattern of respiratory dysfunction.

Coal-worker's pneumoconiosis

CWP is an interstitial lung disease caused by inhaling coal dust. It has two types of pathology:

1. Simple CWP—nodules usually ≤1 mm; not usually associated with any clinically significant impairment of respiratory function, despite focal aggregates of dust-laden macrophages. The condition does not progress if the affected individual leaves the mining industry.
2. Progressive massive fibrosis—nodules >10 mm; large nodules and scarring results in severe respiratory impairment. The upper lobes are predominantly affected and there may be cavitation of the nodules. This condition may progress even after leaving the mining industry.

Silicosis

This is caused by the inhalation of quartz-containing dust (quartz being silicon dioxide), which is abundant in stone and sand.

It is associated with occupations such as slate mining, quarrying and stone masonry.

Pathogenesis—silica are toxic to macrophages, precipitating inflammation with fibrosis and nodule formation.

TB is a common complication of silicosis (silicotuberculosis). This is thought to be because of impaired local defences as a consequence of accumulated silica in macrophages.

Asbestosis

This interstitial lung disease is caused by the inhalation of asbestos, a fibrous silicate mineral that was widely used between 1890 and 1970. It is associated with occupations involving asbestos (mining/processing, building, insulation/fire-resistant material, shipyard and ship's engine-room work). There are two main forms of asbestos:

1. Serpentine asbestos (white asbestos)—this is the most common form; fibres persist in the lung for a limited time.
2. Amphibole asbestos (blue and brown asbestos)—fibres persist in the lung for many years and are the main cause of malignant mesothelioma.

Risk of disease depends on the duration and intensity of exposure, and the type of asbestos (crocidolite—blue fibres >100 μm are pathogenic).

The characteristics of asbestosis are:

- Latent period—25 years before clinical symptoms become evident.
- Basal interstitial fibrosis.
- Asbestos bodies—fibres coated in acid mucopolysaccharides and haemosiderin may be seen histologically (Fig. 10.8).

- Progressive restrictive type lung disease.
- Pulmonary hypertension—cor pulmonale may develop in the late stages.

Discussion of asbestos exposure in mesothelioma is discussed under pleural disease.

CLINICAL NOTE

DISEASES CAUSED BY ASBESTOS EXPOSURE

Diseases caused by asbestos exposure:

- *Pleural plaques*—well-delineated plaques formed of collagen ± calcification as a result of asbestos exposure. Can be seen on chest X-ray
- *Asbestosis*—diffuse pulmonary fibrosis caused by asbestos
- *Lung cancer*—asbestos exposure increases risk of lung cancer
- *Mesothelioma*—primary malignancy of the pleura

Note: asbestos exposure combined with smoking greatly increases the risk of developing lung cancer but not mesothelioma.

Sarcoidosis

Sarcoidosis is a multisystem disease of unknown aetiology characterized by the presence of noncaseating granulomas primarily affecting the lymph nodes and lungs.

Maximum incidence is in people between 30 and 40 years of age, affecting females slightly more than males.

Other affected sites are the skin, lymph nodes, eyes, liver, spleen, nervous system, phalanges, parotid glands and (rarely) the heart.

The aetiology is unknown but is thought to involve a type IV hypersensitivity reaction. The disease seems to be less common in smokers and more common with increasing geographical distance from the equator.

Histology shows noncaseating histiocytic granulomas in the lung interstitium (Fig. 10.9). Patients with lung involvement present with slowly progressive dyspnoea and cough and are found to have lung shadowing on chest radiograph with bilateral hilar lymphadenopathy.

Diagnosis—there are no diagnostic blood tests for sarcoidosis, but there is often hypercalcaemia, raised serum angiotensin-converting enzyme (ACE) and a reduced tuberculin skin test. The definitive diagnosis is histological, requiring a tissue sample, e.g., skin lesion biopsy, transbronchial biopsy.

Other interstitial lung diseases

Other interstitial lung diseases of note are:

- Goodpasture disease—a diffuse pulmonary haemorrhagic syndrome caused by complement activation following autoantibody binding to the basement membrane.

Table 10.5 Causes of hypersensitivity pneumonitis

Disease	Inhaled antigen
Bird-fancier's and pigeon-fancier's lung	Proteins in bird droppings
Farmer's lung (exposure to mouldy hay)	*Saccharopolyspora rectivirgula* *Thermoactinomyces vulgaris*
Malt worker's lung	*Aspergillus clavatus*
Bagassosis (exposure to molasses)	*Thermoactinomyces sacchari*

- Idiopathic pulmonary haemosiderosis—a rare condition with type 2 pneumocyte hyperplasia.
- Rheumatoid disease—granulomatous inflammation of the lung and pleura are seen in 10%–15% of patients (see Chapter 16).
- Hypersensitivity pneumonitis—immune-mediated interstitial granulomatous inflammation caused by inhalation of organic agents (type III and type IV hypersensitivity). Examples include farmer's lung and pigeon-fancier's lung (Table 10.5).

INFECTIONS OF THE LUNGS

Pneumonia

Pneumonia is defined as infection of the lower respiratory tract, resulting in consolidation of lung tissue with an intraalveolar inflammatory exudate.

Pneumonia is the third most common cause of death in the UK in ≥50-year-olds. It is most common in the very young, the elderly and those who are debilitated or immobile.

Clinical features: Fever, shortness of breath, cough, pleuritic pain and sputum (occasionally with haemoptysis). Signs of consolidation include bronchial breathing and/or coarse crackles. Severe infection requires hospital admission.

CLINICAL NOTE

CURB-65

Severity of pneumonia can be assessed using the *CURB-65* score:

Score 1 point each for:

Confusion: new mental confusion

Uraemia: >7 mmol/L blood urea

Respiratory rate: raised ≥30 breaths/min

Blood pressure: hypotensive—systolic ≤90 mmHg ± diastolic ≤60 mmHg

65: ≥65 years old

Total: 0–1: home treatment, ≥2: severe requiring hospital therapy, ≥3: high risk of death.

Predisposing factors: These can be remembered using the mnemonic 'INSPIRATION'.

CLINICAL NOTE

INSPIRATION

Remember **INSPIRATION** for the predisposing factors of pneumonia:

- ***I***mmunosuppression
- ***N***eurological impairment of the cough reflex
- ***S***ecretion retention
- ***P***ulmonary oedema
- ***I***mpaired mucociliary clearance
- ***R***espiratory tract infection (viral)
- ***A***ntibiotics and cytotoxins
- ***T***racheal instrumentation
- ***I***mpaired alveolar macrophages
- ***O***ther
- ***N***eoplasia

Classification

Pneumonia can be classified according to:

- Microbiology: causative organisms may be bacterial, viral, fungal or protozoal (Table 10.6).
- Pattern of infection: either lobar or bronchopneumonia (Table 10.7).
- Clinical classification: according to disease acquisition, i.e., community-acquired, hospital-acquired, disease of immunosuppression or aspiration pneumonia.

Table 10.6 Common pathogenic bacteria in hospital and community-acquired pneumonia

Community-acquired infection	Hospital-acquired infection
Streptococcus pneumoniae (>60%)	*Klebsiella spp.*
Haemophilus influenzae	*Pseudomonas spp.*
Legionella pneumophila	*Acinetobacter spp.*
Staphylococcus aureus	Methicillin-resistant *Staphylococcus aureus* (MRSA)
Mycoplasma pneumoniae	*Escherichia coli*
Chlamydia pneumoniae	*Proteus spp.*
Chlamydia psittaci	*Serratia spp.*
Pneumocystis jirovecii (carinii)	Organisms responsible for community-acquired pneumonia can also occur in a hospital setting (but much less frequently)

Causative organisms

Bacterial infection is the most common type of pneumonia, accounting for 80%–90% of cases. Knowledge of the circumstances in which a person develops pneumonia is a strong clue as to the likely organism causing the infection.

As a general rule of thumb, community-acquired pneumonia is usually caused by Gram-positive bacteria whereas hospital-acquired pneumonias are mainly due to Gram-negative bacteria.

Bronchopneumonia

This condition primarily affects the very young, very old or debilitated patients, usually occurring as a secondary event to another predisposing condition. Infection is centred on the bronchi with extension of the acute inflammatory exudate into the alveoli, causing patchy consolidation of the lung; it is not confined to a specific lobe (Fig. 10.10).

Pathogenesis

Infectious organisms enter via the respiratory tract, or rarely by haematogenous spread, and migrate down the bronchial tree, causing patchy suppurative peribronchial inflammation which is not limited to a single lobe, and is often bilateral.

Macroscopically: multiple areas of consolidation are centred around bronchi/bronchioles in dependent parts of the lung. Affected areas are firm and airless and have a white/yellow appearance. Bronchial mucosa is inflamed and pus can be expressed from the more peripheral airways.

Microscopically: there is acute suppurative inflammation of the bronchi and bronchioles, with extension into the alveolar spaces. Neutrophils are abundant in the exudate. Areas of inflammation are bordered by normal aerated lung parenchyma.

On resolution, the inflammatory exudate is often not completely absorbed; instead, it is organized with residual fibrous scarring and permanent lung dysfunction.

Lobar pneumonia

This condition often affects otherwise healthy adults, primarily between the ages of 20 and 50 years old. Consolidation is confined to a lobe and can be partial or involve the whole lobe (Fig. 10.11). Most cases are caused by *Streptococcus pneumoniae* (Gram-positive diplococci), which is the most common cause of community-acquired pneumonia.

Pathogenesis

Organisms gain entry to distal air spaces without colonization of bronchi. Infection spreads rapidly through the alveolar spaces and bronchioles, causing acute inflammatory exudation into air spaces.

Macroscopically: the whole/partial lobe becomes consolidated and airless. Infection is limited by the pulmonary fissures. There is relative sparing of the bronchioles. Fibrinous pleuritis can be present if the inflammation extends to the pleura.

Table 10.7 Bronchopneumonia versus lobar pneumonia

	Lobar pneumonia	Bronchopneumonia
Affected groups	Healthy individuals	Very young, elderly, debilitated
Distribution	Single lobe	Centred on bronchioles, not restricted to a single lobe
Outcome	Complete resolution and tissue restoration	Incomplete resolution with scarring and tissue destruction
Mortality	Majority recover	Significant risk of death

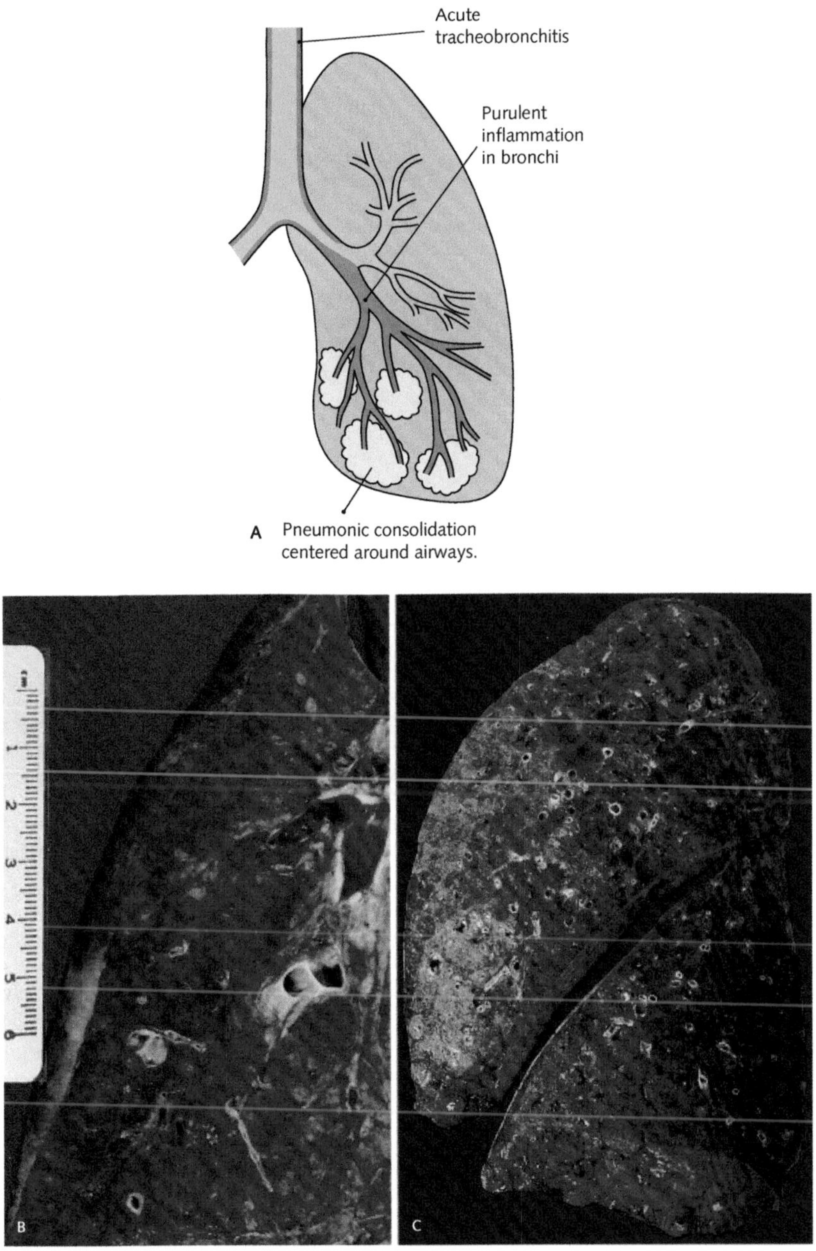

Fig. 10.10 Bronchopneumonia. (A) Bronchopneumonia. (B) Patchy consolidation around small bronchi and bronchioles scattered throughout the lobe. The lesions are grey to red in colour. (C) Confluent grey areas of necrotizing bronchopneumonia centred on the bronchioles with normal intervening lung parenchyma.

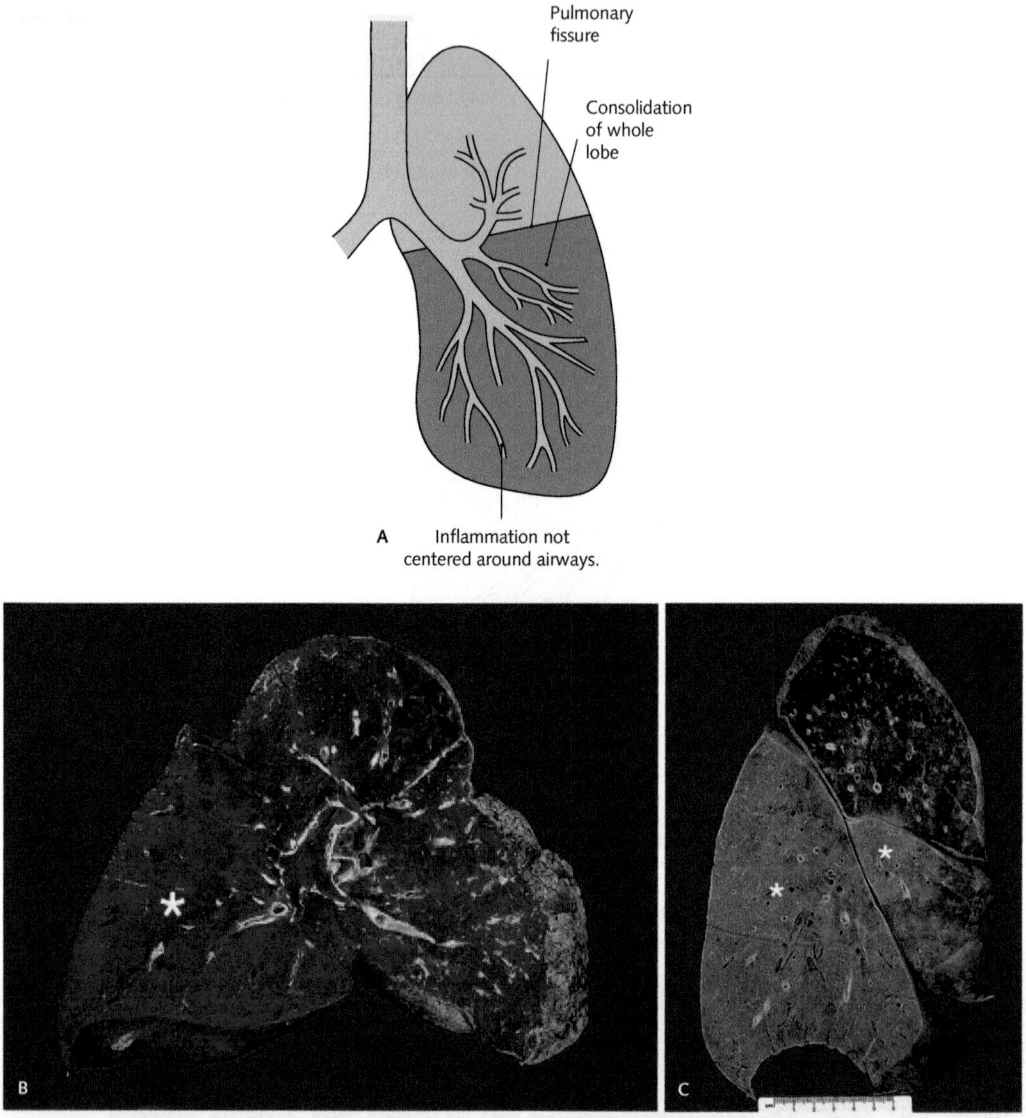

Fig. 10.11 Lobar pneumonia. (A) Lobar pneumonia. (B) Red hepatization. The right lower lobe (asterisk) is inflamed, consolidated and hyperaemic. (C) Grey hepatization showing confluent involvement of two lobes (asterisk) confined by the pleura. The remaining upper lobe is normal.

Microscopically: the alveoli are filled with an acute fibrinosuppurative inflammatory exudate.

Lobar pneumonia evolves through four pathological stages:

1. *Congestion*—acute inflammatory response to an infectious organism with increased alveolar bloodflow, capillary congestion and a protein-rich exudate into the alveoli comprising neutrophils and pathogens.
2. *Red hepatization*—the lobe appears and has the consistency of a piece of liver (hence 'hepatization'). The lobe feels firm and fibrin tags may start to appear on the pleural surface. There is massive accumulation of red cells, neutrophils, bacteria and a fibrin-rich exudate in the alveolar spaces. The alveolar walls are thickened due to oedema and vascular congestion.
3. *Grey hepatization*—the lobe appears grey owing to red cell degeneration and retains the consistency of liver. The alveolar spaces are full of pus, composed of neutrophils and macrophages which are required for fibrin degradation. The alveolar walls remain thickened.
4. *Resolution*—macrophages remove alveolar debris, which is drained via lymphatics and expectorated via the bronchioles and bronchial tree. Most patients recover with their lungs returning to normal structure and function.

Complications and sequelae of pneumonia

- Respiratory failure—usually type 1.
- Hypotension—combination of dehydration and vasodilation secondary to sepsis.
- Atrial fibrillation—common in the elderly.
- Sepsis.
- Bacteraemia—bacterial dissemination of organisms can lead to septicaemia with meningitis, arthritis and endocarditis.
- Lung abscesses—single or multiple areas of suppurative necrosis with cavitation. They are commonly caused by anaerobic bacteria in the context of aspiration pneumonia and are also seen with *Staphylococcus aureus* and *Klebsiella pneumoniae* infections.
- Empyema—a collection of pus in the pleural space owing to extension of underlying parenchymal infection and inflammation into the pleural cavity.
- Jaundice—secondary to sepsis and/or a side-effect of antibiotic use, e.g., co-amoxiclav.
- Pleural effusion—noninfected reactive effusion is common.
- Pericarditis—bacteraemic spread or direct extension of infection to the pericardium.
- Bronchial damage—in bronchopneumonia, imperfect repair of the bronchial mucosa results in scarring of the bronchial wall, with increased predisposition to further infection and bronchiectasis.
- Death—increased risk if pneumonia is severe and particularly if it is a terminal manifestation of debilitating diseases or linked to alcoholism.

Atypical pneumonia

Atypical pneumonia may be caused by a variety of infectious agents, e.g., viruses, fungi, *Mycoplasma*, *Chlamydia* and *Rickettsia* species. It is termed 'atypical' as patients develop a low-grade fever, dry cough and dyspnoea, but have little sputum and few signs of consolidation. In addition, the course is more protracted. It may be patchy or involve an entire lobe. Pleural effusions are uncommon.

The inflammation is centred in the alveolar interstitium and interlobular septa (acute interstitial pneumonitis) with vascular congestion and a mononuclear cell infiltrate. Neutrophils are not a prominent feature. Alveolar consolidation is absent but pink proteinaceous exudate may occur.

The normal architecture of the lung is preserved following resolution of the infection.

Viral pneumonia

This is a common cause of pneumonia in early childhood but is much less frequent in healthy adults. The majority of viral lung infections cause an atypical pneumonia, which is typically self-limiting (e.g., parainfluenza, influenza, respiratory syncytial virus, varicella and adenoviruses). However, these infections can prove fatal in an immunocompromised host.

A minority of viruses cause a much more severe pattern of infection. The influenza viruses can cause an acute fulminating pneumonia with pulmonary haemorrhage; the clinical course may be rapidly fatal.

A common complication is secondary infection with pyogenic bacteria, owing to the stripping of the respiratory epithelium by the initial viral infection preventing mucociliary clearance. This can transform a mild viral lung infection into a severe suppurative bronchopneumonia, particularly after influenza infection.

MOLECULAR

FLU VACCINATION—ANTIGENIC SHIFT AND DRIFT

The influenza virus contains the viral envelope proteins haemagglutinin (H) and neuraminidase (N), of which there are various subtypes, e.g., H2. Small genetic mutations occur over time such that the viruses remain related but are antigenically subtly different, conveying partial immune protection in those previously exposed. This is called antigenic drift and is why the 'flu' vaccine is required yearly as the constituents are modified to mirror the antigenic drift. Pandemics occur because of antigenic shift. Here there is an abrupt change to H and/or N protein subtypes, with the introduction of a new subtype from the animal population, e.g., 'avian flu'—H5N1 influenza virus. In this situation, no immunity exists within the population and the virus spreads rapidly.

Mycoplasma

Mycoplasma species (the commonest is *Mycoplasma pneumoniae*) account for 15%–20% of community-acquired pneumonia. It is more common in children between 5 and 15 years and may occur in epidemics. Infection can also cause extrapulmonary sequelae, including cold agglutinin haemolytic anaemia, thrombocytopenic purpura, erythema multiforme, arthralgias and meningoencephalitis.

Chlamydia and *Rickettsia*

A number of chlamydial and rickettsial infections are complicated by the development of pneumonia. Such infections include typhus, psittacosis *(Chlamydia psittaci)* and Q fever *(Coxiella burnetii)*. Fatal cases are rare, except in psittacosis.

Pneumonia in the immunocompromised

The lungs of immunocompromised patients are extremely prone to infection and it is not uncommon to have coinfection with multiple pathogens. Infectious agents include opportunistic pathogens, i.e., microorganisms that are nonpathogenic to immunocompetent individuals.

Pathogens associated with immunocompromised states include:

- Viruses—cytomegalovirus, respiratory syncytial virus, varicella zoster virus, measles. Cytomegalovirus pneumonitis is particularly common after bone marrow transplantation.
- Fungi—these include *Candida, Aspergillus* and *Pneumocystis.*

Pneumocystis jirovecii: (previously *carinii*) pneumonia (PCP) is common in patients with AIDS. Classically the features are those of a nonproductive cough, increasing shortness of breath, hypoxia on exertion, and bilateral perihilar interstitial infiltrates on chest X-ray. The alveoli are filled with a fine, honeycomb-like proteinaceous material in which small fungal yeasts are seen. This disease has a mortality rate of 10%–20% in those with AIDS.

Candida and Aspergillus: these can both cause widespread areas of necrosis, with the formation of microabscesses containing characteristic fungal hyphae. Mortality is high in invasive pulmonary aspergillosis.

Pulmonary tuberculosis

Pulmonary TB is a chronic granulomatous infection of the lung caused by *Mycobacterium tuberculosis.* It is uncommon in the UK and other developed countries (at about 10 per 100,000, although 26 per 100,000 in London), but extremely common worldwide (up to 500–1000 per 100,000 in parts of Africa and Asia), where it is a leading cause of death.

Rates in the UK are increasing because of HIV infection, an increasingly elderly population, overcrowding, social deprivation, immigrant populations and a reduced priority for control. The development of multidrug-resistant (MDR) tuberculosis has exacerbated this problem.

It should be noted that there are approximately 40 species of mycobacterium, including *Mycobacterium leprae* (causing leprosy), *Mycobacterium bovis* and more opportunistic species such as *Mycobacterium avium-intracellulare* and *Mycobacterium kansasii.*

The classic clinical features of pulmonary TB are fever, night sweats, weight loss and haemoptysis.

Transmission

Transmission is by various means:

- Droplet inhalation of *Mycobacterium tuberculosis* is by far the commonest mode.
- Ingestion of food or unpasteurized milk.
- Inoculation of the skin.
- Haematogenous (usually from intestinal TB).
- Transplacental spread, i.e., congenital TB.

Diagnosis

There are many methods of diagnosis e.g., Ziehl–Neelsen stain (Fig. 10.12), polymerase chain reaction or microbiological culture (which is used to determine antibiotic resistance and sensitivity.).

Risk factors

Risk factors are:

- Close contact with infected individuals—increased risk for those living/working in crowded or unhygienic conditions and for healthcare workers.
- Immunosuppression—the very young, very old, those on immunosuppressive therapy or patients with diseases of immunodeficiency, particularly AIDS.
- Malnourishment.
- Other diseases—preexisting chronic lung disease (especially silicosis), diabetes mellitus and alcoholism.

Pathogenesis

The destructive effects of infection are entirely due to the hypersensitivity reaction of the host directed against bacterial cell wall constituents. The following sequence of events occurs:

1. 0–10 days—mycobacteria excite a transient but marked acute inflammatory response. Neutrophils phagocytose the organisms but are unable to destroy them, as the cell walls are resistant to degradation. Instead, engulfed bacteria are drained into local lymph nodes.
2. After 10 days—development of a T-cell–mediated immune response (type IV hypersensitivity reaction) to the bacterial cell wall constituents results in cytokine release and macrophage activation. Gradually a chronic inflammatory pattern develops, which is dominated by aggregates of epithelioid macrophages, which form variable numbers of granulomas with a central core of necrosis containing viable mycobacteria. Tuberculous granulomas are termed tubercles.

Macroscopically, the granulomas appear as pinhead-sized white or greyish foci (tubercles) in the tissues.

Microscopically, granulomas with a central area of amorphous necrosis are the histological hallmark of TB infection. These granulomas often contain a specific type of multinucleated macrophage called a Langhans giant cell (Fig. 10.13).

The healing of a granuloma occurs slowly, with progressive fibrosis and later calcification. The central necrotic area remains caseous for some time and mycobacteria may remain viable indefinitely within a healed lesion. This is partly due to the ability of *M. tuberculosis* to remain latent within macrophages (inside phagosomes), inhibiting the fusion of lysosomes. Reactivation results in secondary (or postprimary) TB.

TB can be classified into two types, according to the pattern of infection:

1. Primary infection—the first encounter with the organism, resulting in the development of a small parenchymal peripheral focus with a large response in the draining lymph nodes.
2. Secondary infection—reactivation or reinfection of a previously infected individual, resulting in the development of a large, localized, parenchymal reaction but with minimal lymph node involvement.

Primary tuberculosis

The lung is by far the most common site of primary infection, usually occurring in a child or young adult with no specific immunity. Other sites include the pharynx, larynx, skin and intestine.

Inhaled organisms proliferate in the alveoli at the periphery of the lung, often just beneath the pleura. This primary parenchymal tubercle is termed the Ghon focus. It is often associated with enlarged caseous hilar lymph nodes. The combination of lung and lymph node lesions together constitutes the primary complex or Ghon complex.

Primary TB will either resolve or progress as shown below.

Resolution

This occurs in the majority of cases (85%–90%) and the episode is often entirely asymptomatic. The Ghon focus and caseating granulomas in the lymph nodes heal with fibrosis. The disease does not progress owing to the confinement of organisms within a fibrotic shell. However, walled-off bacteria may remain viable within the healed primary complex (latent TB). A tuberculin skin test becomes positive 1–2 months after the onset of infection.

Progression

In patients with poor immunity, the disease is progressive. There is a further spread of mycobacteria with continuing enlargement of the caseating granulomas in the lymph nodes (progressive primary TB). Enlarging nodes spread the infection by eroding into adjacent structures in two ways:

1. Bronchus—erosion of an infected lymph node into a bronchus results in tuberculous bronchopneumonia (Fig. 10.14a). The bacilli pass along the bronchi of one lung where infection can then spread into the opposite lung. There is further spread of infection into the bronchioles and alveoli with the development of extensive, confluent, caseating, granulomatous lesions. This condition is known as 'galloping consumption' and it is usually rapidly fatal.
2. Blood vessel—erosion of an infected lymph node into a blood vessel results in haematogenous spread of mycobacteria to many parts of the body, including the remainder of the lung, causing miliary TB (Fig. 10.14b).

Direct lymphatic spread (i.e., without erosion) may allow spread to the pleura and pericardium.

Secondary tuberculosis

This occurs as a result of the reactivation of quiescent but viable mycobacteria in hosts with weakened immune responses or on immunosuppressive therapy. It results in reinfection by additional organisms. Reactivation occurs in 5%–10% of those with latent infection, usually in the lungs.

Caseous granulomas typically develop in the apical segments of the lungs, spreading directly and locally but without lymph node lesions. Secondary TB will either resolve or spread, as shown below (Table 10.8).

> **HINTS AND TIPS**
>
> **DIFFERENTIATING PRIMARY AND SECONDARY TUBERCULOSIS**
>
> Tuberculosis (TB) is a good example of a chronic inflammatory disease. Remember that primary pulmonary TB has a small granulomatous focus but large lymph node response. By contrast, secondary TB presents with large granulomatous disease (potentially in several different tissues) and minimal lymph node involvement.

Resolution

Spontaneous healing with fibrosis and calcification occurs, although viable organisms may remain without producing any clinical symptoms.

Spread

In adults with poor immune responses, secondary TB progresses locally with direct extension and continuing caseation. Further spread of mycobacteria produces various types of progressive TB:

- Apical cavitation fibrocaseous TB—a direct extension of the infection. Continuing caseation results in the formation of a large caseous mass. If caseous material is expectorated, a cavity results. The lesion can heal at this stage, but it may spread further into the bronchi, bloodstream, directly into the pleura or into the gastrointestinal tract if swallowed. These cavities may be colonized by fungi, especially Aspergillus, forming an aspergilloma.
- Tuberculous pneumonia (see above).
- Miliary TB—the disease becomes widely disseminated with numerous small granulomas in many organs (e.g., kidneys, liver, bone marrow and meninges).
- Complications are often the result of extensive fibrosis involved in the healing process:
    - Pulmonary fibrosis—this is common in relapsing and progressive untreated disease.
    - Pleural fibrosis with obliteration of the pleural space.
- Bronchiectasis—dilatation of the airways can cause secondary infection.

Immunization with the Bacillus Calmette-Guérin (BCG) vaccine is common practice in the UK, with a protective efficacy of 60%–80%.

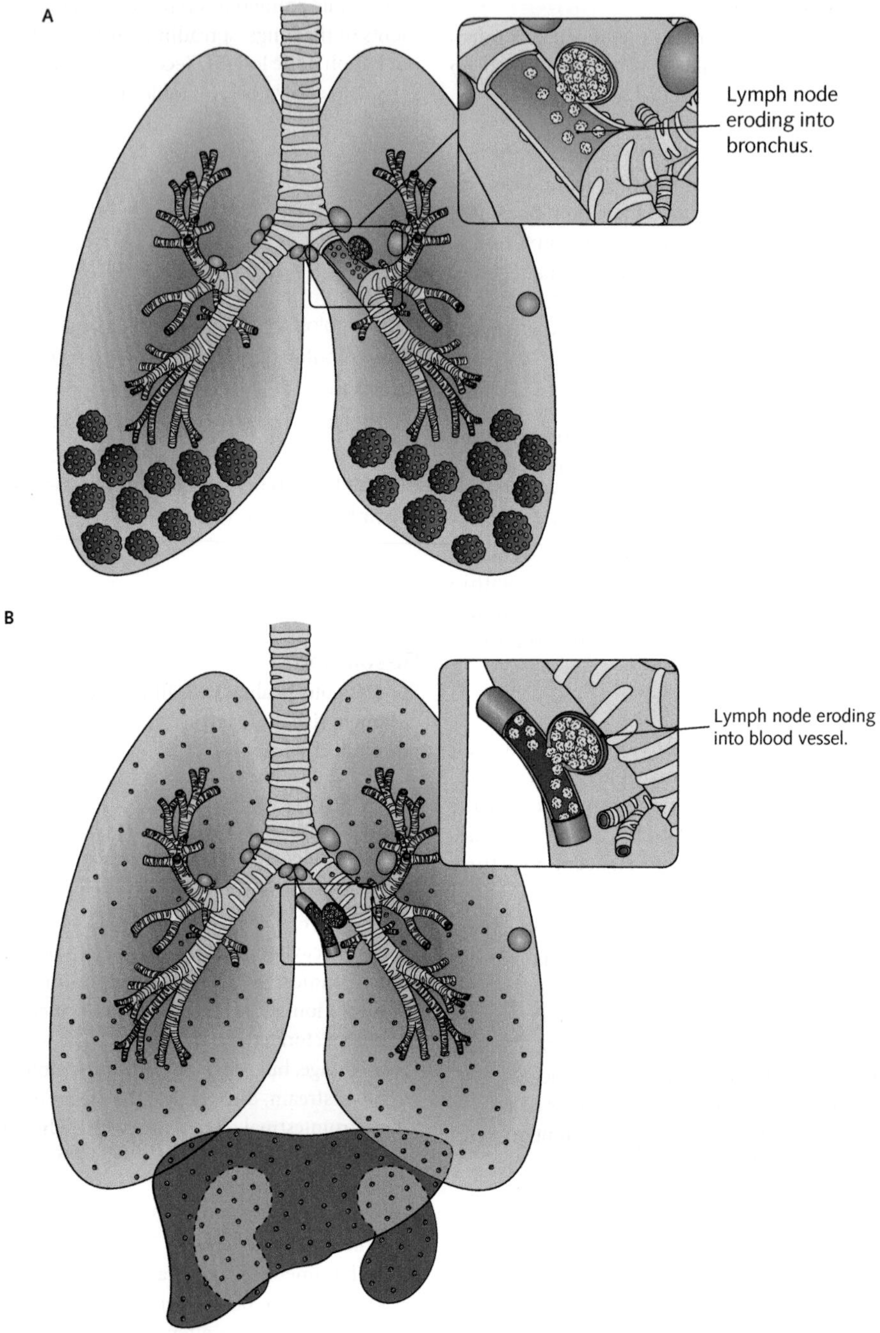

Fig. 10.14 Routes of spread of tuberculosis (TB). Patterns of progressive pulmonary TB. (A) Tuberculous bronchopneumonia. (B) Miliary TB of the lung.

CLINICAL NOTE

IMMUNE RECONSTITUTION

Immune reconstitution or immune reconstitution inflammatory syndrome is the paradoxical relapse of tuberculosis (TB) in a person with HIV after initiation of antiretroviral therapy. It occurs as a result of improvement in CD4+ T cell counts, which allows the patient to mount an immune response to a previously unknown or subclinical TB infection. Therefore, it is important to test all HIV patients for TB prior to initiating therapy.

Table 10.8 Important tuberculosis definitions

Term	Definition
Primary TB	Initial infection in the lung
Ghon focus	Primary parenchymal lung tubercle
Ghon complex	Lung and lymph node lesions in primary TB
Secondary TB	Reactivation of lung TB
Miliary TB	Disseminated haematogenous spread of TB throughout the body

TB, Tuberculosis.

NEOPLASTIC DISEASES OF THE LUNGS

The World Health Organization 2015 classification of lung tumours is based on the tissue from which they are derived:

- Epithelial tumours:
  - Adenocarcinoma
  - Squamous cell carcinoma
  - Neuroendocrine tumours
    - Carcinoid
    - Atypical carcinoid
    - Large cell neuroendocrine carcinoma
    - Small cell carcinoma
- Mesenchymal tumours
  - Pulmonary hamartoma
  - Chondroma
  - Inflammatory myofibroblastic tumour.

A simpler, more clinical approach is to divide the malignant epithelial tumours into non-small cell lung carcinomas (NSCLC) and small cell lung carcinomas (SCLC) as the treatment for each is radically different.

Bronchogenic carcinomas

Bronchogenic carcinomas arise from the epithelium of the bronchi and bronchioles. It is the most common cause of death from neoplasia in the UK, affecting 35,000 people per year. Males are affected more often than females, but there is an increasing incidence in women. The peak incidence is between the ages of 40 and 70 years, reflecting the cumulative exposure to several potential causative carcinogens. The risk factors for lung carcinoma are outlined in Table 10.9.

There are four main histological types of bronchogenic carcinoma (Table 10.10):

1. Adenocarcinoma—35%.
2. Squamous cell carcinoma—30%.
3. Neuroendocrine tumours (including small cell carcinoma)—25%.
4. Large cell lung carcinoma—10%.

A small proportion of tumours are mixed, e.g., adenosquamous carcinoma.

Table 10.9 Risk factors for the development of bronchogenic carcinoma

Risk factor	Comment
Tobacco smoking	Eighty-six percent of lung cancer is caused by smoking Risk is linked to duration and quantity smoked Duration has the most effect on risk Earlier age of commencement increases risk Cigarette smoke contains a large number of carcinogens, e.g., polycyclic hydrocarbons Steady decline in risk if smoking stops
Occupational factors	Exposure to carcinogenic substances: • radioactive material (e.g., plutonium) • asbestos • heavy metals (e.g., cadmium, chromium, nickel, arsenic) • mining: iron oxides and haematite • coal: soot, gas plants, coal-tar pitch
Environmental factors	Radon-22 (a natural radioactive gas in certain geographic areas) Air pollution Diesel exhaust

Table 10.10 Summary of the main histological subtypes of lung cancer

	Small cell carcinoma	Squamous cell carcinoma	Adenocarcinoma
Relative incidence	20%	30%	35%
Sex differences	Males > females	Males > females	Males = females
Associated with cigarette smoking	Yes	Yes	No/less of an association
Most common site	Centrally located	Centrally located	Peripherally located
Chest X-ray	Not seen	Central mass ± cavitation Associated pneumonia common	Focal mass/nodular pattern
Macroscopic appearance	White/tan Soft/friable	Grey/white Irregular spiculate/necrosis ± direct extension into hilar lymph nodes	Tan/white Not associated with large airways Often originate in areas of preexisting lung scarring Entrapped anthracotic pigment
Microscopic appearance	Sheets of cells High N:C ratio Salt and pepper chromatin Absent nucleoli	Sheets of squamous cells ± keratin production	Malignant cells resemble type II pneumocytes Can form acinar, papillary, micropapillary, solid or lepidic patterns.
Nonmetastatic symptoms	ADH secretion	Hypercalcaemia	HPOA
	Ectopic ACTH secretion	HPOA	
	Lambert–Eaton myasthenic syndrome		
Rate of growth	Fast; metastases usually present at diagnosis	Slow-growing; metastasizes late	Slow-growing; metastasizes early

ACTH, adrenocorticotropic hormone; ADH, antidiuretic hormone; HPOA, hypertrophic pulmonary osteoarthropathy.

Tumours may be central (all types) or peripheral (mainly adenocarcinomas).

Central or hilar tumours arise in relation to the main bronchi, extending into the bronchial lumen and invading the adjacent lung. These will present with obstructive symptoms.

Peripheral tumours arise in peripheral airways or alveoli, often occurring in relation to scars and frequently extending to the pleural surface. These can present with pain and pleural effusion.

Metastatic routes:

- Local invasion—central tumours invade locally either through the bronchial wall into the surrounding lung or along the outside of the bronchi (peribronchial spread) to distant parts of the lung. Direct extension into pleura and adjacent mediastinal structures is a feature of advanced disease. Apical lung tumours (Pancoast tumours) may invade local sympathetic ganglia and produce Horner syndrome (ptosis, miosis and anhidrosis).
- Lymphatic spread—carcinomas spread to the ipsilateral and contralateral peribronchial and hilar lymph nodes. Compression of adjacent tissues by infiltrated nodes may then cause symptoms.
- Transcoelomic spread—tumour cells may invade and seed a body cavity (e.g., pleural) causing a malignant effusion.
- Haematogenous spread—most commonly to the brain, bone, liver, adrenal glands and skin.

Histological types

Adenocarcinoma

This is the commonest type of lung cancer. It is derived from glandular cells, resembling mucinous goblet cells, Clara cells or type II pneumocytes. A proportion of adenocarcinomas is thought to originate in areas of preexisting lung scarring or fibrosis (scar adenocarcinomas). Adenocarcinoma has the slowest rate of growth and is the most common form of lung cancer in women. It can be linked to passive cigarette smoking and characteristically develops peripherally.

Microscopically they are classified as mucinous and nonmucinous, and form various patterns, which include acinar, micropapillary, lepidic and solid.

> **HINTS AND TIPS**
>
> **SMOKING AND LUNG CANCER**
>
> Cigarette smoking is the major risk factor for the development of neoplastic diseases of the lung. It is thought to be responsible for approximately 90% of all lung carcinomas. Passive smoking is also linked to lung cancer.

Lepidic adenocarcinoma—Previously called bronchioalveolar carcinoma, this is a separate subtype of adenocarcinoma where atypical cells are seen to grow along septa with preservation of native architecture. Purely lepidic adenocarcinomas have a better prognosis.

Squamous cell carcinoma

Owing to a decline in smoking, this is no longer the commonest type of lung cancer (Fig. 10.15). It is thought to be derived from metaplastic squamous bronchial epithelium, which develops as a result of exposure to noxious agents such as cigarette smoke.

Tumours are typically central and close to the carina, frequently presenting with features related to bronchial obstruction, and are often accompanied by pneumonia. Compared with other types, they are relatively slow-growing and metastasize late; they may be resectable.

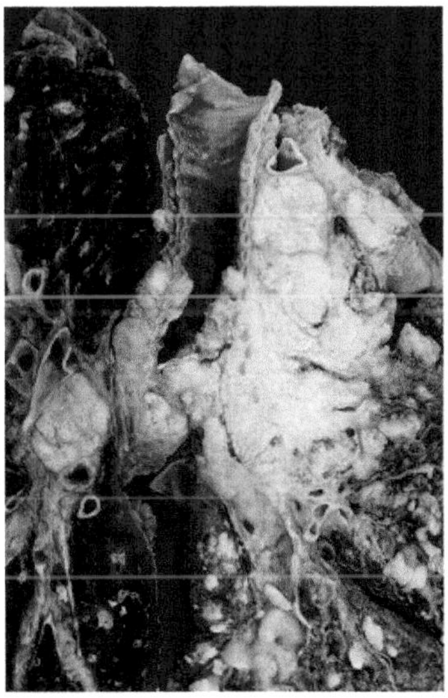

Fig. 10.15 Squamous cell carcinoma. A posterior view of a squamous cell carcinoma of the lung appearing as a white tumour mass. The tumour arises centrally and is invading through the bronchial wall with metastatic deposits to both lungs. The carina is splayed owing to subcarinal lymph node metastatic disease. Tumour is seen to encase the oesophagus at the top of the picture.

Histologically, tumours show a range of differentiation, from well-differentiated lesions producing lots of keratin through to poorly differentiated lesions with only a few keratin-producing cells.

Large cell carcinoma

These are *not* to be confused with large cell neuroendocrine tumours. These are epithelial tumours composed of large undifferentiated cells which lack the appearance of neuroendocrine tumours and cannot be categorised as either squamous cell carcinoma or adenocarcinoma by morphology or immunophenotype. This category is now seldom used as technology has improved diagnostic ability.

Neuroendocrine tumours

Neuroendocrine lung tumours/carcinomas (NET/NECs) arise from the enterochromaffin cells of the bronchial mucosa and occur as a spectrum of tumours which share common characteristics. As a group, they account for 25% of all lung tumours. Division is into low-grade tumours (carcinoid and atypical carcinoid) and high-grade tumours (small cell NEC and large cell NEC), based on the number of mitoses, presence of necrosis, histological appearance and immunohistochemical staining patterns. High-grade tumours are biologically more aggressive.

Small cell carcinoma

These are highly malignant neuroendocrine tumours that tend to be centrally located, grow rapidly and are frequently associated with metastases at the time of diagnosis. Owing to their endocrine nature, they can be associated with paraneoplastic syndromes, e.g., adrenocorticotropic hormone (ACTH) most commonly, or syndrome of inappropriate antidiuretic hormone secretion (SIADH).

Histologically, the cells are round to oval and have little cytoplasm. Characteristically the nuclei mould together with inconspicuous nucleoli and are associated with mitoses and extensive necrosis.

Mesenchymal tumours

Mesenchymal tumours of the lung are rare and together account for a minority of lung tumours. They include inflammatory myofibroblastic tumour, fibroma/fibrosarcoma, haemangioma and leiomyoma/leiomyosarcoma. Haematological malignancies, e.g., lymphoma, can also affect the lung. The most common mesenchymal tumour is a bronchial hamartoma.

Bronchial hamartomas

These are discrete masses of mature pulmonary parenchymal tissue consisting of various proportions of cartilage, smooth muscle, fat, fibrous tissue and entrapped clefts of bronchial epithelium. The term 'pulmonary chondroma' is used when the composition is mainly cartilaginous. Presentation is usually as incidental findings on chest X-rays, appearing as peripheral 'coin lesions' <4 cm in size ± calcification.

If multiple, they may represent part of the Carney triad (extraadrenal paraganglioma, gastrointestinal stromal tumours, pulmonary chondroma).

Secondary tumours of the lung

Metastatic deposits may spread to the lungs from distant primary sites, most often from carcinomas of the breast, kidney, gastrointestinal tract and prostate. Spread is usually via the blood, most commonly resulting in bilateral deposits.

Clinical features of lung cancer

There are no early symptoms of lung cancer and tumours may grow undetected for many years. At presentation 80% have metastatic spread (55% distant, 25% local), leaving the minority (20%) with localized, potentially resectable disease. Ten percent of cases are identified through incidental findings of a lesion on radiological imaging performed for other reasons.

The presentations of lung cancer are outlined in Table 10.11.

Prognosis and staging

Histological types and the stage of lung cancer determine the outcome and its likely response to different treatment modalities. Survival is better for early-stage disease, except for small-cell carcinoma which metastasizes early.

The TNM staging system is used for lung cancer. It varies slightly from other staging systems in that the pleura is also staged, e.g., PL0, PL1 etc.

MOLECULAR

EGFR, ALK AND PDL-1

Molecular testing on lung carcinomas is now standard practice as therapies are available to treat a subset of tumours that contain either *EGFR, ALK* or PD-L1 mutations. The treatments do not cure but can extend life expectancy (months).

Table 10.11 Clinicopathological features of lung cancer

Cause	Clinical features
Pulmonary involvement	
	Cough (80%): infection distal to airway blocked by tumour
	Haemoptysis (60%): ulceration of tumour within the bronchus
	Dyspnoea (60%): local extension of tumour and airway compression
	Chest pain (40%): involvement of pleura and/or chest wall
	Wheeze (15%): narrowing of upper airways (stridor may develop)
	Systemic features: weight loss, anorexia, cachexia and malaise
Local spread	
	Horner syndrome: local invasion of cervical sympathetic ganglion
	Hoarseness: spread to the left apical region may cause recurrent laryngeal nerve palsy
	Pain in T1 dermatome and wasting of intrinsic hand muscles: caused by brachial neuritis as a result of direct invasion of plexus by apical tumours
	Pericardial effusion: owing to direct tumour invasion
	Dysphagia: extension into subcarinal lymph nodes and compression of the oesophagus
	Phrenic nerve palsy: hemidiaphragm paralysis (see on chest X-ray). May cause breathlessness
	SVC syndrome: compression of the SVC causing dyspnoea, facial/arm swelling, hoarseness and stridor
Metastatic spread	
	Pathological fractures
	CNS symptoms (brain metastasis)
	Hepatomegaly or jaundice (liver metastasis)
Nonmetastatic extrapulmonary syndromes	
Endocrine disturbances	SIADH: by small-cell carcinoma and characterized by low sodium and plasma osmolality with high urine osmolality
	Ectopic ACTH secretion: caused by small-cell carcinoma and associated with Cushing syndrome
	Hypercalcaemia: caused by secretion of parathyroid hormone-related peptide by a squamous cell carcinoma

Table 10.11 Clinicopathological features of lung cancer—cont'd

Cause	Clinical features
Neurological syndromes	Peripheral sensory motor neuropathy
	Cerebellar degeneration causing ataxia
	Proximal myopathy
	Dermatomyositis
	Lambert–Eaton myasthenic syndrome: associated with small-cell tumours
Hypertrophic pulmonary osteoarthropathy	Finger clubbing
	Swelling of wrists and ankles with periosteal new bone formation (seen in 2%–3% of squamous cell carcinomas and adenocarcinomas)

ACTH, Adrenocorticotropic hormone; SIADH, syndrome of inappropriate antidiuretic hormone secretion; SVC, superior vena cava.

Treatment

Surgical intervention

Only 10% of all lung tumours are considered operable at diagnosis according to the stage of the disease. For example, distant metastases and advanced local spread are contraindications for surgical resection. Many patients are unsuitable for surgery due to comorbidities (e.g., poor cardiac status). However, 5-year survival rates are as high as 75% in carefully selected patients with early disease (stage 1).

Historically, small-cell carcinoma was deemed inoperable; however, a small subset is now deemed potentially resectable.

Radiotherapy and chemotherapy

The distinction of NSCLC and SCLC is relevant to treatment and prognosis:

1. SCLC—very sensitive to radiotherapy and chemotherapy. Treatment offers good palliation of pain, cough and dyspnoea with a median survival of 11 months.
2. NSCLC—inoperable cases may be treated with radiotherapy depending on clinical circumstances. The role of chemotherapy is limited. Overall prognosis is poor, with only a 50% 2-year survival without spread, 10% with spread.

DISEASES OF VASCULAR ORIGIN

Pulmonary oedema

Pulmonary oedema is defined as the accumulation of extravascular fluid within the pulmonary interstitium (alveolar walls) and the alveolar spaces. This results in decreased lung compliance and decrease in effective lung volume. Oxygenation is reduced, with hypoxaemia, and, if severe, death.

Macroscopically, the lungs are heavy and wet, akin to a saturated sponge. In fatal cases, fluid flows from the cut surface and it can often be seen (and heard!) in the large airways.

Microscopically, the septal blood vessels are congested and the alveoli contain proteinaceous fluid and haemosiderin-laden macrophages known as 'heart failure cells'.

Pathogenesis

Pulmonary oedema arises as a consequence of either:

- An imbalance in Starling forces (hydrostatic/oncotic pressure).
- Increased permeability/damage to the alveolar capillary walls.

Normally, a balance exists between hydrostatic pressure and colloid osmotic (oncotic) pressure within the blood vessels such that only a small amount of fluid passes into the interstitium, which is then drained from the lung via lymphatic channels.

Pulmonary oedema can result from increased hydrostatic pressure (left-ventricular failure) or increased alveolar capillary permeability (inflammatory alveolar reactions) where the lymphatic drainage capacity is exceeded, resulting in a net accumulation of fluid within the interstitium (Table 10.12).

COMMON PITFALLS

PULMONARY OEDEMA VERSUS PLEURAL EFFUSION

Pulmonary oedema and pleural effusions are often confused. They both involve excess fluid accumulation but are separate entities.

- Pulmonary oedema: excess fluid occurs within the lung itself (interstitium and alveoli).
- Pleural effusion: excess fluid occurs within the pleural cavity, i.e., between the chest wall (parietal pleura) and lung surface (visceral pleura).

Table 10.12 Causes of pulmonary oedema

Left-sided heart failure (of any cause) • Aortic/mitral valve disease • Ischaemic heart disease • Hypertension • Cardiomyopathy • Sepsis • Fast atrial fibrillation or ventricular tachycardia
Volume overload, e.g., from intravenous fluids
Pulmonary venoocclusive disease, e.g., pulmonary vein obstruction
Constrictive pericarditis/pericardial effusion
Nephrotic syndrome
Liver disease
Inhaled toxic irritants, e.g., smoke
Aspiration of gastric contents
Allergic reactions
Drowning
Radiation
Blood transfusion reactions

Acute respiratory distress syndrome

Acute respiratory distress syndrome (ARDS) is a clinical syndrome of rapid onset (24–48 hours) and high mortality. It is defined as acute-onset, bilateral radiographic chest infiltrates, hypoxaemia regardless of ventilation and no evidence of left atrial hypertension. Many conditions predispose to ARDS, most commonly sepsis and severe trauma. The causes are listed in Table 10.13.

Histologically the appearance of ARDS is that of diffuse alveolar damage which is widespread and temporally the same. There are three overlapping stages:

1. Acute phase: this is characterized by oedema, haemorrhage and fibrin deposition with cellular debris and the formation of hyaline membranes. There is minimal inflammation. The phase lasts approximately 1 week.
2. Organizing phase: this is characterized by type II pneumocyte hyperplasia and fibroblast proliferation within the interstitial and alveolar space. Hyaline membranes are mostly resorbed.
3. Late fibrotic phase: this is characterized by fibrosis and haphazard collagen deposition. Some cases of ARDS resolve completely whilst others progress to remodelling and lung fibrosis (honeycomb lung).

Mortality in ARDS is usually from sepsis or multiorgan failure rather than a pulmonary cause. Those who survive have significant morbidity with a reduced health-related quality of life.

Fig. 10.16 shows the main events and outcomes in ARDS.

Table 10.13 Causes of acute respiratory distress syndrome

Cause	Clinical features
Indirect injury	Sepsis
	Major trauma, especially associated with raised intracranial pressure and multiple fractures
	Major burns
	Disseminated intravascular coagulation
	Massive blood transfusion
	Amniotic fluid and fat embolism
	Acute pancreatitis
	Cardiac surgery with bypass
	Antitumour chemotherapy
	Paraquat poisoning
Direct injury	Pulmonary aspiration of gastric contents
	Inhalation of toxic fumes or smoke
	Near-drowning
	Pneumonia from many causes requiring ventilation
	Pulmonary contusion

Embolism, haemorrhage and infarction

Pulmonary embolism

Pulmonary embolism (PE) is the occlusion of the pulmonary arterial system, most commonly by a thromboembolism; the vast majority of these arise from deep vein thromboses (DVT) of the lower limb (calf, popliteal, femoral and iliac veins). The pathology of thrombosis is discussed in more detail in Chapter 9.

> **HINTS AND TIPS**
>
> **PULMONARY EMBOLISM AND POSTMORTEM CLOTS**
>
> Postmortem clots are common, lack an internal structure and assume the shape of the pulmonary tree. They are likened to 'chicken fat and redcurrant jelly' both due to their appearance and texture. True thromboemboli assume the shape of the vessel in which they were formed not the vessel they impact. They also have internal structure and, if established, are adherent to the vessel wall.

Clinical features

The annual incidence of PE is approximately 60–70/100,000. The consequences of a PE depend on the extent of the

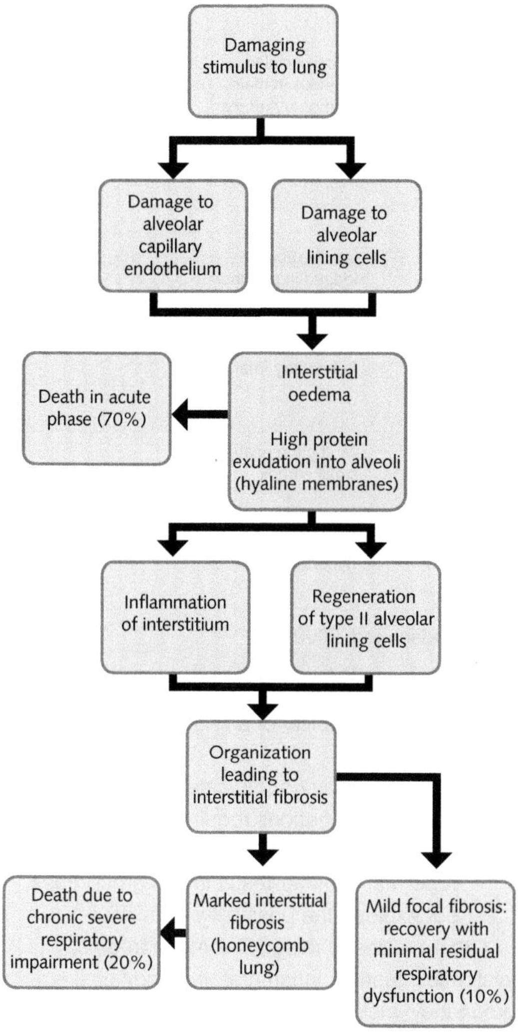

Fig. 10.16 Main events and outcomes in acute respiratory distress syndrome.

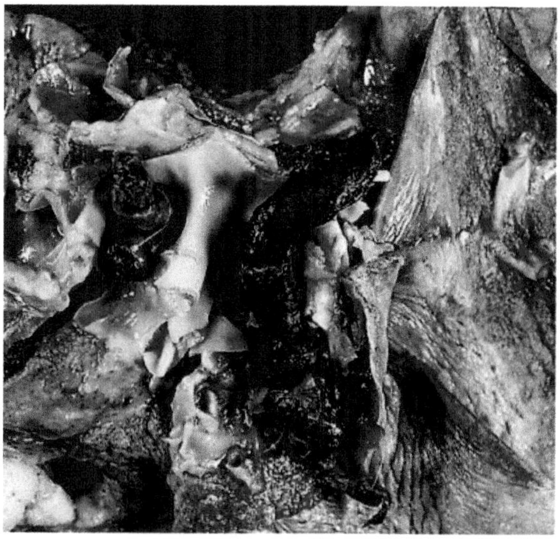

Fig. 10.17 Pulmonary embolism. A coiled firm thrombus is seen occluding the pulmonary trunk (saddle embolism) and main pulmonary arteries.

pulmonary vasculature blockage and the timescale involved (i.e., acute or chronic). They are classified clinically as either massive or submassive based on the respiratory or haemodynamic effects that ensue. Presenting symptoms and signs are variable and include tachycardia, dyspnoea, pleuritic chest pain, hypoxia, haemoptysis, hypotension and cough.

- Massive PE: this is defined as an acute PE with sustained hypotension <90 mmHg systolic for >15 min and/or a PE involving both main pulmonary arteries, or evidence of shock/haemodynamic compromise (altered level of consciousness, oliguria, hypoxia). One example is a saddle embolus at the bifurcation of the left and right pulmonary arteries (Fig. 10.17).
- Submassive PE: this is defined as no sustained hypotension but the presence of right-ventricular dysfunction or myocardial necrosis. Right-ventricular dysfunction is identified by right-ventricular dilatation, ECG change or brain natriuretic peptide elevation. Myocardial necrosis is seen by a raise in troponin I or T.

Pathophysiology

Blockage of pulmonary vasculature leads to both ventilatory and haemodynamic consequences (Fig. 10.18).

- Ventilatory consequences:
  - A ventilation/perfusion (V/Q) mismatch occurs whereby the affected alveoli are ventilated but there is no associated bloodflow to them for gas exchange to occur. They are in essence a dead space. If the area affected is great enough, hypoxaemia arises as insufficient oxygenation occurs. This is further compounded by reduced cardiac output. In a minority of cases pulmonary infarction can occur.
- Haemodynamic consequences:
  - The severity of haemodynamic changes occurs on a spectrum dependent on the location and aggregate size of the obstructing embolus. Emboli impede bloodflow, i.e., increase pulmonary vascular resistance, by reducing the cross-sectional area of the vasculature. This pressure is transmitted back to the right atrium and right ventricle, causing increased right-ventricular work and right heart strain, resulting in reduced cardiac output. If the pulmonary vascular resistance is too high, electromechanical dissociation of the heart occurs, i.e., the heart continues to beat but there is no output, resulting in cardiovascular collapse and rapid death.

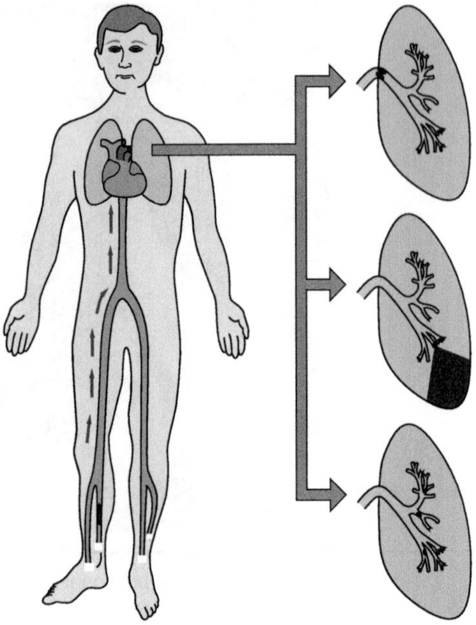

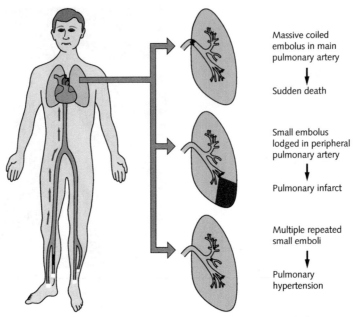

Fig. 10.18 Consequences of a pulmonary embolism. (Adapted from Underwood, 2000.)

Prevention and consequences

The consequences of PE are:

- Pulmonary hypertension, with subsequent right-sided heart strain/cor pulmonale.
- Pulmonary infarction in ~10% of cases.
- Death—the most common preventable cause of death in hospital patients.

Prevention involves:

- Early mobilization following surgery.
- Thromboembolic deterrent stockings.
- Heparin prophylaxis.

COMMON PITFALLS

D-DIMERS

'D-dimers' are the breakdown products of cross-linked fibrin, reflecting the activity of the clotting system. A D-dimer test is often performed inappropriately and misinterpreted.

Low clinical probability of a deep vein thrombosis (DVT) (low Well test score):

- D-dimer assay indicated to exclude DVT.
- A negative result virtually *excludes* the diagnosis of a DVT (a negative result has almost 100% negative predictive value in this situation).
- A positive result is supportive but *not diagnostic* of a DVT; further investigation is required (i.e., a positive result does not confirm a DVT).

High clinical probability of a DVT (high Well test score):

- D-dimer assay *not* indicated.
- Other investigations required, e.g., radiological imaging.
- A normal D-dimer result in this group *does not* exclude the possibility of a DVT.

Other causes of raised D-dimers: trauma, systemic infection, inflammatory conditions, pregnancy, malignancy and postsurgery.

Nonthrombotic emboli

These are rare, but include:

- Fat embolus—following a fracture (especially of long bones), orthopaedic procedures, pancreatitis, soft-tissue trauma.
- Amniotic fluid embolus—during labour.
- Air embolus—after trauma, surgery, therapeutic procedures.
- Decompression sickness (Caisson disease)—rapid decompression (e.g., in deep-sea divers) causes nitrogen to precipitate out of solution and form bubbles with systemic consequences, including pulmonary vessel obstruction.
- Foreign body embolus—talc and starch from intravenous drug use, the legendary 'bullet' from gunshot wounds.
- Tumour embolus—liver, stomach, breast.
- Septic embolus—endocarditic valve leaflets, infected catheters/lines, infection elsewhere in the body.

Pulmonary infarction

Infarction of lung tissue is unusual owing to the dual blood supply of the lung (bronchial and pulmonary circulation) protecting against ischaemia, infarction and necrosis. Infarction is usually caused by embolism occurring in 10%–15% of PE, with 75% of cases involving the lower lobes.

Macroscopic appearance: pulmonary infarcts are typically haemorrhagic (because of blood entering from the bronchial circulation), sharply demarcated and wedge-shaped, with the apex pointing towards the lung hilum and base involving the pleura. Often fibrinous exudate is seen on the overlying pleura as a reactive change which causes chest pain. With time, the infarct becomes organized to form a fibrous scar.

Microscopic appearance: this ranges from preservation of alveolar architecture, with extravasation of blood filling the airspaces and an inflammatory reaction, to ischaemic necrosis.

Pulmonary hypertension and vascular sclerosis

Pulmonary hypertension is an increased arterial pressure within the pulmonary circulation >30/15 mmHg. The aetiology can be primary (rare) or secondary (chronic lung or cardiac diseases). The determinants of pulmonary artery pressure are:

$$PAP = PVR \times CO \times PVP,$$

where *PAP* = pulmonary artery pressure; *PVR* = pulmonary vascular resistance; *CO* = cardiac output; *PVP* = pulmonary venous pressure (which is equivalent to left atrial pressure). Any processes that change/affect any of the variables will affect PAP.

It therefore follows that important secondary causes include:

- COPD—alveolar hypoxia → vasoconstriction and capillary loss/distortion.
- Interstitial fibrosis of the lungs—capillary distortion.
- Left-ventricular failure—increased left atrial pressure → increased back pressure through the lungs to the pulmonary circulation.
- Chronic pulmonary emboli—increased pulmonary arterial resistance secondary to vasospasm and mechanical blockage.

Pulmonary hypertension causes irreversible structural changes to the pulmonary vasculature: medial muscular hypertrophy of the small pulmonary arteries with fibroelastic thickening of the intima and subsequent occlusion. Plexiform lesions may be seen and, in severe cases, fibrinoid necrosis of the vessel walls may occur. This results in progressive right-ventricular dysfunction leading to right-sided heart failure (cor pulmonale) with associated symptoms and signs.

Vasculitic syndromes

Vasculitic syndromes tend to have systemic effects; however, there are some that preferentially, and commonly, affect the lung. These are discussed below.

Granulomatosis with polyangiitis (Wegener granulomatosis)

This is a systemic small-/medium-vessel vasculitis (cytoplasmic anti neutrophil cytoplasmic antibody (cANCA) cANCA-positive) affecting the upper and lower respiratory tract and kidneys, characterized by

- sinusitis
- pneumonia
- necrotizing vasculitis
- glomerulonephritis.

It affects males slightly more often than females, presenting at 40–60 years of age.

Symptoms can include epistaxis, cough, dyspnoea, arthralgia and chest pain. Histologically, necrotizing granulomatous inflammation is present with poorly formed granulomas, giant cells, geographic necrosis and vasculitis. Cavitating lesions on radiological imaging may be seen.

If untreated, the disease is fatal, with most dying of secondary renal and pulmonary complications.

Eosinophilic granulomatosis with polyangiitis (Churg–Strauss)

This is a systemic small-vessel vasculitis (perinuclear anti neutrophil cytoplasmic antibody (pANCA) pANCA-positive) affecting the lungs, skin, heart, gastrointestinal tract and peripheral nerves. It is characterized by the classic triad of:

- asthma
- peripheral blood eosinophilia
- vasculitis.

It affects males and females equally, presenting at 30–50 years of age. There are three recognized phases: prodrome, vasculitic and postvasculitic, with clinical and histological features dependent on the organ systems involved and stage of disease.

Symptoms can include asthma, sinusitis and neuropathy. Histologically, eosinophilic infiltrates are the hallmark of the disease, causing eosinophilic vasculitis, palisaded necrotizing eosinophilic granulomas, gastroenteritis and eosinophilic pneumonia.

Microscopic polyangiitis

This is a multisystemic necrotizing vasculitis of small blood vessels, e.g., capillaries and venules. See Chapter 9 for further discussion.

Diffuse alveolar haemorrhagic syndromes

A few interstitial lung disorders may produce diffuse alveolar haemorrhage. Important examples include:

- Goodpasture syndrome—an autoimmune disease with autoantibodies against collagen IV of the basement membrane, resulting in the breakdown of both lung alveoli and kidney glomeruli (see Chapter 13).
- Granulomatosis with polyangiitis (Wegener granulomatosis).
- Microscopic polyangiitis.
- Idiopathic pulmonary haemosiderosis—a rare disorder of unknown origin causing repeat episodes of diffuse alveolar haemorrhage with haemoptysis. It affects children more often than adults and is characterized histologically by haemosiderin deposition.

DISEASES OF IATROGENIC ORIGIN

Drug-induced lung disease

Many drugs have pulmonary side-effects, causing a wide spectrum of disease. Examples include:

- Diffuse alveolar damage: anticancer (cytotoxic) drugs are the most common, e.g., bleomycin, busulfan, gefitinib.
- Fibrosis: methotrexate, bleomycin, amiodarone.
- Interstitial pneumonia: amiodarone, nitrofurantoin, sulfasalazine, heroin, β-blockers.
- Alveolar haemorrhage: phenytoin, penicillamine, nitrofurantoin, mitomycin C.

Radiotherapy

Radiotherapy, especially to the thorax, can cause radiation-induced lung disease, which has an acute (early) and chronic (late) phase. Complications depend on radiation dosage, tissue volume irradiated and total time of irradiation.

Acute radiation pneumonitis

The onset is 1–2 months after radiation exposure. Diffuse alveolar damage is seen with atypical pneumocytes (type II) and increased numbers of macrophages.

Chronic radiation pneumonitis

The onset is 6–12 months after radiation exposure and it is a progression of acute radiation pneumonitis. Fibrosis occurs.

DISORDERS OF THE PLEURA

Pleural effusion

A pleural effusion is a collection of fluid within the pleural cavity, i.e., between the visceral and parietal pleura. They can be unilateral or bilateral and result from either increased fluid formation or inadequate fluid clearance. Depending on the underlying pathology/mechanism the fluid can either be a transudate or exudate (Fig. 10.19). The various types are discussed below.

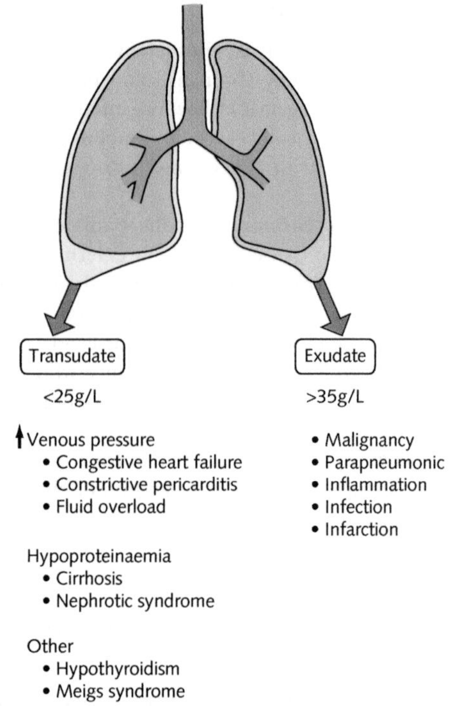

Fig. 10.19 Pleural effusions. The causes of pleural effusions can be grouped into transudates (<25 g/L of protein) or exudates >35 g/L of protein). Additional criteria are required when the protein concentration is equivocal.

Serofibrinous effusion

Acute inflammation of the pleura is accompanied by an accumulation of a protein-rich effusion (>35 g protein/L; exudate) containing fibrinogen/fibrin, most commonly due to infection, infarction or tumour.

Pathogenesis

The effusion is typically unilateral, straw-coloured on aspiration and contains mesothelial cells, macrophages and a variable number of inflammatory cells. In neoplastic diseases, malignant cells may also be identified within the pleural fluid.

The pleural surface is covered by a fibrinous exudate that has a similar appearance to two slices of buttered bread which have been pulled apart, therefore 'bread and butter appearance'.

Sequelae

Common sequelae include:

- Atelectasis—external compression of the lungs causes pulmonary collapse and respiratory impairment.

- Adhesions—formation of fibrous adhesions between the visceral and parietal pleura. May cause the lung to become 'trapped' i.e., unable to fully inflate.
- Fibrosis—obliteration of the pleural space by fibrosis, which is common in longstanding effusions.
- Empyema.

Empyema

This is the accumulation of pus within the pleural cavity. It is typically seen as a complication of pneumonia (including TB) when pathogens invade into the pleural space. It can also complicate thoracic surgery or penetrating chest wall injury.

Common sequelae include septicaemia (haematogenous spread of infection to other organs) and atelectasis. Copious fibrin is produced, causing adhesions and loculated fluid collections preventing adequate drainage.

Hydrothorax

This is a low-protein effusion (<25 g protein/L; transudate) caused by the excess movement of fluid through normal vessel walls owing to an imbalance in Starling forces (hydrostatic and oncotic pressure). They are usually bilateral, with a normal pleura; the aspirated fluid is straw-coloured containing occasional lymphocytes and mesothelial cells.

Common causes are:

- Increased hydrostatic pressure:
  - congestive cardiac failure (most common)
  - constrictive pericarditis
  - fluid overload.
- Decreased oncotic pressure—hypoalbuminaemia.
  - nephrotic syndrome
  - ascites
  - malabsorption.

HINTS AND TIPS

TRANSUDATE/EXUDATE

The difference between 'transudate' and 'exudate' is important. Transudates are characterized by low-protein content in contrast to exudates, which have high-protein content.

Haemothorax

This is accumulation of blood within the pleural cavity. It is most commonly the result of:

- trauma, especially rib fractures
- surgery
- pulmonary infarction
- aortic aneurysm rupture
- intrathoracic malignancy
- coagulopathy, e.g., anticoagulant medication, haemophilia.

If blood remains within the pleural cavity, organization and pleural fibrosis occurs.

Chylothorax

This is the accumulation of chylous fluid within the pleural cavity (Fig. 10.20). This is caused by disruption/laceration of the thoracic duct either traumatically (including surgery) or nontraumatically, e.g., malignant infiltration (lymphoma). Chyle is composed of lymph and emulsified fats, giving the aspirated fluid a milky-white appearance.

Pneumothorax

This is the presence of air in the pleural cavity. Primary pneumothorax occurs in those without any underlying lung disease and secondary pneumothorax occurs as a complication of an underlying lung disease, e.g., COPD. The causes of each are summarized in Table 10.14.

RED FLAG

TENSION PNEUMOTHORAX

This is a life-threatening emergency! Do not order a chest X-ray!

Symptoms and signs:

- Tachypnoea
- Tachycardia
- Hypotension
- ± Hypoxia
- Tracheal deviation away from the side of the pneumothorax
- Hyperresonance on chest percussion
- Reduced expansion and breath sounds
- Distended neck veins.

A tension pneumothorax is a progressive increase in air pressure within the pleural cavity as a result of a one-way valve-like mechanism. Air that enters the cavity on inspiration is unable to escape during expiration. This causes massive collapse of the affected lung, mediastinal shift and compression of the contralateral lung, producing circulatory collapse and cardiac arrest.

Pleural neoplasia

Solitary fibrous tumour of the pleura

This is a rare benign tumour of the pleura occurring in the sixth–seventh decades. The majority arise from the submesothelial parenchyma of the visceral pleura. They are well-circumscribed, pedunculated masses of variable sizes composed of dense fibrocollagenous tissue with fibroblasts. There is no association with asbestos and it does not cause a pleural effusion.

Table 10.14 Causes of pneumothorax

Cause	Type	Clinical features
Spontaneous	Primary[a]	Healthy, no underlying disease
	Secondary	COPD
		Acute severe asthma
		Tuberculosis
		Pneumonia
		Cystic fibrosis
		Pleural malignancy
Traumatic	Chest injury	Penetrating chest wounds
		Rib fractures
		Oesophageal rupture
	Iatrogenic	Subclavian cannulation
		Positive pressure artificial ventilation
		Post thoracocentesis
		Oesophageal perforation during endoscopy
		Lung biopsy

[a] *The cause of primary pneumothorax in some cases is thought to be idiopathic rupture of a subpleural 'bleb'. The risk of a primary pneumothorax is increased in young male smokers and those with tall stature.*
COPD, Chronic obstructive pulmonary disease.

Metastatic neoplasms

These are the most common pleural tumours, most frequently arising from the lungs, breast or ovary, but can arise from any malignant tumour. They are usually associated with a high-protein exudate (see section on 'Pleural effusion' above).

Mesothelioma

This is a rare primary neoplasm of the pleura but is an important cause of death in people previously exposed to asbestos, e.g., in ship building, mining and insulation installation. Mesothelioma can also arise within the peritoneum and pericardium as these too are lined by mesothelial cells. Clinical features include chest pain and breathlessness with recurrent or persistent pleural effusions (blood-stained).

Pathogenesis: there is a latent interval between asbestos exposure and disease presentation of between 25 and 45 years. Crocidolite and amosite fibres (blue and brown asbestos) are thought to be the most important in the development of mesothelioma. Asbestos fibres become trapped in the lung following inhalation and are particularly resistant to macrophage and neutrophil destruction. The exact mechanism is unknown, but it is thought that the resultant chronic inflammation increases oxidative stress, resulting in an accumulation of DNA damage and malignant transformation.

Macroscopic appearance: mesothelioma grows as a thick, white, solid rind encasing the lung and invading thoracic and mediastinal structures (Figs 10.21 and 10.22).

Microscopic appearance: mesotheliomas have three morphological appearances: spindle cells (sarcomatoid type), epithelioid cells (epithelioid type) and a combination of both (mixed/biphasic type). The cells can appear bland or highly malignant, and growth patterns vary from tubuloglandular to sheets and fascicles of tumour cells. Haematogenous and lymphatic metastases are rare.

Disease progression is rapid, with death occurring within 5–20 months of diagnosis (mean ~ 11 months) depending on histological subtype.

CLINICAL NOTE

CYTOLOGY

Cytological specimens from the lung include bronchoalveolar lavage, bronchial brushings and pleural fluid. Diagnostically, they can be very fruitful in identifying lung- and pleural-based malignancies, infections such as pneumocystis pneumonia and inflammatory conditions such as lipoid pneumonia.

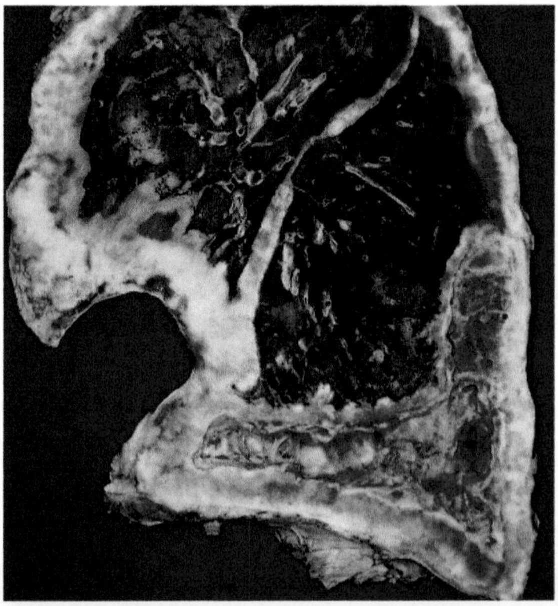

Fig. 10.21 Mesothelioma. A dense, white rind of tumour is seen at the lung periphery and spreading along the interlobar septa. The majority of the lung is encased, with the remaining lung tissue compressed.

Chapter Summary

- Congenital disorders of the lung include bronchogenic cysts, sequestra and congenital pulmonary airway malformations.
- There are many types of diffuse lung diseases, but they can be broadly categorised as obstructive or restrictive.
- Chronic obstructive pulmonary disease is a combination of chronic bronchitis and emphysema.
- Asthma is a common disorder which is divided into extrinsic or intrinsic causes.
- Cystic fibrosis is an autosomal dominant multisystem disease which is characterized by abnormally thick mucus.
- The pneumoconioses include asbestosis, silicosis and coal-worker's pneumoconiosis.
- Sarcoidosis is a multisystem disease characterized by nonnecrotizing granulomas.
- Pneumonia is infection of the lung parenchyma and can be bacterial, viral or fungal.
- The most common cause of pneumonia is bacterial—*Streptococcus pneumoniae*.
- Tuberculosis is most commonly due to infection by *Mycobacterium tuberculosis*. It is characterized by necrotizing granulomas.
- Pleural effusions can be benign or malignant and be comprised of blood, serous fluid, air, chyle or pus.
- Neoplasms of the lung include adenocarcinoma, squamous cell carcinoma and small-cell carcinoma as well as many others. Prognosis is often poor owing to late stage of presentation and metastatic spread.
- Vasculitic syndromes can either be lung-specific or part of multisystemic disease.
- Pulmonary embolism usually arises from the deep veins of the legs and pelvis.
- Primary pleural tumours are rare. The most common is mesothelioma, which grows as a thick rind encasing the underlying lung.
- Asbestos causes a spectrum of lung pathology.

Pathology of the gastrointestinal system 11

DISORDERS OF THE UPPER GASTROINTESTINAL TRACT

The oesophagus

Congenital abnormalities

Oesophageal atresia

In oesophageal atresia, the upper end of the oesophagus is intact, but ends in a blind pouch. Oesophageal atresia affects 1 per 4000 live births, and more than 85% of cases are associated with a tracheooesophageal fistula—an abnormal communication between the lower oesophagus and trachea (Fig. 11.1).

The effects are:

- Fetus—inability to swallow amniotic fluid results in polyhydramnios, the accumulation of an excessive amount of amniotic fluid.
- Neonate—appears healthy initially but swallowed fluid returns through the nose and mouth and respiratory distress occurs. The condition must be surgically corrected in early life but is also associated with other congenital abnormalities.

Webs and rings

These localized constrictions of the oesophagus are caused by mucosal folds or muscular contractions.

In Plummer–Vinson, or Paterson–Brown–Kelly syndrome, upper oesophageal webs are associated with dysphagia in patients with iron-deficiency anaemia, cheilosis and glossitis. This is a rare but important condition because of an association with the development of postcricoid oesophageal carcinoma.

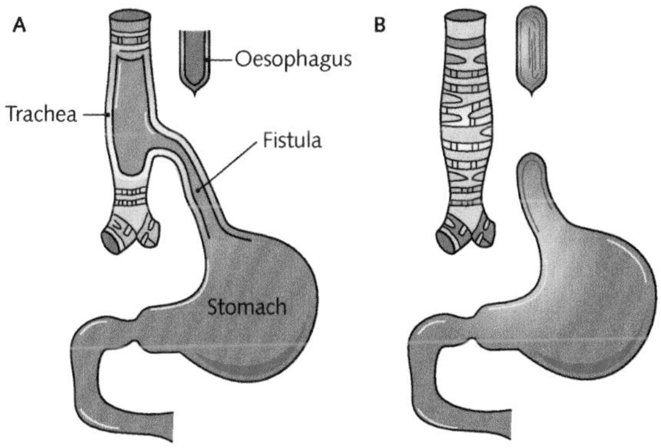

Fig. 11.1 Oesophageal atresia. (A) Blind ending of oesophagus with fistula formed between lower part and trachea. (B) Oesophageal atresia with no fistulous communication: very rare.

Inflammation of the oesophagus (oesophagitis)

Reflux oesophagitis

Inflammation of the oesophagus caused by gastro-oesophageal reflux disease (GORD) is the most common oesophageal abnormality and is caused by reflux of gastric acid through the lower oesophageal sphincter. The condition affects about 5% of adults; it can occur at any age (but with increased incidence over the age of 55 years), and it affects males more often than females.

Table 11.1 lists the predisposing factors of reflux oesophagitis.

Symptoms are a burning pain in the centre of the lower chest commonly known as 'heartburn'.

Complications:

- Peptic ulceration of lower oesophagus—development of small ulcers which become chronic with fibrosis.
- Lower oesophageal stricture—progressive fibrous thickening of the lower oesophageal wall producing difficulty in swallowing (dysphagia).
- Barrett oesophagus—metaplasia of lower oesophageal mucosa, with normal squamous epithelium replaced by glandular columnar epithelium of gastric or intestinal type. This increases the risk of oesophageal adenocarcinoma (see below).

Relevant investigations include endoscopy and 24-hour intraluminal pH monitoring.

Management:

- Lifestyle alterations—weight loss, smoking cessation, avoiding late meals and decreasing alcohol intake.
- Drug therapy—antacids, alginates, H2-receptor antagonists and proton pump inhibitors (severe symptoms).

Table 11.1 Factors predisposing to oesophageal reflux

Factors that increase intraabdominal pressure	Overeating/obesity
	Pregnancy
	Poor posture
Factors that render the lower oesophageal sphincter lax or incompetent	Hiatus hernia
	Smoking
	Alcohol ingestion

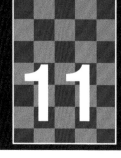

- Surgery—for those not responding to medical therapy, repair of hiatal defects or fundoplication may be appropriate.

Eosinophilic oesophagitis

This is an eosinophil-rich inflammation of the oesophagus endoscopically appearing as corrugated rings (trachealization). Microscopically the squamous epithelium is mosaic-like with >15 eosinophils/high-powered field ± eosinophilic microabscesses. It is associated with atopy.

Other causes

Other less common causes of oesophagitis are:

- Infective agents—*Candida albicans*, herpes simplex and cytomegalovirus may cause acute oesophagitis in the immunosuppressed.
- Physical agents—irradiation or ingestion of caustic agents (e.g., suicide attempts).
- Desquamative skin diseases, e.g., pemphigoid and epidermolysis bullosa may cause oesophageal ulceration, blistering and eventual erosion.

Lesions associated with motor dysfunction

Achalasia

Achalasia is a condition in which there is abnormal peristalsis and lack of relaxation of the lower oesophageal sphincter. This may occur at any age, but it is mainly seen in middle-aged individuals. The cause is unknown but reduced numbers of ganglion cells in the myenteric plexus have been noted in longstanding cases.

The consequences are:

- Dysphagia—increasing slowly over years.
- Regurgitation of undigested food.
- Occasional severe chest pain caused by oesophageal spasm.
- Megaoesophagus—oesophageal distension occurs over a period of time.
- Predisposition to development of squamous cell carcinoma of the oesophagus.

Chagas disease

Infection by *Trypanosoma cruzi* is a cause of secondary achalasia owing to destruction of the myenteric plexus. It is common in South America.

Hiatus hernia

This is a common condition in which the upper part of the stomach herniates through the diaphragmatic oesophageal opening (hiatus) into the thoracic cavity.

It may rarely be caused by a congenitally short oesophagus but is mainly thought to arise from increased abdominal pressure and loss of diaphragmatic muscular tone.

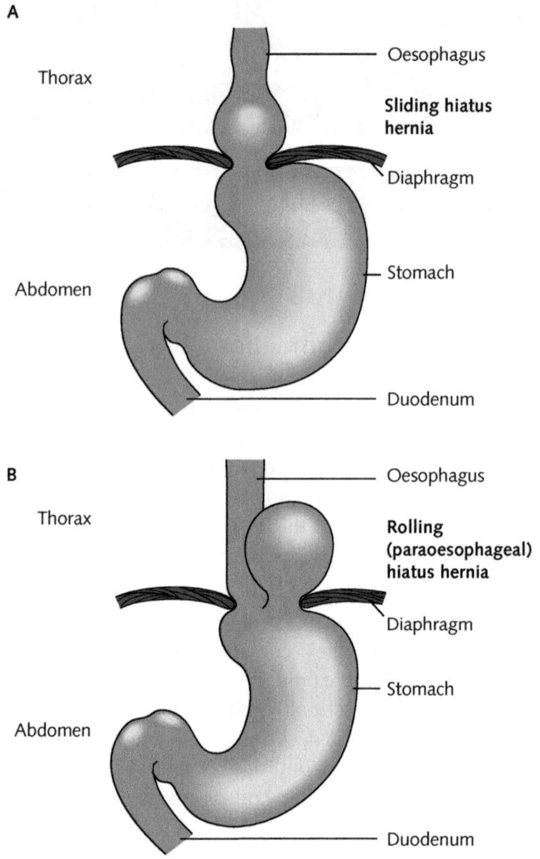

Fig. 11.2 Types of hiatus hernia. (A) Sliding hiatus hernia. (B) Rolling hiatus hernia.

There are two types (Fig. 11.2):

1. Sliding hiatus hernia (90%)—stomach herniates through oesophageal diaphragmatic hiatus, resulting in the gastroesophageal junction moving into the thorax (associated with reflux oesophagitis and peptic ulceration).
2. Rolling (paraoesophageal) hiatus hernia (10%)—the fundus of the stomach protrudes through the hiatus, but the gastrooesophageal junction remains below the diaphragm (less associated with reflux).

Lacerations

Oesophageal perforation is rare, but it may be caused by:

- Traumatic rupture—usually associated with vomiting (Boerhaave syndrome).
- Impaction of a sharp foreign body.
- Intubation of an oesophagus with strictures.

'Mallory–Weiss tear' is a longitudinal oesophageal laceration as a result of severe retching or vomiting. This is most commonly seen in alcoholics, and classically occurs with vomiting of clear fluid (pretearing), followed by vomiting of blood (posttearing).

Oesophageal varices

Oesophageal varices are dilated submucosal veins in the oesophagus.

The condition is caused by portal hypertension (most commonly associated with cirrhosis of the liver).

Pathogenesis

Oesophageal veins normally drain into both systemic and portal venous systems.

Increased pressure in the portal venous system (e.g., as a result of severe diffuse longstanding liver disease) causes dilatation of the oesophageal veins, which often protrude into the lumen.

Rupture of these varices, or ulceration of overlying mucosa, can produce massive haemorrhage into the oesophagus and stomach, often precipitating vomiting of blood (haematemesis).

Management

This involves local measures to control bleeding (e.g., variceal banding) and reduction of portal venous pressure.

Neoplastic disease

Barrett oesophagus

Definition—metaplastic replacement of normal squamous epithelium in the oesophagus with glandular columnar epithelium. It is caused by persistent oesophageal reflux; approximately 10% of these patients will develop Barrett oesophagus.

Barrett oesophagus predisposes to the development of adenocarcinoma. Metaplastic glandular epithelium can progress to intestinal metaplasia, epithelial dysplasia and then to frank adenocarcinoma.

> **HINTS AND TIPS**
>
> **BARRETT OESOPHAGUS**
>
> Barrett oesophagus is a classic example of metaplasia and is a good example to quote in an examination.

Benign neoplastic disease

Benign tumours are uncommon. They arise from normal structures within the oesophagus. The commonest lesions are leiomyomas derived from the smooth muscle of muscularis propria, but many other benign tumours can occur.

Malignant neoplastic disease

The most common malignant tumours of the oesophagus are squamous carcinomas and adenocarcinomas. Oesophageal carcinoma accounts for 2% of cancer cases in the UK each year. They usually arise within the elderly population. Risk factors are:

- Smoking/alcohol.
- Dietary (tannic acid, food colourings, nitrates and nitrosamines).
- Barrett oesophagus
- Corrosives
- Achalasia
- Iron-deficiency anaemia
- Human papilloma virus (HPV) infection—this may have a role in the development of some squamous cell carcinomas (SCCs).

SCCs are more common than adenocarcinomas. They mostly develop in men who are heavy alcohol drinkers or heavy smokers and may be preceded by an epithelial dysplastic change. They usually present late, are located in the middle and lower oesophagus and often cause dysphagia.

Adenocarcinomas mainly occur in the lower oesophagus in areas of metaplasia (Barrett oesophagus). However, some adenocarcinomas are primary carcinomas of the stomach that have infiltrated the lower oesophagus.

Clinical features of oesophageal tumours

- Common—progressively worsening painless dysphagia (of solids then liquids), anorexia, weight loss, anaemia (acute or chronic).
- Rare—hoarse voice (involvement of larynx or left recurrent laryngeal nerve palsy), supraclavicular lymphadenopathy, tracheooesophageal fistula.

Investigations include endoscopy, radiological imaging and biopsy. Management may be palliative to relieve pain and dysphagia (stenting, dilatation, enteral feeding), but combinations of surgery, radiotherapy and chemotherapy (neoadjuvant) may be attempted in early disease. Squamous carcinoma has a slightly better prognosis due to its radiosensitivity, but overall 5-year survival from oesophageal cancer is just 15%.

DISORDERS OF THE STOMACH

Inflammation

Gastritis is the term used to describe inflammation of the gastric mucosa.

Acute gastritis

This superficial acute inflammation is typically caused by ingested chemicals, the most common being alcohol, aspirin and other nonsteroidal antiinflammatory drugs (NSAIDs).

Acute erosive gastritis

Focal loss of the superficial gastric epithelium causes dyspepsia with vomiting and possibly haematemesis if the erosions are numerous.

Causes are:

- NSAIDs.
- Heavy, acute alcohol ingestion.
- Severe stress or shock (e.g., after major trauma or burns).
- Hypotension—acute hypoxia of surface epithelium.

Chronic gastritis

Chronic inflammation of the gastric mucosa is a common condition. It increases with age and is more common in developed countries. Mucosal atrophy occurs with intestinal metaplasia, increasing the likelihood of gastric carcinoma.

The condition is present in over 90% of patients with duodenal ulceration, 70% of those with gastric ulceration and it is also common in those with gastric cancer.

There are three main aetiological types:

- Infectious—gastritis associated with *Helicobacter pylori*.
- Immune—pernicious anaemia and atrophic gastritis without pernicious anaemia.
- Reactive—after gastrectomy or adjacent to erosions/ ulcers.

Helicobacter-associated gastritis

This is the most common form of chronic gastritis, arising at any age and accounting for more than 90% of cases. The pyloric antrum is the most severely affected area, but damage is also seen in the fundus.

Pathogenesis:

- Colonization—*H. pylori* colonizes the surface epithelium. This causes an initial acute neutrophilic gastritis, which gives way to chronic gastritis.
- Urease production—the bacterium produces the enzyme urease, which breaks down urea to give carbon dioxide and ammonia. This can be identified using the urease breath test. Biopsy material can also be added to a *Campylobacter*-like organism (CLO) kit containing urea. If urease is present, ammonia is produced causing the indicator to change colour.
- Inflammatory response—gastritis identifiable on biopsy material with epithelial inflammation and organisms.
- Persistence of infection—once established, infection may persist for years.

Morphological features:

- Mucin depletion leading to damage to the underlying epithelium.
- Atrophy of gastric glands.
- Mixed acute and chronic inflammatory cell reaction in lamina propria and superficial epithelium.
- Intestinal metaplasia—normal gastric epithelium is replaced by a type similar to that of the small intestine.

Autoimmune chronic gastritis

This organ-specific autoimmune disease associated with pernicious anaemia is generally seen in elderly patients with the development of severe mucosal atrophy (atrophic gastritis). It particularly affects the body of the stomach.

Antibodies are of two types:

1. Antibodies against gastric parietal cells (90%)—associated with decreased hydrochloric acid production (hypochlorhydria).
2. Antibodies against intrinsic factor (60%) → failure of absorption of dietary vitamin B12 → interference with normal erythropoiesis in bone marrow → megaloblastic, macrocytic anaemia (pernicious anaemia).

The most common form occurs without pernicious anaemia, even though antibodies of both types are often present. This is due to a residual ability to absorb vitamin B12, which may be lost over time, producing pernicious anaemia.

Morphological features:

- Loss of specialized epithelial cells.
- Fibrosis.
- Infiltrate of plasma cells and lymphocytes.
- Intestinal metaplasia.

Reactive gastritis (reflux/chemical gastritis)

In this pattern of mucosal injury, the dominant feature is epithelial change with minimal inflammatory cell infiltrates. The causes are threefold:

1. Idiopathic—majority of cases.
2. Reflux of alkaline bile-containing duodenal fluid into the lower part of the stomach. This may be caused by motility disturbances (e.g., due to gallstones or cholecystectomy) or pyloric incompetence (as a result of previous surgery to the pyloric area).
3. Drugs—NSAIDs may cause direct damage to the mucus layer.

Morphological features:

- Epithelial desquamation.
- Foveolar hyperplasia.
- Vasodilatation.
- Mucosal oedema.

> **HINTS AND TIPS**
>
> **ABCs OF GASTRITIS**
>
> Remember the ABCs of chronic gastritis:
>
> A—autoimmune/atrophic
>
> B—bacterial (*Helicobacter pylori*)
>
> C—chemical (reflux/reactive gastritis)

Complications of chronic gastritis

Regardless of cause, all forms of chronic gastritis can cause:

- Intestinal metaplasia—more likely to result in dysplasia and eventual carcinoma.
- Peptic ulceration—caused by damage to the gastric lining by acidic gastric secretions.

Gastric ulceration

Peptic ulcers

Peptic ulcers are ulcers of the oesophagus, stomach or duodenum caused by damage to the epithelial lining by gastric secretions, particularly acid.

It is estimated that about 10% of the population of developed countries experience peptic ulceration at some time. Ulcers usually develop in adulthood and have a natural history of repeated healing and relapse over many years.

Sites of peptic ulceration, in order of decreasing frequency, are:

- Duodenum—classically the first portion, due to hypersecretion of acid by the stomach and impaired bicarbonate production in the duodenum.
- Stomach—usually at the antrum, because of regurgitated bile in pyloric incompetence, or surface epithelial damage by *H. pylori* infection or NSAIDs.
- Gastroesophageal junction—caused by gastric reflux onto unprotected mucosa.
- Gastroenterostomy sites.

Aetiology is probably multifactorial but damaging influences include *H. pylori* infection, NSAIDs, alcohol and stress (Cushing and Curling ulcers). Less commonly, peptic ulcers may be associated with acid hypersecretion (e.g., gastrinoma), infection, duodenal obstruction/disruption, vascular insufficiency or radiation.

Other factors, such as chronic gastritis, smoking and genetic predisposition, are also believed to play a role in the pathogenesis.

> **HINTS AND TIPS**
>
> **CUSHING AND CURLING ULCERS**
>
> Cushing ulcers are secondary to raised intracranial pressure—always investigate the cause!
> Curling ulcers are secondary to burns—remember curling irons burn!

Pathogenesis

Upper gastrointestinal (GI) mucosa is normally protected by either squamous epithelium (oesophagus) or an acid-resisting mucous barrier containing neutralizing bicarbonate ions (stomach). Peptic ulceration occurs when the aggressive action of acid and pepsin is not opposed by adequate mucosal protective mechanisms.

Macroscopically, peptic ulcers are typically 1–2 cm in diameter (but they can be much larger) with sharply defined borders surrounding the ulcer crater.

Microscopically, the ulcer crater usually penetrates into the muscularis propria of the stomach and has four histological zones, namely:

- superficial necrotic debris
- nonspecific acute inflammation
- granulation tissue
- fibrosis.

Complete healing of the ulcer leads to fibrous replacement of muscle with regrowth of epithelium over the scar. Clinical features include episodic epigastric pain (alleviated by antacids), which is worsened by eating and may occur with nausea and reflux (oesophageal ulcers).

Sequelae

Complications and sequelae are as follows:

- Healing—slow process hastened by acid-inhibiting agents or mucosal protectants.
- Haemorrhage—may be small and undetected (causing chronic anaemia) or occur as an acute episode of haematemesis.
- Adherence and erosion—ulcer penetrates full thickness of the stomach or duodenal wall, adhering to and eroding into underlying tissue, particularly the pancreas or liver.
- Perforation—may lead to intraabdominal haemorrhage or peritonitis.
- Fibrous strictures—caused by the healing of peptic ulcers, which may obstruct the oesophagus or stomach (acquired pyloric stenosis).
- Malignant change (very rare).

Acute gastric ulcer

Acute peptic ulcers usually develop in areas of erosive gastritis, and they are predisposed by the same factors that promote erosion. In contrast to chronic ulcers, they are generally multiple and shallow with minimal surrounding inflammation or fibrosis.

Acute ulcers may heal without scarring or they may progress to chronicity.

> **RED FLAG**
>
> **NSAIDs AND PPIs**
>
> Consider prescribing a protein pump inhibitor (PPI) with nonsteroidal anti-inflammatory drugs (NSAIDs) to prevent gastric ulceration and its sequelae.

Hypertrophic gastropathy

Ménétrier disease

This rare disease of unknown cause is characterized by gross hyperplasia of gastric pits, atrophy of glands and a marked overall increase in mucosal thickness. It is associated with hypoalbuminaemia as a result of gastric protein loss via superficial ulcerations (a form of 'protein-losing gastroenteropathy').

Hypertrophic gastropathy

An extremely rare condition, this is characterized by acid hypersecretion and gastric protein loss.

Zollinger–Ellison syndrome

This is a gastrin-secreting tumour (gastrinoma) of the pancreatic G cells that results in gastric gland hyperplasia and hypersecretion (see Chapter 14). Multiple peptic ulcers and diarrhoea also occur.

Neoplastic disease

Benign polyps

Benign gastric polyps are rare compared with the incidence of malignant tumours of the stomach. Table 11.2 shows some of the polyps found in the stomach.

Other benign tumours of the stomach are derived from mesenchymal tissues, the most common being leiomyomas. These appear as mucosal or intramural nodules and are usually asymptomatic.

Gastric adenocarcinoma

The vast majority (>90%) of malignant tumours of the stomach are adenocarcinomas derived from mucus-secreting epithelial cells. The incidence of gastric cancer has been falling worldwide, accounting for 2% of new cancer cases in the UK each year. It is more common in the Far East and certain parts of South America, but less so in Western Europe and North America. Males are affected more often than females by a factor of 2:1 (Table 11.3).

Appearance and symptoms are often dependent on the site of the carcinoma:

Table 11.2 Benign gastric polyps

Type	Characteristics
Hyperplastic polyps	Commonest gastric polyp, formed by regeneration of mucosa, often associated with chronic gastritis
Fundic gland polyps	Cystic glandular lesions, female prevalence associated with proton pump inhibitor use.
Peutz–Jeghers polyps	Hamartomatous polyps that occur in Peutz–Jeghers syndrome
Adenomatous polyps	True tumours of the surface epithelium up to 5 cm in size. Very rare, but dysplasia indicates that malignant change is possible

Table 11.3 Risk factors for gastric adenocarcinoma

Risk factors	
Helicobacter pylori infection	Chronic *H. pylori* infection increases gastric carcinoma risk eightfold. This is thought to be the result of chronic gastritis producing intestinal metaplasia, with eventual dysplasia and carcinoma. Chronic inflammation creates reactive oxygen species capable of damaging DNA, along with gland atrophy and hypochlorhydria, which favour further bacterial growth. However, the vast majority of those with *H. pylori* infection do not develop cancer.
Diet	Aetiology is unknown, but dietary factors are suggested to account for geographical variation, e.g., ingestion of smoked and salt-preserved foods.
Lifestyle	Alcohol, obesity and smoking are all associated factors.
Chronic gastritis	Chronic gastritis of any cause, e.g., autoimmune gastritis resulting in intestinal metaplasia, increases the risk of cancer.
Type A blood	Aetiology unknown.
Gastric adenomatous polyps	Up to 3% progress to adenocarcinoma within 10 years.
Postgastrectomy patients	Because of persistent gastric inflammation.
Hereditary gastric cancer	Rare.

- Pylorus—often produce symptoms of gastric outlet obstruction.
- Fundus—typically a fungating, ulcerating mass.
- Cardia—may produce dysphagia.

Unlike chronic peptic ulcers of the stomach, they are not confined to the lesser curvature.

Pathogenesis

The sequence of events in the development of gastric carcinomas is as follows:

Normal mucosa → chronic gastritis → intestinal metaplasia → dysplasia → intramucosal carcinoma (early gastric cancer) → invasive carcinoma

Several genetic changes have been reported in gastric cancer, including alterations of *p53* and *E-cadherin* expression, along with overexpression of oncogenes such as *c-myc*. *E-cadherin* changes appear unique to diffuse type gastric cancer.

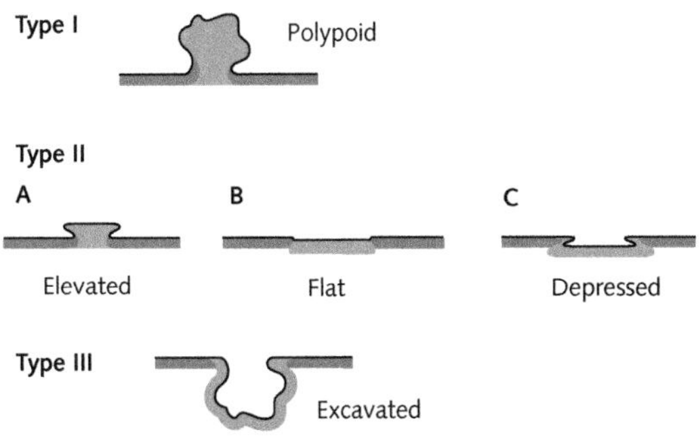

Fig. 11.3 Macroscopic classification of early gastric cancers.

Gastric cancers are classified as either early or advanced according to the extent of their spread through the stomach wall.

Early gastric cancer

This is confined to the mucosa and/or submucosa regardless of whether spread has occurred to regional lymph nodes. It is associated with a good prognosis. The cancer is further divided into three types according to macroscopic appearance (Fig. 11.3).

Advanced gastric tumours

These extend beyond the submucosa and are associated with a poor prognosis. They are further divided into three types macroscopically:

1. Polypoid—protrudes into stomach lumen and presents early because of gastric discomfort and bleeding when traumatized. This is usually amenable to surgical excision and has the best prognosis.
2. Ulcerating (commonest)—similar to benign peptic ulcers but with a raised, rolled edge, necrotic shaggy base and an absence of the rugal folds seen in benign peptic ulcers.
3. Diffuse infiltrative pattern (linitis plastica or 'leather bottle stomach')—presents late and has the worst prognosis. Tumour spreads extensively within mucosa and submucosa producing a shrunken, nonexpansile, rigid stomach. Symptoms are usually nonspecific (e.g., vomiting owing to small stomach capacity) and metastatic spread is common at the time of diagnosis. Surface ulceration is not a prominent feature and so haematemesis is not common until the later stages.

Microscopically, gastric carcinomas are described as diffuse (signet ring) in appearance or of intestinal type (mimicking small bowel epithelium).

Other gastric tumours

These are rare but include:

- Lymphomas (see Chapter 17)—a common site for extranodal non-Hodgkin lymphoma. *H. pylori* infection is associated with a low-grade lymphoma (so-called 'MALToma').
- Neuroendocrine tumours (Chapter 12).
- Gastrointestinal stromal tumours (GISTs)—relatively rare tumours that are thought to arise from interstitial cells of Cajal that control GI peristalsis. GISTs may be benign or malignant; 95% of cases display *c-KIT* mutations.

DISORDERS OF THE INTESTINE

Congenital abnormalities

Meckel diverticulum

This is a true diverticulum of the ileum caused by incomplete regression of the vitelline duct during the embryonic period, occurring in approximately 2% of the population, more commonly in males than females (approximately 3:1).

> **HINTS AND TIPS**
>
> **RULE OF 2s-MECKEL DIVERTICULUM**
>
> Rule of 2s for Meckel diverticulum:
> - Prevalence—2% of the population
> - Site—usually 2 feet (60 cm) from the ileocaecal valve
> - Length—up to 2 inches (5 cm)
> - Most symptomatic by 2 years of age
> - Two tissue types—gastric and pancreatic (usually)

Macroscopically, it is up to 5 cm long and projects from the antimesenteric side of the small bowel around 60 cm from the ileocaecal valve. Microscopically, it is a true diverticulum, consisting of all three layers of bowel: mucosa, submucosa and muscularis propria. About half of cases also contain heterotopic pancreatic or gastric epithelium.

Complications—the majority of these diverticula are asymptomatic; however, the complications include volvulus, inflammation, peptic ulceration from gastric epithelial acid secretion and intussusception (telescoping of one portion of intestine into another; Fig. 11.4).

Small bowel duplication cyst

Duplication cysts are rare congenital anomalies that can occur anywhere along the GI tract with up to half occurring within the small bowel. The majority contain gastric epithelium. They commonly present with obstruction, bleeding or perforation and are diagnosed within the first 2 years of life.

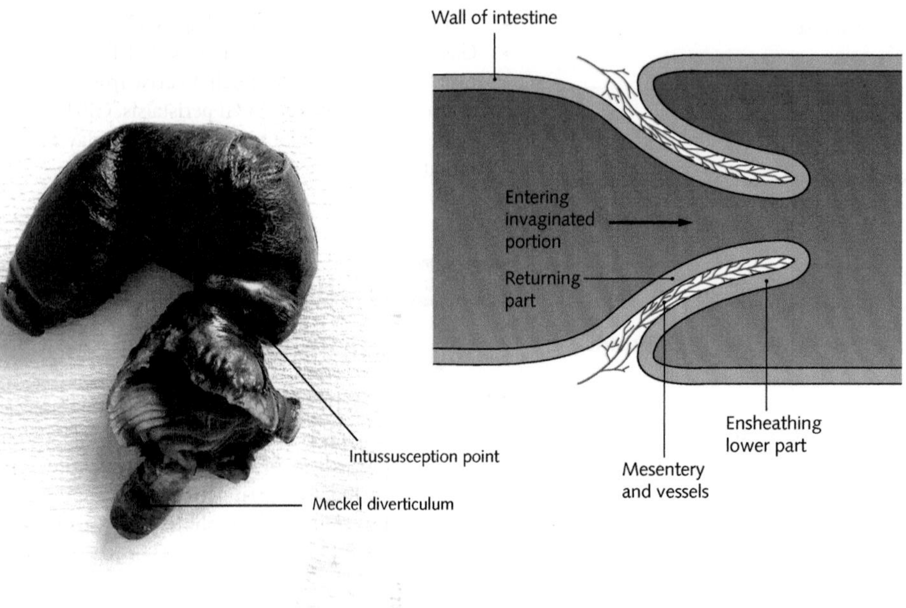

Fig. 11.4 Intussusception and Meckel diverticulum. Intussusception of the terminal ileum secondary to a Meckel diverticulum.

Congenital aganglionic megacolon (Hirschsprung disease)

This congenital condition is characterized by dilatation of the colon owing to the absence of the normal myenteric plexus distal to the dilatation. This condition always involves the rectum and extends proximally for a variable distance along the colon. It results from the failure of neuroblasts to migrate from the neural crest along the length of the developing colon and occurs in 1 per 5000 live births; 80% are in males.

Macroscopically, there is narrowing of the abnormally innervated bowel segment with dilatation and muscular hypertrophy of the proximal bowel segment.

Microscopically, there is an absence of the normal myenteric (Auerbach) and submucosal (Meissner) plexus ganglion cells, and hypertrophy of nerve fibres within the submucosa and muscularis mucosae, with extension of abnormal root-like axons into the lamina propria.

Clinical features—usually early childhood presentation with symptoms of colonic obstruction, i.e., constipation, abdominal distension and vomiting.

Diagnosis—barium enema reveals a small, empty rectum and dilatation above the narrowed segment. A suction biopsy of rectal mucosa will confirm the diagnosis; however, it is important to remember that the first 3 cm of rectum can normally be devoid of ganglion cells.

Treatment is by excision of the aganglionic segments of colon and rectum.

Acquired megacolon

Megacolon can also be a result of acquired disease; however, acquired megacolon differs macroscopically from Hirschsprung disease in that there is no narrowed segment with dilatation extending down to the anus and the rectum is full of faeces.

Causes of acquired megacolon:

- Psychogenic—disregard for the urge to defaecate (usually in children or the depressed).
- Chagas disease—infection by *Trypanosoma cruzi*, with destruction of myenteric plexus. Common in Central and South America.
- Medication—prolonged stimulant laxative abuse—degeneration of myenteric plexus.
- Neurological disorders—Parkinson disease, myotonic dystrophy, diabetic neuropathy and amyloidosis.
- Systemic diseases—lupus, mixed connective tissue disease, scleroderma and dermatomyositis.
- Metabolic diseases—hypothyroidism, hypokalaemia and porphyria.
- Obstruction—usually by neoplasm or inflammatory stricture in the rectum. Rarely, faecal impaction.
- Toxic megacolon—complication of ulcerative colitis (see below), pseudomembranous colitis and cytomegalovirus infection in patients with HIV.

Infections and enterocolitis

Diarrhoea and dysentery

Diarrhoea is hard to define. Many consider it to mean frequent bowel evacuation or the passage of abnormally soft or liquid faeces, although it is clinically defined as the passage of more than 200 g of stool per day.

Dysentery is an inflammatory disorder of the intestinal tract causing severe diarrhoea with blood and mucus.

Classification

Diarrhoea can be classified as:

- Secretory—diarrhoea caused by abnormal ion transport across the intestinal epithelium resulting in excessive intestinal secretions and decreased absorption. Stool volumes may be very high and diarrhoea persists even when there is total fasting.
- Osmotic—diarrhoea caused by the presence of unabsorbed solutes in the colon, which retain water within the lumen by their osmotic effect. Diarrhoea ceases with fasting.
- Exudative—diarrhoea owing to inflammatory exudate consisting of extracellular fluid and pus mixed with blood.
- Deranged motility—diarrhoea as a result of either increased or decreased motility of the small intestine.
- Malabsorption—diarrhoea occurring as a result of malabsorption (see below).

The classification and causes of diarrhoea are described in Table 11.4.

Infectious enterocolitis

Enterocolitis (inflammation of the colon and small intestine) is common and is often a result of infection.

Viral gastroenteritis

Viruses are the most common cause of gastroenteritis in infants and young children; they account for 10% of all food poisoning outbreaks in the UK. Transmission is typically by a faecal–oral route and symptoms are cramps, vomiting, diarrhoea and fever but no blood in stools.

In children most cases are caused by three viruses:

- Rotavirus—causes 50% of infantile diarrhoea and accounts for some adult cases.
- Adenovirus (especially types 40, 41)—the second most common cause (after rotavirus) of acute diarrhoea in young children. It is also a significant cause of diarrhoea in immunocompromised patients (e.g., HIV and posttransplant) and is strongly associated with graft-versus-host disease.
- Astrovirus—most infections occur in childhood and are mild.
- In adults, the Norwalk virus (norovirus) accounts for 30% of cases of gastroenteritis. It is responsible for the 'winter vomiting disease'.

Bacterial enterocolitis

The types of pathogenic mechanisms are as follows:

- Preformed toxin—ingestion of food contaminated with bacterial toxins, e.g., from *Staphylococcus aureus, Bacillus cereus* and *Clostridium perfringens*. Incubation period is very short (1–7 hours).
- Toxigenic organism—ingestion of bacteria that produce toxins in the gut, e.g., *Vibrio cholerae*, enterotoxigenic *Escherichia coli* (ETEC) and *C. perfringens*. So-called 'traveller's diarrhoea' usually occurs by this mechanism and is extremely common.

Table 11.4 Classification and causes of diarrhoea

Type	Causes
Secretory	Infections: bacteria producing enterotoxins, viral diarrhoea, *Giardia*
	Irritants: nonosmotic laxatives, e.g., senna, bisacodyl, bile acids, hydroxyl fatty acids
	Hormonal: vasoactive intestinal peptide, glucagon, medullary carcinoma of the thyroid, Addison disease
	Mucosal infiltration: villous adenoma, lymphoma, collagen diseases
	Congenital: chloridorrhoea
Osmotic	Osmotic laxatives, e.g., lactulose, magnesium sulphate
	Disaccharidase deficiency (lactose intolerance)
	Malabsorption syndromes
	Congenital, e.g., chloridorrhoea (secretory and osmotic), hexose malabsorption
Exudative	Inflammatory diseases, e.g., ulcerative colitis, Crohn disease
	Infections: bacteria causing invasion of the mucosa, i.e., enteroinvasive bacteria such as *Shigella, Campylobacter,* enterohaemorrhagic *Escherichia coli*; and *Entamoeba histolytica*
	Ischaemic colitis
	Radiation colitis
Deranged motility	Decreased motility: systemic sclerosis and other collagen disorders, intestinal pseudoobstruction and diabetic autonomic neuropathy
	Increased motility: carcinoid syndrome, postvagotomy state, thyrotoxicosis and unabsorbed bile salts entering colon
Malabsorption	May be a mixture of secretory, osmotic and exudative diarrhoea (see Table 11.8)

- Enteroinvasive organism—ingestion of bacteria that invade the intestinal mucosa and may cause dysentery as a result of severe inflammation, e.g., *Salmonella typhi*, *Campylobacter jejuni*, *Shigella*, enterohaemorrhagic *E. coli* (EHEC).
- Antibiotic-associated diarrhoea—occurs as a result of overgrowth of one type of bacteria because of disruption of normal gut flora following antibiotic treatment. The main culprit is *Clostridium difficile*; other pathogens include *C. perfringens* and *S. aureus*.
- Necrotizing enterocolitis—this is a rare condition that predominantly affects premature or low birthweight neonates where the bowel becomes inflamed and necrotic with superinfection leading to gas gangrene (pneumatosis cystoides intestinalis). The pathogenesis remains unclear, but it is thought to be due to early oral feeding and intestinal bacterial invasion. It is associated with high morbidity and mortality. Adult cases are related to *C. perfringens* infection.

Table 11.5 provides a summary of common bacterial GI infections.

Clostridium difficile

C. difficile infection most commonly occurs in hospitalized patients secondary to broad-spectrum antibiotic treatment, e.g., ciprofloxacin, co-amoxiclav. This alters the normal intestinal flora, allowing unsuppressed growth of *C. difficile* with the production of the A and B toxins. These cause secretory and bloody diarrhoea, respectively, with fever and abdominal pain. Infection can result in asymptomatic carriage, mild diarrhoea or pseudomembranous/fulminant colitis with significant morbidity and mortality. Treatment is, paradoxically, with metronidazole and vancomycin.

C. difficile produces heat-resistant spores that remain in the environment, requiring isolation of patients and decontamination.

Protozoa

Common protozoal infections include:

- *Trypanosoma cruzi*—infection results in the destruction of the myenteric plexus over a period of years, with resultant dilatation of various parts of the alimentary canal, especially the colon and oesophagus. It is known as Chagas disease and is common in South America.
- *Entamoeba histolytica*/*Entamoeba dispar*—causes amoebic dysentery, which is common throughout the tropics, where it is spread by the faecal–oral transmission of amoebic cysts. The condition follows a chronic course with abdominal pain and alternating periods of diarrhoea and constipation (Fig. 11.5).
- *Giardia lamblia*—infects the small intestine causing giardiasis. Infection occurs by eating food or water contaminated with parasitic cysts. Symptoms include diarrhoea, nausea, abdominal pain and flatulence, as well as the passage of pale, fatty stools. The disease occurs worldwide, and it is particularly common in children (Fig. 11.5).
- Other protozoal infections include *Balantidium coli* (balantidiasis) and *Cryptosporidium* (cryptosporidiosis).

Helminths (worms)

- *Schistosoma mansoni* and *Schistosoma haematobium* (schistosomiasis)—eggs from these worms are laid in the mucosa of small and large bowel and bladder, causing inflammation, ulceration and bleeding.
- *Strongyloides stercoralis* (strongyloidiasis)—a chronic nematode infection that can become a hyperinfection and virulent if the patient becomes immunocompromised (Table 11.6).

Inflammatory disorders of the bowel

The most important of these are idiopathic in origin, namely Crohn disease and ulcerative colitis (together termed

Table 11.5 Summary of common bacterial gastrointestinal infections

Mechanism	Bacterium	Incubation period	Duration (days)	Vomiting	Cramping	Fever	Blood in stool
Preformed toxin	*Staphylococcus aureus*	2–7 h	1	+	+	±	–
	Bacillus cereus	1–6 h	1	+	+	–	–
Toxigenic organisms	*Vibrio cholerae*	2–3 days	Up to 7	+	–	–	–
	Escherichia coli (ETEC)	12 h–3 days	2–4	+	–	–	–
	Clostridium perfringens	8 h–1 day	0.5–1	–	+	–	–
Enteroinvasive bacteria	Non-typhoidal salmonella	8–48 h	4–7	+	±	+	±
	Campylobacter jejuni	2–11 days	3–21	–	+	+	+
	Shigella	1–4 days	2–3	–	+	+	+
	Escherichia coli (EHEC)	1–5 days	1–4	+	+	+	+
Antibiotic-associated bacteria	*Clostridium difficile*	—	—	–	+	+	±

EHEC, enterohaemorrhagic Escherichia coli; ETEC, enterotoxigenic E. coli.

Table 11.6 Summary of colonic infectious agents

Viral	Bacterial	Parasitic
RNA Astrovirus Rotavirus HIV **DNA** Herpesvirus Cytomegalovirus Adenovirus	**Gram-positive** *Clostridium perfringens* *Clostridium difficile* *Bacillus cereus* *Staphylococcus aureus* **Gram-negative** *Chlamydia trachomatis* (lymphogranuloma venereum) *Yersinia enterocolitica* *Neisseria gonorrhoeae* (gonorrhoea) *Vibrio cholera* (cholera) Enterotoxigenic *Escherichia coli* (ETEC) Enterohaemorrhagic *E. coli* (EHEC) *Salmonella typhi* (typhoid) *Campylobacter jejuni* *Shigella* **Mycobacteria** *Mycobacterium tuberculosis* (tuberculosis) *Mycobacterium avium-intracellulare* **Spirochaetes** *Treponema pallidum* (syphilis)	**Protozoa** *Trypanosoma cruzi* (trypanosomiasis, Chagas disease) *Entamoeba histolytica/dispar* (amoebiasis) *Cryptosporidium hominis/parvum* (cryptosporidiosis) *Giardia lamblia* (giardiasis) *Leishmania donovani* (leishmaniasis) *Balantidium coli* (balantidiasis) **Metazoa (helminths)** **Cestodes** *Echinococcus granulosus* (hydatid disease) *Taenia solium* (tape worm—pig) **Trematode** *Schistosoma mansoni* and *S. haematobium* (schistosomiasis) **Nematode** *Ascaris lumbricoides* *Enterobius vermicularis* *Ancylostoma duodenale* *Trichuris trichiura* *Strongyloides stercoralis* (strongyloidiasis)

'inflammatory bowel disease'). These conditions are characterized by chronic, relapsing inflammation of the intestine.

A second group, the microscopic colitides, consists of lymphocytic colitis and collagenous colitis. These are also important causes of inflammation of the bowel.

Crohn disease

A fistulating granulomatous inflammation of unknown cause that affects the full thickness of the bowel wall anywhere in the GI tract from mouth to anus, characterized by a relapsing and remitting course. Its incidence is about 5–7 per 100,000 in the UK but this is increasing.

It usually presents in early adult life, with 90% of patients aged between 10 and 40 years, although a minor secondary peak occurs in the elderly. Females are affected slightly more often than males. There is a higher incidence in northern Europe and the USA than elsewhere.

Clinical features

Symptoms are of abdominal pain, diarrhoea (possibly bloody) and weight loss, with signs of anaemia, clubbing, fever, mouth (aphthous) ulcers and abdominal mass (inflamed bowel loops, abscesses).

Pathogenesis

The cause and pathogenesis are unknown; however, there is an inherited genetic predisposition with mutations in the *NOD2/CARD15* gene on chromosome 16. This gene codes for a protein which facilitates opsonization of gut bacteria. Crohn disease in these patients tends to have a more severe phenotype and is often ileal in location.

Macroscopic appearance

Site—Crohn disease most commonly affects the terminal ileum, but it may affect any part of the GI tract. Two-thirds of cases affect only the terminal ileum, one-sixth affect only the colon and one-sixth are in the terminal ileum and colon.

Pattern:

- 'Skip' lesions—normal bowel areas are present between diseased segments, with a sharp demarcation between the two.
- Haemorrhagic ulcers—initially small and discrete (aphthous), these progress to form deep, linear, fissured ulcers ('rose thorn' ulcers).
- Cobblestone pattern of bowel mucosa caused by submucosal oedema and interconnecting deep fissured ulcers (Fig. 11.6).

Other features:

- Thickened bowel wall due to oedema, fibrosis and muscular hypertrophy.
- Fibrotic strictures.
- Enlargement of mesenteric lymph nodes.

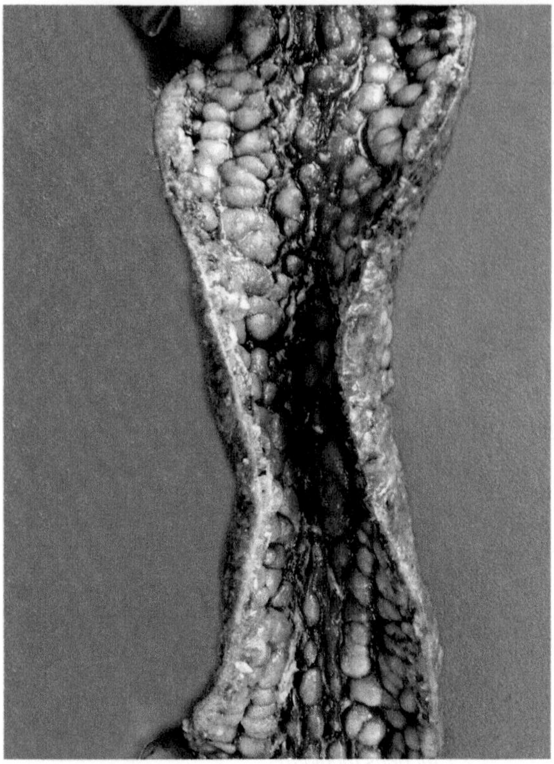

Fig. 11.6 Cobblestone mucosa in small-bowel Crohn disease. A segment of small bowel showing classical cobblestone appearance of the mucosal surface.

- Fistulae.
- External 'fat wrapping'—mesenteric fat extends around the serosal surface.

Microscopic appearance

- Patchy cryptitis and crypt abscess formation adjacent to normal crypts.
- Ulceration/erosions.
- Loss of plasma cell gradient in the lamina propria.
- Transmural inflammation—all layers of the bowel wall are affected, therefore providing the basis of fissures, adhesions, fistulae and sinus formation.
- Lymphoid aggregates develop deep in the bowel wall (Crohn rosary).
- Submucosal oedema.
- Neural hyperplasia.
- Noncaseating epithelioid granulomas present in inflamed bowel wall and mesenteric lymph nodes in approximately 60% of cases.

Complications

The natural history of Crohn disease is one of remitting and relapsing inflammation punctuated by local and systemic complications.

Local complications:

- Strictures and fibrous adhesions leading to intestinal obstruction.
- Fistulae and sinuses—inflammation of the serosal layer leads to the formation of adhesions and sinuses to other bowel loops (enterocolic fistulae), the bladder (enterovesical fistulae), vagina (enterovaginal fistulae) or anterior abdominal wall (enterocutaneous fistulae).
- Anal fissures.
- Inflammatory masses/abscesses/intraperitoneal collections.
- Adenocarcinoma of bowel—4–20-fold increased risk.
- Fulminant colitis (rare).

Extraintestinal complications:

Systemic complications, which develop in 25%–40% of patients with Crohn disease, include:

- Malabsorption/malnutrition—because of diseased bowel or surgical resections.
- Osteoporosis—as a result of malabsorption and repeated use of corticosteroids for treatment.
- Skin disease—pyoderma gangrenosum, erythema nodosum.
- Eye disease—uveitis (episcleritis and iritis).
- Joint disease—polyarthropathy, sacroiliitis, ankylosing spondylitis.
- Chronic liver disease—pericholangitis, primary sclerosing cholangitis.
- Cholelithiasis.
- Finger clubbing.
- Anaemia—of chronic disease and B12 deficiency owing to reduced absorption in the terminal ileum.
- Renal calculi—calcium oxalate stones are the most common.
- Systemic amyloidosis (rare).

COMMON PITFALLS

FISTULA VERSUS FISSURE VERSUS SINUS

Fissure: a linear crack/tear in an epithelial surface where the two apposing sides pull away from each other, e.g., anal fissure.

Fistula: an abnormal connection between two epithelial surfaces consisting of an epithelialized tract connecting either a hollow viscus to skin or to another hollow viscus. Note: epithelialized tracts will not spontaneously heal as the epithelium prevents this.

Sinus: a tract lined by granulation tissue leading from a source of infection to a surface.

Ulcerative colitis

This is a diffuse superficial inflammation of the colorectum of unknown cause characterized by relapses and remissions. It affects about 10 per 100,000 in the UK, with much lower rates in developing countries with warmer climates. Ulcerative colitis has a similar age distribution to Crohn disease but the sex incidence is equal.

Aetiopathogenesis

This is unknown, but the same hypotheses as for Crohn have been proposed, with the exception of smoking, which unusually is associated with a decreased risk. Inappropriate and persistent T-cell activation may play an important role in the pathogenesis.

Macroscopic appearance

Site—ulcerative colitis always involves the rectum (proctitis) and extends proximally for a variable distance. It may affect the whole of the colon (pancolitis), and in severe cases involve the terminal ileum ('backwash' ileitis).

Pattern—the pattern is one of shallow ulceration (which may become confluent), with 'pseudopolyps', hyperaemia and haemorrhage. The diseased bowel is continuous, without gaps of normal tissue.

Microscopic appearance

Inflammation is diffuse and is limited to mucosa, with infiltration of both acute and chronic inflammatory cells. There are numerous crypt abscesses, inflamed crypts (cryptitis), ulceration, crypt atrophy, branching and possible Paneth cell metaplasia.

Clinical features

Clinical features are symptoms of bloody diarrhoea and mucus, cramping discomfort, weight loss with signs of fever, tachycardia, pallor and abdominal tenderness.

Complications

Acute local complications include perforation, dilatation, haemorrhage and dehydration (blood and fluid loss from extensive ulceration).

Toxic megacolon is severe inflammation with dilatation of the colon and passage of bacterial toxins into the bloodstream. There is a risk of bowel perforation which may be life-threatening.

Chronic local complications include strictures, dysplasia and carcinoma (higher cancer risk than Crohn).

Systemic complications are identical to those seen in Crohn disease, except for an additional association with primary sclerosing cholangitis.

A comparison of Crohn disease and ulcerative colitis

Both Crohn disease and ulcerative colitis are examples of inflammatory bowel disease, with many features in common. However, in most cases (about 90%), it is possible to distinguish between these two conditions (Table 11.7 and Figs 11.7 and 11.8).

Diagnosis

The gold standard is colonoscopy: it allows direct visualization of the bowel mucosa and biopsy specimens to be taken

Table 11.7 Comparison of the basic features of Crohn disease and ulcerative colitis

	Crohn disease	Ulcerative colitis
Incidence in UK	~5–7 per 100,000	~10 per 100,000
Site	Any part of gastrointestinal tract but typically terminal ileum	Rectum and colon only
Macroscopic		
Disease continuity	Discontinuous (skip lesions)	Continuous from rectum
Bowel wall	Thickened with strictures and adhesions	Not thickened
Ulcers	Deep fissures form basis of fistulae	Flat bases; do not extend beyond submucosa
Microscopic		
Ulceration	Aphthous and serpiginous fissures	Superficial
Pattern of inflammation	Transmural	Mucosal and submucosal
	Focal/patchy	Diffuse
	Granulomas (in 60% of cases)	No granulomas
Crypt pattern	Little distortion	Distorted in longstanding disease; crypt abscesses
Metaplasia	Possible pyloric gland metaplasia	Possible Paneth cell metaplasia
Anal lesions		
	Present in 75%; perianal fistulae and abscesses, ulceration, chronic fissures, skin tags	Present in <25%
Frequency of fistula		
	10%–20% of cases	Uncommon
Risk of developing cancer		
	Slightly increased	Significantly increased

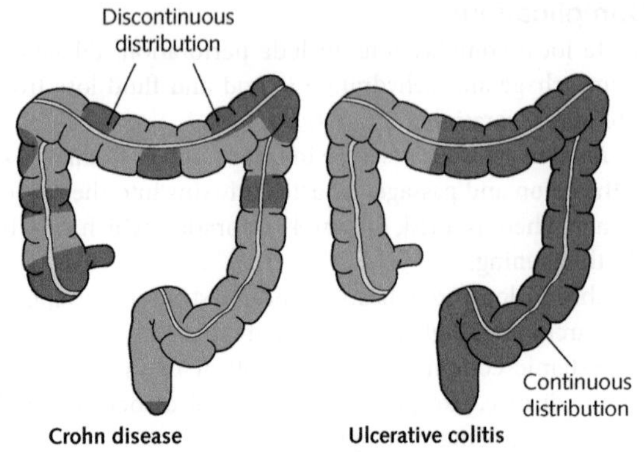

Fig. 11.7 The distribution of Crohn disease and ulcerative colitis.

for histological examination (see Table 11.7). Colonoscopy is also important in the surveillance of patients with long-standing colitis for the early detection of severe dysplasia and invasive cancer.

Management

Management can be medical or surgical.

- ***Medical***—options include corticosteroids, aminosalicylic acid, steroid-sparing agents such as azathioprine and methotrexate and biological therapies, e.g., TNF-α blockers (infliximab, adalimumab).
- ***Surgical***—options include minimal resections for strictures, fistulae or perforations (more common in Crohn disease), colectomies and pouch formation to avoid an end-ileostomy (contraindicated in Crohn disease).

Microscopic colitis

Lymphocytic and collagenous colitis are types of microscopic colitis. Both present with a history of chronic watery diarrhoea and a near normal colonoscopy, rendering the diagnosis a histological one.

Lymphocytic colitis—numerous intraepithelial lymphocytes are present, with increased numbers of lymphocytes and plasma cells within the lamina propria. The crypt architecture is preserved.

Collagenous colitis—is characterized by a thick subepithelial band of collagen in addition to features of lymphocytic colitis.

Malabsorption syndromes

General aspects of malabsorption syndromes

Malabsorption can be caused by disturbances in one or more of the stages of absorption:

- Intraluminal digestion—breakdown of macromolecules (fat, protein, carbohydrate) assisted by, for example, gastric juices and pancreatic digestive enzymes.
- Intraluminal solubilization—liver secretes bile acids required for solubilization and absorption of fats.
- Terminal digestion—enzymes located on the brush border of the small intestinal mucosa hydrolyse large carbohydrate and protein molecules for absorption.
- Transepithelial transport—mucosa is specialized for absorption. Transverse mucosal folds and finger-like villi provide a vast surface area.

Systemic effects of the malabsorption syndromes:

- Weight loss and anorexia.
- Abdominal distension and borborygmi (increased bowel sounds).
- Diarrhoea (chronic, loose, bulky stools).

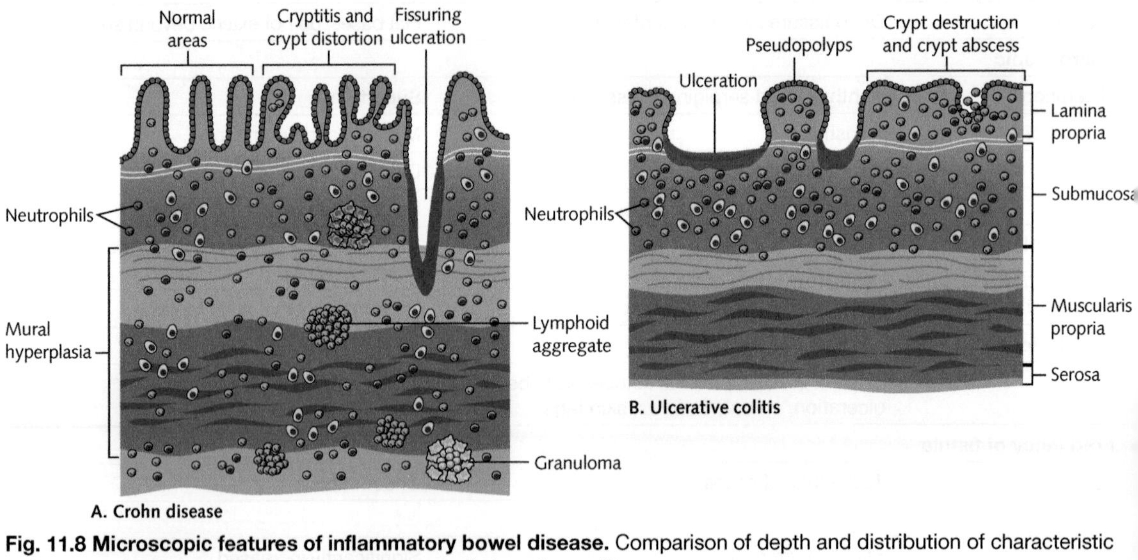

Fig. 11.8 Microscopic features of inflammatory bowel disease. Comparison of depth and distribution of characteristic lesions seen in the bowel wall in Crohn disease and ulcerative colitis.

- Steatorrhoea—malabsorption of fat, producing pale, foul-smelling stools that characteristically float in water.
- Muscle wasting.

Classification of malabsorption syndromes

This is described in Table 11.8.

Coeliac disease

Coeliac disease is a gluten-sensitive enteropathy caused by a chronic inflammatory response to the protein gliadin, a component of gluten (found in wheat, barley and rye). It affects about 1 per 1000 in most white populations of Northern Europe; it is rare in other ethnic origins.

It can present at any age, but it is an important cause of failure to thrive in infants and children. Classically it presents with diarrhoea, steatorrhoea and weight loss; however, nonclassical presentations with vague abdominal symptoms and anaemia have gained prominence.

Definitive diagnosis requires duodenal biopsy showing characteristic histological changes whilst the patient is consuming a gluten-containing diet, with symptomatic resolution occurring on commencement of a gluten-free diet.

The serological markers of anti-endomysial antibodies, IgA antitissue transglutaminase antibodies and antigliadin antibodies are used as a diagnostic aid. Genetically, coeliac disease is strongly associated with HLA-DQ2, which is present in 95% of patients, with the majority of the remainder having HLA-DQ8. There is an increased incidence of disease in first-degree relatives of those affected.

Extraintestinal manifestations can also occur, and these include dermatitis herpetiformis (itchy, blistering skin disease), autoimmune disorders (e.g., type 1 diabetes) and anaemia.

Table 11.8 Causes of malabsorption

Mechanism of malabsorption	Examples
Defective intraluminal digestion or solubilization	Pancreatic insufficiency:
	• Chronic pancreatitis
	• Cystic fibrosis
	• Carcinoma of the pancreas
	Liver disease: failure of bile secretion into duct
Primary mucosal cell abnormalities	Lactase deficiency
Reduced surface area of small intestine	Conditions that cause villous atrophy:
	• Coeliac disease
	• Tropical sprue
	• Crohn disease
	• Malnutrition
	Iatrogenic:
	• Extensive small-intestine resection
	• Jejunal ileal bypass procedures
	• Postradiotherapy
Infection	Postinfective malabsorption
	Giardiasis
	Parasitic infestation of gut
	Bacterial overgrowth in blind loops of diverticula
	Whipple disease
Lymphatic obstruction	Lymphoma
	Primary lymphangiectasia
Drug-induced	Cytotoxic drugs
	Drugs that bind bile salts, e.g., cholestyramine and some antibiotics such as neomycin (which causes steatorrhoea)
Miscellaneous	Thyrotoxicosis—increased gastric emptying and motility
	Zollinger–Ellison syndrome
	Diabetes mellitus—bacterial overgrowth
	Hypogammaglobulinaemia—infection

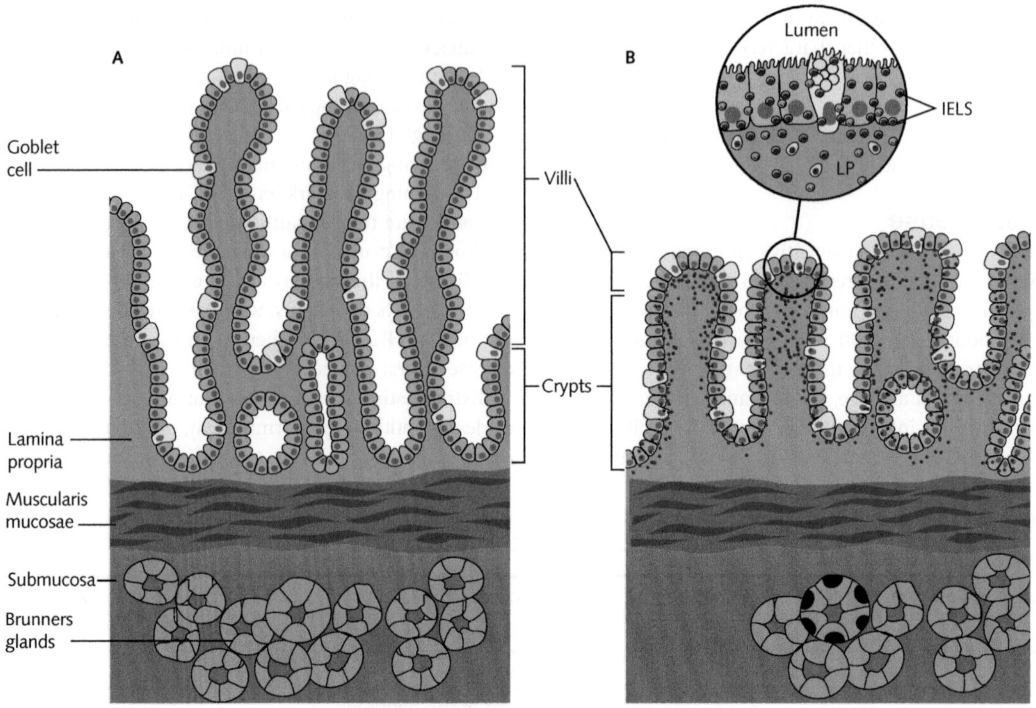

Fig. 11.9 Comparison of duodenal mucosa in (A) normal small bowel versus (B) coeliac disease. *IELS*, intraepithelial lymphocytes; *LP*, lamina propria.

Pathology: macroscopically, the luminal surface becomes flattened, developing a mosaic-like pattern of crypt openings (Fig. 11.9).

Microscopically there is:

- Chronic inflammation of the lamina propria.
- Crypt hyperplasia—increase in the depth of crypts with epithelial cell hyperplasia.
- Increased intraepithelial lymphocytes (cytotoxic CD8+ T-cells).
- Subtotal or total villous atrophy (loss of villous architecture).

Long-term complications are mostly linked with incomplete adherence to a gluten-free diet and include:

- Increased risk of malignant disease:
  - Primary enteropathy associated T-cell lymphoma of the small intestine (EATL).
  - Small-bowel adenocarcinoma (rare).
- Malnutrition with sequelae of vitamin D deficiency, osteoporosis and anaemia.
- Refractory coeliac disease—symptoms of malabsorption despite adherence to a gluten-free diet.

Management is by lifelong strict avoidance of gluten, which leads to gradual recovery of the bowel mucosa.

Tropical sprue

This is an enteropathy resulting in a chronic malabsorption syndrome similar to coeliac disease. The cause is unknown (postulated to be infectious) and almost exclusively affects those who have visited or live in the tropics, i.e., the Caribbean, Southeast Asia, West Africa and India.

Unlike coeliac disease, the distal small bowel is preferentially affected, potentially causing a macrocytic anaemia secondary to B_{12} malabsorption and deficiency.

Whipple disease

Whipple disease is a multisystem disorder involving malabsorption, weight loss, lymphadenopathy and joint pain. The causative agent is the gram-positive bacillus *Tropheryma whippelii.* This rare condition is characterized by tissue infiltration with foamy macrophages that are full of periodic acid-Schiff reagent-positive bacteria.

Bacterial overgrowth syndrome

Malabsorption occurs secondary to excessive bacterial overgrowth in the small intestine, usually the jejunum, the causes of which are outlined in Table 11.9. Clinical features are weight loss, diarrhoea and anaemia (due to vitamin B12 deficiency). Diarrhoea is both secretory (owing to bacterial products affecting mucosa) and osmotic (owing to unabsorbed products and deficiency of disaccharidases because of mucosal damage).

Malabsorption occurs as a result of:

- Deconjugation of bile salts by the bacteria, hence steatorrhoea.
- Damage to the small-intestinal mucosa, probably by bacterial products.

Table 11.9 Causes of small-intestinal bacterial overgrowth

Cause	Example
Excessive entry of bacteria	Achlorhydria
	Infected bile ducts
	Gastrocolic fistula
	Gastric surgery
	Resection of ileocaecal valve
Defective immune mechanisms	Hypogammaglobulinaemia
	Malnutrition
	Old age
Stagnant region	Blind loops
	Enterocolic fistulae
	Jejunal diverticula
	Strictures or other obstruction
	Continent ileostomy
Disturbed motility	Systemic sclerosis
	Intestinal pseudoobstruction
	Diabetic autonomic neuropathy

- Binding of vitamin B12 by bacteria, hence vitamin B12 deficiency.

Management is by antibiotic therapy and surgical resection of a localized abnormality, e.g., stricture, fistula.

Lactase (disaccharidase) deficiency

Lactase is the most important disaccharidase, which is essential for the digestion of lactose (milk sugar). All babies have lactase in their intestines, but the enzyme disappears later in life in about 10% of northern Europeans, 40% of Greeks and Italians, and 80% of Africans and Asians. The presence of undigested lactose in the small intestine (following milk consumption) causes diarrhoea and abdominal pain.

Obstruction of the bowel

Small- and large-bowel obstruction are potentially fatal conditions. The causes are summarized in Table 11.10.

RED FLAG

SYMPTOMS OF BOWEL OBSTRUCTION

The cardinal symptoms of bowel obstruction are:

- Abdominal pain
- Absolute constipation (no faeces or flatus)
- Vomiting
- Abdominal distension.

The presence or absence of the symptom will depend on the level of the obstruction:

- Small bowel ('high obstruction'): vomiting occurs early and frequently, constipation occurs late.
- Large bowel ('low obstruction'): vomiting occurs late, constipation occurs early.

Table 11.10 Major causes of bowel obstruction

Cause	Example
Simple mechanism obstruction	Intraluminal:
	• Foreign bodies
	• Bezoar
	• Gallstone ileus
	• Faecoliths
	• Meconium in cystic fibrosis
	Extramural:
	• Adhesions
	• Hernias
	• Non-intestinal malignancies
	Mural:
	• Colorectal carcinoma
	• Strictures
	• Congenital hypertrophic pyloric stenosis
	• Atresia
	• Imperforate anus
Strangulation obstruction	Intussusception
	Infarction
	Volvulus
	Internal/external hernias
	Bands (adhesions)
Pseudoobstruction (paralytic ileus)	Abdominal causes: postoperative, peritonitis, vascular occlusion, retroperitoneal trauma/bleeding
	Systemic causes: sepsis, electrolyte disturbances, uraemia, hypothyroidism
	Drugs: anticholinergics, opiates

Pathophysiology: distal to the level of obstruction the bowel collapses and proximally dilates owing to accumulation of intestinal secretions (recall that the bowel secretes 9 L of fluid a day!) and swallowed air. The walls become oedematous and then thinned as distension occurs to accommodate the increasing luminal contents. Eventually blood supply is compromised by excessive distension, resulting in ischaemia, loss of wall integrity and translocation of intraluminal bacteria into the peritoneal cavity, causing peritonitis, sepsis and ultimately death.

Major causes of bowel obstruction

Obstruction and pseudoobstruction can be classified as follows:

- Mechanical (simple) obstruction—owing to extramural, mural or intra luminal causes.
- Strangulation obstruction—occlusion of the blood supply by constriction of various causes.
- Pseudoobstruction—abnormal gut motility rather than an organic blockage. This can be acute (Ogilvie syndrome) or chronic. A paralytic ileus is used to refer to an adynamic segment of bowel, which may arise postoperatively.

HINTS AND TIPS

COMMON CAUSES OF SMALL- AND LARGE-BOWEL OBSTRUCTION

Small-bowel obstruction:
- Intraabdominal adhesions—75%
- Hernias—20%

Large-bowel obstruction:
- Colorectal carcinoma in elderly—60%
- Strictures (diverticular disease or ischaemic) —20%
- Volvulus—5%

Hernias

'The protrusion of whole or part of a viscus and its coverings through a defect in its containing compartment into an abnormal position.' They occur at congenital or acquired weakpoints and are very common; about 1 per 100 people have a hernia at some point.

Acquired hernias are:

- Secondary to increased intraabdominal pressure—resulting from cough, straining at defaecation, cysts, carcinoma, pregnancy.
- Iatrogenic—incisional hernias.

Terminology: common sites of abdominal hernias are inguinal (70%), umbilical (10%), incisional (15%) and femoral (5%). Others are epigastric, paraumbilical or linea alba, obturator and Spigelian (Fig. 11.10).

Complications:

- Obstruction—constriction at the neck of the hernial sac causes obstruction of bowel loops within it.
- Strangulation—constriction at the neck of the sac prevents venous return, leading to venous congestion, arterial occlusion and gangrene. This may result in perforation.

Note that strangulation can occur without obstruction if only one wall of the viscus protrudes into the sac (Richter hernia).

Hernias must be repaired because of potential complications. The principles of surgical repair are identification of the sac and contents, mobilization of the sac, reduction of the contents, ligation of the sac and repair of the fascial defect.

Inguinal hernia

This is the most common type of hernia and is substantially more prevalent in men. There are two types: indirect (85%) and direct (15%) inguinal hernias.

- **Indirect:** the hernial sac enters the inguinal canal through the deep ring (lateral to the inferior epigastric artery) and traverses through the canal to the superficial ring; it may eventually reach the scrotum or labia majora. It is the result of a congenital abnormality. Strangulation is a common complication because of the narrow neck of the hernial sac.
- **Direct:** the hernial sac protrudes through a weakness in the fascia transversalis (medial to the inferior epigastric artery) and does not normally descend into the scrotum or labia majora. It originates as a result of weakened abdominal muscles (usually acquired in the elderly). The neck of the sac is wide so strangulation is rare.

Clinically, it is difficult to distinguish between direct and indirect inguinal hernias.

Femoral hernia

The hernial sac protrudes through the femoral canal inferior to the inguinal ligament. There is an increasing incidence with age, and females are affected more often than males by a factor of 2:1 (but inguinal hernia is still more common in both males and females). The most common complication is strangulation owing to the rigid walls of the femoral canal.

Adhesions

Adhesions are areas of fibrosis between adjacent serosal membranes or organs, resulting in their fusion. They are by far the commonest cause of mechanical small-bowel obstruction. The causes can be congenital (e.g., bands in small children) or acquired.

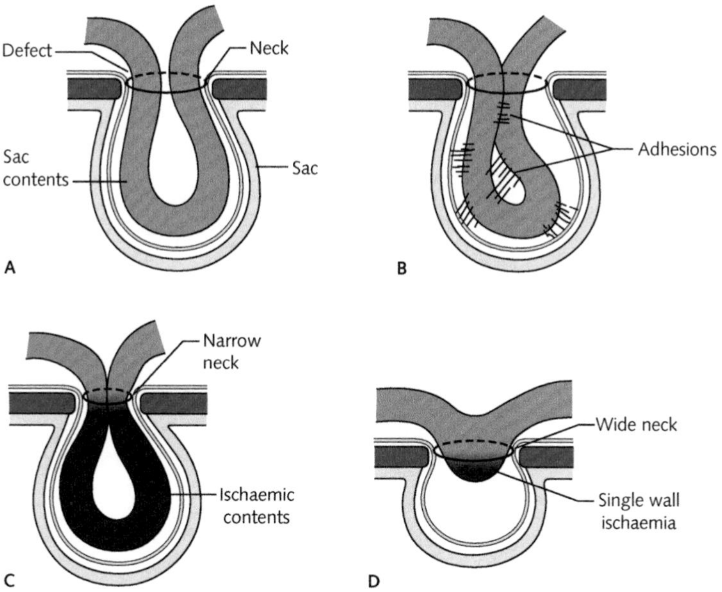

Fig. 11.10 Terminology of hernias. Hernias consist of a sac, sac coverings, sac content and the defect. (A) Reducible—contents of sac can be completely returned to abdominal cavity. (B) Irreducible/incarcerated—content of sac is adherent to itself ± the inner wall of the sac and cannot be completely returned to the abdominal cavity. (C) Strangulated—ischaemia and infarction of the sac contents owing to a compromised blood supply. (D) Richter hernia—a single wall of a viscus protrudes into the sac.

Acquired causes:

- Inflammation, e.g., Crohn disease, sclerosing peritonitis.
- Infection, e.g., appendicitis, diverticulitis, tuberculosis, peritonitis.
- Trauma, e.g., stab wounds.
- Iatrogenic—postsurgery, irradiation.
- Vascular—infarction/gangrene.
- Malignancies.

Intussusception

This is invagination of one part of the bowel into the adjoining segment (Fig. 11.4). The ileocaecal valve is the most common site, with the ileum invaginating into the caecum. It typically affects children under the age of 4 years and is most commonly caused by intestinal lymphoid hyperplasia secondary to viral infection.

Adult cases are extremely rare, and they are almost invariably precipitated by an intraluminal mass (e.g., tumour) or structural abnormality (e.g., Meckel diverticulum) acting as a lead point.

As the contents of the intestine are pushed onwards by muscular contraction, more and more intestine is dragged into the adjoining bowel. The net effect is venous congestion of the invaginated portion, which may suffer infarction if mesenteric vessels are trapped.

Management is by barium reduction in children or by resection in adults because of the high incidence of organic causes, i.e., tumours.

Volvulus

This is a twisting of part of the bowel around its mesenteric pedicle, usually leading to partial or complete obstruction ± venous infarction (strangulation) (Fig. 11.11). It is most commonly seen in redundant loops of the sigmoid colon, but may also occur in the caecum, small intestine and stomach.

Sigmoid volvulus—usually in the elderly with a long, faecally-loaded sigmoid colon.

Caecal volvulus—in younger patients (30–60 years) and associated with developmental failure of peritoneal fixation of the caecum.

Management—may untwist spontaneously, but surgical manipulation is usually performed. Resection of the infarcted segment is required.

Colonic diverticulosis

Definitions

- Diverticulum—a sac or pouch formed at weak points in the wall of the alimentary tract (Fig. 11.12).
  - True diverticulum: contains all the layers of the bowel wall.
  - False diverticulum: involves only mucosa and submucosa.
- Diverticulosis—multiple diverticula are present with no evidence of inflammation.
- Diverticulitis—inflammation of a diverticulum or multiple diverticula.
- Diverticular disease—symptomatic diverticulosis.

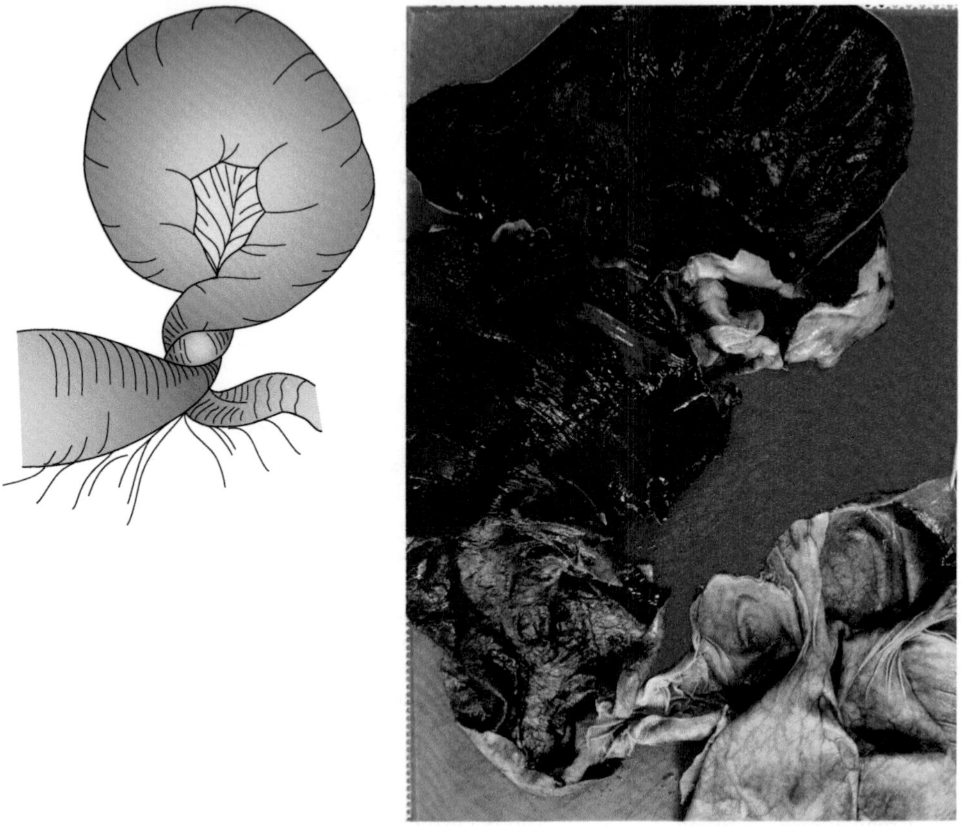

Fig. 11.11 Intestinal volvulus. Colonic volvulus. Resected volvulus demonstrating massive dilatation and infarction with a characteristic sharp transition from viable to infarcted bowel at the point of strangulation. This accounts for 5% of the cases of large-bowel obstruction. Of these, sigmoid volvulus is the most common, followed by caecal volvulus.

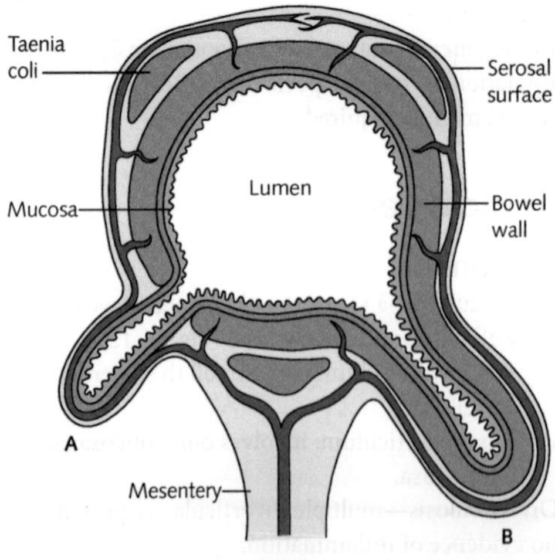

Fig. 11.12 True and false diverticula. *(A)* False diverticulum involves only mucosa and submucosa. *(B)* True diverticulum involves all three layers of the bowel wall.

Aetiopathogenesis of diverticula

Diverticula can be congenital (true diverticula) or acquired (true/false diverticula).

The majority of acquired diverticula are located in the sigmoid colon and typically develop during adult life. Although rare before 35 years of age, by 65 years of age at least one-third of the population of developed countries have diverticula as a result of a chronic lack of dietary fibre. Conversely, diverticula are rare in developing countries with high-fibre diets.

Acquired diverticula are pulsion diverticula formed from increased intraluminal pressure (e.g., straining at the stool), causing protrusion of mucosa at focal points of weakness. Within the colon these are the sites between the mesenteric and antimesenteric taeniae where the neurovascular bundles traverse the bowel wall.

Clinical features

Diverticula are asymptomatic and present when they become inflamed (diverticulitis), causing pain and tenderness in the left iliac fossa, alteration of bowel habit, fever and leucocytosis. A mass may be palpable. Diverticulitis can result in various complications (Table 11.11), with repetitive inflammatory episodes potentially leading to fibrosis and stricture formation.

Vascular disorders of the bowel

Ischaemic bowel disease

Ischaemic bowel disease may affect the small or large bowel, and it is most commonly seen in elderly patients with severe atherosclerosis (Fig. 11.13). The causes are discussed below.

Vessel disease

These are:

- Vascular occlusion—emboli, usually derived from a cardiac mural thrombus, lodge in the superior mesenteric artery, which supplies all the small intestine except for the first part of the duodenum.
- Vascular stenosis (less common)—occurs with thrombosis in a severely atherosclerotic mesenteric artery. It is typically located near its origin from the aorta. The resultant small-bowel infarction is extensive and usually fatal. Patients can present with intestinal claudication.
- Vasculitic syndromes, e.g., polyarteritis nodosa, Henoch–Schönlein purpura, systemic lupus erythematosus.

> **HINTS AND TIPS**
>
> **VASCULOPATHY**
>
> Vasculopathy is not an isolated/localized phenomenon, i.e., if vascular disease presents in one vascular territory then it is likely there is occult vascular disease elsewhere, e.g., heart, periphery.

Table 11.11 Complications of diverticulitis

Complication	Consequences
Perforation	Generalized peritonitis Pericolic abscess Fistula (bladder, vagina, small bowel)
Obstruction/ stricture	Oedema of inflamed segment Fibrosis and stricturing of inflamed segment Adherence of small-bowel loops
Haemorrhage	Acute, perfuse and painless Chronic and occult (most common)
Colorectal carcinoma	Can be identified incidentally when an 'inflammatory mass' is resected

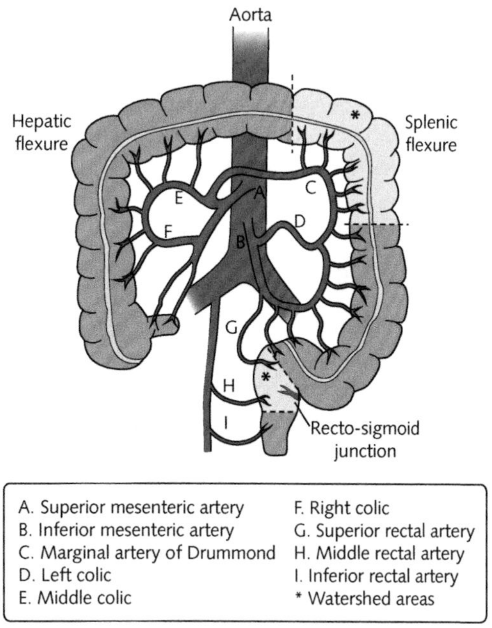

Fig. 11.13 Watershed areas of the colon. The marginal artery of Drummond, formed by the union of the distal branches of superior and inferior mesenteric arteries, provides end-arterial supply to the splenic flexure watershed area (Griffiths point). The superior rectal artery (from inferior mesenteric artery) and middle and inferior rectal artery (from iliac artery) anastomose to provide blood to the rectosigmoid junction (Sudeck point).

Strangulation

Thin-walled veins which drain blood from the small bowel become occluded by extrinsic pressure, e.g., from:

- a loop of bowel in a narrow hernial sac
- intussusception
- volvulus
- adhesions.

Venous occlusion causes congestion and oedema of the bowel wall. Increased pressure prevents entry of oxygenated arterial blood, leading to ischaemic necrosis (also known as mesenteric ischaemia or intestinal angina).

Classification of severity

Ischaemic infarcts are classified according to the depth of involvement:

- Mucosal infarction—transient or reversible infarction which may be followed by complete regeneration. However, increased permeability to toxic substances can cause gradual progression to a transmural infarct.
- Mural infarction—infarction of mucosa and submucosa up to the muscularis propria. The mucosa is ulcerated, oedematous and haemorrhagic. Healing occurs by granulation tissue formation. Mural infarction may lead to the development of fibrotic strictures (occurs in about half of patients with ischaemic bowel disease).

- Transmural infarction—necrosis extends through the muscularis propria. The bowel is flaccid, dilated and liable to perforation. Surgical resection is an option, but many patients already have peritonitis, endotoxaemia and severe circulatory problems at the time of diagnosis, so the prognosis is poor.

HINTS AND TIPS

WATERSHED AREAS

The splenic flexure is a common and early site of ischaemic damage as it is a watershed area where the distal-most branches of the superior and inferior mesenteric arteries meet (Fig. 11.13). Collateralization of blood supply (watershed areas) and solitary arterial supply makes these intestinal regions more sensitive to hypoperfusion and ischaemia. The rectosigmoid junction is also a watershed area.

Angiodysplasia

This is characterized by abnormally dilated and ectatic veins, venules and capillaries that develop in the mucosa and submucosa of the large intestine (typically caecum and right colon), often causing occult or massive intestinal bleeding. It occurs in the elderly and the exact pathogenesis remains unclear.

Table 11.12 Differential diagnosis of melaena and per rectal bleeding

Melaena[a]	Per rectal blood

Gastrointestinal bleeding
• Peptic ulcer disease
• Oesophagitis (severe)
• Small bowel
  ○ Meckel diverticulum
  ○ Angiodysplasia
• Right colon
	Benign
	• Haemorrhoids
	• Diverticular disease
	• Colitis
	• Anal fissure
	• Angiodysplasia (if large volume bleed)

Ingested blood • Epistaxis (nose bleed) • Haemoptysis	Malignant • Left-sided colon cancer • Rectal carcinoma

Bleeding diathesis
• Liver disease
• Thrombocytopaenia
• Haemophilia
• Drugs
  ○ Anticoagulants
  ○ Aspirin
  ○ Nonsteroidal antiinflammatory drugs	

Mimics of 'black' stools • Iron tablets • Bismuth • Charcoal	

[a] *Melaena is the per rectal passage of altered blood and it appears as thick black tar-like stools. For it to be 'altered' it must have arisen in the upper gastrointestinal tract and undergone digestion. Fresh rectal bleeding denotes lower gastrointestinal tract.*

Anorectal disease

Anal fissures

An anal fissure is a longitudinal tear in the anal epithelium below the dentate line. Anal fissures present with severe pain on defaecation, which persists for hours after as a throbbing/gnawing discomfort. Blood characteristically may be seen on the paper (Table 11.12).

Patients are usually constipated, and the fissure is initiated by the trauma of passing a large firm stool. A vicious cycle ensues of anal spasm/high anal resting pressure, causing local hypoperfusion which impedes fissure healing. Ninety percent occur posteriorly in the midline and the majority become chronic. A tag of anal epithelium ('sentinel pile') may develop as a result of overhealing at the end of the fissure.

Anal fistula

A fistula is 'an abnormal connection between two epithelial surfaces'. They are most commonly seen in Crohn disease and present with a mixture of watery discharge, itching (pruritus ani), bubbling on defaecation and possible pain if inflamed. Other causes include bipolar bursting of an intersphincteric abscess, tuberculosis and rectal carcinoma.

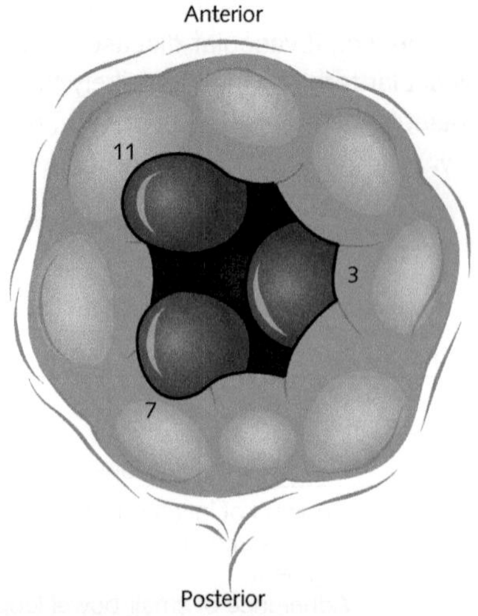

Fig. 11.14 Distribution of haemorrhoids within the anus. Diagram to illustrate the 3, 7, 11 distribution of haemorrhoids around the anus. (Adapted with permission from Ellis H. Lecture Notes in General Surgery, 12th edn. Chichester: Wiley-Blackwell, 2010.)

Haemorrhoids (piles)

Haemorrhoids are an enlargement of the anal cushions, which are highly vascularized areas within the anal canal. They are the most common anal condition, affecting as much as 40% of the population at some point. Presentation is with bright red rectal bleeding on the stools, paper or in the pan. They are painless unless they become ulcerated or strangulated. Pruritus ani and a sensation of a mass protruding through the anus can also be present.

Haemorrhoids develop as a result of increased intraabdominal pressure, e.g., constipation with straining at defaecation and pregnancy. Rarely, raised portal hypertension can cause haemorrhoid formation. They arise above the anorectal margin, most commonly within the 3, 7 and 11 o'clock positions (Fig. 11.14).

Clinical classification

There are four degrees of haemorrhoid:

1. First-degree—present in the lumen but do not prolapse; these tend to bleed.
2. Second-degree—prolapse on defaecation but return spontaneously.
3. Third-degree—remain prolapsed but can be digitally replaced.
4. Fourth-degree—persistently prolapsed, cannot be reduced.

Diagnosis is by proctoscopy (to visualize the haemorrhoids) or by sigmoidoscopy (to exclude coexisting rectal pathology).

Treatment involves reducing constipation and straining with a high-fibre diet or direct therapy to the haemorrhoid with injection sclerotherapy or band ligation. Surgical removal of the haemorrhoid (haemorrhoidectomy) is rarely required.

Perianal haematoma (thrombosed external piles)

This is a blood clot in the subcutaneous haemorrhoidal vein, which presents suddenly as a painful bluish lump at the anal verge. The pain is continuous, reaching a maximal peak at day 2–3. Bleeding is only seen if ulceration occurs.

It is important to recognize perianal haematomas as they are often mistaken for haemorrhoids. Pain can be relieved by incision and expression of the blood clot within the first 1–2 days; otherwise, they regress to form a fibrous tag or spontaneously discharge the clotted blood.

Lymphogranuloma venereum

Lymphogranuloma venereum (LGV) is a sexually transmitted disease cause by *Chlamydia trachomatis* causing proctitis associated with painful inguinal lymphadenopathy (bilateral in a third of patients). It is almost exclusively reported in men who have sex with men, the majority of whom are HIV-positive (70%–96%). Clinically and histologically LGV can mimic inflammatory bowel disease. Thickening and fibrosis can occur in chronic infections, leading to rectal strictures. The most reliable diagnostic test is real-time polymerase chain reaction (PCR) on a fresh rectal swab.

Anal intraepithelial neoplasia

Anal intraepithelial neoplasia (AIN) is a premalignant lesion of the anus (squamous epithelium), akin to cervical intraepithelial neoplasia (see Chapter 15) and is driven by HPV infection. It is classified as low grade (AIN I) when dysplasia affects the basal third of the epithelium or high grade (AIN II and III) when it affects two-thirds or full epithelial thickness. High-grade AIN is a precursor to anal carcinoma, but the natural history of low-grade AIN is not well established.

Anal cancer

The anal canal is lined by a mix of epithelium from glandular (proximal) to squamous (distal). SCCs account for 80% of anal cancers; other types include adenocarcinoma, melanoma and lymphoma. HPV infection is linked to 90% of anal SCCs, making SCC a preventable disease.

The incidence of anal cancer is increasing, although it still accounts for <1% of all cancers. It is more common in females than males, with a survival rate of 64% at 5 years. In women, tumours arise more commonly above the dentate line and usually in the sixth decade and in men more commonly below the dentate line in the third decade. There is an increased incidence in men who have sex with men who are HIV-positive, and those who are immunosuppressed. Other risk factors include smoking and previous vulval or cervical premalignant lesions.

Neoplastic disease of the intestine

Primary tumours of the small intestine are rare; those that do arise are outlined in Table 11.13. In contrast, tumours of the large bowel are extremely common. The colon and rectum are frequently affected by both benign and malignant tumours.

Classification of intestinal tumours

Intestinal tumours can be classified according to Table 11.13.

Neoplastic epithelial lesions

Adenomas

These premalignant tumours are derived from the glandular epithelium of the bowel. Common in older subjects, they are present in up to 50% of persons aged over 60, more males than females by a factor of 2:1.

Aetiology is probably multifactorial. Both genetic and environmental (dietary) factors have been implicated.

There are three types:

1. Tubular—rounded lesions (0.5–2 cm in size). Often pedunculated (i.e., have a stalk of normal mucosa). Microscopically composed of tube-shaped glands.

Table 11.13 Types of intestinal tumour

	Small intestine	Large intestine
Polyps	• Hamartomas	• Hamartomatous polyps ◦ Peutz–Jeghers ◦ Juvenile polyps
	• Juvenile polyps	• Hyperplastic polyps: small, flat, pale lesions typically 5 mm in size, which occur most commonly in the rectum and sigmoid colon
	• Adenomatous polyps (in FAP and Gardner syndrome)	• Inflammatory pseudopolyps (of ulcerative colitis)
	• Inflammatory fibroid polyps	• Premalignant:
		• Adenomas (dysplastic): ◦ Tubular adenoma ◦ Villous adenoma ◦ Tubulovillous adenoma
		• Sessile serrated lesion with dysplasia
Neoplastic epithelial lesions	Adenocarcinomas	Colorectal adenocarcinoma
Mesenchymal lesions	• Benign: lipoma, neurogenic tumours, leiomyoma and haemangioma • Malignant: some smooth muscle tumours (leiomyosarcomas)	Rare: usually incidental findings or at postmortem; seldom responsible for symptoms; lipomas, leiomyomas, haemangiomas, neurofibromas Malignant: some smooth muscle tumours (leiomyosarcomas)
Lymphoma	Common site for primary lymphoma of the GI tract; coeliac disease is a major predisposing factor (enteropathy-associated T-cell lymphoma)	Very uncommon in large bowel
Neuroendocrine tumours (carcinoid tumours)	Most common site for neuroendocrine tumours (ileum>jejunum>duodenum); lesions typically scattered singly throughout GI tract; may secrete hormones, e.g., somatostatin, VIP	Uncommon—most common in the appendix. Do not usually produce functioning hormones

FAP, Familial adenomatous polyposis; GI, gastrointestinal; VIP, vasoactive intestinal polypeptide.

2. Villous—frond-like lesions about 0.6 cm thick, which occupy a broad area of mucosa (1–5 cm in diameter). Microscopically composed of finger-like epithelial projections.
3. Tubulovillous—raised lesions (1–4 cm in size). Pedunculated but composed of both tube-shaped glands and finger-like epithelial projections.

All three types have dysplastic epithelium, which can be low or high grade.

Serrated lesions

Serrated lesions are characterized by serrated glands with branched/dilated crypts. Current UK nomenclature is included for clarity and is as follows:

- Sessile serrated lesions—arise in the right colon and are >10 mm. They are sessile (i.e., not pedunculated) and tend to occur on mucosal folds, characteristically covered by a blob of mucus.
  - Potentially associated with advanced colorectal neoplasia.
  - Can be part of a serrated polyposis syndrome.
- Traditional villous adenoma—rare, 1%–3% of adenomas. Formed of eosinophilic pencillate cells with serrated glands. Commonly found in the rectosigmoid colon.
- Sessile serrated lesion with dysplasia—a sessile serrated lesion with high- or low-grade dysplasia.

Progression from adenoma to carcinoma

Most carcinomas of the colon develop from previous adenomas. Progression from adenoma to carcinoma is the well-established sequence for development of carcinoma of the colon. More recently, a separate genetic pathway has been identified for a subset of colorectal carcinomas called serrated carcinomas, some of which are thought to arise from dysplastic sessile serrated lesions.

Risk of malignant change is greatest where adenomas show the following features:

- Large—less than 1 cm (1% malignant); 1–2 cm (12% malignant); more than 2 cm (30% malignant).
- Villous architecture—more likely to undergo malignant transformation.
- High-grade dysplasia.
- Serrated lesion with dysplasia.

MOLECULAR

GENETICS OF COLORECTAL CANCER

The molecular classification of colorectal cancer is becoming increasingly important as it more accurately predicts behaviour and prognosis and guides management. There are two pathways by which colorectal carcinoma can arise:

- ***Classical pathway:*** Adenoma → carcinoma sequence
  Seventy percent of sporadic cases, involves chromosomal instability with increased copy numbers, loss of heterozygosity and accumulation of mutations in tumour suppressor genes.
  Major genes involved: *APC*, *KRAS*, *TP53* and *SMAD4*.
- ***Serrated pathway:*** Serrated lesion → serrated carcinoma
  Thirty percent of sporadic cases, the majority associated with microsatellite instability which occurs due to mutations in DNA mismatch repair enzymes, e.g., MLH-1 and MSH-2. The major genes involved are *BRAF* and *KRAS*.
  For further discussion see Chapter 6.

Polyposis syndromes

Familial adenomatous polyposis

Familial adenomatous polyposis (FAP) is a rare autosomal dominant condition caused by a mutation in the *APC* gene located on the long arm of chromosome 5. It is characterized by the presence of >100 adenomas of the large bowel from about the age of 25. There is a 100% risk of developing colorectal carcinoma by the age of 45. Extraintestinal manifestations are also possible, which include gastric fundic gland polyps, desmoid tumours and duodenal adenocarcinomas.

Lynch syndrome

Previously known as hereditary nonpolyposis colon cancer, this is the most common form of inherited colon cancer. It arises from mutations in the DNA mismatch repair genes *MSH-2* (50%), *MLH-1*(30%–40%), *MSH-6* (7%–10%) and *PMS2* (<5%), which are associated with microsatellite instability.

Clinically it is characterized by the development of tumours, including colorectal carcinoma, at an early age (40–50 years). Colorectal carcinomas tend to occur on the right side, are poorly differentiated and associated with a prominent inflammatory response. Colorectal adenomas may be present (<10). There is also an increased risk of tumours at other sites, such as endometrium, stomach, small bowel, pancreatobiliary tract and brain. This is important to note as synchronous/metachronous tumours will be present in 30% of cases, therefore the presenting tumour of Lynch syndrome may be a non-colorectal carcinoma e.g. endometrial. (Table 11.14).

Colorectal carcinoma

This adenocarcinoma is derived from the glandular epithelium of the large-bowel mucosa.

It is the third most common cause of death from neoplasia, with a peak incidence between 60 and 70 years of age; it is rare under the age of 40 years.

There is a high incidence in developed countries; 72 per 100,000 males and 56 per 100,000 females in the UK are diagnosed each year, with a higher incidence in Scotland for both sexes. Environmental factors are thought to play a large role in the aetiology of colorectal cancer (Table 11.15).

Macroscopic features—the most common sites for colorectal carcinomas are illustrated in Fig. 11.15. Colorectal carcinomas exhibit different growth patterns, e.g., polypoid (where exophytic tumour can fill the lumen with a small underlying attachment to the wall) or annular (circumferential) with extensive or focal invasion and ulceration. Within the caecum it is typical for the tumour to form a large solid mass.

In advanced cases, serosal invasion can occur, resulting in serosal puckering ± adhesions and fistulae to other organs, e.g., ovary, small bowel.

Microscopic features—98% of colorectal cancers are adenocarcinomas; the majority are well-moderately differentiated, forming recognizable glandular structures. Poorly differentiated carcinomas have lost their glandular architecture and have a poorer prognosis.

Serrated carcinomas have a serrated architecture and are often mucinous with an intense lymphocytic infiltrate.

Presentation:

Right-sided carcinomas (ascending colon):

- Presentation—later than for left-sided carcinomas.
- Anaemia—common sign from chronic occult blood loss in stool.
- Obstruction—late as the caecum is a capacitance vessel so substantial growth can occur occultly.
- Weight loss.

Left-sided carcinomas (descending colon):

Table 11.14 Polyposis syndromes

Syndrome	Inheritance	Age presentation	Polyps	Location	Other associations/ extraintestinal	Genetic mutations	Malignant risk/ colorectal carcinoma
FAP syndrome	AD	10–15 years	Adenomas >100 usually 1000s	Colon	CHRPEs, fundic gland polyps, desmoids (Gardner syndrome[a]: osteomas, dermoid tumours, skin cysts)	*APC*	100%
Attenuated FAP	AD	44–56 years	Adenomas <100	Colon	Same as FAP	*APC*	100%
Lynch syndrome	AD	<50 years	Adenomas <10	Colon	Endometrial, stomach and ovarian carcinomas	*MSH-2*, *MLH-1*	80%
Peutz–Jeghers syndrome	AD	10–15 years	Hamartomatous polyps (1–10s of polyps)	Small bowel and colon most common. Anywhere in the GIT	Mucocutaneous pigmentation. Cancers of GIT, breast, ovary	*STK11/LKB1*	93%

[a] *Gardner syndrome is now considered part of the FAP spectrum.*
AD, Autosomal dominant; CHRPE, congenital hypertrophy of the retinal pigment epithelium; FAP, familial adenomatous polyposis; GIT, gastrointestinal tract.

Table 11.15 Risk factors for colorectal carcinoma
Environmental
• High-fat diet
• Low-fibre diet
• Red and processed meat consumption (high-protein diet)
• Alcohol—risk increases by 7% per unit consumed per day
• Smoking
• Obesity (body mass index >30)
Medical history
• Longstanding and extensive ulcerative colitis
• Previous pelvic radiotherapy
Genetic
• Family history of colorectal cancer, especially at a young age
• Multiple sporadic adenomatous polyps
• Familial adenomatous polyposis (FAP)
• Lynch syndrome

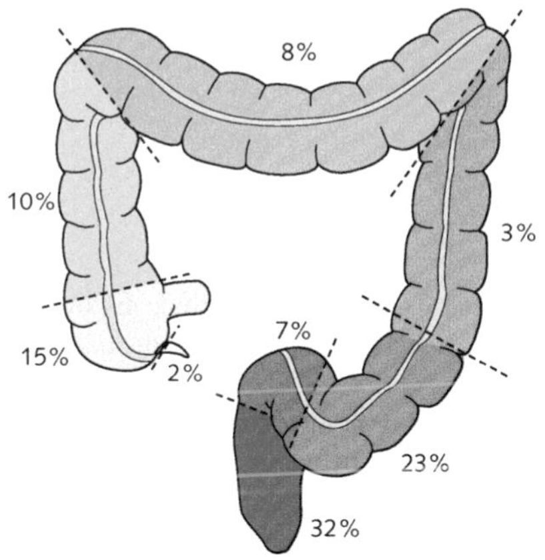

Fig. 11.15 Site and incidence of carcinomas of the large bowel.

- Presentation—earlier than right-sided carcinomas.
- Obstruction—mechanical obstruction occurs early as lesions tend to be annular and inhibit the passage of formed faeces.
- Bleeding—frank blood may be noted mixed in with stools if the tumour is very distally located (Table 11.12).

Prognosis: this relates to stage, which is assessed using the tumour, node, metastasis (TNM) and the modified Dukes classifications (Fig. 11.16). Five-year survival is over 90% in Dukes A cancer, but less than 5% in Dukes D. Dukes C and D cancers (common presentations) require adjuvant chemotherapy and/or radiotherapy after surgical resection. Overall, 5-year survival is around 60%.

RED FLAG

SYMPTOMS AND SIGNS OF COLORECTAL CANCER

Unexplained weight loss—from catabolic effects of cancer
Persistent change in bowel habit—correlates potentially to obstruction
Anaemia—from occult (chronic) blood loss
Blood mixed in with stool
Abdominal pain or discomfort

CLINICAL NOTE

COLORECTAL CARCINOMA SPREAD

- Local—adjacent bowel wall and adherent structures (e.g., bladder)
- Lymphatic—draining mesenteric lymph nodes
- Blood—to liver via portal vein and then elsewhere
- Transcoelomic—through the peritoneal cavity

DISORDERS OF THE APPENDIX

Nonneoplastic conditions

Acute appendicitis

This is inflammation of the appendix, usually secondary to obstruction. Subsequent infection may develop. It occurs most often in teenagers and young adults, with a slight male predominance.

Other

- Infective processes (particularly after obstruction)—the commonest organisms are *Mycobacterium tuberculosis* and *Yersinia*.
- Lymphoid hyperplasia—often seen in children secondary to infection and may mimic acute appendicitis clinically.

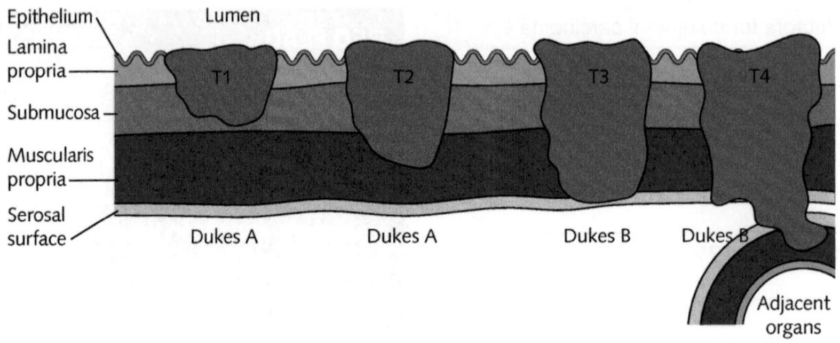

Fig. 11.16 Tumour, node, metastasis (TNM) staging of colorectal carcinoma. TNM staging of colorectal carcinoma with comparative Dukes classification. T1—tumour invades through muscularis mucosae into submucosa; T2—invasion into but not through muscularis propria; T3—invasion through muscularis propria with intact serosal surface; T4—invasion through serosa or invasion into other organs. TNM staging is used over Dukes; however, Dukes (A–D) is still referred. Dukes stage C correlates to any stage with lymph node involvement (N1) and Dukes D correlates to any stage with metastases (M1).

- Crohn disease—can occur anywhere along the GI tract, including the appendix.
- Obstruction of the appendiceal base—may cause retention of intraluminal mucin, forming a mucocele.

Neoplasms of the appendix

Neuroendocrine tumours

The commonest neoplasm of the appendix is a low-grade neuroendocrine tumour. Most are asymptomatic and demonstrate benign behaviour, but intermediate and frankly malignant features can be seen. Treatment is surgical excision.

Mucinous neoplasms

Low-grade appendiceal mucinous neoplasms are the commonest mucinous neoplasm of the appendix. Average age at presentation is 60 years; they may be associated with GI and ovarian adenocarcinoma.

Perforation of mucinous neoplasms can cause accumulation of mucin in the peritoneum (pseudomyxoma peritonei). Complications are seeding of tumour cells, forming epithelial implants, peritonitis and adhesions. Treatment is via surgical excision and chemotherapy.

Metastasis

Breast, gastrointestinal and gynaecological malignancies are the most frequent carcinomas to metastasize to the appendix.

DISORDERS OF THE PERITONEUM

Peritonitis

This is inflammation of the peritoneal lining of the abdominal cavity. The causes may be infective or noninfective (e.g., secondary to trauma or inflamed intraabdominal organ).

Peritoneal infection

This can either be of primary (see Chapter 12) or secondary infection. Primary infection (less common) is seen in patients with peritoneal dialysis, cirrhosis with ascites or abdominal trauma.

Secondary infection (most common) is typically an extension of inflammation from abdominal viscera. For example:

- Appendicitis, cholecystitis, pancreatitis or salpingitis.
- Ruptured ulcers—peptic and ulcerated neoplasms.
- Diverticulitis.
- Chlamydial infection—a complication of female pelvic inflammatory disease that is increasing in incidence.
- Strangulated bowel.
- Tuberculosis.

Organisms involved are typically a mixture of normal gut commensals with a predominance of anaerobic bacteria and coliforms.

Irritation of the peritoneum by leaking bile, gastric juice, pancreatic enzymes or urine produces an exudate that is initially sterile but which usually becomes infected within 6–12 h.

As peritonitis develops, inflammation of visceral and parietal peritoneum produces a purulent exudate; the intestine becomes flaccid, dilated and covered with fibrinous plaques that form adhesions between bowel loops.

Clinical features are:

- Guarding and rebound tenderness.
- Board-like abdominal rigidity.
- Absent bowel sounds (paralytic ileus).
- Tachycardia and pyrexia.

Complications and management

Complications are:

- Hypovolaemic shock.
- Sepsis from absorbed bacterial products.
- Paralytic ileus—paralysis of gut motility caused by serosal inflammation of the small bowel.

- Fibrous adhesions as a result of organization of fibrin by granulation tissue.
- Abscesses, particularly in the paracolic gutters and beneath the diaphragm (subphrenic recesses).
- Localized peritonitis is due to the capacity of omentum to wall off infection.
- Diagnosis is by clinical examination, imaging and microbiological investigations.

Management is by:

- Treatment of shock.
- Antibiotic therapy.
- Surgery—removal of contaminating source, e.g., appendicitis or perforated bowel.
- Peritoneal toilet and lavage.

Retroperitoneal fibrosis

This is dense progressive fibrosis of the peritoneum particularly affecting the visceral peritoneum of the small intestine. In most cases no cause is found, although there are rare associations with some medications (practolol and methysergide). It is also seen in patients who have received radiotherapy or are undergoing long-term continuous ambulatory peritoneal dialysis.

Mesenteric cysts

These are cysts found within the mesentery of the abdominal cavity or attached to the peritoneal lining.

Cystic lymphangiomas (sequestered lymphatic channels)

These cystic developmental abnormalities of lymphatics are typically asymptomatic and discovered incidentally at laparotomy or autopsy.

Pinched-off enteric diverticula (enterogenous cysts)

These common lesions are found either incorporated in the bowel wall or in the mesentery.

Neoplasms

Mesothelioma

A rare condition, this is associated with exposure to asbestos. It corresponds to the much more common pleural mesothelioma (see Chapter 10).

HINTS AND TIPS

PERITONEAL CAVITY AND METASTASIS

The peritoneal cavity is a common site of metastases; malignancy of any organ within the peritoneal cavity may lead to peritonitis.

Metastasis

The most common metastatic tumours to the peritoneal cavity are from the stomach, ovary, pancreas and colon.

Metastases result in protein-rich effusions (i.e., an exudate) containing neoplastic cells, which may also grow as tiny white nodules on the mesothelial surface of the cavity. Nodules eventually coalesce to form sheets of tumour over the surface of the viscera.

Chapter Summary

- Barrett oesophagus is a metaplastic process that has a high risk of progression to adenocarcinoma.
- Gastric ulcers are most commonly associated with *Helicobacter pylori*, nonsteroidal antiinflammatory drugs (NSAIDs) and alcohol.
- *H. pylori* is the commonest precursor of gastric adenocarcinoma, increasing the risk by eightfold.
- Most gastric cancers are adenocarcinomas.
- There are many causes of diarrhoea; the most common are infections but others include enteropathies, inflammatory bowel disease, ischaemia, drugs and many others.
- Coeliac disease is a gluten-sensitive enteropathy; gluten is found in wheat, barley, rye and oats.
- *Clostridium difficile* is a hospital-acquired infection and a major cause of morbidity and mortality in hospitalized patients.
- The commonest causes of bowel obstruction are adhesions (small bowel) and carcinoma (large bowel).
- Inflammatory bowel disease is comprised of ulcerative colitis and Crohn disease.
- In Crohn disease there is patchy transmural inflammation predisposing to fistulae and stricture formation.
- In ulcerative colitis inflammation is confined to the mucosa and extends proximally from the rectum in a continuous pattern.
- Colorectal cancer is the fourth most common form of cancer in the UK, usually occurring after age 40. The vast majority are adenocarcinomas and are left-sided.
- Colorectal carcinoma is now thought to arise from two genetically different pathways: classical and serrated.
- Lynch syndrome is the most common hereditary colorectal cancer syndrome and is caused by mutations in mismatch repair genes.
- Neuroendocrine tumours are the commonest neoplasms of the appendix; however, acute appendicitis is the commonest overall pathology.
- Peritonitis should be diagnosed quickly to prevent generalized inflammation, which has a high mortality rate if untreated.

Pathology of the hepatopancreaticobiliary system

12

GENERAL ASPECTS OF HEPATIC DAMAGE

See Fig. 12.1.

Patterns of hepatic injury

Following hepatic injury, the liver has a limited set of responses:

- necrosis
- inflammation
- regeneration
- fibrosis.

All pathological processes of the liver result in one or more of the above reactions.

Necrosis

Acute hepatocellular injury can result in variable forms of necrosis. The underlying type of necrosis depends on aetiology.

Coagulative necrosis

This is typically a result of ischaemia (see Chapter 3).

Hydropic degeneration

This is the ballooning of individual hepatocytes, generally as a result of viral hepatitis. Mild swelling is reversible, but more advanced changes may progress to necrosis.

Apoptosis

This is programmed cell death, which appears microscopically as cell dropout. Clinically there is no increase in alanine aminotransferase.

Focal necrosis

Necrosis of small groups of hepatocytes occurs in acute viral- or drug-induced hepatitis.

Zonal necrosis

Necrosis confined to certain parenchymal zones is seen with particular conditions, e.g., the centrilobular area (zone 3) is affected in paracetamol toxicity (Fig. 12.2 and see Fig. 12.9).

Submassive necrosis

Necrosis of the majority of hepatocytes occurs with fulminant hepatic damage and is seen in some cases of viral and toxin-induced damage.

Interface (piecemeal) necrosis

Liver cells at the interface between the parenchyma and inflamed portal tracts are destroyed.

Inflammation

Inflammation of the liver is known as hepatitis, and it is a common response to a wide array of damage, e.g., viral infection, autoimmune disorders, drugs and toxins.

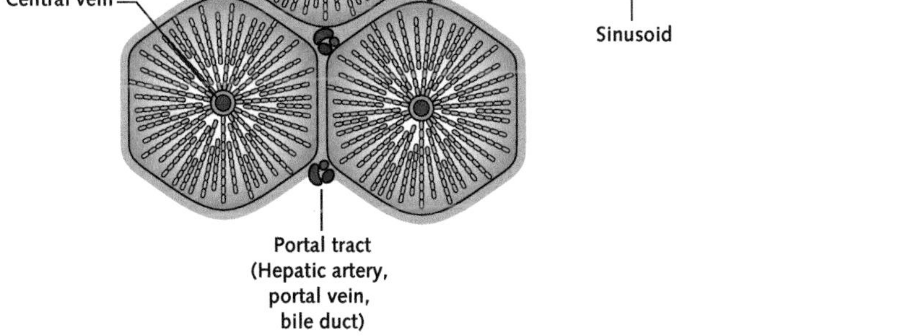

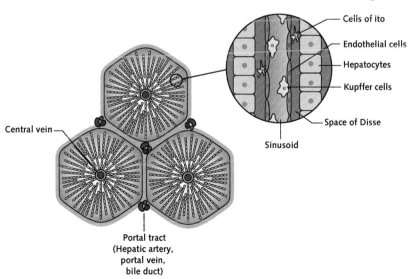

Fig. 12.1 Ultrastrucutre of the liver.
The liver is arranged into functional lobules formed from cords of hepatocytes surrounding central veins. Portal tracts contain a triad of bile duct, artery and vein. Blood percolates through the liver from the portal tracts to the central veins.

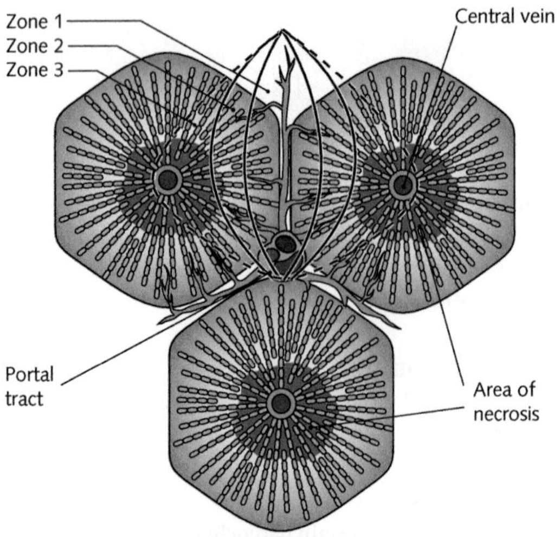

Fig. 12.2 Centrilobular (zone 3) zonal necrosis. Zone 1 is periportal (near the portal vein) with high oxygen concentration; zone 2 is parenchymal; zone 3 is pericentral (near the central vein) which has a low oxygen concentration.

Regeneration

Under normal circumstances there is very little liver cell proliferation. However, following hepatic injury, liver cell regeneration occurs to restore liver function, even if the architectural structure of the liver cannot be restored. This is a crucial phenomenon which allows recovery in patients with fulminant or subfulminant liver failure. The liver has a nodular appearance as regeneration is predominantly in the periportal area (zone 1) where oxygen concentration is highest.

Fibrosis

Repeated chronic damage to the liver can result in fibrosis, which is usually considered an irreversible change. Growth factors produced as part of an inflammatory response are thought to stimulate proliferation and differentiation of mesenchymal cells (the normally inconspicuous fat-storing cells of Ito located in the space of Disse) into collagen-secreting fibroblasts.

Development of fibrosis is an important complication of several liver diseases, and it is one of the characteristic features of cirrhosis.

Cirrhosis

Cirrhosis is an irreversible condition in which the liver's normal architecture is diffusely replaced by nodules of proliferating hepatocytes separated by bands of fibrosis. Cirrhosis represents the end-stage of many processes—it is not a specific disease in itself. It involves:

- Chronic destruction of liver cells.
- Chronic inflammation that stimulates fibrosis.
- Nodular regeneration of hepatocytes.

Macroscopically, the liver is tawny and characteristically knobbly (due to nodules). The cut surface shows parenchyma replaced by nodules of regenerating hepatocytes separated by fine fibrosis.

Microscopically, the nodules of hepatocytes are separated by bands of collagenous tissue. Bile ducts and portal vessels run in the fibrous septa.

Cirrhosis can be classified according to the size of regenerative nodules (Table 12.1) or its aetiology (Table 12.2). Aetiological classification is most useful in determining prognosis and treatment. The clinical features of chronic liver failure and cirrhosis are illustrated in Fig. 12.3.

Consequences of cirrhosis include:

- Liver failure—reduced hepatocyte function (decreased synthesis of proteins, failure of detoxification).
- Portal hypertension and its complications (see below)—a result of impeded bloodflow through the liver.
- Reduced immune competence—increased susceptibility to infection.
- Increased risk of hepatocellular carcinoma.
- Increased risk of portal vein thrombosis.
- Clotting abnormalities—reduced production of factors II, VII, IX and X.

Table 12.1 Classification of cirrhosis according to nodular size

Type	Nodule size
Micronodular	≤3 mm
Macronodular	3 mm to 2 cm
Mixed micronodular and macronodular	Mixture of small and large

Table 12.2 Causes of cirrhosis

Classification of cirrhosis according to incidence in developed countries	
Common	Alcoholic liver disease
	Cryptogenic (no cause found)
	Chronic hepatitis caused by hepatitis B and C viruses
Uncommon	Autoimmune chronic hepatitis
	Primary biliary cholangitis
	Chronic biliary obstruction (biliary cirrhosis)
	Cystic fibrosis
Treatable but rare	Haemochromatosis
	Wilson disease
Rare	α_1-antitrypsin deficiency
	Galactosaemia

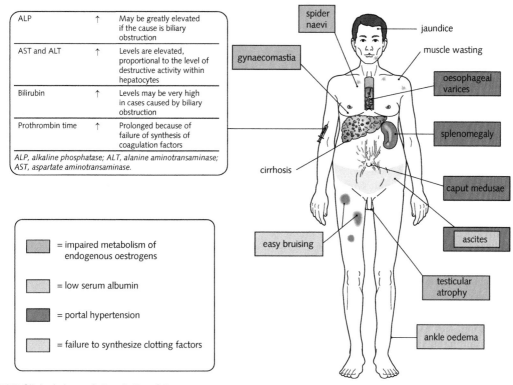

ALP	↑	May be greatly elevated if the cause is biliary obstruction
AST and ALT	↑	Levels are elevated, proportional to the level of destructive activity within hepatocytes
Bilirubin	↑	Levels may be very high in cases caused by biliary obstruction
Prothrombin time	↑	Prolonged because of failure of synthesis of coagulation factors

ALP, alkaline phosphatase; ALT, alanine aminotransaminase; AST, aspartate aminotransaminase.

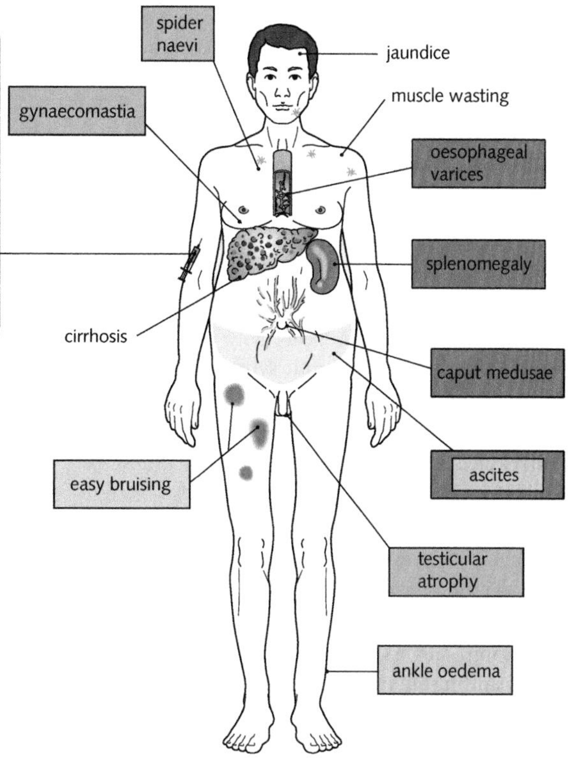

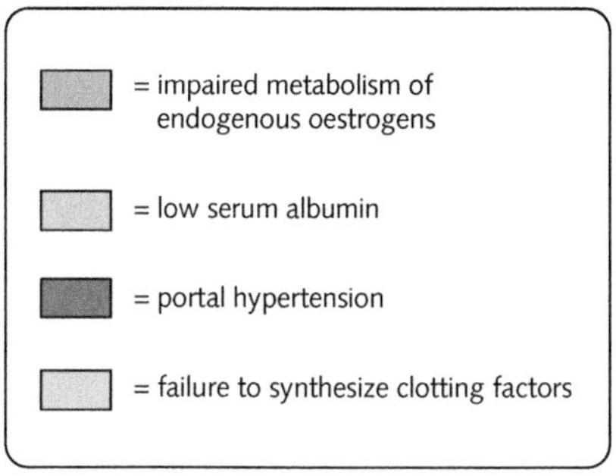

Fig. 12.3 Clinical signs of chronic liver failure

Portal hypertension, ascites and splenomegaly

Portal hypertension

This is a continued elevation in portal venous pressure; normal portal venous pressure being less than 2–5 mmHg. Causes of portal hypertension can be classified according to whether the site of obstruction to flow is:

- prehepatic—blockage of vessels before the hepatic sinusoids
- hepatic—blockage in the hepatic sinusoids
- posthepatic—blockage in the central veins, hepatic veins or vena cava

Table 12.3 lists the causes of portal hypertension.

Complications—portal hypertension causes backpressure in the portal vascular bed, leading to splenomegaly, ascites and varicose venous channels due to portosystemic shunts.

Table 12.3 Classification of portal hypertension

Prehepatic	Portal vein thrombosis
Hepatic	Cirrhosis (most common cause of portal hypertension)
	Idiopathic portal hypertension
	Hepatic fibrosis: caused by schistosomiasis (important cause in endemic areas)
	Venoocclusive disease
Posthepatic	Disease of hepatic veins and branches, e.g., Budd–Chiari syndrome
	Severe right-sided heart failure
	Constrictive pericarditis

Portosystemic shunts

Venous communications that link portal and systemic venous systems become enlarged in portal hypertension. Anastomotic channels become dilated, resulting in the development of varicose venous channels. The four sites of portal-systemic anastomosis are:

- Lower third of the oesophagus—left gastric vein (portal tributary) anastomoses with oesophageal veins (systemic tributary); forms oesophageal varices—may cause severe bleeding.
- Midpoint of the anal canal—superior rectal veins (portal tributary) draining upper half of anal canal anastomose with middle and inferior rectal veins (systemic tributaries); forms rectal varices.
- Paraumbilical veins—connect left branch of the portal vein with superficial veins of anterior abdominal wall (systemic tributaries); forms caput medusae—distension of paraumbilical veins.
- Veins of the ascending colon, descending colon, duodenum, pancreas and liver (portal tributaries) anastomose with renal, lumbar and phrenic veins (systemic tributaries).

Pathogenesis—under normal conditions, portal venous blood traverses the liver and drains into the inferior vena cava of the systemic venous circulation by way of the hepatic veins. In portal hypertension, flow through this direct route is reduced and the portal venous blood is forced through smaller communications that exist between the portal and systemic systems.

Ascites

Ascites is the accumulation of free fluid in the peritoneal cavity. Common causes are:

- peritonitis
- malignancy within the peritoneal cavity
- hypoproteinaemia, e.g., nephrotic syndrome
- portal hypertension—most commonly caused by cirrhosis
- heart failure.

Pathogenesis of ascites in cirrhosis—increased transudation of fluid in ascites occurs as a result of:

- ↑ hydrostatic pressure in portal veins.
- ↑ plasma oncotic pressure (secondary to reduced albumin synthesis by damaged liver cells).

Table 12.4 describes the types of ascites.

Clinical features are abdominal distension with fullness in the flanks, shifting dullness on percussion and fluid thrill.

Prognosis—only 10%–20% of patients survive 5 years from onset of ascites.

Table 12.4 Types of ascites

Transudate low-protein fluid (<30 g/L)	Exudate high-protein fluid (> 30 g/L)
Cirrhosis	Malignancy
Constrictive pericarditis	Peritonitis
Cardiac failure	Pancreatitis
Hypoalbuminaemia, e.g., nephrotic syndrome	Budd–Chiari syndrome
	Hypothyroidism
	Lymphatic obstruction (chylous ascites)

CLINICAL NOTE

SPONTANEOUS BACTERIAL PERITONITIS

Spontaneous bacterial peritonitis is infection of ascitic fluid with no obvious origin. It usually occurs in patients with portal hypertension and cirrhosis. Infection is usually by enteric bacteria, especially *Escherichia coli*. Up to one-third of patients show no/mild abdominal signs; therefore, a high index of suspicion must be maintained.

Splenomegaly

Increased pressure in the portal vein is transmitted to the splenic vein (a branch of the portal vein) resulting in splenomegaly. A variety of haematological abnormalities are associated with splenomegaly (see Chapter 17).

Jaundice and cholestasis

Jaundice

This presents as a yellowing of the skin, sclerae or mucous membranes, indicating excess bilirubin in the blood. It is clinically detectable when plasma bilirubin exceeds 50 μmol/L (3 mg/dL), although the biochemical definition refers to any reading above normal levels (approximately 18–24 μmol/L).

The metabolism of bilirubin is illustrated in Fig. 12.4.

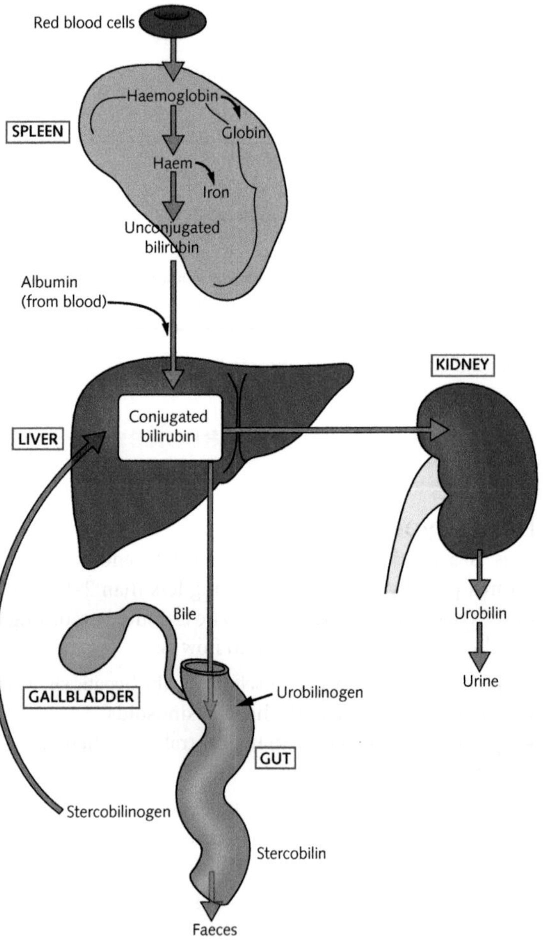

Fig. 12.4 Bilirubin metabolism.
Red cells are removed and broken down by the spleen releasing haemoglobin which is degraded into its constituent haem molecules and globin proteins. Bilirubin is produced from haem and is conjugated within the liver (addition of glucuronic acid for solubilization) before entering the intestines where bacteria convert it to urobilinogen. From here urobilinogen is excreted via the intestines as stercobilin or is reabsorbed into the blood and excreted via the kidneys as urobilin or in bile from the gallbladder.

Causes of jaundice

The easiest way to classify jaundice is by aetiology (Table 12.5):

- Prehepatic—the most common cause is haemolysis-associated jaundice, a mild form of which occurs in many neonates owing to immature liver function in the first weeks of life.
- Intrahepatic—any cause of hepatocellular damage or intrahepatic cholestasis may be responsible. Hereditary enzyme defects may reduce the ability to conjugate bilirubin, producing jaundice. Gilbert syndrome is the most common of these conditions; it is not serious and requires no treatment.
- Posthepatic—any obstruction beyond the liver, e.g., gallstones.

Unconjugated versus conjugated hyperbilirubinaemia

An alternative classification system is based on chemical analysis of bilirubin in the blood (Table 12.5).

Failure of bile flow caused by the obstruction of either small intrahepatic or large extrahepatic bile ducts is termed cholestasis. It results in jaundice as the high concentration of conjugated bilirubin is displaced back into the blood resulting in dark urine (high urobilinogen content), while the lack of bilirubin passing through the liver produces pale faeces. Conjugated bilirubin may be deposited in the skin, causing itching (pruritus).

Unconjugated hyperbilirubinaemia is caused by states such as haemolysis, where the excessive release of bilirubin overwhelms the ability of the liver to conjugate it into a water-soluble form (bilirubin glucuronate). Insoluble bilirubin does not enter the urine and so this remains a normal colour, but faeces are darkened by the increased amount of bilirubin excreted through the gut. Pruritus does not usually occur.

> **HINTS AND TIPS**
>
> **JAUNDICE**
>
> Two important points to note about jaundice:
>
> 1. Liver disease is not the only cause of jaundice; there are other causes, e.g., haemolysis.
> 2. Many patients with significant liver disease are not jaundiced.

Hepatic failure

This is usually the endpoint of longstanding chronic liver disease, when up to 90% of hepatic function has been lost. Sequelae include ascites and oesophageal varices secondary to portal hypertension, bleeding due to coagulopathies, brain, lung and renal impairment.

Hepatic encephalopathy

This is a neuropsychiatric syndrome caused by severe liver disease, occurring most often with cirrhosis but occasionally in acute fulminant hepatic failure.

Pathogenesis is:

- Liver failure—the liver is unable to remove exogenous/endogenous compounds from the circulation. Neurotoxins (e.g., ammonia) accumulate, cross the blood–brain barrier and impair neuronal transmission.

Table 12.5 Causes and classification of jaundice

Site	Bilirubin	Example	Features
Prehepatic	Unconjugated	Haemolysis	Urine: normal Faeces: dark
Intrahepatic	Unconjugated	Impaired bilirubin uptake (Gilbert syndrome) Crigler–Najjar syndrome Drugs, e.g., rifampicin	Increased risk of pigment gallstones No itching (excess urobilinogen with haemolysis)
	Conjugated	Impaired bilirubin excretion into bile: • Dubin–Johnson syndrome • Rotor syndrome	Urine: dark Faeces: pale Itching
		Small bile duct obstruction: • Acute/chronic hepatitis • Cirrhosis • Intrahepatic tumours • Pregnancy-associated cholestasis • Sclerosing cholestasis • Intrahepatic biliary atresia	
Posthepatic	Conjugated	Large bile duct obstruction, e.g., gallstones, strictures, carcinoma	Urine: dark Faeces: pale Itching

- Shunting—in portal hypertension, there is shunting of portal blood past the liver directly into the systemic circulation.

The overall effect is a biochemical disturbance of brain function. The condition is reversible and rarely shows marked pathological changes in the brain.

Hepatorenal syndrome

Renal failure secondary to liver failure occurs in advanced cirrhosis, and almost always in conjunction with ascites.

The kidneys themselves are normal. Renal failure is thought to result from altered systemic bloodflow, including diminished renal flow.

Prognosis—recovery depends on improvement of liver function, but in chronic liver disease this seldom occurs.

DISORDERS OF THE LIVER AND BILIARY TRACT

Congenital errors of metabolism

Haemochromatosis

This condition is caused by excessive iron absorption and deposition within the tissues, including the liver. There are two types:

1. Primary (hereditary)—caused by an autosomal recessive mutation in the *HFE* gene on chromosome 6. The resulting abnormal HFE protein is linked to excessive absorption of iron from the gut via dysregulation of hepcidin and ferroportin. Ninety percent of those affected are male.
2. Secondary (haemosiderosis)—excessive iron accumulation in the tissues caused by other primary diseases (e.g., chronic haemolytic disorders, disorders of ineffective erythropoiesis), parenteral iron overload (e.g., repeated blood transfusion) and others.

Effects of iron accumulation

Iron accumulates as haemosiderin in many tissues, including the liver, pancreas, pituitary, heart and skin, causing them to appear rusty brown. This results in progressive damage and dysfunction of the organ:

- Liver—haemosiderin accumulates in the periportal region and spreads to affect the whole liver, causing hepatocyte necrosis and eventually cirrhosis.
- Heart—infiltration of cardiac muscle can cause arrhythmias and cardiomyopathy with subsequent heart failure.
- Pancreas—damage to pancreatic islets may result in diabetes mellitus.
- Skin—slate grey to bronze pigmentation of skin owing to excess haemosiderin in conjunction with increased melanin production, especially on sun-exposed areas, genitals and skin folds.

Diagnosis—high serum iron and ferritin levels with high transferrin saturation in the blood. Diagnosis is confirmed by a liver biopsy demonstrating heavy iron deposition, hepatic fibrosis or cirrhosis.

Management:

- Regular venesection (bleedings) to remove iron and maintain normal serum ferritin.
- Investigation of first-degree relatives by blood testing and possible genetic screening.

> **HINTS AND TIPS**
>
> **BRONZED DIABETES**
>
> The term 'bronzed diabetes' is often used to describe haemochromatosis owing to the combination of diabetes and hyperpigmentation.

Wilson disease

This autosomal recessive disorder of copper metabolism results in chronic destructive liver disease and presents at a younger age than haemochromatosis (6–40 years).

Normally, dietary copper is taken up by the liver, complexed to ceruloplasmin (a copper-binding protein) and then the whole complex is secreted into the plasma. Circulating ceruloplasmin is subsequently recycled by the liver, with any remaining excess copper being reexcreted into the bile.

In Wilson disease, a mutation in the copper transport ATPase gene (*ATP7B* on chromosome 13) results in failure of the liver to secrete the copper–ceruloplasmin complex into the plasma. The copper complex accumulates within the hepatocytes, saturating the available ceruloplasmin and leaving free copper to spill over into the blood, where it can cause haemolysis or be deposited in various tissues.

- Liver—chronic hepatitis, which progresses to cirrhosis.
- Brain—psychiatric disorders, abnormal eye movements and movement disorders resembling Parkinson disease.
- Eye—development of greenish-brown discoloration around cornea (Kayser–Fleischer rings) due to deposits in the Desçemet membrane.

Diagnosis—low levels of serum ceruloplasmin and high free copper levels with increased copper urinary levels; liver effects confirmed by biopsy.

Management is by copper chelators, e.g., D-penicillamine, trientine and zinc.

Alpha$_1$-antitrypsin deficiency

Alpha$_1$-antitrypsin is a serine protease inhibitor that is normally produced and secreted by the liver to inhibit the activity of protease enzymes. Mutations in the encoding genes prevent its secretion, resulting in damage to the liver (ultimately cirrhosis) and lung parenchyma (causing emphysema). The histological hallmark is periodic-acid Schiff diastase-resistant (PASD+) protein globules within the cytoplasm of periportal hepatocytes.

The gene encoding α_1-antitrypsin is highly polymorphic and located on chromosome 14. Some genotypic variants have no effect and some a very mild effect. The most common genotype is *PiMM*, which can be considered as 'wild-type' for the gene. The most common clinically significant mutation is *PiZZ*, which results in failure to produce α_1-antitrypsin. In heterozygotes, such as *PiMZ*, there is an increased risk of lung damage, especially emphysema in smokers, as expression is codominant.

Manifestations of *PiZZ* are highly variable, ranging from neonatal hepatitis to childhood hepatic fibrosis to subclinical chronic hepatitis, which presents late with cirrhosis.

Others

Reye syndrome

This rare syndrome is characterized by acute encephalopathy with cerebral oedema as a result of sudden severe impairment of hepatic function (associated with microvesicular fatty degeneration) with minimal tissue inflammation. It occurs with high-dose aspirin use in children and adolescents, often following a viral infection, most commonly upper respiratory tract.

Infectious and inflammatory disease

Viral hepatitis

Viral infection is a common cause of acute hepatitis. The main viral hepatitides are a group of hepatotrophic viruses of different viral types that all cause a primary hepatitis.

Clinical features are similar in all forms of acute hepatitis regardless of aetiology. Symptoms include nausea, anorexia, low-grade pyrexia and general malaise. Signs are tender hepatomegaly and jaundice 1 week after onset of symptoms, peaking at about 10 days.

Investigations—raised serum levels of conjugated bilirubin and liver aminotransferases (both aspartate and alanine).

> **HINTS AND TIPS**
>
> **FULMINANT HEPATITIS**
>
> Fulminant hepatitis is distinguished from hepatic encephalopathy occurring as a result of deteriorating chronic liver disease by its occurrence within 8 weeks of onset of the precipitating illness, and in the absence of evidence of preexisting liver disease.

Hepatitis A

This RNA enterovirus is prevalent in tropical countries, but uncommon in developed countries. It is the most common travel-related illness in the UK.

Transmission—faecal–oral route, e.g., from:

- Nurseries or institutions where hygiene levels are inadequate (person-to-person via hand-to-hand contact).
- Recreational activities in waters contaminated by sewage outfalls.
- Ingestion of sewage-contaminated shellfish.
- (Sexual) oral–anal contact.

Time course—illustrated in Fig. 12.5.

Prognosis—the majority of patients recover fully with restoration of normal liver function tests. However, a small minority (1–3 per 1000) develop fulminant hepatic failure, with a mortality rate of 85%.

The disease never causes chronic hepatitis and infection confers subsequent immunity. There is no carrier state. A vaccine is available for long-term immunity.

Hepatitis B

This is a virulent DNA virus of the Hepadnaviridae family that can integrate into host DNA. The highest concentrations are in blood, but it is also present in saliva, semen and vaginal secretions. Transmission can be:

- Blood-borne—IV drug users, tattooing, acupuncture, blood transfusions.
- Sexual intercourse—high risk in unprotected sex.
- Vertical transmission—from mother to child perinatally at the time of birth.
- Family contacts—toothbrushes, nail scissors, razors, etc. that may contain traces of blood.

Hepatitis B is most prevalent in Africa and Asia.

There are three clinical patterns of infection (Fig. 12.6):

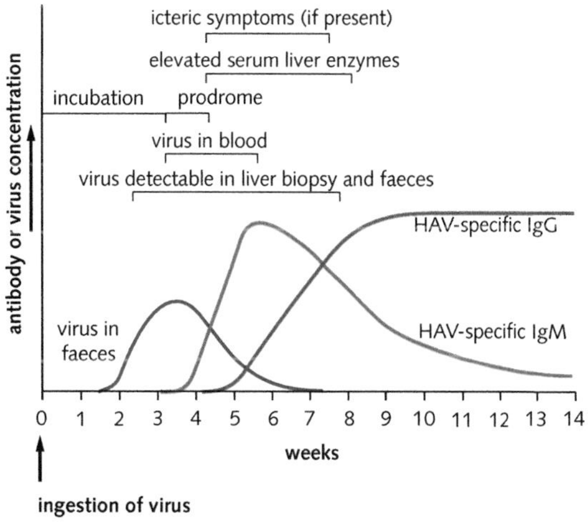

Fig. 12.5 Course of infection in hepatitis A.
HAV, Hepatitis A.

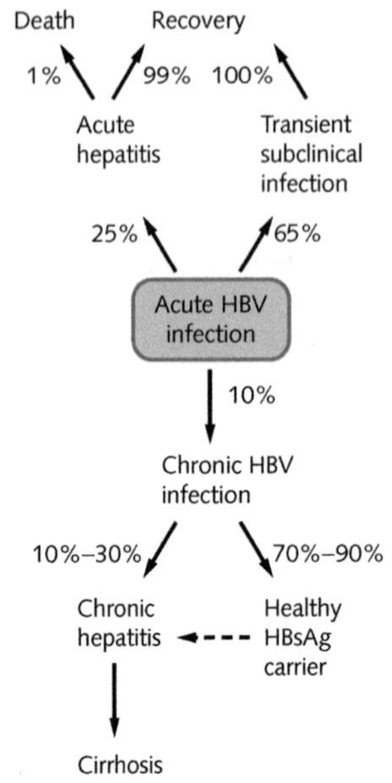

Fig. 12.6 Summary of the possible course of hepatitis B infection.
HBsAg, hepatitis B surface antigen; *HBV*, hepatitis B virus. (Adapted with permission from Kumar P, Clarke M. Clinical Medicine, 7th edn. London: Baillière Tindall, 2009.)

1. Asymptomatic infection (65%)—transient subclinical infection with complete recovery.
2. Acute hepatitis B
   - Self-limiting hepatitis (25%)—symptoms include jaundice, malaise and anorexia, but the majority recover and develop lifelong immunity.
   - Fulminant acute hepatitis (<1%)—massive hepatocyte necrosis.
3. Chronic hepatitis B infection (10%)
   - Inactive carriers—the majority enter an asymptomatic carrier state, which carries a future risk of chronic hepatitis.
   - Active chronic hepatitis B—a minority progress to chronic hepatitis after initial infection. Chronic hepatitis is a strong risk factor for cirrhosis and 3%–5% with chronic hepatitis B infection will develop hepatocellular carcinoma (HCC). Coinfection with HIV and hepatitis C and alcohol consumption also increase the risk. There is typically a latency period of 20–30 years between infection and cancer.

Time course—this is illustrated in Fig. 12.7.

Complications—these are cirrhosis (as a result of chronic hepatitis) and HCC. Carriers of hepatitis B are 200 times more likely to get liver cancer than the general population; however, there is typically a latency period of 20–30 years between infection and cancer.

Treatment—95% of infected adults do not enter a carrier state, in contrast to 90% of infants and 50% of children who will become chronically infected. Treatment is with pegylated interferon-α/β for carriers, potentially in combination with antiviral drugs. Prophylactic vaccination based on the hepatitis B surface antigen (HBsAg) is available, but up to 10% of normal individuals fail to produce protective antibodies.

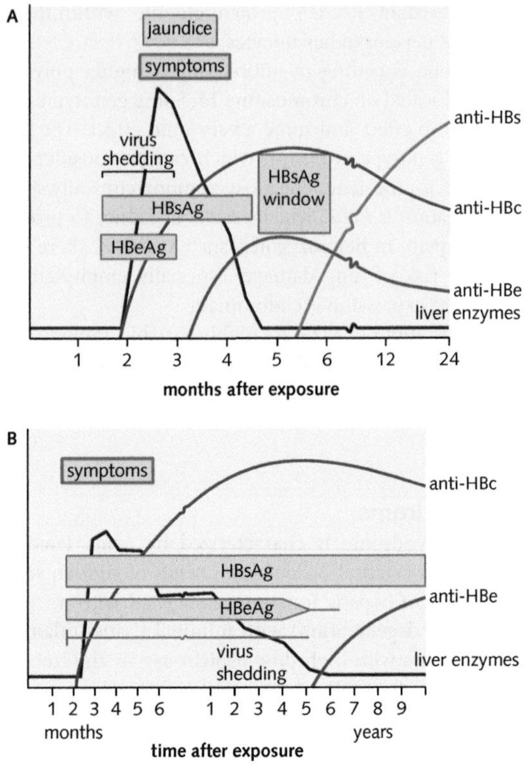

Fig. 12.7 Time course of infection in hepatitis B.
Course of infection in hepatitis B. (A) Acute hepatitis. (B) Chronic hepatitis. HBsAg window is the timepoint where neither HBsAg nor anti-HBs can be detected because of immune complex formation. *anti-HBc*, antibody to hepatitis B core antigen; *anti-HBe*, antibody to HBeAg; *anti-HBs*, antibody to HBsAg; *HBeAg*, hepatitis Be antigen; *HBsAg*, hepatitis B surface antigen.

Hepatitis C

Hepatitis C is an RNA flavivirus of which there are six genotypes. It is a major cause of hepatitis worldwide.

Transmission—predominantly blood-borne spread, although sexual and vertical transmissions do occur. Hepatitis C is widespread among intravenous drug users and was previously spread by blood transfusions before serological screening of donated samples was introduced in September 1991.

The majority of patients develop acute hepatitis (65%–90%); infection is asymptomatic in 10%–35% of cases, although it may progress to the carrier state. Chronic hepatitis develops in 70%–80% of those infected, increasing lifelong risk of cirrhosis and hepatocellular carcinoma.

Treatment—is determined by genotype and is with pegylated interferon-α in combination with an antiviral such as ribavirin.

Hepatitis D

This RNA virus is incomplete and can only cause infection in the presence of hepatitis B virus, forming a Dane particle; transmission is as for hepatitis B virus. Both viruses may be acquired simultaneously or hepatitis D may be acquired later as a superinfection.

The virus increases the severity of chronic hepatitis and accelerates the progression to cirrhosis. It may predispose to the development of fulminant hepatitis.

Hepatitis E

This RNA virus has the same transmission pattern as hepatitis A and a similar clinical picture. It can develop into fulminant hepatitis, especially in pregnant women.

Other viruses

Nonhepatotrophic viruses may also cause hepatitis. Examples include group B arbovirus (yellow fever), Epstein–Barr virus and cytomegalovirus.

Autoimmune hepatitis

Autoimmune hepatitis has a prevalence of about 4 per 10,000 and typically occurs in women (70% of cases) between the ages of 20 and 40 years.

It is a progressive necroinflammatory process driven by T-cell–mediated autoimmunity associated with hyperglobulinaemia (mainly IgG) and serum autoantibodies. It is classified based on the antibody profile:

- Type 1 disease: anti-smooth muscle (SMA) and antinuclear antibodies (ANA).
- Type 2 disease: anti-liver-kidney microsomal antibodies (LKM-1) and anti-liver cytosol 1 (ACL-1).

Type 1 disease (most common) is associated with other autoimmune disorders such as Graves disease, systemic lupus erythematosus and Sjögren syndrome (dry eyes and mouth).

Clinically, there is insidious onset of anorexia, malaise and fatigue accompanied by abdominal distension and mild jaundice (with dark urine and itching). The disease may run a relapsing and remitting course, but it progresses inexorably to fibrosis and cirrhosis.

Microscopically, plasma cells are seen at the interface between portal tracts and liver parenchyma.

Complications are cirrhosis, liver failure and HCC.

Treatment is with corticosteroids; azathioprine may help to reduce steroid dosage.

Prognosis—patients who do not respond to treatment will almost always progress to cirrhosis. However, many patients develop cirrhosis despite having a response to treatment. If end-stage liver disease develops, liver transplantation is an effective procedure.

Fulminant hepatitis

This rare syndrome of hepatic encephalopathy results from sudden severe impairment of hepatic function. It is caused by acute, severe liver damage such as:

- Viral infections (most common cause), e.g., hepatitis B.
- Drugs and poisons, e.g., paracetamol overdose, carbon tetrachloride.
- Nonviral infections, e.g., Leptospira, *Toxoplasma gondii*, *Coxiella burnetii*.
- Metabolic—Wilson disease, pregnancy.
- Ischaemic—shock, severe cardiac failure, Budd–Chiari syndrome.

The pathogenesis of hepatic encephalopathy has already been described (see previous).

Clinical features are:

- Cerebral disturbance (mental changes progressing from confusion to stupor and coma).
- Weakness, vomiting and nausea.
- Rapidly developing jaundice with fetor hepaticus (distinctive breath odour).
- Asterixis—flapping tremor.
- Ascites and oedema.

The liver may enlarge initially, but later it shrinks and becomes impalpable owing to hepatocyte destruction; disappearance of hepatic dullness on percussion indicates shrinkage and is a poor prognostic sign.

Complications:

- Oedema—this may be cerebral (causing raised intracranial pressure) or pulmonary (contributing to respiratory failure).
- General vasodilatation—hypotension and hypothermia.
- Infection.
- Coagulation disorders.
- Pancreatitis.
- Renal failure—deterioration parallels that of liver failure.
- Metabolic—hypoglycaemia, hypokalaemia, hypocalcaemia, hypomagnesaemia, acid–base disturbance.

There is no specific treatment. Management is by close observation, treating complications as necessary.

Prognosis:

- Sixty-six percent of patients with minor signs survive.
- Ten percent of patients with coma survive.
- Those who recover from fulminant hepatic failure usually regain normal hepatic structure and function.

Liver abscess

This is a localized collection of pus within the liver that is walled off and surrounded by damaged and inflamed liver tissue. Liver abscesses are rare but important, as they are inevitably fatal if untreated. They can be caused by bacteria, fungi or parasites.

Pyogenic abscesses

The most common causative organisms are *Escherichia coli*, various streptococci and other enterobacteria.

Mode of infection:

- Haematogenous spread—usually solitary abscesses:
  - Portal vein (intraabdominal infections, e.g., appendicitis, diverticulitis) are the most common cause.
  - Hepatic artery (bacteraemia, e.g., from dental infection, bacterial endocarditis).
- Direct extension—almost always predisposed by biliary obstruction resulting in ascending cholangitis or gallbladder empyema. Usually causes multiple small abscesses.
- Penetrating trauma (including liver biopsy).

Symptoms of infection (swinging fever, night sweats) and right upper quadrant pain (± radiation to the right shoulder) are common, along with hepatomegaly and mild jaundice.

Investigations include ultrasound imaging. Needle aspiration at this time can confirm the diagnosis in addition to providing material for culture.

Management is by prolonged antibiotics and drainage of the abscess.

Prognosis—the mortality of patients with liver abscesses is 20%–40%, usually through failure to make the diagnosis.

Amoebic abscess

Amoebic abscess is the commonest cause of liver abscesses worldwide, although rare in the UK. The usual causative organism is *Entamoeba histolytica,* which is transmitted from the bowel to the liver via the portal venous system, resulting in an abscess composed of central necrotic material with a rim of trophozoites. Eighty percent are solitary and occur within the right hepatic lobe. Endemic areas include Africa, Asia and South America.

Hydatid cyst

This results from the accidental ingestion of ova from the dog tapeworm (*Echinococcus granulosus*), which hatch into larvae and invade the bowel wall, accessing the portal venous system. They can invade any organ; however, the liver and lung are the most common sites. The larvae become encysted and develop into worms. Presentation is with hepatomegaly and pain, or the result of a complication, including intraperitoneal/thoracic rupture, bile duct obstruction and secondary infection of the cyst.

Alcohol, drugs and toxins

Alcoholic liver disease

Alcohol use is the most common cause of liver disease in developed countries. Women are more prone to alcohol-induced liver damage than men.

Alcohol is metabolized almost exclusively in the liver, and liver damage is related to daily alcohol intake. Toxicity of ethanol is probably caused by the generation of its metabolic breakdown product, acetaldehyde, which binds to liver proteins and damages hepatocytes. Alcohol also stimulates collagen synthesis in the liver, leading to fibrosis.

Alcoholic liver disease (ALD) is a spectrum of diseases, which include fatty liver, alcoholic steatohepatitis, acute hepatitis and cirrhosis.

Fatty liver (hepatic steatosis)

Fatty liver is the most common manifestation of ALD; however, there are many other causes of steatosis. The condition is characterized by the accumulation of fat (triglyceride) globules within the cytoplasm of hepatocytes. It is reversible on cessation of alcohol ingestion. Macroscopically the liver is heavy, greasy and pale yellow.

It is thought that alcohol stimulates hepatocyte triacylglycerol production, while impairing its excretion from the liver. The condition reflects severe metabolic derangement and it may affect a few or almost all hepatocytes.

Alcoholic steatohepatitis

Alcoholic steatohepatitis is steatosis with inflammation in the context of excess alcohol consumption. Microscopically it is a triad of ballooning degeneration of hepatocytes, neutrophilic lobular inflammation and steatosis. Eosinophilic accumulations called Mallory–Denk bodies (Mallory hyaline) and perivenular or pericellular 'chicken-wire' fibrosis may also be present. It is almost indistinguishable from nonalcoholic steatohepatitis—history is key. The risk of progression to cirrhosis is increased.

Acute alcoholic hepatitis

This is acute hepatitis with focal necrosis of liver cells. At high concentrations, alcohol causes toxic injury to hepatocytes, evoking a neutrophil-dominant inflammatory reaction, which is reversible on abstinence. Mallory–Denk bodies may be seen on liver biopsy. Continued alcohol consumption causes the development of fibrosis around central veins. The result is hepatic fibrosis/cirrhosis.

The illness resembles acute viral hepatitis, and liver function tests show raised levels of aminotransferases and γ-glutamyltransferase.

Alcoholic cirrhosis

This is irreversible architectural disturbance as a result of sustained alcoholic liver injury.

Alcoholic cirrhosis may develop after episodes of acute alcoholic hepatitis or may be insidious in its onset, presenting only as end-stage liver disease. It is macroscopically and microscopically identical to cirrhosis of any cause (see previous). It carries an increased risk of HCC.

Nonalcoholic fatty liver disease/ nonalcoholic steatohepatitis

Fatty change is commonly associated with obesity and type 2 diabetes. There is predominantly a macrovesicular steatosis (large fat globules), although conditions such as pregnancy may show a microvesicular steatosis (small fat globules). In a minority of cases accompanying steatotic inflammation is seen, causing a nonalcoholic steatohepatitis. This has the same risk of progression to cirrhosis as alcoholic hepatitis.

Drugs and toxins

The liver is the main organ of drug metabolism and, consequently, drugs (including herbal compounds) are a common cause of liver damage and must always be considered in the evaluation of liver disease. Hepatotoxic drugs may be divided into two main groups: intrinsic hepatotoxins and idiosyncratic hepatotoxins.

Intrinsic hepatotoxins

These have dose-dependent, predictable toxic effects. They are responsible for a high incidence of toxic damage to the liver via direct toxicity of an unmetabolized drug or its metabolite. The best-known example is paracetamol (Fig. 12.8).

Idiosyncratic hepatotoxins

These have non-dose-dependent, unpredictable toxic effects. They cause liver disease in a small percentage of exposed individuals as a result of hypersensitivity (drug-mediated autoimmunity) or abnormal drug metabolism. Phenytoin is a good example of this.

Circulatory disorders of the liver

Overview

Vascular disorders of the liver (Table 12.6) can be classified into one of three categories depending on their pathogenic mechanisms:

1. Obstruction to outflow—hepatic vein obstruction.
2. Lobular compromise.
3. Obstruction to inflow—obstruction of portal vein or hepatic artery occlusion.

Diseases causing obstruction to outflow (hepatic vein obstruction)

Budd–Chiari syndrome—obstruction occurs in the larger hepatic veins.

Cardiac disease—right-sided cardiac failure causes engorgement of the inferior vena cava resulting in passive hepatic congestion.

Clinical manifestations depend on the cause and speed with which obstruction develops, but congestive hepatomegaly and ascites are features in all patients.

Budd–Chiari syndrome

This rare condition is caused by occlusion of more than two branches of the main hepatic veins or (more rarely) the hepatic portion of the inferior vena cava (Table 12.7).

Obstruction of the hepatic vein causes severe hepatic congestion with atrophy and/or necrosis of liver cells in the affected areas. Fibrous scarring eventually occurs in areas of hepatocyte necrosis. True cirrhosis supervenes in a minority of cases.

Clinical manifestations—patients with severe acute disease present with:

- painful hepatomegaly
- acute portal hypertension
- rapid development of ascites
- jaundice.

In the acute form, death results unless a surgical portosystemic vascular shunt is created. Chronic onset can be asymptomatic and carries a lower mortality rate.

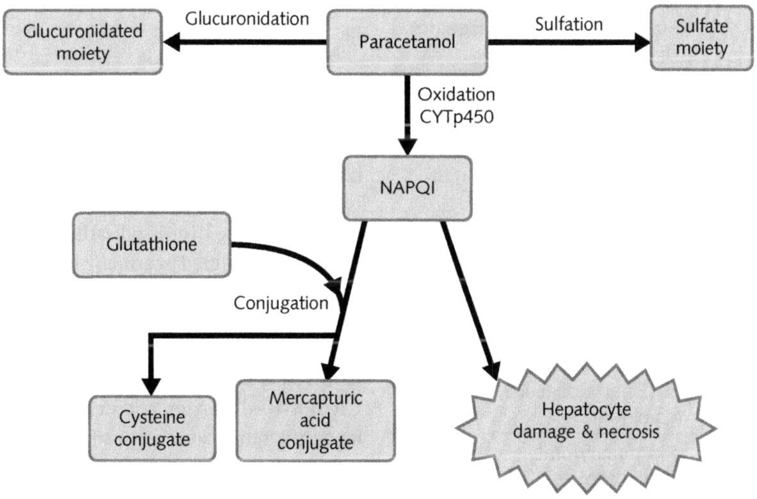

Fig. 12.8 Paracetamol metabolism.
The majority of paracetamol is metabolized and detoxified by sulphation and glucuronidation. A small proportion is oxidized to N-acetyl-p-benzoquinone imine (*NAPQI*) (toxic) via the cytochrome p450 enzymes. This is rapidly detoxified to soluble cysteine and mercapturic acid conjugates and excreted in urine. Paracetamol overdose saturates these pathways, NAPQI rises and binds to proteins and nucleic acids, causing centrilobular necrosis. Conditions where glutathione is decreased lower the toxic dose of paracetamol. *CYTp450*, Cytochrome p450.

Table 12.6 Vascular disorders of the liver

Cause	Example
Outflow (hepatic vein) obstruction	Veno-occlusive disease
	Budd–Chiari syndrome
	Right-sided cardiac failure
Lobular compromise	Cirrhosis
	Noncirrhotic fibrosis:
	• Infective, e.g., schistosomiasis
	• Drugs, e.g., alcohol, hypervitaminosis A, vinyl chloride, arsenic
	• Congenital, e.g., congenital hepatic fibrosis, infantile polycystic disease
	• Nodular regenerative hyperplasia
	Systemic circulatory disturbances, e.g., shock
Inflow obstruction	Extrahepatic:
	• Portal vein obstruction:
	○ Portal vein thrombosis
	○ Extrinsic compression of portal vein
	○ Congenital stenosis
	• Hepatic artery occlusion:
	○ Hepatic artery thrombosis
	○ Embolism, e.g., infective endocarditis
	Intrahepatic:
	• Occlusion of intrahepatic portal vein branches

Table 12.7 Aetiology of Budd-Chiari syndrome

Idiopathic	Underlying cause unknown in 10% of cases
Thrombotic causes	Haematological diseases, for example:
	• Myeloproliferative disorders (e.g., polycythaemia rubra vera)
	• Paroxysmal nocturnal haemoglobinuria
	• Deficiencies of antithrombin III, factor V Leiden, proteins C and S
	Antiphospholipid syndrome
	Intraabdominal malignancy, e.g., hepatocellular carcinoma
	Pregnancy/oral contraceptives
Local compression of hepatic vein (rare)	Obstruction due to tumours, e.g., liver, kidneys or adrenals
	Congenital venous webs
	Inferior vena cava stenosis

Passive congestion

Congestive cardiac failure causes venous outflow obstruction in the liver because of back pressure transmitted as described below:

Inferior vena cava → hepatic vein → central veins → centrilobular congestion

Centrilobular sinusoids are dilated by blood and the centrilobular hepatocytes undergo atrophy and necrosis (centrilobular necrosis), giving rise to the appearance of what is described as a 'nutmeg liver' (chronic passive venous congestion).

The condition is common in tricuspid valve incompetence where the liver is pulsatile.

Shock/left-sided cardiac failure may cause hepatic hypoperfusion, potentially resulting in centrilobular coagulative necrosis.

Diseases resulting in lobular compromise

Cirrhosis—distortion and destruction of the hepatic vascular architecture causes sinusoid occlusion.

- Noncirrhotic fibrosis—where fibrotic damage to the liver does not amount to true cirrhosis, e.g., schistosomiasis infection.
- Systemic circulatory disturbances—shock from any source causes severe hypoperfusion, resulting in zonal necrosis.
- Sinusoidal occlusion—can occur in sickle cell disease and disseminated intravascular coagulation.

Diseases resulting in obstruction to inflow

Extrahepatic:

- Portal vein obstruction—thrombosis, extrinsic compression
- Hepatic artery compromise—thrombosis, embolism.

Intrahepatic:

- Intrahepatic portal vein branches—occlusion causes areas of venous infarction.

Portal vein obstruction

Obstruction of the portal vein results in portal hypertension and its associated complications, e.g., oesophageal varices. The causes may be thrombotic or nonthrombotic.

Thrombotic conditions (those that predispose to portal vein thrombosis) are:

- Cirrhosis—leads to portal hypertension and stasis.
- Inflammatory—thrombophlebitis and intraabdominal sepsis (e.g., appendicitis, pancreatitis, diverticulitis).
- Neoplastic—e.g., HCC, pancreatic carcinoma and haematological malignancies (e.g., myeloproliferative disorders: polycythaemia rubra vera and essential thrombocytosis), which can directly invade or compress the portal vein.
- Hypercoagulable states—splenic vein thrombosis (often secondary to pancreatitis) may propagate into the portal vein.
- Others—trauma, postsurgery, idiopathic.

Non-thrombotic conditions are external compression (e.g., by tumour masses, porta hepatis lymphadenopathy) and cirrhosis.

Liver infarction

True infarction of the liver is rare because of its dual blood supply and rich anastomosis of bloodflow through the sinusoids. However, hepatic bloodflow may be compromised in the following conditions:

- Surgical trauma or accidental ligation of the hepatic artery.
- Therapeutic arterial embolization of the liver or therapeutic hepatic arterial ligation (performed to treat isolated neoplastic masses).
- Bacterial endocarditis—embolism.
- Eclampsia.
- Polyarteritis nodosa—a necrotizing vasculitis.

Neoplasms of the liver

Benign tumours/lesions

Hepatic adenomas

These typically affect premenopausal women, especially those taking oestrogen-containing oral contraceptives. Other associations are obesity, alcohol and steroid use.

The macroscopic appearance is of a well-circumscribed nodule up to 20 cm in size.

The microscopic appearance closely resembles that of normal liver, except that portal tracts are absent.

Complications—the majority of lesions are asymptomatic, but subcapsular adenomas can spontaneously rupture, leading to intraabdominal haemorrhage, which is a surgical emergency.

Focal nodular hyperplasia

This lesion is commonly found in middle-aged women and is characterized by nodular parenchyma with a central stellate scar and radiating fibrous septa containing thick-walled blood vessels. The lesion is often subcapsular, circumscribed and usually <5 cm.

Bile duct hamartomas

These are very common lesions (also known as von Meyenburg complexes) composed of focal proliferations of abnormal bile ducts in a collagenous stroma. They appear as small white nodules, often beneath the liver capsule, and may be mistaken for metastatic tumour deposits at laparotomy.

Haemangioma

These are common hamartomas composed of abnormal vascular channels in a collagenous stroma. They are often found incidentally at autopsy in 2%–5% of the population and are typically seen just beneath the capsule as a dark lesion (usually <4 cm in size).

Malignant

Hepatocellular carcinoma

Carcinoma of hepatocytes is the commonest primary tumour of the liver. Although incidence is increasing, HCC is still uncommon in the UK (approximately 1 per 100,000). It is up to 100 times more common in parts of Africa and the Far East, probably because of the higher incidence of hepatitis B and contaminating mycotoxins. Males are affected more often than females.

Predisposing factors are:

- Cirrhosis—independent of cause.
- Hepatitis B or C infection—with chronic carrier state.
- Mycotoxins—these contaminate certain foods, e.g., aflatoxins produced by the fungus *Aspergillus flavus*.

Tumours may consist of a single mass or multiple nodules. HCCs often produce α-fetoprotein (elevated in 60%–80% of cases), which is secreted into the blood and is useful as a diagnostic marker. Prognosis is very poor, with 10% overall 5-year survival rate.

Cholangiocarcinoma

This is an adenocarcinoma arising anywhere in the biliary tree. Within the liver, it may originate from the intrahepatic bile duct epithelium, accounting for 5%–10% of all cases of primary liver tumours.

Many cases are of unknown origin, but predisposing factors include:

- Chronic inflammatory disease of the intrahepatic biliary tree, particularly sclerosing cholangitis.
- Disease caused by Chinese liver flukes *(Clonorchis sinensis).*

Lesions tend to be detected late and are associated with a very poor prognosis; most patients do not survive more than 6 months from diagnosis.

Hepatoblastoma

This is the commonest hepatic neoplasm in children and is associated with syndromes in one-third of cases. They are usually solitary and have increased α-fetoprotein. Poorer prognosis is associated with large lesions and age under 1 year.

Angiosarcomas

These highly malignant tumours are derived from vascular endothelium and are characterized by multifocal haemorrhagic nodules within the liver. The tumours are rare but can be associated with exposure to substances such as vinyl chloride monomer (used to make polyvinyl chloride) and anabolic steroids.

Secondary tumours

The majority of malignant liver tumours are metastatic. The most common primary carcinomas that metastasize to the liver are colorectal, breast, lung and stomach. However, any cancer may spread to the liver, including leukaemia, lymphomas and melanomas.

Mode of spread is haematogenous, through the portal vein (tumours of the gastrointestinal tract) and the systemic circulation (other tumours). There are usually multiple nodular deposits with a central area of necrosis.

Clinically, the liver is enlarged, hard and craggy on palpation.

Extensive metastases can cause compression of the intrahepatic bile ducts leading to obstructive jaundice.

Disorders of the biliary tree

Disorders associated with biliary cirrhosis

Biliary cirrhosis is the result of the longstanding obstruction of bile ducts leading to the development of obstructive jaundice, liver cell necrosis and fibrosis with regenerative nodules. The main causes are:

- Primary biliary cholangitis—intrahepatic bile duct destruction of unknown aetiology.
- Secondary biliary cirrhosis—unrelieved obstruction of the main extrahepatic bile ducts.
- Primary sclerosing cholangitis—inflammation and fibrosis of bile ducts (both intrahepatic and extrahepatic).

Biliary obstruction causes oedema and expansion of intrahepatic portal tracts with portal tract fibrosis. Bile droplets develop in biliary canaliculi, which may rupture and cause death of adjacent hepatocytes (so-called 'bile infarct'). Over a long period of time, liver cell death, regeneration and fibrosis result in cirrhosis.

Primary biliary cholangitis

This cholangitis (formerly called primary biliary cirrhosis) occurs as a result of progressive chronic destruction of intrahepatic bile ducts. Approximately 20,000 people in the UK live with primary biliary cholangitis, typically among the middle-aged population. Females are affected more often than males by a factor of 10:1.

Aetiology is unknown, but it is thought to be autoimmune—antimitochondrial antibodies are present in more than 90% of cases. There is often an association with other autoimmune diseases, e.g., rheumatoid arthritis, thyroiditis, systemic lupus erythematosus, scleroderma and Sjögren syndrome.

Pathogenesis is progressive, chronic, granulomatous and inflammatory. Inflammatory damage with fibrosis may spread from portal tracts to the liver parenchyma. The condition eventually leads to cirrhosis and its complications over a period of about 10 years.

There are four stages:

1. Florid bile duct lesion—noncaseating granulomatous deposits.
2. Ductular proliferation (periportal) upstream from damaged bile ducts.
3. Scarring (bridging fibrosis).
4. Cirrhosis.

CLINICAL NOTE

PRIMARY BILIARY CHOLANGITIS

Initially, primary biliary cholangitis causes fatigue, arthralgia, pruritus and mild jaundice. This progresses following cirrhosis to:

- jaundice
- severe pruritus
- hepatosplenomegaly
- malabsorption
- xanthelasma and possible xanthomata.

Investigations involve:

- liver function tests—features of cholestasis (raised alkaline phosphatase, cholesterol and bile acids)
- antimitochondrial antibodies
- liver biopsy—histological proof
- endoscopic retrograde cholangiopancreatography (ERCP)—rules out obstructive causes of cirrhosis.

No specific therapy is available; liver transplantation is often necessary.

Secondary biliary cirrhosis

This occurs as a result of prolonged mechanical obstruction to bile flow in large ducts outside the liver or within the porta hepatis. Causes are:

- Gallstones—impacted in common bile duct (most common cause).
- Tumours—e.g., carcinoma of bile duct, carcinoma of the pancreas.
- Strictures—usually following surgery.
- Congenital diseases—choledochal cyst, extrahepatic biliary atresia.

Histological features—bile pigment accumulates in hepatocytes, in dilated biliary canaliculi and in Kupffer cells. Prolonged obstruction causes:

- 'Bile infarcts'—extravasated bile from canaliculi causing hepatocyte death.
- 'Bile lakes'—pool of bile outside of the canaliculi.
- Cirrhosis.

Complications are cholangitis (inflammation of the bile ducts, usually as a result of superimposed infection) and those of cirrhosis.

Primary sclerosing cholangitis

Chronic inflammation and obliterative fibrosis of bile ducts with stricture formation causes progressive obstructive jaundice. Peak incidence is between 25 and 40 years, in males more so than females. Aetiology is unknown but is probably autoimmune in nature. Patients may have elevated immunoglobulin levels and up to two-thirds of patients are positive for perinuclear antineutrophilic cytoplasmic antigen (p-ANCA).

Ulcerative colitis is present in 60% of patients with primary sclerosing cholangitis.

The effects are:

- Large intrahepatic and extrahepatic bile ducts—development of fibrous strictures with segmental dilatation causing a 'beaded' appearance on endoscopic retrograde cholangiopancreatography (ERCP).
- Medium-sized ducts and ducts in portal tracts—inflammation with concentric 'onion-skinning' fibrosis around ducts.
- Small bile ducts in portal tracts—replaced by collagenous scarring (vanishing bile ducts).

Clinical features—patients develop cholestatic jaundice (pale stools, dark urine and pruritus) with progression to cirrhosis over a period of about 10 years. There is an increased risk of developing cholangiocarcinoma.

Table 12.8 summarizes the differences between primary biliary cholangitis and primary sclerosing cholangitis.

Ascending cholangitis

Obstruction of the bile duct, usually from gallstones, strictures or carcinoma, can result in infection of the biliary tree. The commonest organisms are Gram-negative bacteria, especially *E. coli* and *Klebsiella*.

Clinical features—most patients present with fever, jaundice or abdominal pain. A small proportion of patients present with all three; this is known as Charcot triad.

Diseases of the gallbladder

See Fig. 12.9 for the anatomy of the biliary tree.

Gallstones (cholelithiasis)

Gallstones (stones formed in the gallbladder) are the most common cause of disease affecting the biliary tree. They occur in 10% of all adults in the UK, females more often than males by a factor of 2.5:1. The number of stones per patient has varied from 1 to 26,000. However, despite the high incidence of gallstones, only about 1% of patients with gallstones develop complications.

Table 12.8 Comparison of primary biliary cholangitis and primary sclerosing cholangitis

	Primary biliary cholangitis	Primary sclerosing cholangitis
Sex association	Females > males by 10:1; middle-aged population	Males > females; peak incidence 25 and 40 years
Aetiology	Unknown, probably autoimmune	Unknown
Bile duct changes	Progressive chronic granulomatous inflammatory damage with fibrosis	Narrowing and obliteration of intrahepatic and extrahepatic bile ducts
	Eventual cirrhosis	Eventual cirrhosis
Laboratory findings		
Liver function tests	Features of cholestasis (increased alkaline phosphatase, cholesterol and bile acids)	Features of cholestasis (increased alkaline phosphatase, cholesterol and bile acids)
Serology	Antimitochondrial antibodies	Hypergammaglobulinaemia and p-ANCA
ERCP	Patent and nondilated biliary tree	Fibrous strictures with segmental dilation → 'beaded' appearance

ERCP, Endoscopic retrograde cholangiopancreatography; p-ANCA, perinuclear antineutrophilic cytoplasmic antigen.

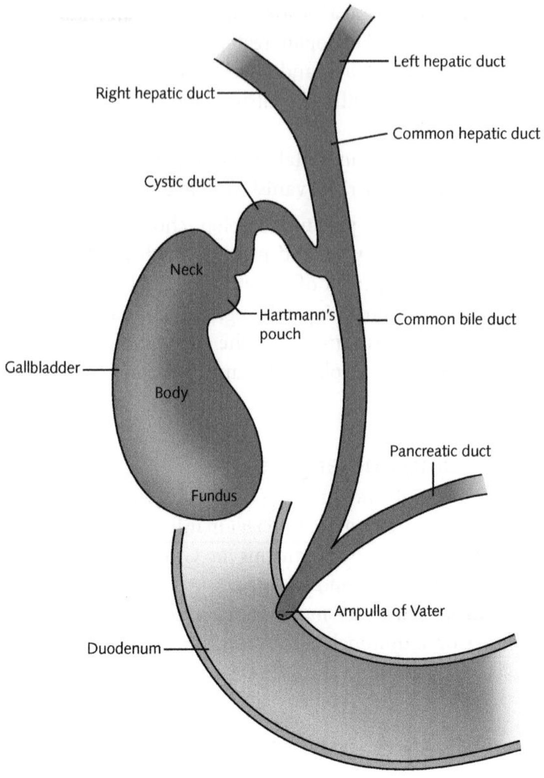

Fig. 12.9 Anatomy of the biliary tree.

There are three main types of gallstone: mixed stones, accounting for 80%, cholesterol stones (10%) and pigment stones (10%), all of which contain varying quantities of calcium salts (Fig. 12.10).

Mixed stones

Mixed stones are composed of varying proportions of cholesterol, calcium bilirubinate and calcium carbonate. They are multifaceted and often laminated with concentric light and dark rings on their cut surface. These are associated with chronic cholecystitis.

Cholesterol stones

Cholesterol stones can be large and single (solitaire) or mulberry-like. They are the consequence of cholesterol crystallization within the gallbladder when cholesterol reaches levels beyond the solubilizing capacity of bile salts (supersaturation). This may occur because of:

- Hypersecretion of cholesterol (most common mechanism).
- Decreased secretion of bile salts, due to either defective bile synthesis or excessive intestinal loss of bile salts (promotes crystallization).
- Abnormal gallbladder function, usually hypomotility.

Risk factors for cholesterol stones are shown in Table 12.9.

Pigment stones

The major constituent of these stones is bile pigment (calcium bilirubinate). They are typically found in patients with haemolytic disorders, such as sickle cell disease and thalassaemia, due to increased bilirubin production, hence pigment stones are typically black, small, multiple and gritty.

Complications, investigations and management

Gallstones may be asymptomatic (80% of cases), symptomatic (pain and other symptoms) or complicated.

Complications include:

- Biliary colic—temporary spasm of the gallbladder causing pain when the gallstone temporarily obstructs the cystic duct.
- Cholecystitis—chemical inflammation of the gallbladder owing to bile stagnation as a result of stone impaction into the neck of the gallbladder or cystic duct.
- Jaundice—impaction of a stone in the common bile duct (choledocholithiasis), leading to biliary obstruction and escape of bile into the circulation.

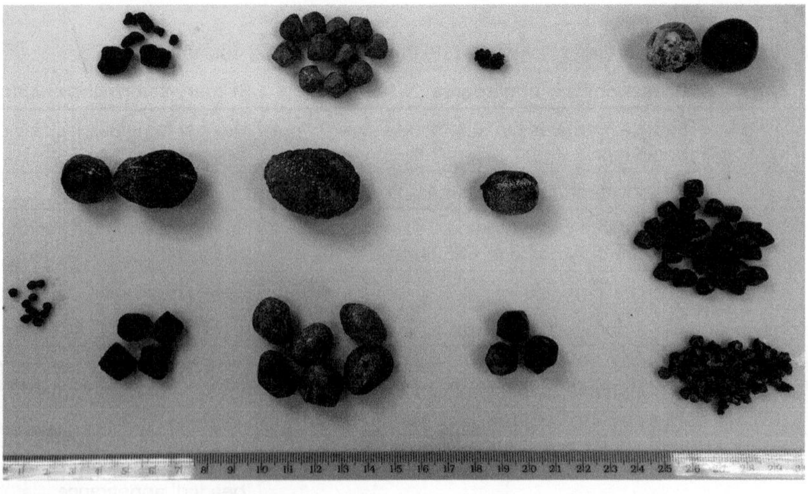

Fig. 12.10 Gallstones.
Gallstones come in all shapes, sizes and colours.

Table 12.9 Risk factors associated with cholesterol stones

Age	↑Cholesterol secretion
Female	↑Cholesterol secretion
Pregnancy	↑ Cholesterol secretion
	↓ Bile secretion
	Impaired gallbladder motility
Obesity	Altered cholesterol secretion
Rapid weight loss	Altered cholesterol secretion
Ethnic origin	May ↑ cholesterol secretion
Gallbladder stasis	Impaired gallbladder motility
Parenteral therapy	
Spinal cord injury	

- Cholangitis—inflammation of the bile duct, usually as a result of biliary obstruction complicated by bacterial infection (pus in the bile duct).
- Pancreatitis—impaction of a stone distal to the opening of the pancreatic duct.
- Mirizzi syndrome—rare cause of jaundice by extrinsic compression of the extrahepatic bile ducts by a gallstone impacted in the cystic duct or Hartmann pouch.
- Gallstone ileus—accounts for 0.5% of mechanical small-bowel obstruction when gallstone(s) enter the bowel via a biliary–enteric fistula and impact within the bowel, causing obstruction.
- Predisposition to carcinoma of the gallbladder.

Investigations are:

- Ultrasound (most useful).
- Abdominal X-ray—10%–20% of stones are visible due to calcification (in contrast to renal stones, where 90% are radioopaque).
- Oral cholecystography and CT scanning.

Management is by:

- Surgery (cholecystectomy).
- Extracorporeal shock-wave lithotripsy and ERCP—useful for those patients unsuitable for surgery.

HINTS AND TIPS

RULE OF Fs

Rule of thumb to remember the causes of gallstones:

*F*at
*F*emale
*F*ertile
*F*orty
*F*air

Cholecystitis

This is inflammation of the gallbladder. Aetiology is almost always associated with gallstones. There are two types, acute and chronic.

Acute cholecystitis

This acute inflammation of the gallbladder is precipitated by the chemical effects of concentrated static bile. It is typically caused by obstruction of outflow by stones at the gallbladder neck or cystic duct, and it may be exacerbated by secondary infection with enteric organisms such as *E. coli*.

In severe cases, an empyema may develop whereby the lumen distends with pus, causing increased risk of perforation and peritonitis.

Chronic cholecystitis

Chronic cholecystitis is invariably associated with gallstones. The wall of the gallbladder is thickened and rigid from fibrosis and muscular hyperplasia and may contain mucosal outpouches (Rokitansky-Aschoff sinuses) with a variable chronic inflammatory infiltrate of the mucosa and submucosa.

Porcelain gallbladder

Porcelain gallbladder refers to diffuse calcification of the gallbladder wall, rendering it brittle with a blueish tinge macroscopically. The pathogenesis is unclear, but there is a strong link to the presence of gallstones and chronic inflammation. Porcelain gallbladder is significant as it is associated with a 6% risk of gallbladder carcinoma.

Cholesterolosis

Lipid-laden 'foamy' macrophages can accumulate in yellow streaks beneath the luminal epithelium (cholesterolosis). Macroscopically this is described as a 'strawberry gallbladder' as the pattern is reminiscent of a strawberry skin.

Mucocele

The gallbladder fills and distends with sterile mucin as a result of obstruction to the gallbladder neck in the absence of inflammation.

Carcinoma of the gallbladder

Carcinoma of the gallbladder accounts for less than 1% of all cancers and is usually an adenocarcinoma, invariably associated with gallstones and chronic cholecystitis. Most cases are seen in women over the age of 70 years. There is a poor prognosis due to liver invasion and metastasis at presentation.

Remember Courvoisier's law: 'in the presence of jaundice, a palpable gallbladder is most likely due to malignant obstruction of the bile duct *not* gallstones'.

DISORDERS OF THE EXOCRINE PANCREAS

Acute pancreatitis

This acute inflammation of the pancreas is caused by the destructive effect of enzymes released from pancreatic acini. It is relatively common, affecting 10–20 per 100,000 per year in developed countries. By far the most common causes of acute pancreatitis are gallstones (50% of cases) and alcohol ingestion (20%) (Table 12.10).

Pathogenesis

Duct obstruction

Impaction of a gallstone distal to the site of union of the common bile duct and pancreatic duct results in:

- Reflux of bile along the pancreatic duct → toxic injury to pancreatic acini.
- Increased intraductal pressure → enzymatic leakage from pancreatic ducts.

Pancreatic proenzymes (zymogens) are inappropriately activated at some stage in this process, allowing autodigestion of pancreatic tissue. It is believed that the conversion of trypsinogen to trypsin is central to an activation cascade.

Note—chronic alcohol ingestion may also produce increased intraductal pressure owing to production of a protein-rich pancreatic fluid, which can form solid plugs in smaller pancreatic ducts.

Direct acinar injury

Less common causes of pancreatitis (e.g., viruses, drugs and trauma) may produce direct acinar damage.

> **HINTS AND TIPS**
>
> **I GET SMASHED**
>
> A useful mnemonic for memorizing the causes of pancreatitis is **I GET SMASHED: *I***diopathic, ***G***allstones, ***E***thanol, ***T***rauma, ***S***teroids, ***M***umps, ***A***utoimmune (polyarteritis nodosa), ***S***corpion stings (rare in the UK!), ***H***yperlipidaemia (also hypercalcaemia and hypothermia), ***E***RCP and ***D***rugs (e.g. Azathioprine, sulfasalazine, valproic acid.).

Table 12.10 Diagnosis of acute pancreatitis

Pancreatic enzymes	Increased serum lipase and/ or amylase
Imaging	Pancreatic swelling on ultrasound or CT
Deranged liver function tests	↑ bilirubin, ↑ alkaline phosphatase, ↓ albumin

Patterns of injury

Irrespective of the cause of pancreatitis, acinar damage leads to the liberation of lytic enzymes (proteases and lipases), causing necrosis of normal tissue. The three patterns of pancreatic necrosis are:

- Periductal—necrosis of acinar cells adjacent to ducts. Typically caused by duct obstruction, particularly associated with gallstones and alcohol.
- Perilobular—necrosis of the periphery of lobules. Caused by poor vascular perfusion, usually as a result of shock.
- Panlobular—necrosis affects all portions of the pancreatic lobule. This often develops from initial periductal or perilobular necrosis.

A vicious circle of necrosis occurs in which enzymatic release results in further acinar damage and further enzyme release:

- Lipases → fat necrosis and decreased calcium due to saponification.
- Proteases → destruction of pancreatic parenchyma. Endocrine destruction results in hyperglycaemia.
- Elastase and other enzymes → vascular damage with haemorrhage into pancreas or peritoneum. Extensive haemorrhage is known as acute haemorrhagic pancreatitis.

Clinical features

- Symptoms—severe central abdominal pain of sudden onset (often radiating through to the back), nausea, vomiting.
- Signs—tachycardia, fever, jaundice, shock, rigid abdomen, discoloration around the umbilicus (Cullen sign) or in the flanks (Grey Turner sign) secondary to intraabdominal haemorrhage.

Complications, investigations and management

Management is by physiological support and treatment of shock, respiratory failure and pain (Table 12.11).

Prognosis

Mortality is about 10%–15% (negligible in mild cases, but up to 50% in cases with severe haemorrhagic pancreatitis). Several classification systems (e.g., Ranson criteria,

Table 12.11 Complications of acute pancreatitis

Local	Pancreatic pseudocyst, abscess formation
Gastrointestinal	Gastric and duodenal erosions, bleeding, intestinal ileus
Systemic	Shock, renal failure, acute respiratory distress syndrome, hyperglycaemia, hypocalcaemia, peritonitis

Glasgow criteria, APACHE score) exist to determine severity and prognosis.

Death may be from shock, renal failure, sepsis or respiratory failure, with contributory factors being protease-induced activation of complement, kinin and the fibrinolytic and coagulation cascades.

Chronic pancreatitis

This is chronic inflammation and fibrosis of the pancreas with a relapsing and remitting course, causing irreversible damage.

It is a relatively rare disease but with increasing incidence because of a rise in the incidence of alcoholism. Typically, it occurs between the ages of 35 and 45 years, in males more often than females. It is associated with increased risk of developing pancreatic carcinoma.

Aetiology—the main causes of chronic pancreatitis are outlined in Table 12.12.

Pathogenesis—thought to be similar to the mechanisms involved in acute pancreatitis. However, there is permanent impairment of function.

Morphological features:

- Chronic inflammation with parenchymal fibrosis.
- Loss of pancreatic parenchymal elements.
- Duct strictures with formation of intrapancreatic calculi (stones).

Clinical features:

- Recurrent bouts of severe abdominal pain.
- Malabsorption owing to reduced exocrine function (decreased lipase and protease secretion)—steatorrhoea (fat in faeces).
- Diabetes mellitus (destruction of pancreatic parenchyma)—this occurs in advanced disease.

Table 12.12 Main causes of chronic pancreatitis

	Cause	Pathogenesis
Common	Chronic alcoholism (majority of cases)	Protein plugs form in ducts and become calculi; ducts are obstructed, inflamed and scarred
	Biliary tract disease	Gallstones or anatomical abnormalities of pancreatic ducts
	Idiopathic chronic pancreatitis	Pathogenesis uncertain
Rare	Cystic fibrosis	Protein plugs in ducts
	Familial pancreatitis	Autosomal dominant
	Autoimmune pancreatitis	IgG4-related disease

Episodes of acute pancreatitis may complicate chronic pancreatitis.

Relevant investigations include imaging (by plain radiograph for calcification of the pancreas, ultrasound, CT and ERCP) and functional tests.

Management is based on alcohol abstinence, pain relief, dietary fat restriction and surgery for correctable causes.

Pseudocysts

Pseudocysts are the commonest cysts in the pancreas and are localized collections of fluid and necrotic inflammatory debris caused by release of pancreatic enzymes. They are not 'true' cysts because they have no epithelial lining; instead, they are surrounded by a zone of inflammatory granulation tissue. They communicate into the pancreatic duct system and occur in both acute and chronic forms of pancreatitis.

Although many pseudocysts spontaneously resolve, there is a risk of infection, compression or perforation.

Neoplasms of the pancreas

Cystic tumours

These are mostly benign, well-circumscribed masses composed of multiple cystic cavities lined by either serous or mucin-secreting epithelium. Serous cystic neoplasms can be associated with von Hippel–Lindau syndrome.

Carcinoma of the pancreas

This tumour accounts for 5% of cancer deaths in the UK. Most are adenocarcinomas arising from the pancreatic ducts. Incidence rises with age.

Associations include cigarette smoking, chronic pancreatitis, a diet high in fat and carbohydrate, and diabetes in women. Around 10% of cases have a clear genetic association (e.g., hereditary pancreatitis, multiple endocrine neoplasia).

The development of pancreatic cancer follows an adenoma–adenocarcinoma sequence similar to that seen in colonic cancer (see Chapter 4). Precursor lesions with the potential to form adenocarcinomas are termed pancreatic intraepithelial neoplasias (PanIN). Several genetic mutations are associated with development of pancreatic carcinoma.

MOLECULAR

PANCREATIC CARCINOMA

Ninety percent of pancreatic carcinomas have *KRAS* mutations.

Up to 75% of pancreatic carcinomas show inactivation of *p53* and *SMAD4* tumour suppressor genes.

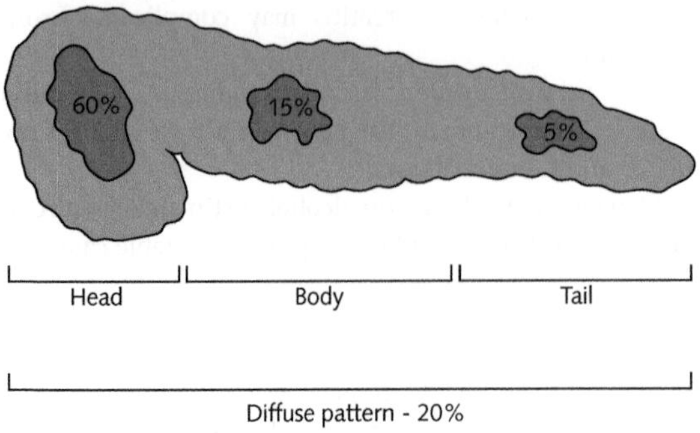

Fig. 12.11 Location of pancreatic cancer.

Macroscopic appearance—gritty, hard, grey nodules invading adjacent gland and local structures.

Tumours arise with different frequencies in different parts of the pancreas (Fig. 12.11).

Microscopic appearance—tumours are typically moderately differentiated adenocarcinomas composed of glandular spaces in a fibrous stroma.

Routes of spread:

- Local—causes obstructive jaundice or invasion of the duodenum.
- Lymphatic—spread to adjacent lymph nodes.
- Blood—spread to the liver.

Clinical features:

- Weight loss, anorexia and chronic persistent pain in the epigastrium radiating to the back.
- Obstructive jaundice with painless palpable distension of gallbladder (Courvoisier law). Carcinoma in the head of the pancreas tends to present early with obstructive jaundice. As a result, tumours are on average smaller at diagnosis than in other sites.
- Rarely, there may be vomiting (duodenal obstruction), venous thrombosis (migratory thrombophlebitis), acute pancreatitis or diabetes mellitus (destruction of islets of Langerhans with carcinoma).

HINTS AND TIPS

TROUSSEAU SIGN

Trousseau sign—migratory thrombophlebitis, occurs secondary to venous thromboembolism in malignancy. Increased cell turnover in tumour cells activates procoagulative factors and thrombin, resulting in an intrinsic hypercoagulable state. It is commonly associated with pancreatic cancer.

Management:

- Curative resection (Whipple procedure)—rarely possible.
- Palliative surgery—often performed to bypass obstruction of the bile duct (relieving jaundice) and obstruction of the duodenum.

Prognosis is extremely poor—5-year survival is just 5%.

Refer to Chapter 14 for discussion of islet cell (endocrine) tumours of the pancreas.

Chapter Summary

- The liver has a limited number of responses to injury although the causes of liver injury are numerous and diverse.
- Cirrhosis—nodular regeneration and fibrosis of the liver—is the terminal endpoint of chronic liver conditions regardless of cause. Can become decompensated and cause ascites and encephalopathy.
- Cirrhosis is irreversible and predisposes to development of hepatocellular carcinoma.
- Hepatitis can be caused by infection, drugs and toxins (including alcohol), congenital metabolic errors and autoimmunity.
- Alcoholic liver disease is a spectrum of steatosis, steatohepatitis, acute hepatitis and cirrhosis.
- Haemochromatosis and Wilson disease are autosomal recessive conditions of iron and copper deposition, respectively, primarily affecting the liver and causing chronic damage.
- The minority of patients with hepatitis B enter a chronic carrier state (10%) versus the majority in hepatitis C. This is significant as there is an increased risk of progression to cirrhosis.

- Amoebae are the commonest cause of liver abscess worldwide; bacteria are the commonest cause in the UK.
- Jaundice is subclassified based on site (e.g., prehepatic causes) or conjugation state of bilirubin.
- Hepatic adenomas are associated with oral contraceptive and steroid use.
- Metastases are the commonest malignant tumours in the liver.
- Primary biliary cholangitis commonly affects young women and primary sclerosing cholangitis commonly affects young men.
- Gallstones are common and vary in their constituents, size, appearance and number.
- Recurrent pancreatitis predisposes to development of pancreatic carcinoma.

Pathology of the kidney and urinary tract

13

ABNORMALITIES OF KIDNEY STRUCTURE

Congenital abnormalities of the kidney

Congenital abnormalities of kidneys are common, affecting 3%–4% of newborn infants.

Agenesis of the kidney

Unilateral

Unilateral agenesis occurs in 1 in 1000 births. It may occur alongside other congenital diseases, most commonly those of the genitourinary system, e.g., abnormal uterus, seminal vesicle cysts. It can be associated with chromosomal abnormalities, e.g., trisomy 21, 22q11 microdeletion and Turner syndrome, or part of a more complex syndrome, e.g., VACTERL (vertebral anomalies, cardiac anomalies, tracheooesophageal fistula, renal agenesis and limb deformities).

The solitary kidney undergoes marked compensatory hypertrophy and is susceptible to infections, stones and progressive glomerulosclerosis. It affects males more often than females by a factor of 2:1; the left kidney is usually the absent one.

Bilateral

Bilateral renal agenesis occurs in 1 in 5000 births and is incompatible with life, usually due to pulmonary hypoplasia. Characteristically, there is oligohydramnios in pregnancy as the kidneys are not present to contribute to amniotic fluid volume (absence of fetal urine), which in turn results in pulmonary hypoplasia. Infants also have other abnormalities, which include hand and feet deformities, absent genitourinary structures, e.g., uterus and gastrointestinal malformations.

It can occur as part of Potter sequence (pulmonary hypoplasia with characteristic facies: low-set ears, flattened nose, recessed chin and prominent epicanthic folds).

Hypoplasia

Kidneys fail to reach the normal adult size. May be unilateral or bilateral. True developmental hypoplasia is rare as shrinkage is more likely to have been acquired as a result of chronic infection or other insults in early life.

Horseshoe kidney

The poles of two normally functioning kidneys are fused, usually inferiorly, to form a large U-shaped (horseshoe) kidney. This is the most common congenital abnormality of the kidney, affecting ~1 in 800 people. It is typically asymptomatic; however, the horseshoe kidney has an increased predisposition to disease owing to its abnormal anatomy. Examples include hydronephrosis, ureteropelvic junction obstruction, stone formation and infection. The incidence of Wilms tumours and carcinoid tumours is also higher in horseshoe kidneys.

Cystic diseases of the kidney

Overview of cystic kidney disease

This heterogeneous group of diseases comprises:

- Hereditary disorders.
- Developmental (but not hereditary) disorders.
- Acquired disorders.

Each disease is distinguished by a characteristic distribution of cysts, illustrated in Fig. 13.1.

Table 13.1 provides a summary of cystic diseases of the kidney. Accurate diagnosis of cystic diseases is important for two reasons:

1. Appropriate patient management to delay onset of renal failure.
2. Appropriate genetic counselling in the case of hereditary cystic diseases.

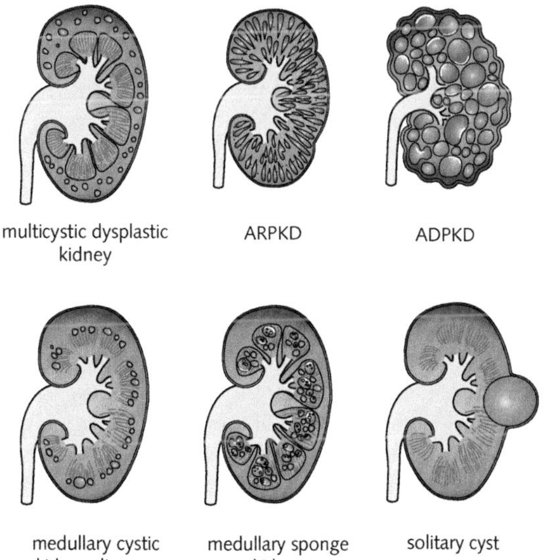

Fig. 13.1 Cystic diseases of the kidney.
ADPKD, autosomal dominant polycystic kidney disease; *ARPKD*, autosomal recessive polycystic kidney disease.

Table 13.1 Summary of cystic diseases of the kidney

Type of cystic disease	Clinical features
Hereditary	
Autosomal dominant polycystic disease	Chronic renal failure and hypertension
Autosomal recessive polycystic disease	Chronic renal failure and hypertension
Medullary cystic disease (autosomal dominant)	Early-onset chronic renal failure
Juvenile nephronophthisis (autosomal recessive)	End stage renal failure at a young age
Medullary sponge kidney (occasionally familial)	Renal stones predispose to renal colic and infection
Developmental	
Multicystic renal dysplasia	Typically asymptomatic
Acquired	
Simple renal cysts	Typically asymptomatic
Dialysis-associated cystic disease	

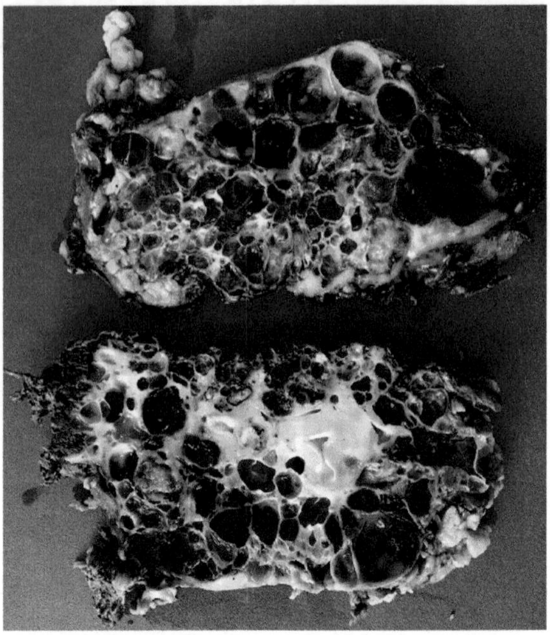

Fig. 13.2 Macroscopic appearance of adult polycystic kidney disease.
Multiple cysts of varying sizes are present, replacing the entire parenchyma of the kidney. Some contain consolidated secretions or show evidence of haemorrhage.

Multicystic renal dysplasia

This results from abnormal metanephric differentiation of the embryonic kidney. This is usually unilateral but can be bilateral. The renal tissue is formed of multiple noncommunicating cysts of varying sizes with intervening dysplastic parenchyma. No pelvicalyceal system is present owing to abnormal interactions with the ureteric bud and the kidney is nonfunctional.

The condition is often detected on antenatal scans or presents as an abdominal mass in the newborn. It can remain occult until adulthood. The contralateral kidney may have anomalies in 40% of cases.

Autosomal dominant (adult) polycystic kidney disease

Autosomal dominant (adult) polycystic kidney disease (ADPKD) is a hereditary disease that presents at between 40 and 60 years of age with an abdominal flank mass, haematuria or renal insufficiency/failure. Incidence is 1 per 1000 live births and accounts for 10% of all end-stage renal disease (ESRD). Both sexes are equally affected.

Aetiology—ADPKD is genetically heterogeneous, with mutations occurring in the *PKD1* and *PKD2* genes, affecting the proteins polycystin 1 and 2, respectively. Eighty-five percent of cases are linked to *PKD1* and 15% to *PKD2*, which has a slower onset. The condition is asymptomatic at first but eventually replacement and compression of the functioning renal parenchyma over many years by enlarging cysts leads to progressive impairment of renal function.

Macroscopically—the kidneys are asymmetrically enlarged and heavy. The parenchyma is completely replaced by numerous large cysts (up to 5 cm in diameter). These contain clear, brown or haemorrhagic fluid (Fig. 13.2).

Microscopically—the cysts arise anywhere along the nephron and are lined by various types of flattened epithelium. They communicate with nephrons and calyces and become disconnected as the disease progresses. The surrounding parenchyma shows extensive fibrosis interspersed with residual nephrons.

Complications and associations:

- Chronic renal failure and uraemia.
- Nephrolithiasis.
- Hypertension.
- Mitral valve prolapse.
- Liver cysts—40% of cases.
- Pancreatic, splenic and pulmonary cysts (less common).
- Berry aneurysms within the circle of Willis.
- Subarachnoid haemorrhage (10% of cases): secondary to berry aneurysms or hypertensive haemorrhage.

Autosomal recessive (childhood) polycystic kidney disease

Autosomal recessive polycystic kidney disease (ARPKD) is a rare autosomal recessive condition (1 per 10,000 live births) in which there is bilateral cystic replacement of the kidneys present at birth. Congenital hepatic fibrosis with ductal plate malformations and fibrosis of all portal tracts is always present. Heterogeneous mutations in the *PKHD1* gene that codes for fibrocystin are responsible for the condition.

Macroscopically—bilateral symmetrical renal enlargement with smooth external surfaces. The cut surfaces show loss of corticomedullary differentiation with replacement of the parenchyma by small (3 mm) medullary cysts. The cysts are uniformly distributed and appear elongated and cylindrical, arranged radially such that they are perpendicular to the cortex.

Microscopically—the cysts arise from the collecting ducts and, as such, are lined by cuboidal cells. Nephrons are present between the cysts; however, glomeruli are difficult to identify.

Prognosis—prognosis is governed by the severity of the disease. Those severely affected are stillborn or do not survive the neonatal period. Those surviving longer may have respiratory problems secondary to pulmonary hypoplasia, renal failure and portal hypertension.

Cystic diseases of the renal medulla

The classification of cystic diseases is complicated, with morphological and clinical overlap. The situation is improving, however, with the improved understanding of the pathological aetiology and underlying genetic mutations.

Medullary sponge kidney

This is a sporadic congenital disease presenting in adulthood as either an incidental finding on imaging or from a complication of the condition. Renal function is not usually impaired and the main clinical problem is the development of renal stones (60% of cases) that predispose to renal colic and infection. Haematuria can also be seen. The disease is bilateral in 70% of cases.

Macroscopically, the kidneys are not enlarged. The cut surface shows small (1- to 7 mm) cysts limited to the medulla and renal papillae. Microscopically, the cysts arise from the collecting tubules and are in continuity with the collecting ducts. They are lined by cuboidal epithelium. The interstitium usually shows chronic inflammation. Renal failure is not associated with this condition.

Nephronophthisis and medullary cystic disease

This is a group of hereditary diseases characterized by development of cysts at the corticomedullary junction of the kidney arising from the distal tubules and collecting ducts. Cyst size is variable, up to several centimetres. These diseases are associated with tubular atrophy and interstitial fibrosis which ultimately lead to glomerulosclerosis and renal failure. The kidneys are usually normal or slightly small in size with granular surfaces. They differ by the age of onset and the underlying genetic mutations.

Nephronophthisis—This is a group of autosomal recessive conditions affecting children and adolescents, causing early onset end-stage renal failure (ESRF) (4–20 years). They are one of the frequent causes of ESRF in children and adolescents. Three forms are recognized: juvenile, adolescent and infantile. Juvenile and adolescent forms are associated with mutations in *NPHP1* and *NPHP3* genes, which code for nephrocystin proteins. The infantile form is associated with the *NPHP2* gene and inversin protein, and is distinguished clinically from the other forms by severe hypertension and onset of ESRF around 4 years of age.

Extrarenal manifestations are seen within this group in contrast to medullary cystic disease where they are not. Examples include retinal dystrophy, cerebellar aplasia and hepatic fibrosis.

Medullary cystic kidney disease—This group of diseases presents in adults with ESRF around 50 years of age. Inheritance is autosomal dominant and involves the genes *MUC1*, coding for mucin 1 in type 1 disease, and *UMOD*, coding for uromodulin in type 2 disease. The hallmark of type 2 disease is hyperuricaemia.

Cystic diseases of the cortex

Simple cortical cysts

These common lesions occur as solitary or occasionally multiple cystic spaces in otherwise normal kidneys. Incidence increases with age and they are rare before 40 years of age.

The abnormality is widely believed to be acquired, but the cause is unknown.

Macroscopically, cysts are of variable size (generally <5 cm) and they contain clear watery fluid. Microscopically, they are lined by flattened cuboidal epithelium and surrounded by a thin fibrous capsule.

Cysts have no effect on renal function; however, they require clinical differentiation from cystic tumours and other cystic disorders. Suspicious features include thickened, irregular walls, vascular septa and enhancement with contrast on imaging.

DISEASES OF THE GLOMERULUS

Overview of glomerular disease

Glomerular diseases are typically caused by damage to one or more of the components that form the glomerulus (Fig. 13.3):

1. Endothelial cells lining the capillary loops.
2. Glomerular basement membrane (GBM).
3. Mesangium—the supporting tissue of the capillary loops, comprising phagocytic cells (mesangial cells) and extracellular material (mesangial matrix).
4. Podocytes (epithelial cells)—located within the Bowman capsule and line the outer surface of the GBM, forming a series of foot processes.

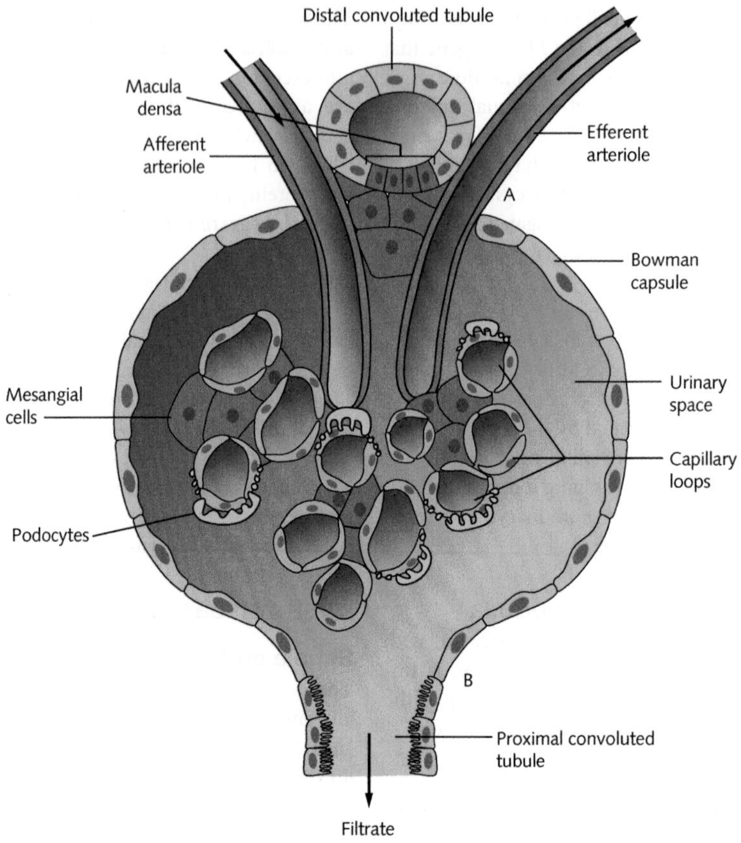

Fig. 13.3 Structure of the glomerulus.
The start of the nephron is the Bowman capsule, which wraps around the glomerular capillaries entering at the vascular pole *(A)*. The capillaries form loops supported by the mesangial matrix and mesangial cells. The podocytes (epithelial cells) surround the external surface of the capillary loops and produce foot processes to from part of the glomerular basement membrane. Blood entering the capillary loops is filtered, with the effluent passing into the urinary (Bowman) space and down the proximal convoluted tubule at the renal pole *(B)*, along the nephron and into the renal pelvis.

HINTS AND TIPS

UNDERSTANDING GLOMERULAR DISEASE CLASSIFICATION

The classification of glomerular disease can appear overwhelming. It can be described:

- Clinically—by the type of syndrome it produces, e.g., nephrotic syndrome, nephritic syndrome, rapidly progressive.
- Histologically—by the microscopic appearance, e.g., focal segmental glomerulonephritis.
  It is helpful to appreciate that the histological 'diagnosis' does not necessarily correlate with a single disease, but rather a pattern of disease that has several causes. For example, 'glomerulosclerosis' can be caused by diabetes, systemic lupus erythematosus and HIV. It is helpful to identify the histological process to guide treatment and inform prognosis.

Patterns of glomerular disease

Glomerular disease can also be described by its distribution, either within a single glomerulus or within the kidney as a whole:

1. Segmental—part of glomerulus.
2. Global—whole glomerulus.
3. Focal—some glomeruli.
4. Diffuse—all glomeruli.

Thus a glomerular disease may be described as one of 'diffuse global', 'diffuse segmental', 'focal global' or 'focal segmental'. The vast majority are either 'diffuse global' or 'focal segmental' (Fig. 13.4).

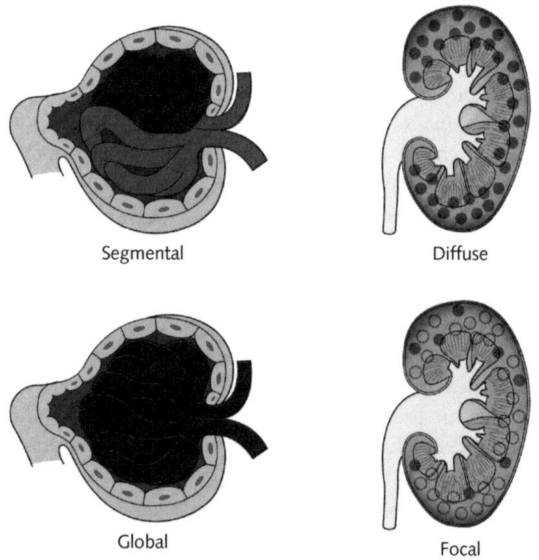

Fig. 13.4 Patterns of glomerular disease.
Glomerular disease can be described by its distribution in relation to the glomerular capillary (segmental or global) or in relation to the distribution of the disease (diffuse or focal).

Aetiology of glomerular diseases

The aetiology of glomerular diseases is extensive. It may be classified as:

- Primary (majority)—idiopathic (Fig. 13.5).
- Secondary—disease process is secondary to systemic disease (Table 13.2).
- Hereditary—Alport syndrome, Fabry syndrome and congenital nephrotic syndrome.

Clinical manifestations of glomerular disease

Glomerular pathology produces a spectrum of presentations from pure proteinuria (reflects injury to podocytes and architecture) to pure haematuria (inflammation of the glomeruli). Many diseases lie somewhere along this spectrum, with differing degrees of mixed proteinuria and haematuria (Tables 13.3 and 13.4).

Five key syndromes cover most presentations. These are described below.

Asymptomatic haematuria

This is haematuria without significant proteinuria, which may be continuous or intermittent, varying in severity from macroscopic to microscopic.

Asymptomatic proteinuria

This is proteinuria (>0.3 g every 24 h) without haematuria, which may be continuous, orthostatic (postural) or transient. It is typically detected at a routine medical examination.

Acute nephritic syndrome

This presents with sudden onset of haematuria, proteinuria (often with urinary casts) and hypertension. Loin pain and headache may be present and the patient will often feel unwell.

Nephrotic syndrome

In nephrotic syndrome there is proteinuria (usually >3.5 g every 24 h) with hypoalbuminaemia (serum albumin <3.0 g/L) and oedema. There is also hypercholesterolaemia, increased infection risk and a prothrombotic state. It may be due to primary or secondary glomerular disease.

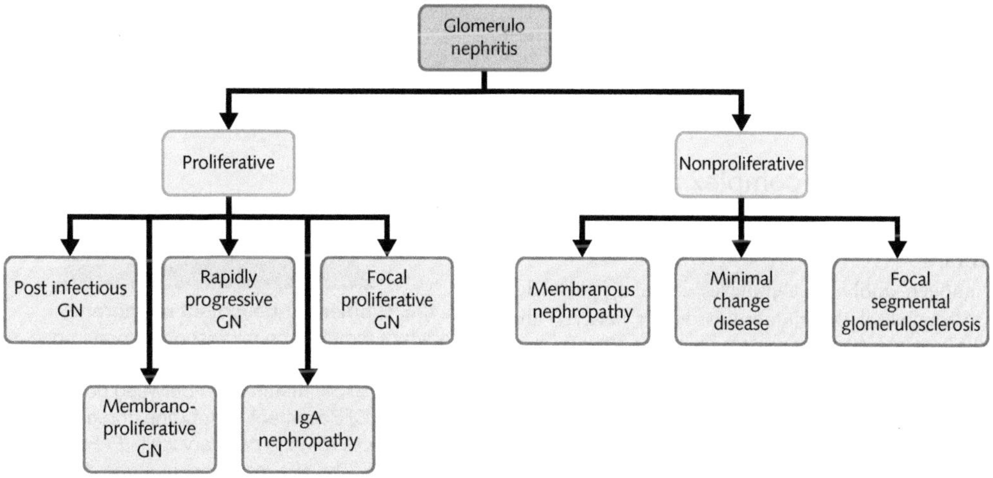

Fig. 13.5 Classification of glomerulonephritis.
Glomerulonephritis *(GN)* can be divided in many ways. Histologically it can be divided into proliferative disease (proliferation of mesangial and epithelial cells within the glomerulus) and nonproliferative disease.

Table 13.2 Secondary causes of glomerular disease

Aetiology	Example
Immune complex-mediated conditions	Systemic lupus erythematosus
	Henoch–Schönlein purpura
	Infective endocarditis Methicillin-resistant *Staphylococcus aureus*
Metabolic conditions	Diabetes mellitus
	Renal amyloidosis
	Multiple myeloma
Vascular conditions	Polyarteritis nodosa
	Granulomatosis with polyangiitis (Wegener granulomatosis)
	Haemolytic uraemic syndrome
	Idiopathic thrombocytopaenic purpura
	Disseminated intravascular coagulation

Chronic renal failure

This is an irreversible deterioration in renal function caused by progressive destruction of individual nephrons over a long period of time. Impairment of excretory, metabolic and endocrine functions of the kidney leads to the clinical syndrome of uraemia.

The mechanism of glomerular injury

Many glomerular diseases are caused by immune-mediated damage. Different patterns of immune-mediated damage point to different diagnoses. It is therefore important to identify the site, type and pattern of immune complex and complement deposition within the glomerulus by immunofluorescence and electron microscopy.

The four main mechanisms of immune-mediated damage are described below.

Circulating immune complex nephritis

This is the most common pattern of immunological disease.

Mechanism

Soluble antigen–antibody complexes circulating in the blood are trapped at the glomerulus, either between the mesangium and endothelial cells (subendothelial) or between the GBM and podocytes (subepithelial). Complexes activate the complement cascade via the classical pathway and leucocytes via the Fc portion of antibodies. Activated components of complement bring about the characteristic acute inflammation of glomerulonephritis by attracting neutrophils, increasing vascular permeability and causing membrane damage. Immunofluorescent subendothelial and subepithelial granular deposits are seen within the mesangium or along the GBM (Fig. 13.6).

Example

Systemic lupus erythematosus (SLE): depending on the size and charge of the immune complexes, these may get trapped at the endothelial, intramembranous or subepithelial regions of the GBM or mesangium.

Immune complex deposition

Mechanism

Circulating antibodies target antigens which have become 'implanted' or trapped within the glomerulus from the circulation, or preexisting intrinsic tissue antigens. Immune complexes are therefore formed within the glomerulus itself with little complement and no inflammatory or proliferative responses. Antigens include bacterial or viral products, or endogenous components of the GBM.

Example

Poststreptococcal glomerulonephritis: streptococcal antigens are implanted into the GBM during infection.
Goodpasture syndrome: in which autoantibodies target a domain on the α3 type IV collagen chain within the GBM. These antibodies may cross-react with collagen in the lung, simultaneously producing lung and kidney disease.

Cytotoxic antibodies

Mechanism

Antibodies against cellular components of the glomerulus, e.g., mesangial and endothelial cells can cause cytotoxic destruction of these cells.

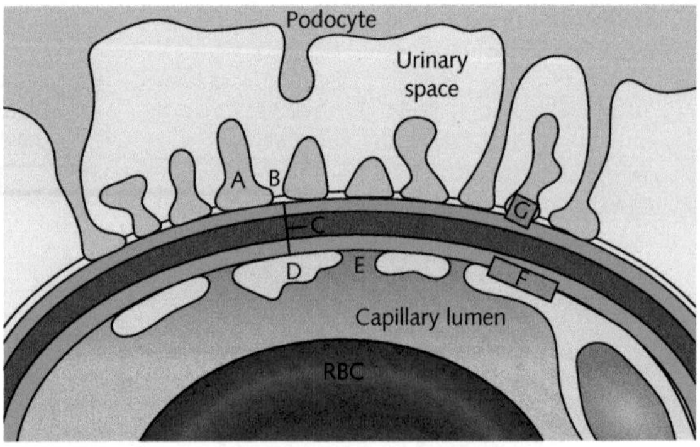

Fig. 13.6 Glomerular basement membrane. Diagram of the electron microscopic appearance of the glomerular basement membrane. *(A)* Podocyte foot processes. *(B)* Slit membranes between podocyte foot processes. *(C)* Basement membrane (three layers). *(D)* Endothelial cell forming capillary wall. *(E)* Fenestration in capillary wall. The spaces where immune deposits can be located are subendothelial space *(F)* and subepithelial space, *(G)* as well as in the basement membrane. *RBC*, red blood cell.

Activation of the alternative complement pathway

Mechanism

The alternative complement pathway is normally activated by the presence of bacterial cell walls, and it is independent of immune complex formation. However, in certain disease conditions, the alternative pathway can be activated by different mechanisms.

Example

In dense deposit disease (a C3 glomerulopathy), circulating autoantibody (termed 'C3 nephritic factor') stabilizes the alternative pathway C3 convertase (C3bBb), which usually has a short half-life. C3 is persistently activated by the action of the alternative C3 convertase, resulting in reduced serum concentration of C3.

Proliferative glomerulonephritis

This group of disorders is characterized histologically by varying degrees of proliferation of mesangial and epithelial (and sometimes endothelial) cells within the glomerulus (Table 13.5).

The majority of cases of glomerulonephritis (over 70%) belong to this group.

Proliferative glomerulonephritis can be divided according to histological appearance into:

- postinfectious (diffuse) proliferative
- rapidly progressive
- membranoproliferative.

However, it must be emphasized that these subdivisions are not diagnoses but rather describe a pattern of reaction caused by a glomerular insult.

Table 13.5 Examples of proliferative glomerulonephritis

Condition	Features
Goodpasture syndrome	A proliferative glomerulonephritis The Goodpasture antigen is a domain of type IV collagen in the basement membrane; this is a target for autoantibodies
MPGN	An immune-complex disease thought to involve a disorder of complement, characterized by subendothelial deposits There is a persistently low serum C3
C3 glomerulopathy	An autoimmune-mediated abnormality of complement. There is marked thickening of the capillary walls owing to deposition of C3 (dense deposit disease)

MPGN, Membranoproliferative glomerulonephritis.

Postinfectious (diffuse) glomerulonephritis

Diffuse, global, acute inflammation of glomeruli is caused by the deposition of immune complexes in the glomeruli. Presentation is usually with nephritic syndrome.

Aetiology is as follows:

- Poststreptococcal (most common)—onset is 1–2 weeks after a primary pharyngeal or skin infection with group A β-haemolytic streptococci.
- Nonstreptococcal (less common)—a range of bacterial, viral and parasitic infections can also cause this pattern of disease.

Immune complexes are formed against circulating or implanted antigen within the GBM and are filtered out, producing characteristic histological changes:

1. Leucocytes within the glomerulus—numerous neutrophils are predominantly seen, with a later infiltration of lymphocytes and macrophages.
2. Endothelial and mesangial cell proliferation.
3. Large granular deposits of IgG and C3 along the capillary loops seen on immunofluorescence.
4. Immune complex deposition—appear as subepithelial humps on the GBM.

Rapidly progressive glomerulonephritis (crescentic glomerulonephritis)

Rapidly progressive glomerulonephritis (RPGN) is the clinical manifestation of severe glomerular injury characterized by the formation of cellular crescent-shaped masses within the Bowman space in >50% of the glomeruli. It can lead to renal failure within weeks to months and may arise from other types of glomerulonephritis, occurring in a small percentage of patients with poststreptococcal glomerulonephritis.

Severe damage to the glomerular capillaries causes fibrin and blood to leak into the Bowman space, stimulating crescent formation and inflammatory infiltration. Crescents are cellular masses of epithelial cells, macrophages and layers of fibrin. The crescents enlarge to fill the Bowman space, leading to compression of the glomerular capillaries, glomerular ischaemia and ultimately permanent glomerular damage.

Pathologically RPGN is classified into three categories:

1. Anti-GBM disease—this accounts for ~3% of RPGN cases. It is characterized by smooth, linear IgG ± C3 immunofluorescent staining along the capillary loops. Goodpasture syndrome is present when there is associated haemoptysis/pulmonary haemorrhage. Here the autoantibody is directed towards the α3 chain of collagen type IV, which is accessible within the alveolar and glomerular basement membranes.
2. Immune complex disease—this accounts for 45% of RPGN cases and may complicate any of the nephritides caused by immune-complexes, e.g., SLE, Henoch–Schönlein purpura (HSP), IgA nephropathy. Granular staining with one or more immunoglobulins is present.
3. Pauci-immune—this accounts for 50% of cases of RPGN. Characteristically there is a lack of immune complex

deposition demonstrated by negative immunofluorescent stains for all type of immunoglobulins. Pauci-immune RPGN can be idiopathic or occur as part of a systemic vasculitis, e.g., granulomatosis with polyangiitis (Wegener granulomatosis). In both situations most patients are positive for antineutrophil cytoplasmic antibodies (ANCA) (see Chapter 17).

Membranoproliferative glomerulonephritis

Membranoproliferative glomerulonephritis (MPGN), also known as mesangiocapillary glomerulonephritis, is a histological pattern of disease and a diagnosis. Historically, MPGN was divided into types I, II and III; it is now classified as:

- MPGN – caused by immune complex deposition
- C3 glomerulopathies – dense deposit disease (DDD) and C3 glomerulonephritis.

The light microscopic appearances are of diffuse, global lesions characterised by mesangial and endocapillary proliferation and GBM thickening. Silver stains show a "tram track" appearance due to subendothelial deposits causing reduplication of the GBM. Immunofluorescence (IMF) and electron microscopy (EM) differentiate the conditions.

MPGN: IMF shows chunky staining for IgG, IgM and C3 within the capillary walls and mesangium. EM reveals subendothelial dense deposits.

Dense deposit disease: is a distinct disease affecting adolescents. IMF shows chunky mesangial and capillary staining for C3. IgG and IgM are negative. EM demonstrates large electron dense GBM and mesangial deposits

C3 glomerulonephritis: affects adults of ~ 30 years. IMF shows granular capillary and mesangial staining for C3. EM deposits, located within the mesangium or subendothelial space, are not electron dense.

Presentation is with nephrotic/nephritic syndrome and low serum complement. Idiopathic MPGN is more common in children/young adults. MPGN associated with diseases (e.g., lupus nephritis, cryoglobulinaemia and viral hepatitis) is more common in adults.

> **CLINICAL NOTE**
>
> NEPHROTIC AND NEPHRITIC SYNDROME
>
> **Nephrotic syndrome**
>
> Proteinuria >3.5 g/day
> Hypoalbuminaemia
> Oedema
> Hypercholesterolaemia
>
> **Nephritic syndrome**
>
> Hypertension
> Haematuria
> Urinary red cell casts
> (± Proteinuria and oedema)

IgA nephropathy

IgA nephropathy is the most common cause of glomerulonephritis in adults. It is characterized by microscopic haematuria with variable proteinuria and possible intermittent macroscopic haematuria. It is thought to have a generally benign course; however, slow progression to ESRD is seen in approximately 15% of cases.

Microscopically, mesangial proliferation with increased mesangial cells and matrix is seen. Immunofluorescence shows large mesangial deposits of IgA with electron-dense deposits on EM.

Systemic diseases can also be associated with IgA deposition such as SLE, hepatitis and dermatitis herpetiformis.

Membranous glomerulonephritis

This is a common cause of nephrotic syndrome in adults; however, patients may present with proteinuria less than the nephrotic range or haematuria initially. Proteinuria is nonselective, in contrast to minimal change disease where it is selective. All age groups are affected, but the highest incidence is between the fifth and seventh decades. Males are affected more often than females.

The glomeruli show diffuse thickening of the capillary wall. Unlike proliferative types of glomerulonephritis, membranous glomerulonephritis has no associated inflammation or endothelial/epithelial cell proliferation, although the mesangial cell population may be slightly increased. Silver staining shows spikes protruding from the basement membrane and immunofluorescence shows diffuse granular staining for C3 and IgG along the capillary loops. Subepithelial deposits are seen on EM.

Aetiology:

- Primary—80%–90% of cases are apparently idiopathic; however, recently 60%–80% of adults in these cases have been found to have autoantibodies against the phospholipase A2 receptor (anti-PLA2R) on podocytes.
- Secondary—membranous glomerulonephritis is found in association with a number of conditions, which are listed in Table 13.6. It is therefore important to exclude secondary causes of the disease at the time of diagnosis.

There are four pathological stages:

1. In-situ formation of immune complexes on the epithelial side of the GBM (diffuse, global pattern) seen as dense deposits on EM.
2. Mild mesangial increase.
3. New basement membrane is laid down around the deposits of immune complex such that they are incorporated into a thickened basement membrane.
4. The basement membrane becomes 'lacy' on EM as the deposits become lucent.

Over many years, gradual hyalinization of the glomeruli (glomerulosclerosis) occurs, with death of individual nephrons. Prognosis is variable and related to cause, but as a rule of thumb: one-third of patients undergo spontaneous

Table 13.6 Conditions associated with membranous glomerulonephritis

Type	Example
Infections	Malaria
	Syphilis
	Hepatitis B and C
Malignancy	Carcinoma (lung, breast, gastrointestinal tract)
	Lymphoma
Drugs	Nonsteroidal antiinflammatory drugs, gold, mercury, penicillamine, captopril
Systemic disease	Systemic lupus erythematosus (10% of renal involvement is of the membranous pattern)

remission without treatment, one-third are stabilized with persisting proteinuria and one-third progress to develop chronic ESRF.

Minimal change disease

This is the most common cause of nephrotic syndrome in children, with males affected more often than females. It is less common in adults, accounting for ~15% of cases of nephrotic syndrome. There is no associated renal insufficiency, haematuria or hypertension. Proteinuria is selective for albumin.

Minimal change disease is characterized by a normal appearance of glomeruli on light microscopy, with effacement of the podocyte foot processes on EM. Immunofluorescence is negative for immune complex deposition. Cells of the proximal tubules may show accumulation of lipid and protein, giving rise to the alternative name of 'lipoid nephrosis'.

Pathogenesis—aetiology is unknown, although in some cases an association with respiratory infection has been noted.

Pathogenesis is postulated to be immunologically related because of the near universal response to corticosteroid therapy. T-cells are implicated in cytokine release with damage to the podocytes. Subsequently, loss of the GBM polyanionic charges occurs, which is required to prevent the filtration of macromolecules such as albumin.

Prognosis in children is good, with no permanent renal damage; however, relapses are common. In adults, the outlook is variable.

Focal segmental glomerulosclerosis

This is a common cause of nephrotic syndrome in adults, presenting with nonselective proteinuria or nephrotic syndrome with or without renal insufficiency. Microscopic haematuria can also be present in up to 50% of patients.

Segments of the glomeruli are partially replaced by sclerotic (hyaline) material, which, in most cases, is excess mesangial matrix. Initially the disease is focal and favours the corticomedullary glomeruli. Later the disease progresses to become diffuse and global. Immunofluorescence is entirely negative or shows weak focal mesangial IgM or C3 deposition. Epithelial foot process effacement is seen on EM, with wrinkling of the GBM.

Aetiology and pathology is variable and related to age:

- Primary (most common)—idiopathic disease affecting children and young adults. Focal deposition of IgM is seen at biopsy.
- Secondary—clinical correlation is required to exclude secondary causes in adults, such as HIV, hepatitis B and drug toxicity, including heroin and analgesics.

Focal segmental glomerulosclerosis is a progressive disease which can lead to ESRF, especially if proteinuria is high and the disease is refractory to treatment.

HINTS AND TIPS

GLOMERULONEPHRITIS SYNDROMES

It is useful to remember that the clinical syndromes of glomerulonephritis broadly relate to histological findings:

- Asymptomatic proteinuria and nephrotic syndrome are associated with basement membrane thickening as a result of either structural change or deposition of excessive mesangial matrix, e.g., membranous glomerulonephritis, glomerulosclerosis.
- Asymptomatic haematuria and nephritic syndrome are associated with proliferation of the endothelial or mesangial cells, e.g., diffuse, global glomerulonephritis.
- Mixed nephritic/nephrotic syndrome is associated with combined damage to the basement membrane and cell proliferation, e.g., membranoproliferative glomerulonephritis.

Hereditary glomerulonephritis

Alport syndrome

This syndrome is characterized by the clinical triad of glomerulonephritis, deafness and ocular lesions. The genes affected encode collagen IV chains found in the basement membranes of the kidney, ear and eye.

Inheritance can be:

- X-linked—85% of cases: mutation of the *COL4A5* gene.
- Autosomal recessive—15% of cases: mutation of the *COL4A3/COL4A4* genes.

- Autosomal dominant—rare: mutations in the *COL4A3/COL4A4* genes.

The clinical presentation includes:

- Glomerulonephritis—usually presents as microscopic or gross haematuria ± proteinuria in childhood or early adulthood.
- Deafness—sensorineural.
- Ocular disease—occurs in only severely affected patients and includes anterior lenticonus (conical shape deformity of the lens) and dot and fleck retinopathy.

ESRF occurs in nearly all males with X-linked disease and a variable portion of females. Risk is governed by the type of mutation and the degree of proteinuria, with heavy proteinuria precipitating a more rapid onset of ESRF.

The glomeruli have a variable appearance microscopically, appearing normal or with segmental sclerosis. Immunofluorescent stains are negative for immunoglobulins and complement. In men a loss of collagen IV α5 chain is seen, with a mosaic staining pattern in women in the X-linked form. The characteristic lesion on EM is splitting of the GBM, with irregular areas of thickening and thinning.

Fabry syndrome

Fabry syndrome is a rare X-linked recessive lysosomal storage disorder. Metabolism of glycosphingolipid is impaired owing to deficiency of the enzyme galactosidase A. It is a multisystemic syndrome with progressive disease in the kidney characterized by hypertension and proteinuria. Presentation in males is in childhood or late adulthood. Only 1% of female carriers are affected by renal disease.

Chronic glomerulonephritis

Chronic glomerulonephritis is the third leading cause of chronic kidney disease (CKD) and is the consequence of many diseases affecting the kidney, particularly proliferative types of acute glomerulonephritis. Renal damage accumulates over time, with progression to CKD and ultimately ESRF as glomerular filtration rate (GFR) declines with loss of nephron mass. The rate of progression to ESRF is dependent on cause (Table 13.7).

Macroscopically - affected kidneys are small and contracted with a granularity to the external surface, reflecting fine scarring caused by nephron hyalinization. The pelvicalyceal system is normal, an important distinction from cases of ESRF due to chronic pyelonephritis.

Microscopically - there is hyalinization of the glomeruli, tubular atrophy and interstitial fibrosis. In patients who present for the first time with chronic glomerulonephritis, it is often not possible to ascertain the cause because of diffuse global glomerular destruction.

Transplantation is the only method of fully correcting the loss of renal function in chronic renal failure. Renal replacement therapy (e.g., haemodialysis) maintains low levels of blood purification, but cannot fully replace the metabolic functions of a kidney.

GLOMERULAR LESIONS IN SYSTEMIC DISEASE

Systemic lupus erythematosus

Around half of all patients with SLE will display renal involvement within 5 years of diagnosis. The majority of these cases are glomerular lesions, which may be of numerous histological patterns. Clinically, there is a wide spectrum, from minor abnormalities such as asymptomatic proteinuria, to severe glomerular disease leading to renal failure. Features of nephritic syndrome, nephrotic syndrome or a mixed picture may occur.

The basis of glomerular damage is immune-complex deposition in the basement membrane (leading to basement membrane thickening) or in the mesangium (leading to mesangial expansion).

Patterns of glomerular damage are based on the International Society of Nephrology and Renal Pathology Society classification. Six classes of glomerular disease are described (Table 13.8).

Table 13.7 Symptoms and signs of renal failure

Symptoms	Signs
General malaise	Uraemia
Breathlessness on exertion	Anaemia
Nausea and vomiting	Metabolic bone disease (renal osteodystrophy)
Disordered gastrointestinal motility	Hypertension
Headaches	Acidosis
Pruritus	Neuropathy
Pigmentation	Generalized myopathy
	Endocrine abnormalities

Table 13.8 Simplified International Society of Nephrology and Renal Pathology Society 2003 classification of lupus nephritis

Class	Features
I	Renal glomeruli normal on light microscopy, but immunofluorescence shows mesangial deposits
II	Mesangial disease on light microscopy
III	Focal glomerulonephritis
IV	Diffuse glomerulonephritis
V	Membranous glomerulonephritis
VI	Advanced sclerosis

Immune complexes

The immune complexes of SLE are characterized by the presence of IgG, IgA, IgM, C3 and C1q (known as a 'full-house' pattern). The detection of this pattern and location of immunoglobulins and complement factors is important in distinguishing lupus glomerulonephritis from nonlupus patterns.

Note that, although glomerular lesions are the main abnormalities of renal involvement in SLE, there may also be extraglomerular vascular abnormalities and tubular damage, particularly interstitial nephritis.

Henoch–Schönlein purpura

This immune-complex–mediated systemic vasculitis affects small arteries in the skin, joints, intestine and kidneys (see Chapter 17). Immunofluorescence reveals mesangial IgA deposits.

Significant renal damage occurs in over one-third of cases, ranging from proteinuria, possibly with nephrotic syndrome, to RPGN.

Diabetic glomerulosclerosis

Diabetic glomerular damage causes an increase in the permeability of the GBM, leading initially to asymptomatic proteinuria and then nephrotic syndrome and renal failure.

The pathogenesis of basement membrane changes is probably related to the persistent insulin deficiency and/or hyperglycaemia of the diabetic state. This stimulates biochemical alterations in the composition of the basement membrane, most notably a deficiency of proteoglycans with an excess of collagen IV and fibronectin. Glomerular hypertrophy may occur in response to hyperfiltration (increased glomerular bloodflow in diabetes). Increased glycosylation of proteins contributes to glomerular damage by increasing extracellular matrix.

Histologically, three types of glomerular lesions occur, representing a continuous spectrum of increasing severity:

1. GBM thickening.
2. Diffuse mesangial expansion—excess mesangial matrix formation in an even pattern throughout the glomerulus combined with capillary thickening eventually encroaches on the capillaries (diabetic microangiopathy and proteinuria occur).
3. Nodular glomerulosclerosis (Kimmelstiel–Wilson nodules)—nodular expansion of the mesangium at the tips of the glomerular lobules is characteristic of diabetic nephropathy.

There is progressive hyalinization of glomeruli with obliteration of afferent arterioles, capillary loops and death of individual nephrons. Over a period of years this leads to chronic renal failure.

Prognosis—approximately 10% of all people with diabetes die in renal failure. This rises to 50% if patients develop diabetes in childhood (type 1 diabetes mellitus).

Amyloidosis

This is a condition in which amyloid—extracellular protein fibrils—are deposited in a variety of tissues (see Chapter 17) and is an important cause of nephrotic syndrome in adults.

Amyloid is deposited in the GBM and in the mesangium of the kidney, resulting in membrane thickening and increased mesangial matrix formation. The net result is the development of:

- Proteinuria—membrane thickening leads to an increase in membrane permeability.
- Nephrotic syndrome—increased deposition of amyloid causes progression of protein loss.
- Chronic renal failure—combined effect of amyloid deposition and increased mesangial matrix formation eventually leads to expansion of the mesangium, causing compression of the glomerular capillary system and transition into chronic renal failure.
- Amyloid is also deposited in the walls of intrarenal vessels, particularly the afferent arterioles. Congo red staining highlights amyloid deposition.

Polyarteritis nodosa

Polyarteritis nodosa is a systemic disease characterized by inflammatory necrosis of the walls of small and medium-sized arteries (see Chapter 9). Necrosis of medium-sized arteries causes small infarcts in the kidney; necrosis of arterioles and the glomerular tuft produces glomerular infarction, which is segmental or global.

Granulomatosis with polyangiitis

Previously known as Wegener granulomatosis, this immune-complex–mediated systemic necrotizing vasculitis primarily affects the nose, upper respiratory tract and kidneys (see Chapters 9 and 10). Renal involvement is of variable severity, causing one of the following:

- Focal segmental glomerulonephritis (asymptomatic haematuria or nephritic syndrome).
- Rapidly progressive crescentic glomerulonephritis (rapidly progressive acute renal failure with crescent formation in the glomeruli).

This condition usually responds to immunosuppressive therapy.

DISEASES OF THE TUBULES AND INTERSTITIUM

Acute tubular necrosis

Necrosis of the renal tubular epithelial cells produces acute, but usually reversible, renal failure. It results from ischaemic, metabolic or toxic insults (Table 13.9).

Table 13.9 Causes of acute tubular necrosis

Type	Causes
Ischaemic	Major surgery
	Extensive acute blood loss
	Severe burns
	Haemorrhage
Toxic	Endogenous products: haemoglobinuria and myoglobinuria (e.g., from crush injuries)
	Heavy metals: lead, mercury
	Organic solvents: chloroform, carbon tetrachloride
	Drugs: antibiotics, nonsteroidal anti-inflammatory drugs, ciclosporin
	Others: paraquat, phenol, ethylene glycol, poisonous fungi

The aetiology is:

- Ischaemic (most common)—caused by failure of renal perfusion, typically the result of hypotension and hypovolaemia in shock.
- Toxic—drugs, e.g., nonsteroidal anti-inflammatory drugs (NSAIDs) or, less commonly, heavy metals and organic solvents.

Clinical features are oliguria (less than 500 mL urine output per day) with symptoms of renal failure.

There are three phases to acute tubular necrosis (ATN):

1. Oliguric phase—necrosis of renal tubular cells and interstitial oedema causes tubule blockage by casts and reduced glomerular bloodflow, and therefore filtration.
2. Polyuric phase—tubules slowly open as phagocytic cells begin to remove necrotic material. Polyuria is caused by the temporary loss of the medullary concentration gradient (hypernatraemia in tubules) as regenerated renal tubule cells are initially undifferentiated.
3. Recovery phase—regenerated tubular cells restore renal function.

The morphological features are:

- Ischaemic ATN—kidneys are pale and swollen. Histology reveals flattened, vacuolated epithelial cells along the entire length of the tubules.
- Toxic ATN—kidneys are red and swollen. Histology reveals flattened, vacuolated epithelial cells restricted to proximal tubular cells, those of the distal tubule being spared.

Acute pyelonephritis

This is acute suppurative inflammation of the tubules and interstitium caused by bacterial infection. Susceptibility is highest in childhood, pregnancy, immunosuppression and in the elderly.

Most cases of infection are caused by enterobacteria from the patient's faecal flora (e.g., *Escherichia coli*, *Proteus* and *Klebsiella* species) or by staphylococci from (perineal) skin flora. The organism may enter the kidney by one of two routes: ascending infection from the lower urinary tract (promoted by pregnancy, glycosuria in diabetes, stasis of urine) or via the blood in bacteraemia/septicaemia.

Macroscopically - the condition is characterized by numerous abscesses throughout the kidney:

- Cortical abscesses—small, yellowish-white abscesses, usually spherical, less than 2 mm in diameter and sometimes surrounded by a zone of hyperaemia. They are most prominent on the subcapsular surface.
- Medullary abscesses—yellowish-white linear streaks that converge on the papilla. Pelvicalyceal mucosa is hyperaemic or covered with a fibrinopurulent exudate.

Microscopically - there is focal inflammation with infiltration of tubules by neutrophils, interstitial oedema and tubular necrosis.

Clinical features are classically the triad of fever, rigors and pain in the back.

Acute pyelonephritis may resolve with or without scarring or chronic infection. In severe cases, pyonephrosis (pus-filled kidney associated with obstruction), renal papillary necrosis, perinephric abscess or death may occur. Untreated, infection may spread to cause Gram-negative septicaemia with shock.

Diagnosis is by examination of midstream urine, with culture to determine the causative organism and antibiotic susceptibility.

Chronic pyelonephritis

Chronic inflammation of the tubules and interstitium is associated with nephron destruction and coarse scarring of the kidneys. It may be reflux-associated, often due to ureteric or urethral obstruction.

Reflux-associated chronic pyelonephritis

Reflux of urine from the bladder into the ureter predisposes to recurrent bouts of inflammation. It is most common in childhood and early adult life, with males affected more often than females.

Normally, the ureter enters the bladder obliquely so that contraction of the bladder wall during micturition closes the ureteric orifice. In patients with vesicoureteric reflux, the terminal portion of the ureter is short and orientated at approximately 90 degrees to the mucosal surface. Contraction of the bladder tends to hold the ureteric orifice open, thus facilitating reflux of urine, enabling organisms to gain access to the kidney from the bladder.

Macroscopically - the kidneys have irregular, depressed areas of scarring, 1–2 cm in size, most commonly sited in

Table 13.10 Diseases of the tubules and interstitium

Condition	Features
Toxic and drug-induced	Inflammation of the renal interstitium and tubules (tubulointerstitial nephritis) owing to exposure to toxic agents. There are two types: acute and chronic
Urate nephropathy	Affects a small group of patients with hyperuricaemia
Hypercalcaemia and nephrocalcinosis	Hypercalcaemia causes calcification of the renal parenchyma and tubular damage
Multiple myeloma	Some types of myeloma are characterized by proliferating plasma cells, which produce monoclonal free light chains (Bence Jones proteins), which can be detected in the urine. These cause physical obstruction and damage to the tubules

the renal calyces at the poles of the kidney. Involvement may be either bilateral or unilateral.

Microscopically - kidneys have irregular areas of interstitial fibrosis with chronic inflammatory cell infiltration (chronic interstitial nephritis). Tubules are atrophic or dilated and contain proteinaceous casts. Glomeruli show periglomerular fibrosis and many demonstrate complete hyalinization.

Clinical features are symptoms of urinary tract infection and uraemia.

Diagnosis is by:

- Intravenous urography—reveals reduction in kidney size and focal scarring associated with clubbing of the adjacent calyces.
- Urine culture—for identification of infecting organism.

Prognosis—the course is usually long and punctuated by acute exacerbations.

Other diseases of the tubules and interstitium are shown in Table 13.10.

Tubulointerstitial nephritis

This is inflammation of the tubules and interstitium which is characterized histologically by an eosinophilic infiltrate in the renal parenchyma indicating an allergic component. It is commonly associated with a hypersensitivity picture (usually to NSAIDS, penicillins or sulpha drugs) but may also occur secondary to infection (pyelonephritis).

Renal papillary necrosis

This is coagulative necrosis of the renal papillae secondary to ischaemia of the renal medullary vasculature. It is associated with sickle cell disease, diabetes mellitus, analgesics (especially NSAIDs) and pyelonephritis. Disease ranges from involvement of a single papilla to diffuse bilateral involvement. Consequences include infection, metabolic imbalance and renal failure.

DISEASES OF THE RENAL BLOOD VESSELS

Benign nephrosclerosis

This is the most common form of nephropathy, and is found in approximately 75% of autopsies of people over the age of 60 years. It is characterized by hyaline sclerosis of the arterioles and small arteries of the kidney and is associated with longstanding benign hypertension and worsened by diabetes mellitus. Chronic renal failure is one of the major sequelae.

In longstanding benign hypertension, there is reduced flow of blood to the glomeruli caused by vascular changes that affect:

- Branches of the renal artery—thickening of arterial walls owing to fibroelastic intimal proliferation, internal elastic lamina reduplication and muscular hypertrophy of the media. It results in focal areas of ischaemia with scarring.
- Afferent arterioles—undergo hyalinization (arteriolosclerosis), their muscular walls being replaced by a rigid and inelastic amorphous material.

A progressive reduction in bloodflow to the nephrons leads to chronic ischaemia with slow conversion of individual glomeruli into a mass of hyaline tissue devoid of capillary lumina (Fig. 13.7).

Blood supply to the tubules is also derived from glomerular bloodflow. There is, therefore, eventual ischaemic destruction of the associated tubule, with gradual destruction of individual nephrons over many years.

Clinical features—there are no clinical symptoms initially, although a gradual increase in blood levels of urea and a reduction in GFR occur.

Eventually, critical numbers of nephrons become dysfunctional and the patient develops manifestations of chronic renal failure.

Prognosis—less than 5% of patients with well-developed benign nephrosclerosis die from renal failure. Death in the great majority of cases of benign hypertension occurs from congestive heart failure, coronary insufficiency, cerebrovascular accidents or the development of malignant hypertension.

Malignant nephrosclerosis

Renal disease is associated with malignant, accelerated hypertension. This form of hypertension usually develops in individuals with preexisting benign hypertension.

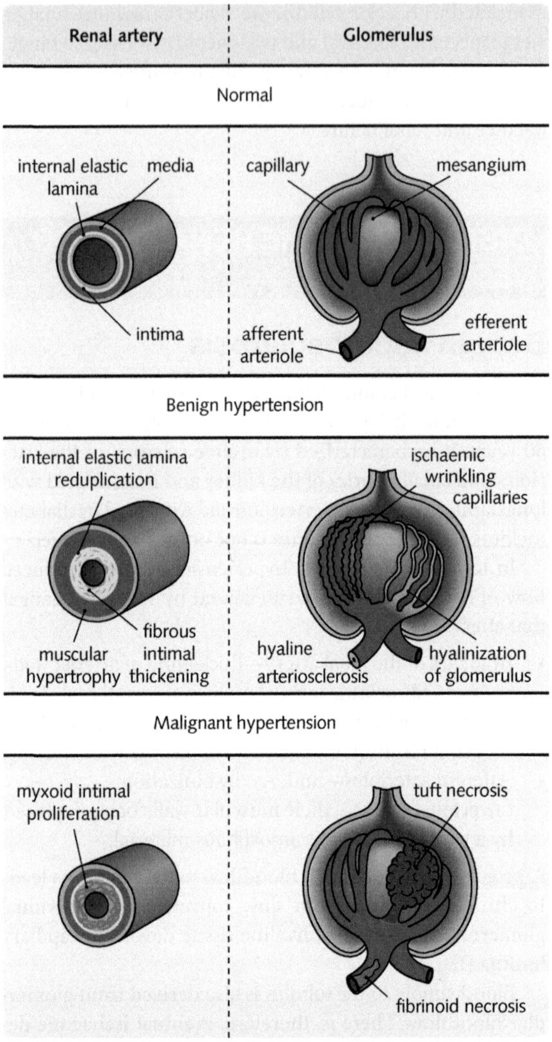

Fig. 13.7 Vascular changes associated with hypertensive renal disease.

Pathogenesis—in accelerated hypertension, the rise in blood pressure is very rapid, causing a pattern of renal damage that differs from that seen in benign hypertension:

- Larger muscular vessels undergo fibroelastic proliferation of the intima, but no muscular hypertrophy. This is stimulated by factors such as platelet-derived growth factor.
- Afferent arterioles frequently undergo fibrinoid necrosis following exposure to the sudden high pressures.
- Glomerular capillary network—segmental fibrinoid necrosis of the glomerular tuft.

The patient develops acute renal failure when sufficient nephrons are rendered nonfunctional. Afferent arteriole necrosis stimulates the renin-angiotensin system, which contributes to ischaemia by promoting intrarenal vasoconstriction.

The renal changes seen in benign and accelerated hypertensive nephrosclerosis are summarized in Fig. 13.7.

Untreated accelerated hypertension causes death from renal failure in 90% of cases, usually with marked rapidity. However, if hypertension is treated adequately, before there is evidence of impairment of renal function by a raised blood urea, then prognosis is good and subsequent renal failure is unusual.

Renal artery stenosis

This narrowing of the renal arteries is typically caused by generalized atherosclerosis but may rarely be caused by arterial fibromuscular dysplasia.

Atherosclerotic occlusion of the renal artery is usually most severe at its origin from the aorta. Renal artery stenosis at this point can lead to two main pathological processes:

1. Chronic ischaemia of the affected kidney—reduction in function of all nephrons on that side produces an end-stage shrunken kidney. However, the contralateral kidney undergoes compensatory hypertrophy so that renal function is largely unaffected.
2. Renovascular hypertension—inadequate perfusion of the kidney may lead to hyper-reninism and subsequent abnormal activation of the renin-angiotensin system (see Chapter 14). This condition is important as it is a rare, but recognized, cause of hypertension which is amenable to surgical correction.

HINTS AND TIPS

RENAL ARTERY STENOSIS

A useful diagnostic pointer for renal artery stenosis is to look for associated features of:

- Vascular disease elsewhere
- Severe or drug-resistant hypertension
- Abdominal bruits (over the kidneys).

Thrombotic microangiopathies

Haemolytic uraemic syndrome

Haemolytic uraemic syndrome (HUS) is a complex syndrome of disordered platelet function that is characterized by the triad of thrombocytopaenia, haemolysis and acute renal failure.

There are three subtypes of HUS: childhood, adult and secondary.

Childhood haemolytic uraemic syndrome

This usually affects children under 4 years of age. Many cases are associated with intestinal infection by verocytotoxin-producing *Escherichia coli* (notably type O157:H7). The immediate prognosis is better than for adult and secondary types, but future risk of renal disease is increased.

Adult haemolytic uraemic syndrome

This is more frequently fatal than childhood HUS and is associated with the following conditions:

- Pregnancy—occurring postpartum, even several months after delivery.
- Oestrogen therapy—contraceptive pills or oestrogen therapy for men with prostatic carcinoma.
- Infections, e.g., typhoid, viruses and shigellosis.
- Chemotherapeutic and immunosuppressive therapy, e.g., ciclosporin.

Secondary haemolytic uraemic syndrome

This occurs as a complication of:

- Malignant hypertension.
- SLE (often as a result of antiphospholipid syndrome).
- Transplant rejection.

Pathogenesis

Platelets adhere to damaged endothelium of small vessels, including the glomerular capillaries, where they undergo aggregation and trigger fibrin deposition. Reduced prostaglandin and nitric oxide production from the damaged endothelium promotes platelet aggregation. Fibrin strands form a tight mesh that deforms erythrocytes as they are forced through the obstruction (microangiopathic haemolysis).

Morphological features within the kidney are:

- Endocapillary proliferation—in response to fibrin and platelet deposition in glomerular tufts.
- Luminal narrowing—arterioles and small arteries show fibrin and erythrocytes in the walls, often with thrombosis which, when extensive, can result in cortical necrosis.

Clinical features and prognosis

Clinical features are:

- Sudden onset of oliguria with haematuria.
- Gastroenteritis.
- Anaemia with schistocytes (fragmented erythrocytes).
- Thrombocytopaenia.
- Hypertension in 50% of cases.

In childhood HUS, symptoms are often preceded by a prodromal episode of diarrhoea or flu-like illness lasting for 5–15 days.

Prognosis depends on the severity of attack, but mortality may be as high as 40%.

Thrombotic thrombocytopaenic purpura

Thrombotic thrombocytopaenic purpura (TTP) and HUS are thought to represent the same disease process, but with a different distribution of thrombotic lesions. In TTP, occlusive plugs lead to widespread ischaemic organ damage, often affecting the brain more than the kidney, resulting in early neurological abnormalities and progressive renal impairment.

Renal infarcts

There are two mechanisms of renal infarction: embolic infarction and diffuse cortical necrosis.

Embolic renal disease

Renal infarcts are usually due to the passage of emboli along renal arterial branches. The most common causes are:

- Embolization of atheromatous material.
- 'Cholesterol emboli'—these are showers of cholesterol microemboli that may occur as a complication of arterial interventions (e.g., arteriography) in those with severe atheromatous disease.
- Mural thromboemboli from the left side of the heart following myocardial infarction.
- Bacterial vegetation from infective endocarditis.

Resultant infarcts may be clinically silent or may result in haematuria and loin pain. Macroscopically, infarcts are pale or white and they have a characteristic wedge shape with the apex directed towards the hilum.

Diffuse cortical necrosis

This rare pattern of renal infarction is associated with conditions resulting in severe hypotension (and therefore global hypoperfusion and ischaemia), the most common of which are hypovolaemic shock, septic shock and eclampsia of pregnancy.

The pathogenesis is uncertain, but diffuse spasm of renal blood vessels is thought to play a major part in precipitating ischaemic damage.

Macroscopically, necrosis is confined to the outer part of the renal cortex, which in the acute stages is pale and focally haemorrhagic.

This condition results in acute renal failure and prognosis depends on the extent of the damage.

NEOPLASTIC DISEASE OF THE KIDNEY

Benign tumours of the kidney

Angiomyolipoma

These mesenchymal tumours of the kidney are composed of blood vessels, smooth muscle and fat in varying proportions, which blend together and have characteristic appearances on imaging. They have no malignant potential but are clinically significant owing to the risk of spontaneous haemorrhage with increasing size, which may be fatal. Discovery is usually incidental, and they can occur sporadically or in association with tuberous sclerosis.

Oncocytoma

Classically, these tumours are usually unencapsulated, solitary lesions with a tan/mahogany brown cut surface and central, white, stellate scar. They are formed of large epithelioid eosinophilic cells with small round nuclei. Presentation is around 50 years of age with flank pain or haematuria; clinically they are difficult to differentiate from renal cell carcinomas so are excised. Oncocytomas are associated with tuberous sclerosis and Birt–Hogg–Dubé syndrome.

Papillary adenoma

These are benign epithelial tumours derived from renal tubular epithelium. Macroscopically, they are discrete yellow/grey nodules, usually <5 mm in diameter, situated in the renal cortex.

Microscopically, cuboidal cells line complex branching papillae resembling renal cell carcinoma. A diagnosis of papillary adenoma versus renal cell carcinoma is arbitrarily governed by size of the lesion: if <1.5 cm then they are regarded as adenomas, if >1.5 cm they are regarded as papillary renal cell carcinomas. In practical terms, all papillary adenomas are treated.

Malignant tumours of the kidney

Renal cell carcinoma

This is an adenocarcinoma derived from the renal tubular epithelium in adults. This tumour accounts for around 85% of primary malignant renal tumours and ~3% of all carcinomas. It is usually seen after the age of 50 years with a higher incidence in males.

Risk factors include tobacco smoking (double the relative risk of nonsmokers), obesity and hypertension. The majority of renal carcinomas are sporadic, but familial forms exist which include von Hippel–Lindau syndrome and hereditary clear cell/papillary carcinomas.

Clinical features: renal cancers can be asymptomatic, allowing them to attain a large size and metastasize before they are identified.

- Common presenting symptoms—haematuria (most reliable), flank pain, flank mass, constitutional symptoms (fever, malaise, weight loss).
- Symptoms from metastatic disease, e.g., bone or brain.
- Paraneoplastic syndromes—hypercalcaemia, hypertension and polycythaemia.

Macroscopically—they are commonly round, expansile, well-circumscribed masses occurring most commonly within the upper pole of the kidney. Size ranges from a few centimetres to over 20 cm. The cut surface shows a yellow/tan variegated appearance with areas of haemorrhage and necrosis. Extension into the renal vein may be seen macroscopically, with growth as a solid core into the inferior vena cava and eventually the right atrium (Fig. 13.8).

Microscopically—the classic microscopic appearance is that of polygonal cells with optically clear cytoplasm (clear cell carcinoma) arranged in nests and trabeculae with centrally located nuclei (Fig. 13.9). Tumour grade is based on

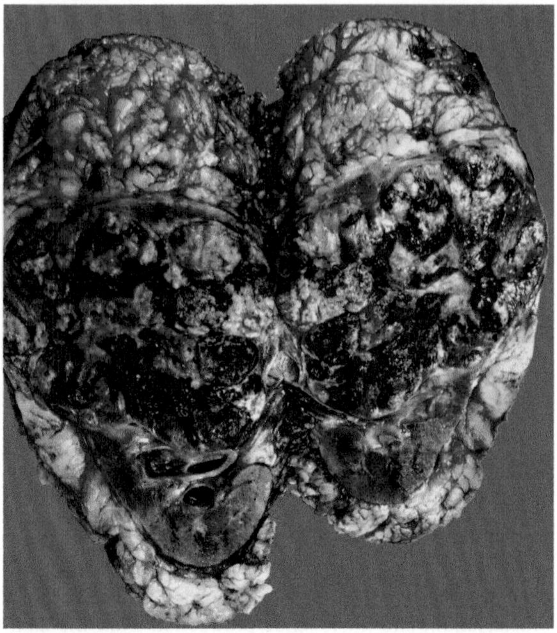

Fig. 13.8 Renal cell carcinoma.
Macroscopic appearance of renal cell carcinoma. Here a kidney has been opened in the coronal plane towards the renal hilum and shows a well-circumscribed fleshy tumour. There is expansile growth with distortion of, but not invasion into, the renal capsule. The cut surface is characteristically variegated in appearance, with haemorrhagic yellow and tan areas. Perinephric fat surrounds the kidney.

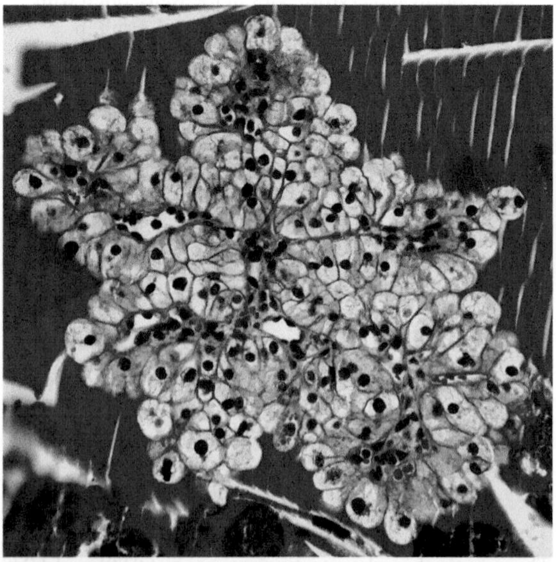

Fig. 13.9 Microscopic appearance of clear cell renal cell carcinoma.
The cells are cuboidal to polygonal in shape, with optically clear cytoplasm and well-demarcated borders. The nuclei are round and centrally located with inconspicuous nucleoli. The appearance of the nuclei determines the grade of renal cell carcinomas.

the appearance of the nuclei from small, round and uniform (low-grade) to pleomorphic and irregular with prominent nucleoli (high-grade). Clear cell carcinoma is the most common type of renal cell carcinoma; however, other types exist (Table 13.11):

- **Papillary renal cell carcinoma:** these account for 10% of renal epithelial neoplasms and macroscopically appear as white masses with haemorrhagic and cystic change. Microscopically, they are formed of papillae lined by eosinophilic or clear cells associated with foamy macrophages at the cores of the papillae.
- **Chromophobe renal cell carcinoma:** these account for 5% of renal epithelial neoplasms. Microscopically, they are composed of polygonal cells with eosinophilic cytoplasm, raisinoid nuclei and a plant-like (thick) cell membranes.

Spread is by:

- Direct invasion—erosion through the renal capsule into perinephric fat, Gerota fascia or the ipsilateral adrenal gland.
- Lymphatic invasion—to paraaortic and other regional lymph nodes.
- Haematogenous—commonly the lungs, bone, brain and adrenal glands. Metastatic deposits are often round and are referred to as 'cannon ball' due to their appearance.

Prognosis depends on the stage at presentation. Stage is governed by the size of the tumour and invasion outside of the kidney into local structures. In early stage disease 5-year survival is around 80%; this drops dramatically to 5% with invasion of the ipsilateral adrenal gland and the presence of metastatic disease.

CLINICAL NOTE

DIFFERENTIAL DIAGNOSIS OF UNILATERAL RENAL ENLARGEMENT

Differential diagnosis of unilateral renal enlargement is:

- Hydronephrosis
- Acute pyelonephritis
- Compensatory hyperplasia
- Tumour
- Renal vein thrombosis.

Table 13.11 Comparison of renal neoplasms

Feature	Oncocytoma	Renal cell carcinoma	Renal pelvis urothelial carcinoma	Wilms tumour (nephroblastoma)
Macroscopic appearance	Parenchymal location. Tan/mahogany brown with a white central stellate scar. Unencapsulated. Well-demarcated. No areas of necrosis	Spherical. Parenchymal location. Expansive and distorts renal capsule. Variegated yellow/tan with haemorrhagic foci	Cream/grey. Exophytic and friable masses. Located in renal pelvis	Malignant. Grey/white. Expansile. Lobulated. Central necrosis and haemorrhage common
Microscopic appearance	Sheets of eosinophilic cells with finely granular cytoplasm. Indistinct cell borders	Polygonal cells usually with optically clear cytoplasm and central nuclei	Majority transitional epithelium and papillary. Squamous carcinoma possible	Triphasic: blastema, stroma and epithelial cells
Percentage of renal tumours	5%	80%	5–10%	85%[a]
Age of onset	55 years	50–70 years	60–70 years	1–4 years
Clinical	Generally benign behaviour. Associations with tuberous sclerosis and Birt-Hogg-Dubé syndrome	Malignant. Propensity to invade the renal vein. Associated with paraneoplastic syndromes. Seen in von Hippel–Lindau syndrome	Malignant. Early presentation due to frank haematuria, hydronephrosis and flank pain due to their location. Synchronous or metachronous tumours of bladder or ureter	Malignant. Pulmonary metastases are usually present at time of diagnosis. 6% of childhood cancers. Abdominal mass commonest presentation. Tumour can exceed the size of the kidney

[a] *Of paediatric renal lesions.*

Urothelial carcinoma of the renal pelvis

This malignant tumour accounts for 10% of all renal tumours. It is derived from the transitional cells of the urothelium and is histologically identical to urothelial carcinoma/transitional cell carcinoma (TCC) of the bladder. Owing to field effect changes to the urothelium, tumours can be multicentric or occur within the contralateral kidney. Fifty percent of patients will develop a subsequent bladder carcinoma.

Renal pelvis urothelial carcinomas are rare before 40 years of age and affect men more often than women. Tumours generally present early with haematuria or obstruction due to their location. Risk factors include smoking, exposure to petrochemicals, aniline dyes, coal/coke and chronic pyelonephritis with renal calculi.

Wilms tumour (nephroblastoma)

This is the fourth commonest childhood malignancy and the most common childhood urological malignancy, occurring between the ages of 1 and 4 years. Ninety percent of cases arise before 6 years of age; males and females are equally affected. Most cases are sporadic; however, some form part of syndromic states, e.g., WAGR (Wilms tumour, aniridia, genitourinary abnormalities, retardation), Denys–Drash and Beckwith–Wiedemann syndromes.

At least three different types of genes are important in Wilms tumour. The most characteristic of these is *WT1* (chromosome 11), which has dual roles in nephrogenesis and as a tumour suppressor gene. Other genes include *WT2* and *P53*.

Clinical presentation—the majority present with asymptomatic large abdominal masses, which may be accompanied by abdominal pain, haematuria and hypertension. Metachronous or synchronous tumours occur in up to 10% of cases.

Macroscopically—Wilms tumours occur as large solitary masses which extensively replace the renal parenchyma. The cut surface is a homogeneous tan/grey, soft, fleshy mass with a lobular appearance. Necrosis, haemorrhage and cysts may also be seen. Extension beyond the renal capsule into perinephric fat and base of mesentery is frequent. Lung metastasis occurs early and is identified in a high proportion of cases at the time of diagnosis.

Microscopically—classically the tumour is triphasic and is composed of:

1. Blastemal tissue—small round blue cells which resemble developing fetal metanephric tissue.
2. Epithelial elements - usually tubule formation.
3. Stroma—fibroblast-like, myxoid or heterologous elements such as cartilage and skeletal muscle.

Skeletal muscle cells may be present, as well other heterologous elements such as cartilage and smooth muscle. It is important to identify areas showing anaplasia microscopically, as these are poor prognostic indicators regardless of stage.

Prognosis is related to tumour stage at diagnosis; however, the 5-year survival rate has increased to 80%.

DISORDERS OF THE URINARY TRACT

Congenital abnormalities of the urinary tract

Ureteric abnormalities

These occur in up to 3% of people, although they have no clinical significance in most cases.

Double and bifid ureters

These are the most common ureteric abnormality and often occur in association with duplication of the renal pelvis. They may be associated with vesicoureteric reflux and are predisposed to recurrent infections.

Ureteropelvic junction obstruction

This is the most common cause of hydronephrosis in children. It is usually caused by a stricture that may be either intrinsic (within the wall of the ureter) or extrinsic (associated with external factors, e.g., an aberrant vessel). This ureteric obstruction provides a barrier to the conduction of a wave of contraction.

Bladder abnormalities

Diverticula

Congenital diverticula are rare and are more often acquired as a result of bladder outlet obstruction. Symptoms are due to urinary stasis and the resultant infection.

Urethral abnormalities

Hypospadias

The urethra opens on to the underside of the penis, either on the glans (glandular hypospadias), at the junction of the glans with the shaft (coronal hypospadias) or on the shaft itself (penile hypospadias).

Epispadias

The urethra opens on to the dorsal (upper) surface of the penis. All varieties can be corrected surgically.

Posterior urethral valves

This condition in males is caused by congenital formation of posterior urethral membranes causing urethral obstruction of varying degrees of severity. Bladder muscle hypertrophy may occur secondarily. Patients are predisposed to infection, incontinence and renal failure.

Urinary tract obstruction

This is obstruction of urine at any level within the urinary tract after leaving the kidney. Obstruction may be caused by either a structural lesion (majority) or congenital neuromuscular defects that prevent contraction waves, and thus the flow of urine.

Structural lesions can be classified into:

- Intrinsic lesions—within the urinary tract, e.g., stones, caseous or necrotic debris, fibrosis (following trauma or infection) or tumour.
- Extrinsic lesions—causing pressure from outside the urinary tract, e.g., tumours of the rectum, prostate, uterus or ovaries, aberrant renal arteries, retroperitoneal fibrosis and pregnancy.

Causes vary according to the site of the obstruction (Table 13.12).

Pathogenesis—obstruction at any point in the urinary tract causes increased pressure proximal to the blockage, resulting in dilatation of proximal structures, e.g., renal pelvis, calyces, ureter:

- Obstruction at the pelviureteric junction → hydronephrosis.
- Obstruction of the ureter → hydroureter with subsequent development of hydronephrosis.
- Obstruction of the bladder neck or urethra → bladder distension with hypertrophy of its muscle (seen on cystoscopic examination as trabeculation) with subsequent development of hydroureter and hydronephrosis.

Hydronephrosis

Hydronephrosis (renal distension by urine) may be:

- Unilateral—caused by unilateral obstruction anywhere above the bladder. It is typically detected late, because renal function is maintained by the nonobstructed kidney. Renal parenchyma becomes severely atrophic and renal function is permanently impaired (end-stage hydronephrosis).
- Bilateral—caused by obstruction at the level of the bladder or urethra. Obstruction is typically detected at an earlier stage, as renal failure develops before severe atrophy of both kidneys.

In both forms, urinary tract obstruction predisposes to cystitis and pyelonephritis, as well as stone formation.

Table 13.12 Sites of urinary tract obstruction

Site	Cause
Renal pelvis	Calculi, tumours
Pelviureteric junction[a]	Stricture, calculi, extrinsic compression
Ureter	Calculi, extrinsic compression (pregnancy, tumour, fibrosis)
Bladder neck[a]	Tumour, calculi
Urethra[a]	Prostatic hyperplasia or carcinoma, urethral valves, urethral stricture

[a] *Indicates commonest sites.*

Effects of hydronephrosis

The net result of hydronephrosis is that fluid entering the collecting ducts cannot empty into the renal pelvis and intrarenal resorption of fluid occurs.

If the obstruction is removed at this stage, then renal function returns to normal. However, persistence of obstruction leads to atrophy of the renal tubules and promotes interstitial inflammation, which leads to glomerular hyalinization and fibrosis.

Clinical features depend on the cause and site of the lesion. Obstruction proximal to the bladder will either cause renal colic characterized by acute onset of pain, or hydronephrosis characterized by dull flank pain. The clinical feature of obstruction below the bladder is difficulty in micturition. This occasionally results in bladder distension ± progression to bilateral hydronephrosis.

Superimposed infection causes malaise, fever, dysuria, haematuria and sometimes septicaemia. Management is by removal of the obstruction and treatment of the infection.

Urolithiasis (urinary calculi)

This is the formation of stones in the urinary tract. It affects 1%–5% of the population in the UK and onset is typically after 30 years of age, with males affected more often than females.

Stones can form anywhere in the urinary tract, but the most common site is within the renal pelvis.

Composition of stones:

- Calcium oxalate (70%–75%).
- Triple phosphates/struvite (15%)—magnesium ammonium phosphate stones.
- Uric acid (5–10%).
- Cysteine (2%).

> **HINTS AND TIPS**
>
> **RADIOPAQUE STONES**
>
> Ninety percent of urinary calculi are radioopaque compared with 10% of gallstones and therefore can be appreciated on plain abdominal X-rays. Uric acid stones are radiolucent.

Aetiology is:

- Acquired—as a result of obstruction, persistent infection (nitrogen-splitting bacteria like *Proteus* spp. produce byproducts which increase stone formation), or reduced urine volume.
- Inherited—primary metabolic disturbances, e.g., cystinuria.

The mechanism of stone formation is not well understood, but it is thought to involve an excess of solute in the urine (owing to either a primary increase in metabolite or to stasis) or reduced solubility of solute in the urine (owing to persistently abnormal urinary pH).

Calculi vary greatly in size, from sand-like particles to large round stones, or even staghorn calculi, which take the shape of the renal pelvis and calyceal system (Fig. 13.10).

The condition may present with:

- Renal colic (often with nausea and vomiting)—caused by the passage of small stones along the ureter.
- Dull ache in the loins—due to the presence of stones in the kidney.
- Recurrent and intractable urinary tract infection, haematuria or renal failure.

Cytological assessment of urine containing crystals can suggest the presence of urinary calculi (Fig. 13.11). Occasionally, the condition is asymptomatic and discovered only during radiological examination for another disease.

HINTS AND TIPS

LOCATION OF RENAL CALCULI

Calculi are commonly found in order of frequency in the:

- Kidney
- Ureter
- Ureteropelvic junction
- Ureterovesical junction
- Bladder

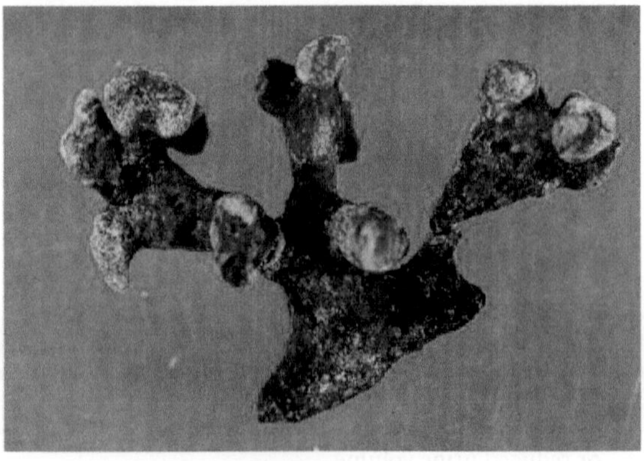

Fig. 13.10 Staghorn calculus.
Macroscopic image of a staghorn calculus. The calculus has assumed the shape of the pelvicalyceal system.

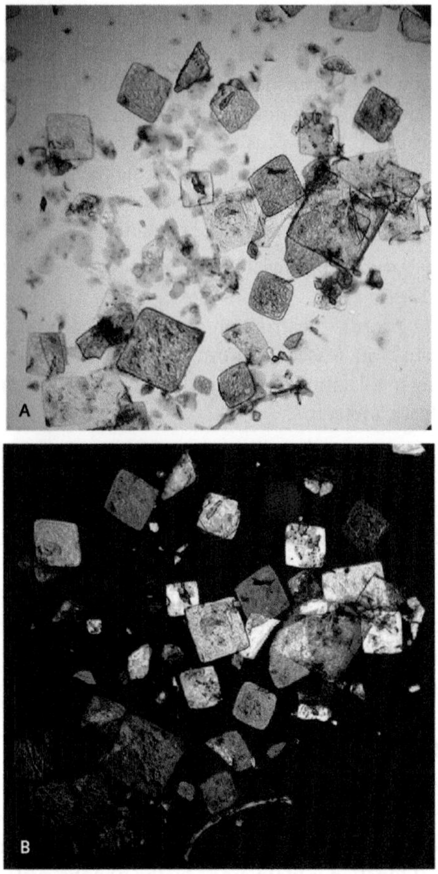

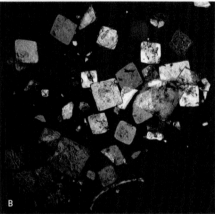

Fig. 13.11 Urinary crystals.
(A) Microscopic image of urine cytology showing urinary crystals. (B) Microscopic image of the same urinary crystals under polarized light, demonstrating their birefringent nature.

Inflammation and infection of the urinary tract

Acute pyelonephritis

Acute pyelonephritis is discussed above.

Cystitis

This is inflammation of the bladder and it is extremely common. Females are affected more often than males because they have a shorter urethra (i.e., shorter distance for bacteria to travel).

Aetiology

The condition is most commonly due to infection, but it is occasionally caused by physical agents, e.g., radiation or mechanical irritants. Infective causes are:

- Bacterial (most common)—usually Gram-negative coliform bacilli, e.g., *Escherichia coli* and *Proteus* species, but *Streptococcus faecalis*, *Pseudomonas aeruginosa* and staphylococci are also common.

- Viral—adenovirus may cause haemorrhagic cystitis in children, polyomavirus (BK virus) in those who are immunosuppressed.
- Parasitic—*Schistosoma haematobium*, which is common in Africa.
- Fungal—*Candida*.
- Tuberculosis—usually secondary to renal mycobacterial disease.
- Therapy-related—Bacillus Calmette-Guérin (BCG) therapy (used in the treatment of bladder cancer) or radiation-induced.

Risk factors are:

- Urinary retention—due to obstruction, bladder paralysis, bladder diverticula, calculi, foreign bodies (e.g., urinary catheters), tumours or uterine prolapse.
- Infection of adjacent structures, e.g., prostatitis, urethritis and diverticular disease of the colon.
- Diabetes mellitus—glycosuria favours infection.
- Pregnancy.
- Trauma, e.g., catheterization.

Infection normally ascends from the urethra but may descend from the kidney in some cases of renal infection (e.g., renal tuberculosis). Direct spread from adjacent organs (e.g., colonic diverticulitis) may occur, but haematogenous and lymphatic spread are rare.

Macroscopically, there is acute inflammation, with oedema, erythema and later ulceration of bladder mucosa.

Microscopically, there is infiltration of mucosa with acute inflammatory cells.

Clinical features—the classic triad of increased urinary frequency, lower abdominal pain and dysuria are common. Systemic effects of inflammation (e.g., fever) may also occur.

Sequelae:

- Resolution (common).
- Chronicity if the underlying cause is untreatable.
- Development of pyelonephritis and associated complications.

> **HINTS AND TIPS**
>
> **HAEMORRHAGIC CYSTITIS**
>
> Haemorrhagic cystitis may be drug-induced. The commonest causative agent is cyclophosphamide.

Ureteritis

This is inflammation of the ureter and is usually due to an ascending urinary tract infection.

Causative organisms are the same as for cystitis; an acute bacterial cystitis may lead to an ascending ureteritis.

Complications—organisms may gain access to the renal parenchyma to produce acute pyelonephritis, with the formation of abscesses in the renal medulla and cortex.

NEOPLASTIC DISEASE OF THE URINARY TRACT

Bladder metaplasia

Glandular metaplasia (cystitis cystica et glandularis)

This is cystic dilatation or glandular metaplasia of von Brunn nests in the lamina propria. Some show metaplasia from transitional epithelium to an intestinal variant of cystitis glandularis, lined by colonic, mucin-secreting epithelium. It is quite common and often seen in normal bladder.

Adenomatous metaplasia (nephrogenic adenoma)

This benign condition is characterized by either metaplasia of the urothelium to resemble collecting tubules of the kidney or shedding of renal tubular cells into the urothelium. It is associated with trauma, stones and genitourinary surgery.

Squamous metaplasia

There are two types:

1. Keratinizing squamous metaplasia (leucoplakia)—the bladder mucosa develops white plaques, which are often secondary to chronic irritation, e.g., calculi. A proportion (~20%) progress to squamous cell carcinoma of the bladder.
2. Nonkeratinizing squamous metaplasia (vaginal metaplasia)—white plaques are seen on the trigone. This only occurs in women, is associated with oestrogen production and has no pathological significance.

Neoplasms of the bladder

Benign

Urothelial papilloma

These are benign tumours of the bladder that appear as frond-like exophytic growths of normal urothelium attached to the mucosa by a fibrovascular stalk. They may also have an endophytic growth pattern whereby they grow downwards into the lamina propria (inverted papilloma).

Malignant

Carcinoma in situ

Carcinoma in situ (CIS) is a flat high-grade malignancy of the surface urothelium. Cystoscopy shows red patches on the mucosal surface caused by underlying telangiectatic blood vessels. It may become invasive. Approximately half of cases of CIS have a synchronous invasive urothelial carcinoma.

Urothelial carcinoma

Previously known as transitional cell carcinoma (TCC), these are tumours of the urothelium. They are the tenth most common cancer in the UK and account for 3% of all cancer deaths. They are most commonly found in those aged 60–70 years, with males affected more often than females by a factor of 3:1. They are strongly linked to cigarette smoking.

Aetiology:

- Chemicals—exposure to environmental agents excreted in high concentrations in the urine. Known carcinogens are associated with cigarette smoking, aniline dyes and the rubber industry, to name a few.
- Leucoplakia (see above)—associated with bladder stones.
- Bladder diverticula.

Most tumours are at the base of trigone and around the ureteric orifices.

Morphological types:

- Papillary (most common)—warty masses projecting into the lumen, often with little or no invasion of the bladder wall. Only a small percentage evolve into invasive carcinoma.
- Solid—tumours grow directly into the bladder wall and are often ulcerated or encrusted. Most are invasive from the outset.
- Mixed papillary and solid.

> **COMMON PITFALLS**
>
> **UROTHELIAL CARCINOMAS**
>
> The majority of urothelial cancers are caused by exposure to environmental agents. Therefore, bladder tumours are often multifocal and may be found in conjunction with urothelial tumours at other sites of the lower urinary tract, e.g., renal pelvis, ureters or urethra.

Other tumours of the bladder

Only a small proportion of bladder cancers are of squamous origin (squamous cell carcinoma). They are most often associated with schistosomiasis infection. Adenocarcinomas and mesenchymal tumours are rare. Secondary tumours usually occur following direct invasion from the cervix, prostate or rectum.

Grading and staging of bladder carcinomas

The degree of differentiation (grade) and extent of spread (stage) are important indicators for prognosis.

Formerly, papillary urothelial carcinomas were graded as I–III (well–poorly differentiated). Currently, tumours are classified as low grade or high grade based on the degree of nuclear atypia and mitoses present. Tumour, node, metastasis (TNM) staging follows the same principles as other cancers (Fig. 13.12). Tumours that invade through the muscularis propria are treated more aggressively than superficial tumours.

Spread is as follows:

- Local—to pelvic structures.
- Lymphatic—to iliac and paraaortic lymph nodes.
- Haematogenous—to liver and lung.

Clinically, the disease classically presents with painless haematuria, but symptoms of recurrent urinary tract infections may occur. Rarely, it may present with hydronephrosis (from ureteric obstruction), pneumaturia from a vesicocolic fistula or urinary incontinence from vesicovaginal fistula.

Treatment usually involves transurethral resection of bladder tumours, with the potential for intravesical chemotherapy (BCG immunotherapy) in multifocal tumours. Radical cystectomy may be considered for patients with invasive disease.

Prognosis depends on the histological type of the tumour and extent of spread. Papillary noninvasive tumours have an excellent prognosis, whereas solid, invasive, urothelial tumours have an overall 5-year survival rate of only 35%.

pTa	Noninvasive papillary carcinoma
pTis	Carcinoma in situ (CIS)
pT1	Tumour invades lamina propria
pT2	Tumour invades muscularis propria
pT3	Tumour invades perivesical tissue
pT4	Tumour invades adjacent structures

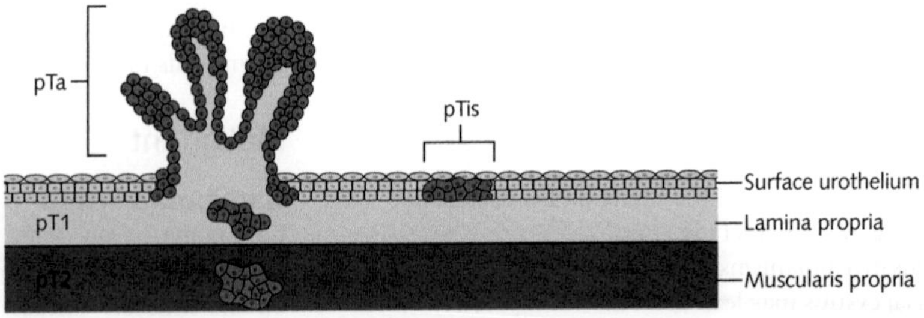

Fig. 13.12 Staging of bladder cancer.
Diagram showing the early stages of bladder cancer and key summarizing the tumour, node, metastasis (TNM) staging system.

COMMON PITFALLS

pTa vs pTis

Papillary carcinoma (pTa tumours) and carcinoma in situ (pTis tumours) are non-invasive and are limited to the surface urothelium. Carcinoma in situ is classified as a high-grade lesion and therefore has a worse prognosis compared with pTa tumours.

Chapter Summary

- Cystic renal diseases can be congenital, hereditary or acquired, and range from solitary cysts to multiple cysts completely replacing the parenchyma.
- Glomerular disease can affect any constituent of the glomerulus: capillary endothelial cells, mesangial cells, glomerular basement membrane or podocytes (epithelial cells).
- Glomerular disease can be categorised by the clinical syndrome produced, e.g., nephrotic syndrome, nephritic syndrome, asymptomatic haematuria.
- The most common cause of nephrotic syndrome in adults is focal segmental glomerulosclerosis.
- The most common cause of nephrotic syndrome in children is minimal change disease.
- There are six classes of lupus nephritis, a condition characterized by a 'full house' of immune complex deposits.
- Kimmelstiel–Wilson nodules are pathognomonic of diabetic glomerulosclerosis.
- Like diabetes mellitus, amyloidosis causes nephrotic syndrome and nodular deposits in glomeruli. Unlike diabetes mellitus, these stain with Congo red.
- Ischaemia is the commonest cause of acute tubular necrosis.
- Nephrosclerosis is characterized by fibromuscular hypertrophy and hyalinization of afferent arterioles.
- Haemolytic uraemic syndrome is characterized by the triad of haemolysis, thrombocytopaenia and acute renal failure.
- Benign renal tumours include angiomyolipoma, papillary adenoma and oncocytoma.
- Malignant renal tumours include clear cell renal cell carcinoma, papillary renal cell carcinoma, chromophobe carcinoma, Wilms tumour and urothelial carcinoma of the renal pelvis.
- Ninety percent of urinary tract stones are radioopaque.
- Acute pyelonephritis is commonly associated with Gram-negative bacterial infection (e.g., *Escherichia coli* or *Proteus* spp.).
- Carcinoma in situ of the bladder is always a high-grade lesion.
- Urothelial carcinoma is the commonest malignancy of the bladder and is associated with smoking and aniline dyes.
- Squamous cell carcinoma of the bladder is associated with schistosomiasis infection.

Pathology of the endocrine system 14

DISORDERS OF THE PITUITARY

The pituitary (hypophysis) is a small (500–1000 mg), bean-shaped gland lying within a recess of the sphenoid bone called the sella turcica. The pituitary is composed of two parts:

1. Anterior lobe (adenohypophysis): derived from the buccal cavity: synthesizes and secretes various hormones that mostly act on other endocrine glands (Fig. 14.1).
2. Posterior lobe (neurohypophysis): a down growth of tissue from the hypothalamus that remains in direct continuity with it via the pituitary stalk. It stores and secretes two hormones synthesized in the hypothalamus: antidiuretic hormone (ADH; vasopressin) and oxytocin.

The hypothalamus controls hormonal secretion of the pituitary:

- directly via neuroendocrine cells—posterior pituitary;
- indirectly via the secretion of releasing hormones into the median eminence—anterior pituitary.

Secretion of pituitary hormones is regulated by neural and chemical stimuli from the hypothalamus, diseases of which cause secondary abnormalities in pituitary function.

This cooperation between the nervous system and endocrine apparatus is referred to as neuroendocrine signalling. Neuroendocrine cells are defined as those that release a hormone in response to a neural stimulus. Important examples include:

- neurones of the supra-optic nucleus (projecting into the posterior pituitary), which release ADH or oxytocin;
- chromaffin cells of the adrenal medulla, which release adrenaline.

Figure 14.2 exemplifies the neuroendocrine signalling showing the integration of signals between the

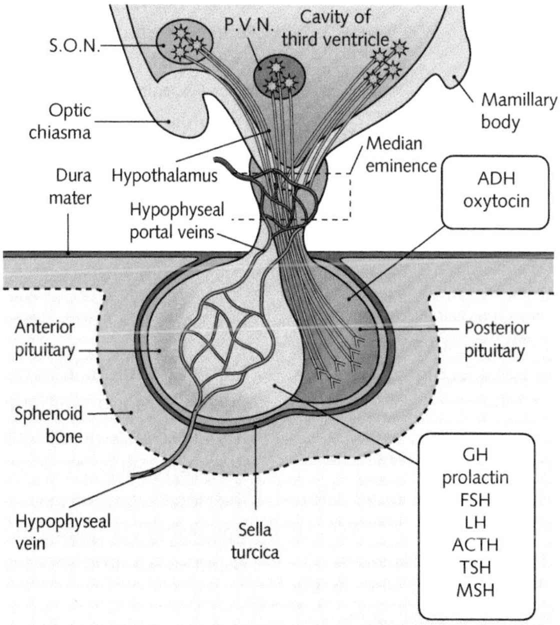

Fig. 14.1 Pituitary gland. Pituitary gland in relation to the hypothalamus. ***Anterior pituitary***: hormones are produced within the hypothalamic nuclei, whose terminal branches end within the median eminence. Here the hormones gain access to the hypothalamic–hypophyseal portal system and travel to the anterior pituitary, causing anterior pituitary hormone release. ***Posterior pituitary:*** hormones are produced within the cell bodies of the neurons located in the supra-optic nuclei (SON) and paraventricular nuclei (PVN) of the hypothalamus. Their terminal branches end directly within the capillaries of the posterior pituitary, i.e., not via the median eminence. *ACTH*, Adrenocorticotrophic hormone; *ADH*, antidiuretic hormone; *FSH*, follicular-stimulating hormone; *GH*, growth hormone; *LH*, luteinizing hormone; *MSH*, melanocyte-stimulating hormone; *TSH*, thyroid-stimulating hormone.

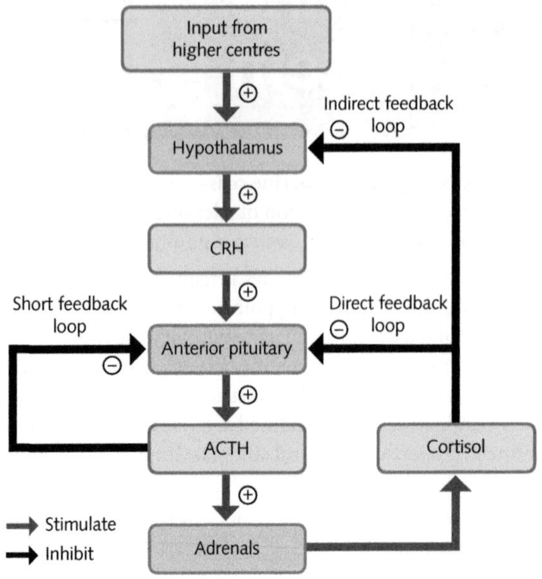

Fig. 14.2 Negative feedback loops. Schematic representation of the integration between the higher brain centres, hypothalamus, pituitary and target organ signalling. The example is for cortisol, highlighting the negative feedback loops that control hormone release at each level. Similar feedback loops exist for the other pituitary hormones. *ACTH*, Adrenocorticotrophic hormone; *CRH*, corticotropin-releasing hormone. (Redrawn with permission from Dr P. Xiu.)

hypothalamus, pituitary and adrenal gland in the release and regulation of adrenal hormones.

The anterior pituitary: hyperpituitarism

Hyperpituitarism is defined as excessive secretion of one or more of the pituitary hormones. The most common cause is a functioning (hormone-secreting) adenoma. Adenomas occur most commonly in young adults.

Anterior lobe adenomas

Anterior lobe adenomas comprise about 13% of all intracranial tumours (posterior lobe adenomas do not occur). These tumours do not usually metastasize, but cause significant morbidity because of their location and excess hormone secretion. They are classified as: microadenomas (<10 mm) and macroadenomas (>10 mm) regardless of their functional status.

Microscopically they are composed of a monomorphic population of cells with finely granular cytoplasm, round to oval nuclei with stippled chromatin and inconspicuous nucleoli. Mitoses are not a feature and architecturally pseudoacini can be present.

Effects of pituitary adenomas

Effects can be physical, i.e., the consequences of a space-occupying lesion (compression of adjacent structures) or disturbances in endocrine function. Compression can affect:

- the remainder of the pituitary → hypopituitarism;
- optic chiasm → visual field defects, notably bitemporal hemianopia;
- brain (large tumours) → distortion of the midbrain obstructing cerebrospinal fluid flow causing raised intracranial pressure and hydrocephalus;
- dura → headaches;
- cavernous sinus → cranial nerve III, IV or VI palsies.

The endocrine effects depend on which hormone is being excessively secreted (see later).

Types of functioning adenomas

Functioning adenomas may produce any of the anterior lobe (adenohypophyseal) hormones, but the majority produce prolactin (prolactinomas, lactotroph adenomas), growth hormone (GH) (somatotroph adenomas) or adrenocorticotrophic hormone (ACTH) (corticotroph adenomas). Table 14.1 gives an overview of consequences of excess or inadequate hormone secretion.

Prolactinomas

These account for 60%–75% of all pituitary adenomas occurring between 20–60 years of age, most commonly in women. Serum prolactin levels are abnormally elevated (>6000 mU/L) with associated amenorrhea and galactorrhoea (women), and ejaculatory failure or impotence (men). Mild prolactin increases can be seen with any large adenomas due to the 'stalk effect' (see box below). Unlike other anterior lobe hormones, prolactin secretion is regulated by tonic inhibition from the hypothalamus through dopamine.

> **COMMON PITFALLS**
>
> **PROLACTIN AND THE STALK EFFECT**
>
> Large adenomas can compress the pituitary stalk and thus reduce the amount of dopamine reaching the anterior pituitary via the hypothalamic–hypophyseal portal system. As prolactin is under the negative control of dopamine, reduced dopamine concentrations result in the release of suppression and prolactin levels rise.

Somatotroph adenoma

This is the second commonest pituitary tumour (5%), resulting in hypersecretion of growth hormone (GH), the effects of which depend on the developmental stage of the individual (Fig. 14.3) resulting in either giagantism or acromegaly.

Table 14.1 Clinical features of hyperpituitarism (adenomas) and hypopituitarism

Pituitary hormone	Target organ hormone	Hormone excess	Hormone deficiency
Corticotrophin	Cortisol	Cushing disease	Features of primary hypoadrenalism but with decreased pigmentation (rather than an increase)
Thyrotropin	Thyroxine	Thyrotoxicosis	Hypothyroidism
Gonadotrophins	LSH and FSH	Precocious puberty	Prepubertal: • failure to enter puberty • undescended testes • eunuchoidism Postpubertal: • infertility • amenorrhoea • oligospermia • progressive loss of secondary sex characteristics (hypogonadism)
Somatotropin	Growth hormone	Children: gigantism Adults: acromegaly	Children: failure of longitudinal growth Adults: tendency to hypoglycaemia
Prolactin	None	Hyperprolactinaemia Galactorrhoea Infertility Gynaecomastia	Inadequate lactation

ACTH, Adrenocorticotrophic hormone; FSH, follicle-stimulating hormone; GH, growth hormone; LH, luteinizing hormone; TSH, thyroid-stimulating hormone.

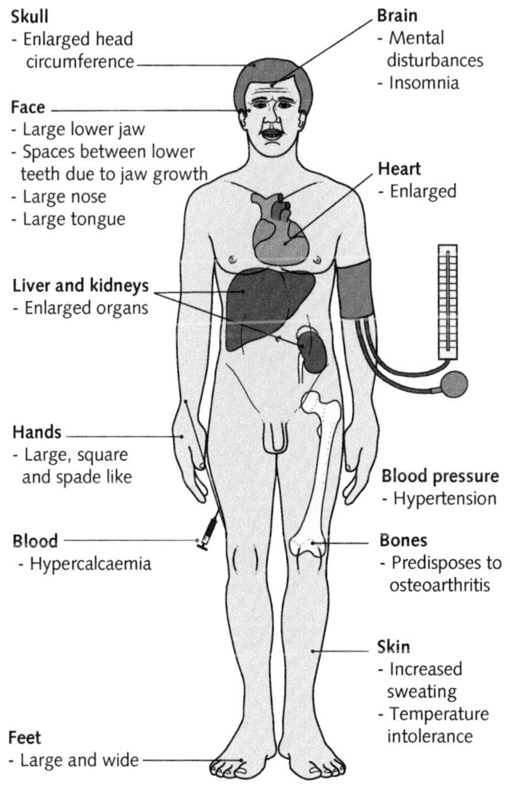

Fig. 14.3 Features of acromegaly.

- Growth plates are open (preepiphyseal union—prepubertal): leads to gigantism, i.e., excessive vertical growth in a regular and initially well-proportioned manner.
- Growth plates are closed (postepiphyseal union—adults): leads to acromegaly, which is characterized by enlargement of the hands, feet and head. Presentation may also be with secondary diabetes or cardiovascular disease due to the effects of IGF-1, which is secreted by the liver when GH levels are high. The average age of diagnosis is 40 years.

HINTS AND TIPS

ACROMEGALY

In acromegaly it is often difficult for the patient to appreciate small changes over time. Helpful objective indicators of soft tissue growth are old photographs of the patient and enquiry as to whether their ring size, shoe size or glove size has increased.

Corticotrophin adenoma

Overproduction of ACTH by a pituitary adenoma causes adrenal hyperplasia, resulting in the excessive secretion of glucocorticoids causing Cushing disease, the effects of which are described later (Fig. 14.11).

Other functioning adenomas

Other functional secreting adenomas, e.g., thyroid-stimulating hormone (TSH), gonadotrophs (luteinizing hormone (LH) and follicle-stimulating hormone (FSH)), are extremely rare.

The anterior pituitary: hypopituitarism

This is insufficient production and secretion of pituitary hormones with a prevalence of ~4.2/100,000 per year. Hormones are lost in a characteristic order; however, it is rare for all hormones to be lost.

1. Gonadotrophins
2. GHs
3. Thyrotropin
4. Corticotrophin
5. Prolactin—uncommon.

The clinical features depend on the patient's age, type of hormone deficiency and rate of onset.

Hypopituitarism can be caused by either hypothalamic lesions or pituitary lesions resulting in a lack of functioning tissue. The most common cause is a pituitary adenoma.

Hypothalamic lesions:

- *Idiopathic deficiency:* one or more of the releasing hormones, e.g., gonadotrophin-releasing hormone (GnRH; Kallmann syndrome—genetic isolated gonadotrophin deficiency with anosmia, low testosterone and failure to go through puberty), growth hormone-releasing hormone (GHRH) or, more rarely, thyrotropin-releasing hormone (TRH) or corticotrophin-releasing hormone (CRH).
- *Infarction.*
- *Inflammation:* e.g., sarcoidosis, tuberculous meningitis.
- *Suprasellar tumours:* e.g., craniopharyngioma or, more rarely, pinealoma, teratoma or a metastatic disease, which can grow and impinge on the pituitary.
- *Malnutrition.*

Pituitary lesions:

- *Idiopathic deficiency*: one or more of the pituitary hormones.
- *Infection*: tuberculosis, syphilis, meningitis.
- *Granulomatous diseases*: sarcoidosis, histiocytosis, granulomatosis with polyangiitis.
- *Pituitary apoplexy*: infarction or haemorrhage of the pituitary gland usually occurring in the presence of an adenoma. Presents with sudden onset severe headache, visual disturbance and altered mental state.
- *Sheehan syndrome*: ischaemic necrosis of the anterior pituitary due to hypotensive shock secondary to obstetric haemorrhage.
- *Empty sella syndrome*: an enlarged, empty sella turcica. This may be a primary anatomical variant whereby the arachnoid herniates into the sella effacing the pituitary against bone, or it may follow spontaneous infarction, surgery, or radiotherapy.
- *Trauma:* either direct to the pituitary or the stalk. Includes surgery, radiotherapy and basal skull fractures.

The posterior pituitary

Diseases of the posterior pituitary are much less common than those of the anterior pituitary and are usually the result of damage to the hypothalamus by infarction or tumour invasion. Posterior pituitary diseases typically cause disorders of inappropriate ADH secretion and diabetes insipidus. There are no known effects of abnormal oxytocin secretion.

Diabetes insipidus

Diabetes insipidus (DI) is a rare condition characterized by the persistent excretion of excessive quantities of dilute urine (polyuria) and constant thirst (polydipsia).

There are two types:

1. Cranial DI—caused by the failure of ADH production.
2. Nephrogenic DI—distal tubules of the kidney are refractory to the water resorptive action of ADH.

Clinical features—irrespective of aetiology, in DI reabsorption of water from the glomerular filtrate in the renal collecting ducts does not occur, resulting in polyuria (up to 20 L per day is possible) and high risk of body water depletion. DI is potentially lethal without appropriate therapy.

Syndrome of inappropriate antidiuretic hormone secretion

ADH (vasopressin) is normally secreted in response to increased plasma osmolality and/or reduced arterial blood pressure. In the syndrome of inappropriate antidiuretic hormone secretion (SIADH) the plasma concentration of ADH is inappropriate for the plasma osmolality. Excess ADH results in water retention (decreased serum osmolality), inappropriate urine concentration (increased urine osmolality) and hyponatraemia in a euvolaemic patient. Hyponatraemia in this situation is the result of haemodilution, not sodium deficiency.

Symptoms are related to the severity of the hyponatraemia with weakness, reduced mental function and, in severe cases, cerebral oedema, impaired consciousness, coma and death. Body oedema is not usually seen as free water, rather it is evenly distributed to all body compartments. Box 14.1 outlines the causes of SIADH.

Craniopharyngioma

A tumour most commonly found in children, occurring above the sella turcica arising from remnants of Rathke pouch. It accounts for 5%–10% of all childhood tumours, and 1%–3% of adult intracranial tumours. Presentation is

BOX 14.1 CAUSES OF SIADH

The causes, and therefore differential diagnosis, of syndrome of inappropriate antidiuretic hormone secretion (SIADH) are numerous. Note that primary hypersecretion of ADH is not a recognised cause.

Causes of SIADH

Paraneoplastic syndromes:

- bronchial carcinoma (especially small-cell carcinoma)
- prostate carcinoma
- pancreatic carcinoma
- thymoma
- intracranial tumours
- Hodgkin lymphoma

Thoracic pathology:

- pneumonia
- empyema
- tuberculosis

Intracranial pathology:

- skull fracture
- haemorrhage
- encephalitis
- meningitis

Drugs

- chlorpropamide, carbamazepine, chlorpromazine
- tricyclic antidepressants

Other

- hypothyroidism
- Guillain–Barré syndrome
- systemic lupus erythematosus

with visual disturbances (bitemporal hemianopia, loss of visual acuity), endocrine dysfunction (hypothyroidism, growth retardation and DI) or symptoms and signs of raised intracranial pressure. Macroscopically, craniopharyngiomas are ~3 to 4 cm in size, cystic/solid and characteristically contain calcification. Microscopically, islands of epithelial cells containing central stellate cells and peripheral palisaded cells are seen. Prognosis worsens with increasing age.

Pineal gland tumours

These are rare tumours accounting for 1% of adult and 3%–8% of childhood intracranial tumours. They can arise from developmental rests of embryonic germ cells or from the pineocytes themselves. Pineocyte-derived tumours include: pineocytomas, pineal tumours of intermediate grade and pineoblastomas.

THYROID DISORDERS

Congenital disorders of the thyroid

Thyroglossal cysts

As the embryo grows, the thyroid gland descends into the neck remaining connected to the tongue by a narrow canal, the thyroglossal duct. This eventually closes and regresses.

Cystic remnants of parts of the thyroglossal duct are known as thyroglossal cysts (Fig.14.4). These cysts may form anywhere along the course of descent but are always located near or in the midline of the neck. Cysts usually develop as painless, progressively enlarging masses which move upward on protrusion of the tongue. There is no alteration in thyroid function.

Lingual thyroid

Lingual thyroid is ectopic thyroid tissue at the base of the tongue. It occurs when there is failure of descent during embryogenesis.

Thyrotoxicosis (hyperthyroidism)

This syndrome is caused by the excessive secretion of thyroid hormones—typically both thyroxine (T_4) and tri-iodothyronine (T_3). Symptoms include tachycardia, sweating, tremor, anxiety, increased appetite, weight loss diarrhoea and heat intolerance (Fig. 14.5).

Primary hyperthyroidism is caused by:

- Graves disease (exophthalmic goitre)—the most common cause of thyrotoxicosis, characterized by a diffusely enlarged thyroid gland that is stimulated to produce excess hormone by an immunoglobulin G (IgG) autoantibody.
- Toxic multinodular goitre—second most common cause of hyperthyroidism.
- Adenoma (Plummer disease)—solitary thyroid nodule producing excess hormone with remainder of the thyroid gland being suppressed.

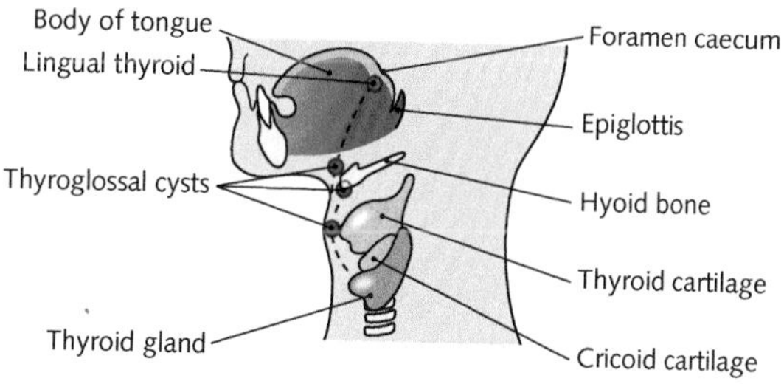

Fig. 14.4 Path of descent of thyroid gland. Path of descent of thyroid gland *(broken line)* and localization of thyroglossal cysts.

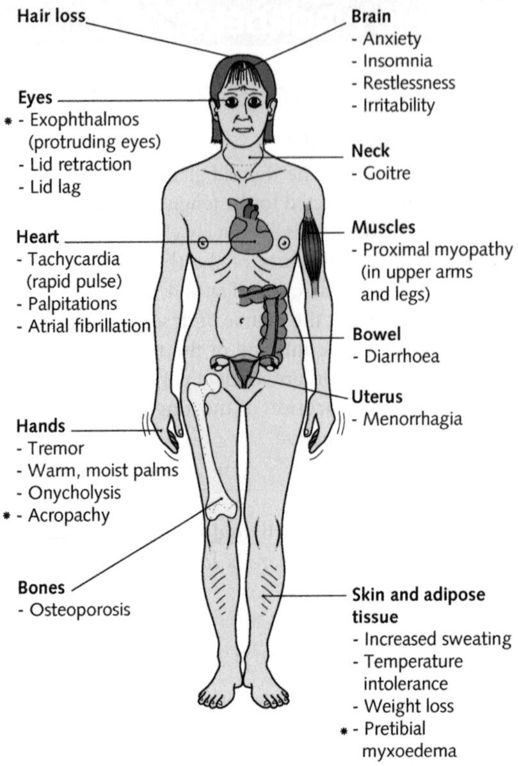

Fig. 14.5 Features of thyrotoxicosis. Summary diagram illustrating features of thyrotoxicosis. (*additional features seen only in Graves disease.)

- Thyroiditis—inflammation of the thyroid causing hyperthyroidism (e.g., De Quervain thyroiditis). Note that thyroiditis is more commonly associated with hypothyroidism (see later).
- Drugs—either direct ingestion of large doses of thyroid hormone (thyrotoxicosis factitia) or through iodide-inducing drugs (e.g., amiodarone).

Graves disease

Graves disease is an autoimmune disorder that results in thyrotoxicosis due to overstimulation of the thyroid gland by autoantibodies. It is the most common form of thyrotoxicosis, females being affected more often than males by a factor of 8:1. It is usually associated with a diffuse enlargement of the thyroid.

Pathogenesis—IgG-type immunoglobulins (thyroid-stimulating immunoglobulins) bind to TSH membrane receptors and cause prolonged stimulation of the thyroid, lasting for as long as 12 hours (cf. 1 hour for TSH). The autoantibody binds at a site different to the hormone-binding locus and is termed the TSH-receptor autoantibody (TRAb); 95% of Graves disease patients are positive for TRAbs.

Histologically, the gland shows diffuse hypertrophy and hyperplasia of acinar epithelium, reduction of stored colloid (giving follicles a scalloped appearance) and lymphoid follicle formation.

The clinical features of Graves disease are similar to those of general thyrotoxicosis but with some additional features (see Fig. 14.5), namely:

- Exophthalmos (protrusion of the eyeballs in their sockets)—due to the infiltration of orbital tissues by fat, mucopolysaccharides and lymphocytes as a result of autoimmune cross reactivity. This may cause compression of the optic nerve, and hence blindness. However, only about 5% of Graves patients show signs of exophthalmos.
- Thyroid acropachy—enlargement of the fingers and clubbing.
- Pretibial myxoedema—accumulation of mucoproteins in the deep dermis of the skin resulting in nonpitting oedema.

Hypothyroidism

Decreased activity of the thyroid gland results in decreased production of thyroid hormones. There are two forms:

1. Hypothyroidism present at birth → congenital hypothyroidism
2. Hypothyroidism in adults → myxoedema.

Hypothyroidism in adults (myxoedema)

This common clinical condition is associated with decreased function of the thyroid gland and a decrease in the circulating level of thyroid hormones. It affects 1% of people in the United Kingdom, with females affected more often than males by a factor of 6:1. It can present at any age but most commonly presents between 30 and 50 years of age.

The causes of primary hypothyroidism are:

- Autoimmune thyroiditis—atrophic form, e.g., primary atrophic thyroiditis, and goitrous form (such as Hashimoto thyroiditis).
- Graves disease—approximately 5% of patients with thyrotoxicosis develop hypothyroidism in later years, unrelated to treatment. Probably caused by a spectrum of antithyroid antibodies, some of which stimulate TSH receptor and some of which are destructive.
- Treatment of hyperthyroidism—surgical ablation, radioiodine or drug treatment.
- Severe iodine deficiency—rare in the United Kingdom, but common worldwide.

Myxoedema—If severe hypothyroidism is left untreated, the patient may develop life-threatening myxoedema coma.

The effects of hypothyroidism are shown in Figure 14.6.

HINTS AND TIPS

A reminder of the differences between primary and secondary hyperthyroidism and hypothyroidism:

- primary hyperthyroidism—↑ thyroid hormones, ↓ TSH
- secondary hyperthyroidism—↑ thyroid hormones, ↑ TSH (excess TSH production due to pituitary tumour)
- primary hypothyroidism—↓ thyroid hormones, ↑ TSH
- secondary hypothyroidism—↓ thyroid hormones, ↓ TSH (failure of TSH production due to pituitary disease)

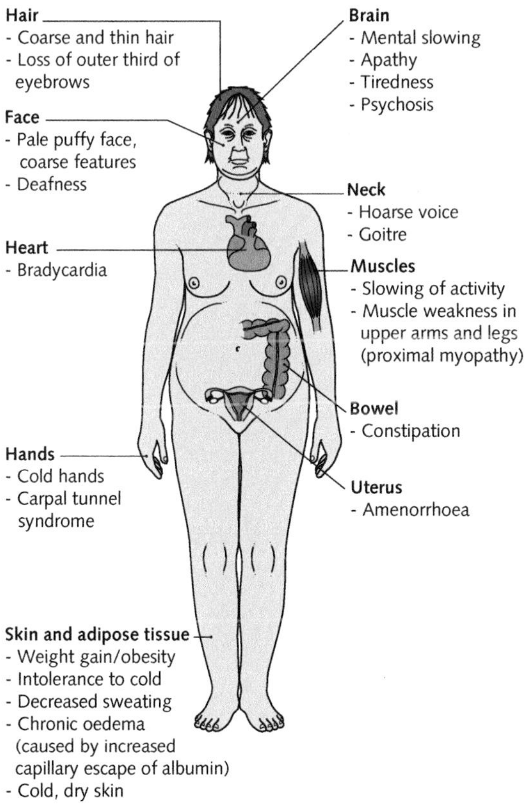

Fig. 14.6 Features of hypothyroidism. Summary diagram illustrating features of hypothyroidism in the adult.

Thyroiditis

This inflammation of the thyroid gland can have a viral or autoimmune aetiology and result in either hypothyroidism or hyperthyroidism.

Hashimoto thyroiditis (most common cause of hypothyroidism)

This autoimmune disease results in a destructive thyroiditis. It can occur at any age, but typically affects the middle-aged, and females more often than males by a factor of 12:1.

Thyroid peroxidase antibodies (TPO) are most commonly found in the serum of affected individuals (90% of cases). The disease is associated with the HLA-DR5 and HLA-B8 haplotypes, and patients with Hashimoto disease (and Graves disease) show a high incidence of other autoimmune diseases.

Macroscopically, the thyroid gland is usually:

- diffusely enlarged (typically 2–5 times normal size)
- firm in consistency
- white or grey cut surface as a result of the disappearance of thyroglobulin-containing colloid.

Microscopically, the thyroid gland shows:

- small thyroid follicles infiltrated by lymphocytes;
- lymphoid follicle formation and increased fibrous tissue stroma;
- sometimes follicles lined by eosinophilic (mitochondrial-rich) epithelial cells known as Hürthle cells;
- reduced colloid content of disrupted acini.

The patient may present with this condition because of goitre formation or because of the symptoms of hypothyroidism. The hypothyroid state tends to develop slowly. However, damage to thyroid follicles may lead to the release of thyroglobulin into the circulation causing transient thyrotoxicosis. Some cases proceed to primary atrophic thyroiditis. Furthermore, there is an increased incidence of non-Hodgkin lymphoma originating in the thyroid of patients with Hashimoto thyroiditis.

De Quervain thyroiditis

A rare, viral thyroiditis seen in young and middle-aged women, often presenting as a slightly diffuse tender swelling of the thyroid; this is also known as subacute, giant cell or granulomatous thyroiditis. It is associated with viral infections, usually Coxsackie, mumps and adenovirus.

Characteristic features are:

- painful enlargement of the thyroid (about twice normal size; normal weight is 20–30 g);
- transient febrile illness of short duration.

Histological examination shows:

- inflammation with a giant cell granulomatous reaction engulfing leaked colloid (hence the synonyms giant cell or granulomatous thyroiditis);

- degeneration of follicles with inflammatory cell infiltration (neutrophils, plasma cells, lymphocytes and histiocytes);
- fibrous scarring (late).

The illness is usually self-limiting and settles in a few weeks. Transient hyperthyroidism can result from the release of thyroglobulin and excessive amounts of thyroid hormone.

Severe thyroiditis may be fatal in the elderly and debilitated.

Subacute lymphocytic thyroiditis

This form of autoimmune thyroiditis is associated with amiodarone and lithium therapy.

Histological changes are similar to those in Hashimoto thyroiditis, but they are focal rather than diffuse, hence its other name: focal lymphocytic thyroiditis. The disease is less severe than Hashimoto thyroiditis, and it is often asymptomatic. It may also present with the symptoms of hyperthyroidism.

A comparison of the main types of thyroiditis is provided in Table 14.3.

Riedel thyroiditis

Is a chronic inflammatory condition characterized by replacement of normal thyroid tissue with dense woody fibrosis. It is usually self-limiting and, in general, has a good prognosis.

Thyroid goitres

Definitions

A goitre is any enlargement of the thyroid gland. There are two types:

1. Toxic goitre, i.e., goitre associated with thyrotoxicosis.
2. Nontoxic goitre, i.e., goitre associated with normal (euthyroid) or reduced levels of thyroid hormones.

Toxic goitre

Graves disease

This is the most common cause of toxic goitre (described previously).

Toxic multinodular goitre

This results from the development of hyperthyroidism in a multinodular goitre (see later).

Nontoxic goitres

Diffuse nontoxic goitre (simple goitre)

This diffuse enlargement of the thyroid gland is classified into:

- Endemic goitre—due to iodine deficiency.
- Sporadic goitre—caused by goitrogenic agents (substances that induce goitre formation) or familial in origin. Examples of goitrogenic agents include certain cabbage species, because of their thiourea content, and specific drugs or chemicals, such as iodide, paraminosalicylic acid and drugs used in the treatment of thyrotoxicosis. Familial cases show inherited autosomal recessive traits, which interfere with hormone synthesis via various enzyme pathways.
- Physiological goitre—enlargement of the thyroid gland in females during puberty or pregnancy.

Multinodular goitre

This is the most common cause of thyroid enlargement and is seen particularly in the elderly (nearly all simple goitres eventually become multinodular). The exact aetiology is uncertain but it may represent an uneven responsiveness of various parts of the thyroid to fluctuating TSH levels over a period of many years.

Morphological features are irregular hyperplastic enlargement of the entire thyroid gland due to the development of well-circumscribed nodules of varying size. The nodules contain brown, gelatinous colloid; consequently, it is often termed multinodular colloid goitre.

Most patients are euthyroid and generally seek treatment for cosmetic reasons (an unsightly swelling in the neck) or compression symptoms, e.g., pressure on the trachea producing stridor or pressure on the recurrent laryngeal nerve producing hoarseness.

However, toxic changes occasionally occur in a multinodular goitre resulting in hyperthyroidism, when it is termed a toxic multinodular goitre.

Neoplasms of the thyroid

Tumours of the thyroid are generally benign. Carcinomas are uncommon and lymphomas are rarer still.

Table 14.3 Summary of the features of thyroiditis

	Hashimoto thyroiditis	De Quervain thyroiditis	Subacute lymphocytic thyroiditis
Aetiology	Autoimmune	Viral	Autoimmune
Histological features	Diffuse lymphocytic infiltration of thyroid	Giant cell granulomatous inflammatory reaction	Focal lymphocytic infiltration of thyroid
Hypothyroidism	Common	Rare	Rare

Benign tumours

Follicular adenoma

These are usually encapsulated, solitary, solid nodules. Compression of the adjacent gland is a common feature, and the centre may show areas of haemorrhage and cystic change. Histologically, follicular adenomas are comprised of microfollicle formation and lack capsular or vascular invasion.

Rarely, follicular adenomas may synthesize excess thyroid hormones ('toxic adenomas/Plummer disease'), causing thyrotoxicosis.

CLINICAL NOTES

FNA OF A THYROID MASS

Fine needle aspiration (FNA) of the thyroid is frequently performed for clinically and radiologically suspicious lesions. However, it should be noted that it is not possible to differentiate a follicular adenoma from a follicular carcinoma based on cytology, as the differentiating features are capsular and vascular invasion. In these cases, a histological diagnosis is made after excision.

Malignant tumours

These rare tumours account for less than 1% of total cancer deaths in the United Kingdom, with females affected more often than males by a factor of 3:1. Types of malignant thyroid tumours and their basic features are outlined in Table 14.4.

Papillary thyroid carcinoma

This is the most common thyroid cancer. It is a well-differentiated tumour most commonly found in younger patients, has a female predominance and can be found incidentally. It presents as a nonencapsulated infiltrative mass.

Histologically, it consists of epithelial papillary projections into gland-like spaces and calcified spherules may be present (psammoma bodies). Diagnosis is based on characteristic nuclear features, e.g., intranuclear inclusions and grooves, or nuclear clearing (described as 'Orphan Annie nuclei').

It is a slow-growing tumour with an excellent prognosis. Metastatic spread is via the lymphatics.

Follicular carcinoma

Characterized histologically by uniform microfollicles, and differentiated from an adenoma by the presence of capsular and/or vascular invasion. Metastatic spread is usually haematogenous to bones, lungs and brain.

Many of these tumours retain the ability to take up radioactive iodine (^{131}I), which may be used as a highly effective targeted form of radiotherapy, usually after surgical thyroidectomy. The prognosis is therefore good.

Anaplastic carcinoma

This highly malignant, undifferentiated adenocarcinoma usually presents in the elderly as a diffusely infiltrative mass. In about half of cases there is a history of multinodular goitre.

The prognosis is very poor due to rapid invasion of local structures such as the trachea, producing respiratory obstruction.

Medullary carcinoma

This rare neuroendocrine tumour arises from parafollicular C cells, which commonly synthesize and secrete calcitonin but which may also secrete 5-hydroxytryptamine (serotonin), various peptides of the tachykinin family, ACTH and prostaglandins.

High levels of serum calcitonin are useful diagnostically but produce no clinical effects.

Although medullary carcinoma is most common in the elderly, it also occurs in younger individuals. Here it is commonly associated with other endocrine tumours, such as phaeochromocytoma as part of the multiple endocrine neoplasia (MEN) syndromes 2a and 2b (see later). Amyloid deposition is an associated finding in these tumours.

Table 14.4 Types and features of malignant thyroid tumours

Tumour type	Origin of tumour	Frequency (%)	Typical age range (years)	Spread	Prognosis (% for 10-year survival)
Papillary	Follicular cells	70	20–40	Lymphatic	95
Follicular	Follicular cells	10	40–60	Haematogenous	60
Anaplastic	Follicular cells	5	>60	Aggressive local invasion; Haematogenous	1
Medullary carcinoma	Parafollicular C cells	5–10	>40 (unless associated with MEN)	Local, lymphatic and haematogenous	50 (but very variable)
Lymphoma	Lymphocytes	5–10	>60	Lymphatic	10

MEN, Multiple neuroendocrine neoplasia.

MOLECULAR

MOLECULAR ASSOCIATIONS OF THYROID CANCER

More than 90% of thyroid cancers are associated with genetic mutations; some mutations are more common in certain subtypes:

Papillary thyroid carcinoma: BRAF, RET
Follicular thyroid carcinoma: RAS, PTEN
Medullary thyroid carcinoma: RET

HINTS AND TIPS

BONES, STONES, GROANS AND PSYCHIC MOANS

For symptoms of hypercalcaemia remember 'bones, stones, abdominal groans and psychic moans':

Bones: bone pain, pain from pathological fractures
Stones: renal stones, nephrocalcinosis
Abdominal groans: abdominal pain, vomiting/constipation, anorexia, peptic ulcer, and rarely pancreatitis
Psychic moans: depression, emotional lability, tiredness, lassitude

Lymphomas

Most thyroid lymphomas are regarded as tumours of mucosa-associated lymphoma tissue (MALT lymphoma). Interestingly, non-Hodgkin B-cell lymphomas occasionally arise in long-standing, autoimmune thyroiditis, especially Hashimoto disease.

PARATHYROID DISORDERS

Parathyroid hormone

Parathyroid hormone (PTH) is a polypeptide (84 amino acid residues) secreted by the chief cells of the parathyroid glands. The main action of PTH is to increase serum calcium and decrease serum phosphate.

In bone, PTH stimulates osteoclastic bone resorption and inhibits osteoblastic bone deposition. The net effect is the release of calcium from bone.

In the kidney, PTH has the following effects:

- increases calcium reabsorption
- decreases phosphate reabsorption
- increases 1α-hydroxylation of 25-hydroxyvitamin D (i.e., activates vitamin D) which causes increased gastrointestinal calcium absorption.

Hyperparathyroidism

Hyperparathyroidism is excessive secretion of PTH resulting in hypercalcaemia. There are three types:

1. Primary—hypersecretion of PTH is caused by hyperplasia or neoplasia of the parathyroid glands.
2. Secondary—physiological increase in PTH secretion in response to hypocalcaemia of any aetiology.
3. Tertiary—generation of an autonomous hypersecreting adenoma in long-standing secondary hyperparathyroidism.

Primary hyperparathyroidism

This is the most common type of parathyroid disorder, characterized by a raised or inappropriately normal PTH in the presence of hypercalcaemia. More than 90% of patients are over 50 years of age and the condition affects females more often than males by nearly 3:1. The aetiology and pathology of primary hyperparathyroidism are outlined in Table 14.5. It can also occur as part of the MEN 1 syndrome. It is an important cause of hypercalcaemia.

Secondary hyperparathyroidism

This is compensatory hyperplasia of the parathyroid glands as a physiological response to chronic low serum calcium concentration or increased serum phosphate.

Its causes are:

- chronic renal failure (most common cause)
- small bowel malabsorption syndromes
- vitamin D deficiency

Morphological changes of the parathyroid glands are:

- hyperplastic enlargement of the parathyroid glands (classically all), but to a lesser degree than in primary hyperplasia
- increase in 'water clear' cells and chief cells of the parathyroid glands, with loss of stromal fat cells
- increased number of parathyroid cells in a diffuse or nodular pattern.

Tertiary hyperparathyroidism

The development of autonomous hyperplasia in one or more parathyroid glands after long-standing secondary hyperparathyroidism. This condition results from chronic overstimulation of the parathyroid glands.

Table 14.5 Pathology of primary hyperparathyroidism

Pathology	Frequency	Macroscopic features	Microscopic features	Clinical features
Adenoma	80%	Tan-brown lesion Encapsulated Usually <1 cm Solitary, affecting only one gland Other glands are normal or atrophic	Loss of stromal fat Delicate fibrous capsule Compressed rim of adjacent normal tissue Polygonal chief cells, central nucleus Occasional nests of oxyphil cells	Serum [PTH] drops intraoperatively after removal
Hyperplasia	15%–20%	Diffuse enlargement of some or all glands Combined weight usually <1 g	Predominantly chief cells Islands of oxyphil cells ± delicate fibrous strands around nodules Nodular or diffuse pattern	Maybe sporadic or part of MEN syndrome
Carcinoma	2%–3%	Appears similar to adenoma but tend to be larger Affects one gland Difficult to remove at surgery (adherent and infiltrative) Pale and solid Large, 2–10 g or more	Chief cells Capsular/vascular invasion Metastasis Thick fibrous capsule Fibrous septae extending into the gland	Serum [$Ca2^{+}$] is very high Serum [PTH] is high Metastases to liver, lungs and lymph nodes

MEN, Multiple neuroendocrine neoplasia; PTH, parathyroid hormone.

Table 14.6 Comparison of primary, secondary and tertiary hyperparathyroidism

	Primary	Secondary	Tertiary
Serum PTH and Ca^{2+}	↑PTH; ↑Ca^{2+}	↑PTH; normal or ↑/↔Ca^{2+}	↑PTH; ↑Ca^{2+}
Aetiology	Adenoma	Chronic renal failure	Autonomous hyperplasia of a gland precipitated by chronic overstimulation in secondary hyperparathyroidism
	Hyperplasia	Malabsorption	
	Carcinoma	Pregnancy and lactation	
Predominant effects	Hypercalcaemia	Increased bone resorption Osteomalacia and rickets	Hypercalcaemia and increased bone resorption

PTH, Parathyroid hormone.

Table 14.6 gives a comparison of primary, secondary and tertiary hyperparathyroidism.

Hypoparathyroidism

Hypoparathyroidism is a condition of reduced or absent PTH secretion, resulting in hypocalcaemia and hyperphosphataemia. It is far less common than hyperparathyroidism.

The causes are:

- removal or damage of the parathyroid glands, e.g., during thyroidectomy, autoimmune parathyroid disease (usually occurs in patients who have another autoimmune endocrine disease, e.g., Addison disease);
- congenital deficiency (DiGeorge syndrome)—rare, congenital disorder caused by arrested development of the third and fourth pharyngeal pouches, resulting in an almost complete absence of the thymus (see Chapter 17) and parathyroid gland.

DISORDERS OF THE ADRENAL GLAND

Hormones of the adrenal gland

The adrenal gland is composed of two structurally and functionally distinct endocrine components, the cortex and medulla, which are derived from different embryonic tissue Fig. 14.8.

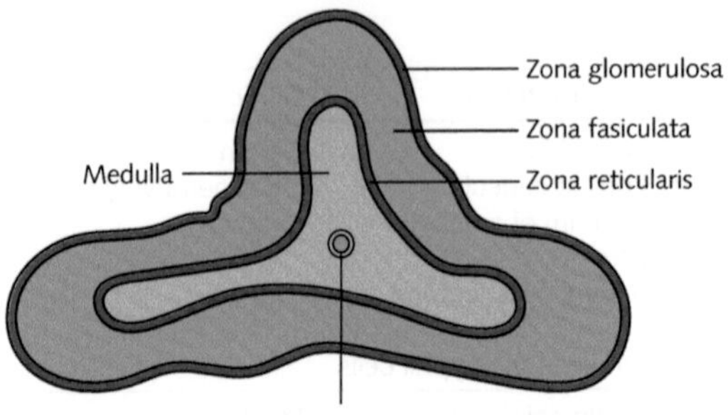

Fig. 14.8 Adrenal gland. Diagram of the adrenal gland showing the cortex, composed of zona glomerulosa, reticularis and fasciculata and the medulla with central vein.

HINTS AND TIPS

SALT, SWEET, SEX

Remember 'GFR: salt, sweet, sex' when you are trying to recall the layers of the adrenal cortex and the hormones they produce:

*G*lomerulosa
*F*asciculata
*R*eticularis

Salt: Aldosterone (mineralocorticoid)—regulates sodium concentration—zona glomerulosa.

Sweet: Cortisol (glucocorticoid)—regulates sugar—zona fasciculata.

Sex: Oestrogens and androgens (sex steroids)—zona reticularis.

COMMON PITFALLS

CUSHING SYNDROME VERSUS DISEASE

Avoid confusing **Cushing disease** and Cushing syndrome. **Remember**:

Cushing disease is used specifically to describe Cushing syndrome secondary to excessive pituitary ACTH secretion, i.e., an adenoma.

Cushing syndrome can arise due to any other cause of raised glucocorticoids; e.g., 'steroid' administration, such as prednisolone, is a common cause of the features of Cushing syndrome.

Cortex

This is the outer part of the gland and is derived from the mesoderm. It synthesizes, stores and secretes various cholesterol-derived hormones, namely:

- mineralocorticoid hormones, e.g., aldosterone (zona glomerulosa)
- glucocorticoid hormones, e.g., cortisol (primarily zona fasciculata)
- sex steroids, i.e., oestrogens and androgens (zona reticularis).

Medulla

This is the inner part of the gland and is embryonically derived from the neural crest, forming part of the sympathetic nervous system. Chromaffin cells synthesize and secrete the vasoactive catecholamines adrenaline (epinephrine) and noradrenaline (norepinephrine).

Hyperfunction of the adrenal cortex

Hyperaldosteronism

Excessive production of aldosterone by the zona glomerulosa of the adrenal cortex results in increased Na^+ retention and increased K^+ loss.

The aetiology is as follows:

- Primary hyperaldosteronism: autonomous hypersecretion of aldosterone independent of the renin-angiotensin system. The causes include:
  - Adrenocortical hyperplasia—most common cause (66%). Bilateral nodular hyperplasia is seen.
  - Adrenal cortical neoplasms (33%):
    - Adenomas (Conn syndrome)—solitary and small (<2 cm) composed of mature cortical cells which may contain spironolactone bodies (Fig. 14.9);
    - Adrenal cortical carcinomas—rare.
- Secondary hyperaldosteronism: hypersecretion of aldosterone secondary to increased serum renin. This is more common than the primary form of the disorder and may be precipitated by renal artery stenosis, diuretics, congestive cardiac failure and hepatic failure.

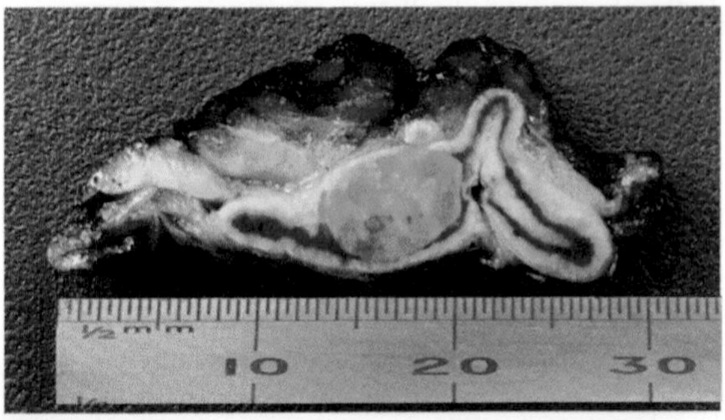

Fig. 14.9 Adrenal adenoma. Macroscopic photograph of the adrenal gland containing a cortical adenoma. The cortex and medulla are clearly demarcated. The orange/yellow coloration is due to the storage of large quantities of hormones which are derived from cholesterol.

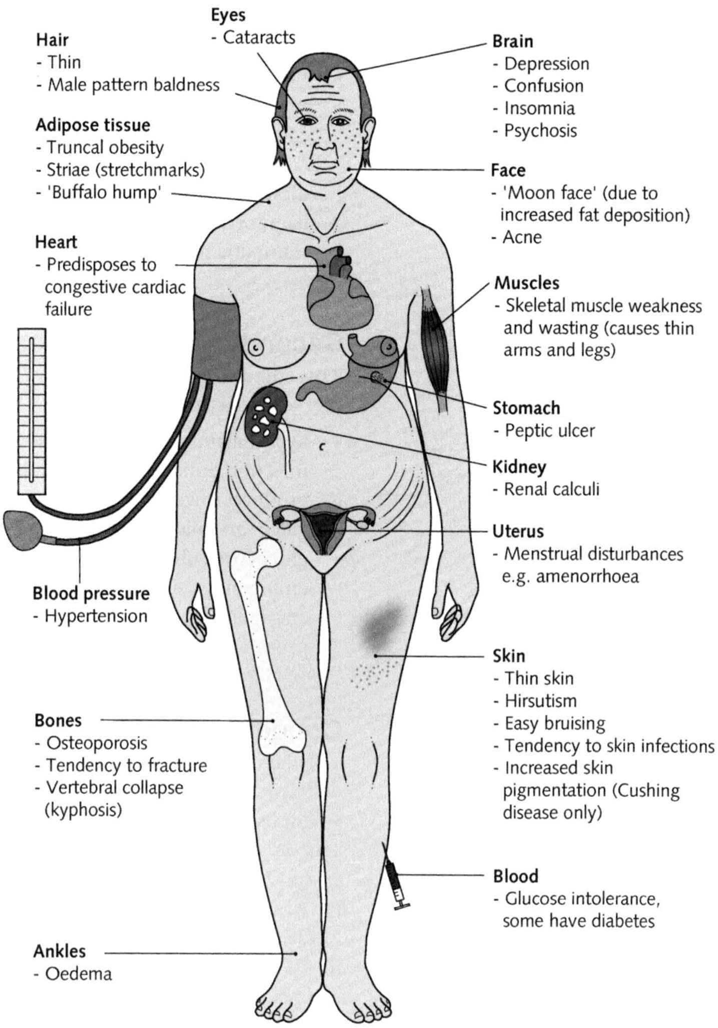

Fig. 14.11 Systemic effects of Cushing syndrome. lemon on sticks. The overall habitus of a person with Cushing syndrome is likened to a "lemon on sticks".

Cushing syndrome

The symptoms and signs of Cushing syndrome are associated with prolonged inappropriate elevation of free corticosteroid levels (Fig. 14.11). The aetiology and classification are summarized in Table 14.7.

Table 14.7 Aetiology and classification of Cushing syndrome

Type[a]	Cause
ACTH dependent	Iatrogenic (ACTH therapy)
	Pituitary hypersecretion of ACTH by corticotroph adenoma (Cushing disease)
	Ectopic ACTH production (benign or malignant nonendocrine tumour)
Non-ACTH dependent	Iatrogenic, e.g., steroid therapy
	Adrenal cortical adenoma
	Adrenal cortical carcinoma

[a] *Cushing syndrome can be classified into two groups depending on whether the aetiology is ACTH dependent or independent. ACTH, Adrenocorticotrophic hormone.*

Hypofunction of the adrenal cortex

Addison disease

This is a rare condition of primary adrenal cortical insufficiency with a concomitant decrease of glucocorticoids and mineralocorticoids.

The clinical features outlined in Table 14.8 are a result of glucocorticoid and mineralocorticoid insufficiency, loss of adrenal androgen production and increased ACTH secretion.

Table 14.8 Clinical features of Addison disease

Hormonal abnormality	Clinical features
Glucocorticoid insufficiency	Vomiting and loss of appetite
	Weight loss
	Lethargy and weakness
	Postural hypotension
	Hypoglycaemia
Mineralocorticoid insufficiency	↓serum Na^+, ↑serum K^+
	Chronic dehydration
	Hypotension
Increased ACTH secretion	Brownish pigmentation of skin and buccal mucosa
Loss of adrenal androgen	Decreased body hair

ACTH, Adrenocorticotrophic hormone.

Aetiology:

- Autoimmune destruction of the cortex—most common cause in the United Kingdom.
- Tuberculosis—most common cause in developing countries. Other infections can also cause adrenal cortical destruction, e.g., *Histoplasma capsulatum.*
- Metastatic cancers.

Primary acute adrenocortical insufficiency (adrenal crisis)

The aetiology includes:

- Iatrogenic—abrupt cessation of prolonged high-dose therapeutic corticosteroids (prolonged corticosteroid therapy produces lowered endogenous steroid production, leading to atrophy of the adrenal cortex).
- Bilateral massive adrenal haemorrhage and infarction (Waterhouse–Friderichsen syndrome)—caused by Gram-negative septicaemia (usually *Neisseria meningitidis*) producing haemorrhage and disseminated intravascular coagulation. Adrenal haemorrhage is also seen in neonates following a traumatic birth.

RED FLAG

ADRENAL CRISIS

Clinical features of an adrenal (Addisonian) crisis are:

- profound hypotension and hypovolaemic shock
- hypoglycaemia
- hyponatraemia
- vomiting/diarrhoea
- abdominal pain
- low grade pyrexia

This is a medical emergency and requires intravenous hydrocortisone and fluid replacement. The precipitating cause should be sought and if possible treated.

Secondary adrenocortical insufficiency

This adrenocortical insufficiency is caused by adrenal atrophy secondary to:

- hypothalamic or pituitary disease (tumours, infection, infarction, surgical destruction), which produces lowered ACTH, hence lowered endogenous glucocorticoids and aldosterone
- glucocorticoid therapy, which suppresses endogenous ACTH production and hence lowers endogenous glucocorticoids and aldosterone production.

Congenital adrenal hyperplasia

This autosomal recessive disorder is usually caused by a deficiency of the enzyme 21-hydroxylase, required for the synthesis of both cortisol and aldosterone. 21-hydroxylase acts on 17OH-progesterone and, consequently, raised levels of 17OH-progesterone are measured in the blood of affected individuals; this is routinely tested in the first week of life. Failure of cortisol production produces an increase in ACTH secretion by the pituitary and hyperplasia of the adrenal cortex.

Production of androgens by the adrenal cortex does not require 21-hydroxylase. Consequently, adrenal hyperplasia causes excessive secretion of androgens resulting in masculinization of females and precocious puberty in males. Aldosterone deficiency is serious, causing a life-threatening hypotensive salt-losing crisis ('salt-wasting syndrome') unless replacement therapy is given.

The adrenal medulla

Phaeochromocytoma

This is a rare tumour (paraganglioma) of the chromaffin cells of the adrenal medulla causing 1 in 1000 cases of hypertension. The majority are sporadic and benign but approximately 25% are familial and 5% are malignant.

Clinical features relate to the effects of adrenaline and noradrenaline hypersecretion namely: sweating, tachycardia, severe headaches, hypertension, pallor and anxiety.

Macroscopic appearance: Circumscribed lobulated grey and tan with possible haemorrhagic areas. Compressed rim of normal adrenal gland may be present.

> **HINTS AND TIPS**
>
> **RULE OF 10 PHAEOCHROMOCYTOMA**
>
> Historically, phaeochromocytomas were known as 'rule of 10' tumours: 10% extra-adrenal, 10% familial, 10% malignant, 10% bilateral. This now no longer holds true as behaviour (benign/malignant) and occurrence are governed by the underlying genetic defect. Familial occurrence is now thought to be in the order of 30%.

Microscopic appearance: This can be variable; however, typically, phaeochromocytomas are composed of polygonal cells with granular cytoplasm arranged in a nest-like 'Zellballen' pattern. The nests are surrounded by sustentacular cells best visualized with immunohistochemical stains (Fig. 14.14). Nuclear hyperchromasia and pleomorphism are variable and are not indicators of malignancy. Scoring systems exist to help predict malignant behaviour, however metastases are deemed by some to be the only absolute criterion.

Other familial syndromes are associated with phaeochromocytomas. These include:

- MEN 2 syndrome
- neurofibromatosis type 1
- von Hippel–Lindau syndrome

Diagnosis is by increased amounts of urinary catecholamines and their metabolites, such as vanillylmandelic acid.

Extraadrenal paragangliomas

Paragangliomas are tumours of the paraganglia (composed of neuroendocrine cells and supporting cells) occurring adjacent to sympathetic and parasympathetic ganglia throughout the body. They can secrete a variety of compounds, dependent on location, and respond to neural or chemical stimuli.

Neuroblastomas

Neuroblastomas are rare tumours that produce catecholamines and are derived from neural crest cells. The adrenal medulla is the most common site of occurrence and can also arise within the paraspinal sympathetic ganglia. They are almost exclusively tumours of children, rarely occurring over the age of 5, and present with fever, weight loss and an abdominal mass.

DISORDERS OF THE ENDOCRINE PANCREAS

Diabetes mellitus

Diabetes mellitus (DM) is a multisystem disease of an abnormal metabolic state characterized by hyperglycaemia due to inadequate insulin action/production. It can be classified into primary and secondary.

Primary DM is a disorder of insulin production/action. It accounts for 95% of diabetic cases.

In 5% of cases, diabetes may be secondary to:

- pancreatic diseases, e.g., chronic pancreatitis
- hypersecretion of hormones that antagonize the effects of insulin, e.g., glucocorticoids in Cushing syndrome, GH in acromegaly, adrenaline (epinephrine) in phaeochromocytomas.

Primary DM is by far the most important cause of diabetes and it is further classified into:

- Type 1, also known as insulin-dependent DM (IDDM) or juvenile-onset diabetes (absolute insulin deficiency)
- Type 2, also known as noninsulin-dependent DM (NIDDM) or mature-onset diabetes (relative insulin deficiency/resistance).

The basic features of these two types of diabetes are described in Table 14.9.

Type 1 diabetes mellitus

Aetiology and pathogenesis—type 1 DM (T1DM) is an organ-specific, autoimmune disorder characterized by antibody-mediated destruction of the β-cell population of the islet of Langerhans.

Two main factors are thought to predispose to autoimmunity:

1. Genetic predisposition—90%–95% of patients with T1DM are HLA-DR3 or HLA-DR4 positive, a feature that is also seen in other organ-specific autoimmune diseases. However, identical twins show a 40% concordance in the development of the disease, indicating the additional importance of environmental factors.

Table 14.9 Table comparing type 1 and type 2 diabetes mellitus

Type 1	Type 2
Childhood/adolescent onset	Middle-aged/elderly onset (usually)
1/3 of primary diabetes	2/3 of primary diabetes
Females = males	Females = males
Acute/subacute onset	Gradual onset
Thin	Obese
Ketoacidosis common	Ketoacidosis rare
Plasma insulin absent or low	Plasma insulin normal or raised
Insulin sensitive	Insulin insensitive (end-organ resistance)
Autoimmune mechanism (islet cell antibodies present)	Nonautoimmune mechanism (no islet cell antibodies)
Genetic predisposition associated with HLA-DR genotype	Polygenic inheritance

2. Viral infection—viral infection may trigger the autoimmune reaction; viruses implicated include mumps, measles and Coxsackie B.

One postulated mechanism is that viruses induce mild structural damage to the islet cells, thereby releasing previously shielded β-cell antigens leading to the recruitment and activation of lymphocytes in the pancreatic tissue.

Histologically, the pancreas shows lymphocytic infiltration and destruction of the insulin-secreting β cells within the islets of Langerhans. This results in insulin deficiency with hyperglycaemia and other secondary metabolic complications.

Type 2 diabetes mellitus

Aetiology and pathogenesis—the precise aetiopathogenesis of type 2 diabetes (T2DM) is unclear but the following factors are thought to be involved:

- Genetic factors—familial tendency with up to 90% concordance rate amongst identical twins. However, there are no HLA associations and inheritance is considered to be polygenic.
- Insulin resistance—impairment in the function of insulin receptors on target cells results in inability to respond to insulin. This is associated with obesity, sedentary lifestyle and poor diet; it is increasingly being seen in younger (even adolescent) individuals.
- Relative insulin deficiency—reduced secretion compared with the amounts required, possibly related to islet cell ageing.

> **HINTS AND TIPS**
>
> **IMPORTANCE OF RECOGNIZING COMPLICATIONS OF DIABETES MELLITIS**
>
> The complications of DM are important; 80% of adults with diabetes die from cardiovascular disease and patients frequently develop serious renal and retinal disease.

Complications of diabetes mellitus

Acute complications

Acute complications in decreasing order of frequency:

- Hypoglycaemia—complication of overtreatment with insulin.
- Diabetic ketoacidosis (DKA)—common in type 1 diabetes due to ↑ breakdown of free fatty acids → ↑ production of ketones → ketoacidosis → dehydration and impaired consciousness.
- Hyperosmolar hyperglycaemic state (HHS), also known as hyperosmolar nonketotic (HONK) state —↑ plasma glucose concentration → ↑ plasma osmolarity → cerebral dehydration → coma. More common in T2DM.
- Lactic acidosis—increased concentrations of lactic acid (produced as an end product of glycolysis instead of pyruvate) may cause coma.

Chronic complications

In recent years, with the advent of insulin therapy and various oral hypoglycaemic agents, morbidity and mortality associated with DM are more commonly the result of chronic rather than acute complications (Fig.14.15).

The complications of diabetes are macrovascular (affecting large and medium-sized muscular arteries) involving accelerated atherosclerosis. Microvascular (microangiopathy) involves small arterioles and capillaries which undergo hyaline arteriosclerosis whereby there is wall thickening secondary to expansion of the basement membrane.

The most important chronic complications of diabetes are:

- macrovascular: accelerated atherosclerosis increasing stroke and myocardial infarction risk;
- microvascular: disease affecting the eyes, kidneys and peripheral nerves;
- predisposition to infections.

Macrovascular complications

Compared with nonaffected people of the same age and sex, individuals with diabetes suffer from an increased severity of atherosclerosis, probably due to increased plasma levels of cholesterol and triglycerides.

The main clinical sequelae include:

- heart → ischaemic heart disease
- brain → cerebral ischaemia/infarction
- legs and feet → peripheral vascular disease leading to intermittent claudication, and gangrene—ischaemia of toes and areas on the heel is a characteristic feature of diabetic gangrene.

Microvascular complications

Microvascular complications are not isolated phenomena. If patients have microvascular pathology affecting one organ, they are highly likely to have microvascular complications in other organs.

Diabetic nephropathy—Diabetes is now one of the most common causes of end-stage renal failure. Associated renal disease can be divided into three forms:

1. Vascular disease
   a. Macrovascular: atherosclerosis affecting aorta and renal arteries → ischaemia.

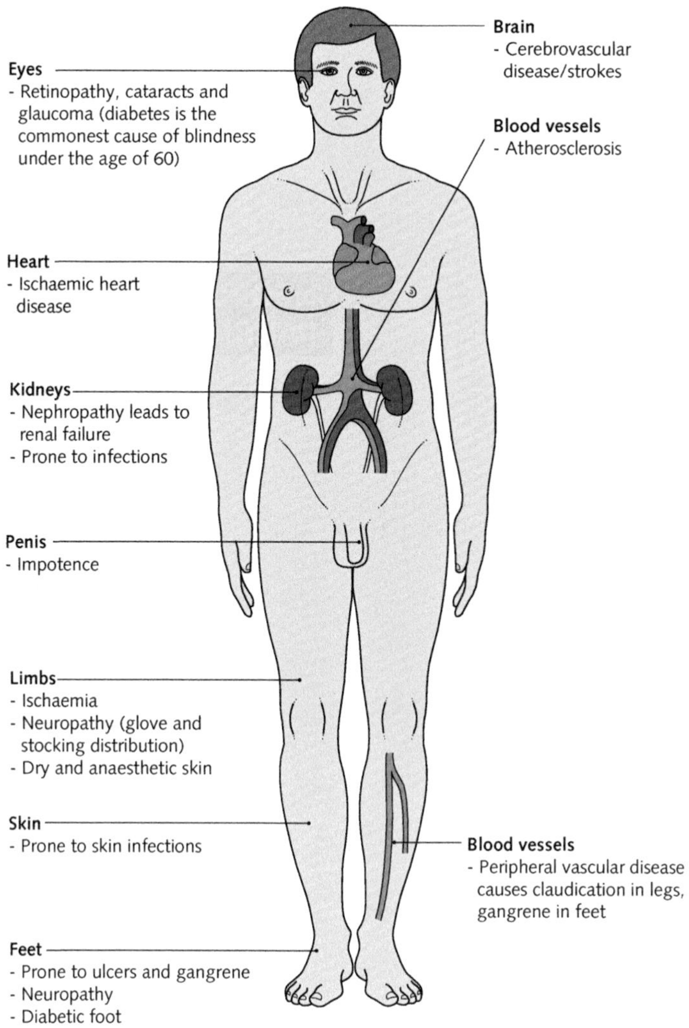

Fig. 14.15 Chronic complications of diabetes mellitus.

b. Microvascular: glomerular capillary basement membrane thickening (hyaline arteriolosclerosis) → ischaemic glomerular damage.

2. Diabetic glomerulosclerosis (diffuse and nodular types): ↑ leakage of plasma proteins through capillary wall into glomerular filtrate → proteinuria and progressive glomerular hyalinization with eventual chronic renal failure.
3. Infection: increased susceptibility to infections due to the relative immunosuppression of diabetes together with reduced neutrophil function. Acute pyelonephritis is a common complication of DM. It may progress to renal papillary necrosis.

Diabetic retinopathy—Diabetes is the most common cause of acquired blindness in the developed world. It can affect the eyes in six main ways:

1. Background retinopathy—small vessel abnormalities in the retina leading to hard exudates, blot haemorrhages and microaneurysms. Does not usually affect acuity.
2. Pre-proliferative retinopathy—cotton wool spots (soft exudates), large blot haemorrhages, venous beading and looping.
3. Proliferative retinopathy—extensive proliferation of new fragile capillaries in the retina. Sudden deterioration in vision may result from vitreous haemorrhage as a consequence of proliferating new vessels or from the development of retinal detachment.
4. Maculopathy—caused by oedema, hard exudates or retinal ischaemia near the macula and results in a marked reduction of acuity.

> **CLINICAL NOTES**
>
> **DIABETIC FOOT**
>
> The sequelae of diabetes mellitus are classically seen in the foot of patients with diabetes. Chronic ischaemia and neuropathy in the feet can result in injury, which may go unnoticed, leading to infection, painless ulceration and possible amputation.
>
> Aetiology of neuropathy:
>
> 1. Motor neuropathy—intrinsic muscle weakness results in limited joint mobility and changes in pressure distribution (especially to the metatarsal head).
> 2. Sensory loss—lack of pain when walking on abnormal pressure points results in damage and development of Charcot joints.
> 3. Autonomic denervation—loss of control of vasomotor tone increases risk of ischaemia and decreased healing; loss of sweat glands leads to dry, scaly skin which is prone to cracks and ulceration.

5. Cataract formation—greatly increased incidence in individuals with diabetes.
6. Glaucoma—increased incidence in those with diabetes due to neovascularization of the iris (rubeosis iridis).

Diabetic neuropathy—Clinically, most cases of diabetic neuropathy affect the peripheral nervous system, although central nervous system pathology does occur. The main effects are:

- microvascular thickening of basement membrane and microthrombi formation in small vessels supplying peripheral nerves;
- axonal degeneration with patchy, segmental demyelination;
- thickening of Schwann cell basal lamina.

The presentation may be of polyneuropathy (classically 'glove and stocking' sensory impairment), mononeuropathy (e.g., carpal tunnel syndrome, pupil-sparing cranial nerve III palsy) or autonomic neuropathy (especially of the gastrointestinal tract, bladder and heart; including symptoms of postural hypotension, nausea, vomiting, impotence and gustatory sweating).

Predisposition to infections—Patients with diabetes have an increased tendency to develop infections, usually of a bacterial or fungal nature. Persistent glycosuria in individuals with poorly controlled diabetes predisposes to urinary and genital infection.

The main organs affected are:

- skin—folliculitis, erysipelas, cellulitis and superficial fungal infections
- oral and genital mucosae—especially with *Candida*
- urinary tract—increased predisposition to acute pyelonephritis, often associated with recurrent lower urinary tract infections.

NEOPLASMS OF THE ENDOCRINE PANCREAS

Islet cell tumours

These tumours are rare compared with those of the exocrine pancreas. They occur most commonly in individuals aged 30–50 years.

For a summary of islet cell tumours see Table 14.10.

Insulinomas

Insulinomas are the commonest islet cell tumour, derived from pancreatic β-cells.

- They cause hypoglycaemia through hypersecretion of insulin.
- They may produce attacks of confusion, stupor and loss of consciousness.
- C-peptide is characteristically increased (commercial insulin preparations remove C-peptide).

Gastrinomas

A syndrome of gastric acid hypersecretion, multiple peptic ulcers and diarrhoea is caused by a gastrin-secreting tumour (gastrinoma) of the pancreatic G cells. Tumours are

Table 14.10 Summary of islet cell tumours

Islet cell tumour	Occurrence	Clinical features
Insulinoma	70%–75%	Hypoglycaemia
Gastrinoma	20%–25%	Zollinger–Ellison syndrome: gastric hypersecretion, multiple peptic ulcers and diarrhoea
VIPoma	Rare	Watery diarrhoea, hypokalaemia and achlorhydria
Glucagonoma	Rare	Secondary diabetes mellitus, necrolytic migratory erythema and uraemia
Somatostatinoma	Rare	Diabetes mellitus, cholelithiasis and steatorrhoea

multiple in 50% of cases, with 10%–20% occurring at other sites, e.g., the duodenum. They are often malignant.

They may be part of the Zollinger–Ellison syndrome or part of the MEN 1 syndrome (see later).

VIPomas

These produce vasoactive intestinal polypeptide (VIP), resulting in a syndrome of *w*atery *d*iarrhoea, *h*ypokalaemia and *a*chlorhydria (WDHA).

Glucagonomas

These glucagon-secreting tumours are derived from pancreatic α-cells and cause secondary DM (usually mild), necrolytic migratory erythema (skin rash) and uraemia.

Somatostatinomas

These somatostatin-producing tumours derived from pancreatic δ-cells are associated with DM, cholelithiasis and steatorrhoea.

Multiple endocrine neoplasia syndromes

Compared with those with single sporadic endocrine tumours, patients with MEN develop multiple endocrine tumours at a younger age, have multiple organ involvement and usually have a strong family history of endocrine neoplasia. The majority of MEN mutations are autosomal dominant, making it important to screen relatives as there is a significant chance that they will have undiagnosed disease/pathology.

There are three main types of MEN syndrome:

1. MEN 1 (Wermer) syndrome.
2. MEN 2a (Sipple) syndrome.
3. MEN 2b (sometimes called MEN 3) syndrome.

MEN 1 syndrome

MEN 1 syndrome is caused by a germ-line mutation in the MEN-1 tumour suppressor gene. It may also occur sporadically from new mutations. Life expectancy is reduced, with 50% of patients dying before 50 years old, mostly from malignant neuroendocrine tumours.

Patients usually show a combination of:

- Primary hyperparathyroidism: 90% of patients (chief cell hyperplasia and adenomas).
- Pancreatic tumours: second commonest manifestation. Tend to be multicentric, unlike non-MEN neuroendocrine tumours. Gastrinomas, insulinomas and nonfunctioning tumours are the most common, however all varieties are possible.
- Pituitary adenomas: tend to be macroadenomas and are usually more infiltrative than their non-MEN counterparts. The most frequent are prolactinomas or growth hormone-secreting tumours.

Rarely, there may also be thyroid tumours and adrenal cortical adenomas.

> **HINTS AND TIPS**
>
> **MEN 1**
>
> Remember the three Ps for organs affected in MEN 1:
>
> *P*ituitary
> *P*ancreas
> *P*arathyroid

MEN 2 syndromes

MEN 2a and 2b syndromes have been linked to mutations in the *RET* proto-oncogene, with near 100% disease penetrance. These conditions are characterized by phaeochromocytomas and medullary carcinomas of the thyroid together with other endocrine abnormalities. Medullary thyroid carcinomas arise from C-cell hyperplasia. Genetic screening of at-risk family members in MEN 2 families now allows prophylactic thyroidectomy for those with RET mutations to avoid the near certainty of medullary carcinoma.

MEN 2a syndrome

Patients have a combination of:

- Medullary carcinoma of the thyroid—typically bilateral and multicentric, presenting in the second or third decades;
- Phaeochromocytoma: present within 50% of patients, bilateral in 60%–80% and nearly all benign;
- Hyperparathyroidism due to parathyroid hyperplasia.

MEN 2b (MEN 3) syndrome

In contrast to MEN 2a, hyperparathyroidism is not a feature. Patients have a combination of:

- phaeochromocytoma
- medullary carcinoma of the thyroid: more aggressive than that seen in MEN 2a
- mucosal neuromas: commonly oral or ocular
- marfanoid-like body habitus
- intestinal ganglioneuromatosis

Chapter Summary

- The pituitary gland is composed of an anterior and posterior lobe.
- Anterior pituitary adenomas are classified as micro- (<10 mm) or macroadenomas (>10 mm) and can be functioning, i.e., produce hormones, or nonfunctioning.
- Pituitary adenomas can have space-occupying effects or endocrine effects.
- Prolactinomas are the most common pituitary adenomas.
- Hypopituitarism can be caused by pathology within the hypothalamus or pituitary gland.
- Diseases of the posterior pituitary include diabetes insipidus and syndrome of inappropriate antidiuretic hormone secretion (SIADH).
- Thyroglossal cysts are remnants of the thyroglossal duct; they are located in the midline and move with protrusion of the tongue.
- Graves disease is an autoimmune condition causing hyperthyroidism.
- Hashimoto disease is an autoimmune condition causing hypothyroidism.
- Goitres may be toxic (associated with thyrotoxicosis) or nontoxic.
- Capsular invasion and vascular invasion differentiate follicular adenomas from follicular carcinomas.
- Papillary thyroid carcinomas are diagnosed by their distinctive nuclear features.
- Hyperparathyroidism can be primary, secondary or tertiary.
- In primary hyperparathyroidism, one parathyroid gland is involved (adenoma); in secondary hyperparathyroidism, classically all the parathyroid glands are involved.
- Hyperfunction of the adrenal cortex can result in hyperaldosteronism and Cushing syndrome.
- Hypofunction of the adrenal cortex results in Addison disease and adrenocortical insufficiency.
- Phaeochromocytomas are tumours of the adrenal medulla and can be associated with the familial syndromes of multiple endocrine neoplasia type 2 (MEN 2), neurofibromatosis type 1 (NF1) and von Hippel–Lindau syndrome (VHL).
- Diabetes mellitus is a common chronic condition due to either insulin deficiency or resistance; it causes multisystem disease secondary to macrovascular and microvascular changes.
- Macrovascular complications mainly affect the brain, heart and legs.
- Microvascular complications mainly affect the eyes, kidneys and peripheral nervous system.
- Islet cell tumours are tumours which arise from the endocrine pancreas.
- MEN 1 syndrome is caused by mutation in the MEN 1 tumour suppressor gene and MEN 2 caused by mutations in the RET proto-oncogene.
- MEN syndromes are characterized by multiple endocrine tumours in different organs, with a younger age of onset compared with sporadic tumours, which tend to be solitary and present at a later age.

Pathology of the reproductive system 15

DISORDERS OF THE VULVA, VAGINA AND CERVIX

Nonneoplastic lesions of the lower genital tract

Bartholin cyst

This common, benign, mucus-secreting cyst on the vulva is derived from obstruction of Bartholin glands (mucus-secreting glands in the posterior part of the labia majora). Frequently there is superimposed infection, termed a Bartholin abscess.

Infections

Certain viral, bacterial, protozoal and fungal infections can frequently occur in the genital tract. The commonest infections are summarized in Table 15.1. Further discussion is seen in Chapter 5.

Dysplastic and neoplastic disorders of the vulva and vagina

Tumours of the vulva

Extramammary Paget disease

Paget disease is an intraepithelial neoplasm arising from cells within the epidermis. It can mimic melanoma in morphological appearance. It usually arises de novo, but can be associated with underlying malignancy. These cases have a poorer prognosis.

Table 15.1 Organisms that cause infections of the lower genital tract

Infection	Organism
Viruses	HPV HSV
Bacteria	*Gardnerella vaginalis* *Chlamydia trachomatis* (lymphogranuloma venereum) *Treponema pallidum* (syphilis)
Protozoa	*Trichomonas vaginalis*
Fungi and yeast	Dermatophytes, *Candida albicans*

HPV, Human papilloma virus; HSV, herpes simplex virus.

Vulval intraepithelial neoplasia

This is dysplastic epithelium of the vulva, generally seen in patients younger than those with invasive tumours. There are two subtypes of vulval intraepithelial neoplasia (VIN)—usual type and differentiated type. Usual-type VIN is the commonest, accounting for 90%–95% of cases and is associated with human papillomavirus (HPV) infection (especially serotypes 16 and 18), usually with visible warty change in the affected and adjacent epithelium.

This form rarely progresses to invasive carcinoma. Differentiated VIN is usually seen in elderly women and is often preceded by lichen sclerosus and atrophy. Approximately 30% of cases progress to invasive squamous cell carcinoma. Like cervical dysplasia (see Neoplasms of the cervix below), VIN is graded based on the degree of atypia within surface epithelium (VIN 1, 2 and 3).

Squamous cell carcinoma

This is the most common malignant tumour of the vulva, typically occurring in elderly women and often showing extensive local invasion and metastases to inguinal lymph nodes. The majority of cases appear to arise de novo, but some form from VIN (usually the differentiated subtype).

Tumours of the vagina

Vaginal intraepithelial neoplasia

Vaginal intraepithelial neoplasia (VaIN) is rare compared with cervical intraepithelial neoplasia (CIN). Most cases are found in young women and are associated with HPV infection. Women often have a history of CIN or invasive cervical cancer. Most low-grade cases regress. High-grade cases can progress to invasive carcinoma if untreated.

Neoplasms

Primary malignant tumours of the vagina are extremely rare, but include squamous cell carcinomas, adenocarcinomas and mesenchymal tumours.

Secondary tumours are also rare. Commonest metastases are from malignant tumours of the cervix, endometrium and ovary. Vaginal bleeding after hysterectomy for uterine or ovarian malignancy should always be investigated and biopsied because of the frequency of metastatic tumour in the residual vaginal vault.

Inflammation of the cervix

Acute and chronic cervicitis

Acute and chronic inflammation of the cervix is particularly common in the presence of an intrauterine contraceptive device. Acute cervicitis is characterised by neutrophilic inflammation and chronic cervicitis is characterized by a heavy plasma cell and lymphocytic infiltrate. Causes may be noninfectious or infectious (e.g., herpes simplex virus, *Trichomonas*, *Candida*, Gardnerella and gonococcal species.

Endocervical polyps

These common abnormalities derived from the endocervix affect up to 5% of women. Large polyps may protrude from the cervix through the external os and can cause intermenstrual bleeding from erosion and ulceration.

Macroscopically, these polyps are smooth and rounded, about 1–2 cm in diameter.

Microscopically, the surface of the polyp may show ulceration and inflammation, often accompanied by squamous metaplasia.

Neoplasms of the cervix

Cervical intraepithelial neoplasia

CIN is the preneoplastic (dysplastic) proliferation of epithelium of the transformation zone of the cervix (Fig. 15.1).

Aetiology—there is a strong association with HPV infection, particularly serotypes 16 and 18, which have been identified in 70% of cervical carcinomas.

Risk factors are:

- sexual intercourse—very low incidence in virgins, with increased risk in those who have had multiple sexual partners and first intercourse at an early age.
- HPV—high-risk HPV serotypes: 16, 18, 31, 33 and 45. Proteins produced by HPV are thought to inactivate products of tumour suppressor genes thereby facilitating tumour development. New HPV vaccines targeted against serotypes 16 and 18 can reduce HPV infection and CIN development (see Chapter 4).
- combined oral contraceptive pill—prolonged use is associated with an increased risk in those who carry HPV infection.
- smoking.
- immunosuppression—predisposes to carcinoma of the cervix, e.g., HIV patients.

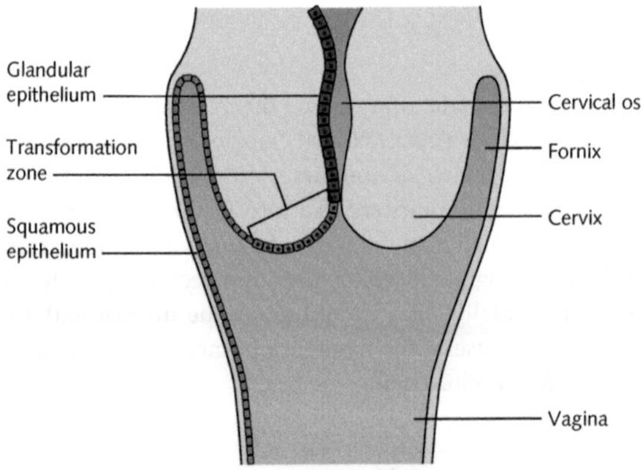

Fig. 15.1 Diagram of the transformation zone.

Classification

Three grades of severity are recognized. Grading depends on the proportion of the cervical epithelium wall that is replaced by atypical cells:

1. CIN I (mild dysplasia)—upper two-thirds of the epithelium normal, basal third atypical cells.
2. CIN II (moderate dysplasia)—upper third of the epithelium normal, atypical cells occupy the lower two-thirds.
3. CIN III (severe dysplasia)—corresponds to carcinoma in situ. Atypical cells extend throughout the full thickness of the epithelium with minimal differentiation and maturation on the surface.

Some classification systems classify dysplasia as low-grade or high-grade squamous intraepithelial lesions (LSIL or HSIL). LSIL corresponds to CIN I and HSIL corresponds to CIN II and III.

Progression

CIN is associated with a risk of progression to an invasive carcinoma, the risk for CIN I being lowest (most cases regress) and for CIN III being the highest.

The natural history of CIN is important as it determines how often screening is required to detect progression of the disease.

Squamous cell carcinoma

The vast majority of cervical carcinomas are squamous cell carcinomas arising from the transformation zone or ectocervix.

There are around 3000 cases of cervical cancer in the United Kingdom each year, with 900 deaths. This equates to a lifetime risk of around 1% (similar across the developed world), compared with 5% in parts of the developing world where screening programmes do not exist. This type of carcinoma occurs in all ages from late teens, but the average age is 45 years.

The carcinoma is preceded by the preinvasive phase of CIN (see previously). Risk factors are as for CIN.

Macroscopically, tumours demonstrate early areas of granular irregularity of the cervical epithelium, with progressive invasion of the stroma causing abnormal hardness of the cervix and late fungating ulcerated areas, which destroy the cervix.

Microscopically, lesions may be keratinizing or nonkeratinizing.

The common presenting symptom is vaginal bleeding in the early stages. Advanced, neglected tumours may cause

Table 15.2 Stages and prognosis for carcinomas of the cervix

Stage	5-year survival (%)	Degree of local invasion
I	85–90	Confined to cervix
II	60	Invasion of upper part of vagina or adjacent parametrial tissues
III	40	Spread to pelvic side wall, lower vagina or ureters
IV	15	Invasion of rectum, bladder wall or outside pelvis

urinary obstruction due to ureter and bladder involvement and may result in hydroureter and hydronephrosis.

In-situ and invasive adenocarcinomas arising from endocervical glands can also occur.

Invasive carcinomas are managed according to the degree of local invasion and survival is related to the stage of the disease (Table 15.2).

Early invasive carcinoma is usually managed by radical hysterectomy and/or radiotherapy, whereas advanced disease is usually only amenable to radiotherapy and/or chemotherapy.

Involvement of the para-aortic lymph nodes is associated with a very poor prognosis.

CLINICAL NOTES

FIGO AND CERVICAL CARCINOMA

Staging of cervical cancers is via the FIGO (International Federation of Gynaecology and Obstetrics) and tumour, node, metastasis (TNM) staging systems.

DISORDERS OF THE UTERUS

Disorders of the endometrium

Pyometrium (pyometra)

This is an accumulation of pus within the endometrial cavity due to compromised drainage through the cervix. This can occur secondary to cervical os stenosis (senile atresia, postradiotherapy), congenital abnormalities and malignancy. Retained intrauterine contraceptive devices are also risk factors. It primarily affects postmenopausal women (60–80 years of age). The commonest symptoms are postmenopausal bleeding, vaginal discharge and abdominal pain; however, 50% of cases are asymptomatic and, surprisingly, fever is present only in the minority. Rarely, pyometra is complicated by spontaneous uterine rupture.

Chronic endometritis

Inflammation of the endometrium is typically associated with menstrual irregularities often found in women who are being investigated for infertility. Patients are usually asymptomatic.

Microscopically, a plasma cell infiltrate within the endometrium is seen associated with lymphocytes and lymphoid follicle formation. There is a mixed microbial population commonly comprised of *Ureaplasma urealyticum*, group B streptococcus and chlamydia.

Risk factors—the majority of cases are associated with a definite clinical risk factor for developing inflammation:

- recent pregnancy; miscarriage or instrumentation (50% of cases)
- chronic pelvic inflammatory disease, e.g., following chlamydial infection (25% of cases)
- use of an intrauterine contraceptive device (about 20% of cases)
- tuberculosis in developing countries (5% of cases).

Endometriosis

This is defined as the presence of endometrial glands and stroma outside of the uterus, which is still capable of responding to cyclical hormonal stimulation. Phases of proliferation and breakdown are associated with the development of the fibrous adhesions and accumulation of hemosiderin pigment. This affects 1 in 15 women of reproductive age. There are numerous sites:

- Common—ovaries, fallopian tubes, pelvic peritoneum, round ligaments, uterosacral ligament, pouch of Douglas.
- Less common—intestinal wall (recto-sigmoid), appendix, bladder, ureter, umbilicus, laparotomy scars.
- Rare—lung, brain, kidney.

Theories of origin

The aetiopathogenesis of endometriosis remains unclear but three main theories operate to various degrees:

1. Retrograde menstruation—fragments of sloughed endometrium migrate through the fallopian tubes during menstruation and implant at distant sites.
2. Metaplasia of peritoneal epithelium—differentiation of peritoneal epithelium into endometrium through hormonal factors.
3. Immune dysfunction—defective immune surveillance allowing the implantation and growth of endometrial tissue within the peritoneum.

Macroscopically, the foci of endometriosis appear as cystic and solid masses, which are characteristically dark brown because of accumulated iron pigment from repeated episodic bleeding.

Microscopically, endometriosis is composed of endometrial glands and stroma, hemosiderin containing macrophages and fibrosis.

Endometriosis may present with chronic cyclical pelvic pain, dysmenorrhoea, dyspareunia and infertility.

Complications

- Infertility (about 30% of cases)—often due to adhesions and blockages affecting ovulatory pathways.
- Bowel obstruction—due to fibrous adhesions between adjacent organs.
- Chocolate cysts—the whole of the fallopian tube and ovary may be converted into a cystic mass containing altered blood, the appearance of which is reminiscent of liquid chocolate.

Endometriosis is oestrogen dependent for continued growth and proliferation. The disease becomes inactive after oophorectomy or the onset of the menopause, therefore induction of a hypooestrogenic state by suppression of ovulation is an effective treatment in many cases (e.g., continuous progesterone therapy).

Endometrial polyps

These localized overgrowths of endometrial glands and stroma are very common and are typically seen in the perimenopausal age range. They are caused by inappropriate glandular proliferation in response to unopposed oestrogenic stimuli, which includes the use of tamoxifen (tamoxifen polyps).

Macroscopically, they are found in the uterine fundus projecting into the endometrial cavity; their size is variable, but they are usually 1–3 cm in diameter. They have a firm, smooth, nodular appearance and occasionally prolapse through the cervical os. They may ulcerate or undergo torsion.

Microscopically, they are composed of cystically dilated endometrial glands within a fibrous spindled stroma containing thick-walled blood vessels.

Clinical features are associated with menstrual abnormalities and dysmenorrhoea.

Endometrial hyperplasia

Endometrial hyperplasia is defined as an increase in the endometrial glands-to-stroma ratio. This can be present with or without cytological (cellular) atypia. Hyperplasia arises in response to oestrogenic stimulation of the endometrium in the absence of progesterone and typically occurs in postmenopausal women, or perimenopausally if ovulation does not occur regularly or if other risk factors, such as obesity, exist. It presents with menorrhagia or postmenopausal bleeding but the severity or frequency is not related to the degree of pathological change. Endometrial hyperplasia with atypia is associated with a 28% risk of progression to malignancy.

> **HINTS AND TIPS**
>
> **ENDOMETRIAL HYPERPLASIA**
>
> Endometrial hyperplasia with atypia is regarded as a premalignant lesion as it is associated with an increased risk of progression to endometrial adenocarcinoma.

Endometrial carcinoma

Adenocarcinomas of the endometrium are the commonest gynaecological malignancy. The mean age of presentation is 56 years and 80% of women are postmenopausal.

Endometrial carcinoma is associated with:

- hyperoestrogenic state—obesity, diabetes, late menopause, prolonged use of unopposed oestrogens, oestrogen-secreting tumours.
- previous pelvic irradiation.
- lower parity.

Although an imperfect categorization, endometrial carcinomas can be thought of as two types (Fig. 15.2):

Type 1 *(Hyperoestrogenic tumours)*—these are associated with a generally good prognosis. They occur in patients close to the menopause and are associated with abnormal oestrogenic stimulation of the endometrium and endometrial hyperplasia. Most tumours are adenocarcinomas (60%) and are graded (I–III) according to the amount of glandular and solid pattern within the tumour. High-grade tumour is associated with a worse prognosis.

Type 2 *(Nonhyperoestrogenic tumours)*—these are more often associated with a poor prognosis, occur in older postmenopausal women and are not associated with oestrogenic stimulation or endometrial hyperplasia.

Macroscopically, there are:

- small tumours—diffuse, solid areas or polypoid lesions in the endometrium.
- larger tumours—fill and distend the endometrial cavity with soft, white, friable tissue.

Microscopically, they are seen as:

- Type 1 tumours—typically well-differentiated adenocarcinomas (endometrioid type) composed of hyperplastic endometrial glandular tissue with only superficial myometrial invasion at diagnosis.
- Type 2 tumours—typically less differentiated with deep myometrial invasion. Included in this group are serous, clear cell and carcinosarcomas.

Clinical features—The condition classically presents as postmenopausal bleeding.

The main route of spread is by local invasion to the cervix, adnexa, bladder and rectum.

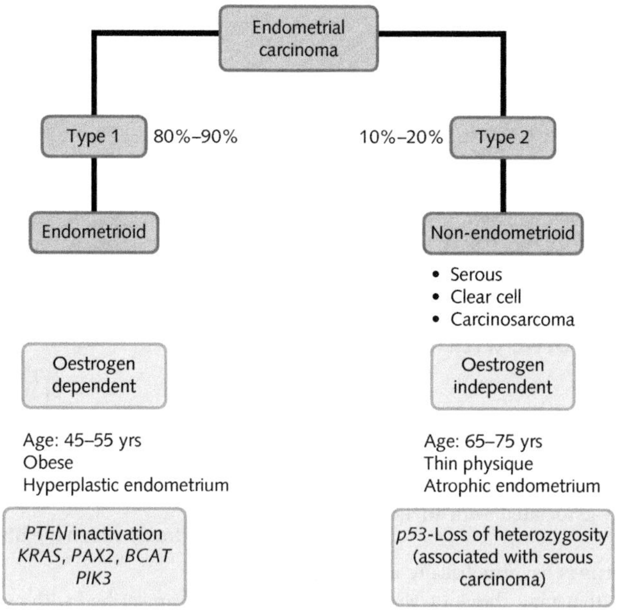

Fig. 15.2 Subtypes of endometrial carcinoma.

If venous and lymphatic invasion occurs, there may be involvement of the vagina and para-aortic nodes. Widespread haematogenous metastasis is uncommon except with papillary serous carcinomas and clear cell carcinomas.

The amount of direct invasion into the myometrium is closely correlated with prognosis.

The prognosis of uterine carcinoma is related to stage (Table 15.3).

Endometrioid carcinoma

Endometrioid carcinoma is the most common type of endometrial cancer and can arise from a background of endometrial hyperplasia. It presents most commonly in women >40 years of age and is characterized by angular, complex glands with hard luminal edges which may form solid areas.

Table 15.3 FIGO staging of endometrial cancer[a]

Stage	Proportion of cases (%)	Degree of invasion	5-year survival (%)
I	75	Corpus of uterus only	85
II	10	Corpus and cervix	65
III	10	Invasion confined to pelvis	40
IV	5	Invasion outside pelvis or involves bladder or rectal mucosa	10

[a] Gynaecological malignancies are staged using the FIGO system, which correlates to the TNM system.
FIGO, International Federation of Gynaecology and Obstetrics; TNM, tumour, node, metastasis.

It can be low or high grade depending on architectural features and the degree of nuclear atypia.

Serous carcinoma

Arises on a background of atrophic endometrium in older women, usually over 55 years old. It is an aggressive endometrial cancer as it is high grade by definition. Three-quarters of woman will have extrauterine disease at presentation and therefore a poor overall outcome. The cancer is composed of numerous papillae forming a slit-like architecture with pleomorphic, bulging (hobnail) nuclei. Psammoma bodies (laminated balls of calcification) are present in some.

Clear cell carcinoma

Similar to serous carcinoma, as they are associated with an older age group (mean age 65–69 years), these present at an advanced stage with a poor prognosis and arise on the background of atrophic endometrium. They can have solid, papillary or tubulocystic architecture and are high grade by definition, with pleomorphic nuclei and clear cytoplasm. The stromal cores tend to be hyalinized.

Mucinous carcinoma

Pure mucinous carcinoma is a rare form of endometrioid carcinoma occurring in 47–89-year-olds. It more commonly occurs in conjunction with an endometrioid component. Characteristically it is formed of mucin-filled epithelial cells.

Carcinosarcoma

Previously known as malignant mixed Müllerian tumours, these tumours are highly malignant endometrial carcinomas that have developed a sarcomatous (mesenchymal) component. They can exhibit heterologous differentiation, e.g., cartilage and skeletal muscle formation.

MOLECULAR

PTEN MUTATION

PTEN tumour suppressor gene is the most frequently mutated gene in type 1 endometrial carcinomas (endometrioid type).

Disorders of the myometrium

Adenomyosis

This is a condition in which endometrial glands and stroma are present deep within the myometrium (rare in post-menopausal women). It can be focal (nodular adenomyosis) or diffuse and is sometimes associated with menorrhagia and dysmenorrhoea.

Macroscopically, the uterus is asymmetrically enlarged by myometrial hypertrophy that may show a trabeculated cut surface. Small, irregular, haemorrhagic lesions—some of which are cystic—may be seen within the affected myometrium.

Microscopically, irregular nests endometrial stroma are found deep within uterine wall. These can be involved in hyperplasia and carcinoma.

Fibroids (leiomyomas)

These are benign smooth muscle tumours that arise in the wall of the uterus (myometrium). They are the most common of all pelvic tumours, affecting over half of all women over the age of 30, usually becoming symptomatic in the decade before the menopause. Their cause is unknown but risk factors include:

- age—rare under 30 years
- race—more common in Afro-Caribbean populations
- parity—more common in nulliparous and women with low fertility
- genetic—often a family history.

Leiomyomas have the following features:

- oestrogen sensitivity
- fast growth in pregnancy
- shrinking at menopause or with antigonadotrophic hormone therapy.

Sites within the uterus (Fig.15.3) are:

- subserosal—just beneath the peritoneum on the outer uterine surface
- intramural (most common)—surrounded by smooth muscle within the uterine wall
- submucosal—lying immediately below the endometrium.

Macroscopically, they are:

- white/cream, rounded, rubbery, pale nodules with a whorled cut surface.

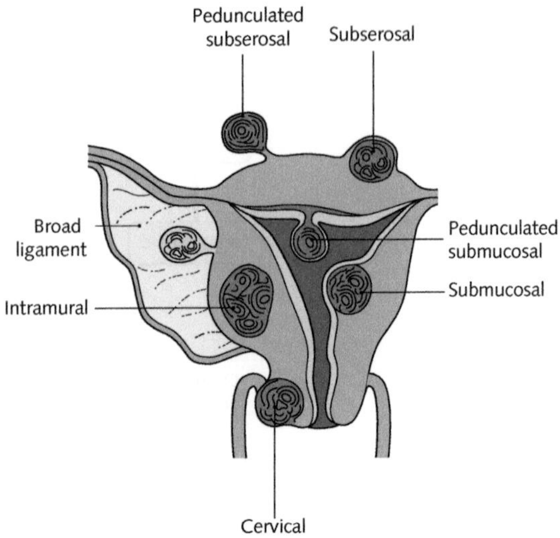

Fig. 15.3 Fibroids within the uterus.

- well-circumscribed with pseudocapsule. They may become pedunculated forming polyps.
- variable size. Most common are 2–4 cm but they range from <1 cm to 20–30 cm in diameter.
- typically multiple.

Microscopically they are seen as:

- nodules of smooth muscle cells forming bundles and fascicles with intervening collagenous stroma.
- lacking cellular atypia with very few mitoses and no areas of necrosis or haemorrhage (compared with malignant leiomyosarcomas).

Malignant change in leiomyomas is considered extremely rare.

Clinical features—leiomyomas may present with abnormal menstrual bleeding, dysmenorrhoea and infertility.

Complications occur following ischaemic (red) degeneration, pregnancy and compression.

Investigations are by ultrasound and laparoscopy.

Management is:

- surgical—women who no longer wish to conceive usually undergo hysterectomy.
- medical—uterine leiomyomas may be shrunk by gonadotrophin-releasing hormone (GnRH) agonists, which induce hypooestrogenism. They are used prior to surgery for easier surgical removal by myomectomy. Prolonged use will cause osteoporosis.

COMMON PITFALLS

FIBROIDS AND FIBROMAS

Remember that fibroids are not fibromas. Fibroids are benign tumours of smooth muscle (leiomyomas).

Leiomyosarcoma

This is a malignant tumour of smooth muscle cells. It is the most common uterine sarcoma but is rare, overall accounting for 1%–2% of all uterine malignancies. It occurs in older women (mean age 54 years) and is not thought to arise from fibroids.

Macroscopically, it appears as a large (>5 cm), bulky, fleshy tumour with necrosis, haemorrhagic areas and invasion. Unlike leiomyomas, they are solitary not multiple.

Microscopically, they are characterized by atypical, pleomorphic smooth muscle cells with numerous mitoses and areas of necrosis. Prognosis is poor, approximately 40% survival at 5 years, as the tumour is locally aggressive and reoccurrence is common.

Endometrial stromal sarcoma

This is a very rare uterine sarcoma which accounts for 0.2% of all uterine malignancies. It occurs in 42–58 year olds, a younger age group compared with that of leiomyosarcomas, and present with abnormal uterine bleeding. Microscopically, they are composed of sheets of endometrial stromal-like cells that form sharply defined tumour islands extensively penetrating the myometrium and lymphatics. Prognosis if confined to the uterus is 54%–100% survival at 5 years, if beyond the uterus there is 30% survival at 5 years.

DISORDERS OF THE OVARY AND FALLOPIAN TUBE

Inflammatory disorders and infections

Salpingitis

Inflammation of the fallopian tube(s).

Acute salpingitis

Aetiology—it is almost always caused by ascending infection from the uterine cavity.

Predisposing factors are:

- following pregnancy and endometritis
- following insertion of an intrauterine contraceptive device (IUCD)
- sexually transmitted diseases *(Mycoplasma, Chlamydia* and gonococci).

Macroscopically, tubes are distended and congested with a red and granular serosal surface due to vascular dilatation.

Microscopically, tubal epithelium shows neutrophil infiltration and the lumen may contain pus.

Chronic inflammation may supervene, with sequelae of fibrosis and occlusion of the tubal lumen on resolution.

Complications

- Infertility—fibrosis causes distortion and fusion of mucosal plicae causing occlusion of the tubal lumen.
- Ectopic (tubal) pregnancy.
- Pyosalpinx—massive distension of tubal lumen by pus.
- Tubo-ovarian abscess—resulting from spread of tubal inflammatory exudate.
- Peritonitis—from rupture and expulsion of the inflammatory contents of the abscess.
- Hydrosalpinx—dilatation of a fallopian tube by clear watery fluid (product of the proteolysis of pus on resolution of an infection).

Pelvic inflammatory disease

Pelvic inflammatory disease (PID) is a combined infection of the upper female genital tract including fallopian tubes, ovaries and peritoneum, which primarily affects young sexually active women. It is typically a result of ascending infection from the cervix or, less commonly, postoperative infection. Predisposing factors are as for suppurative salpingitis (see previously) and sexually transmitted diseases.

Neisseria gonorrhoeae and *Chlamydia trachomatis* are the most common responsible organisms, although anaerobic organisms are often found in pelvic abscesses.

Inflammation is initially acute and, without prompt treatment, may progress to chronic PID, which often results in tubal infertility and increases the risk of ectopic pregnancies.

Clinical features are:

- symptoms—gradual onset of pelvic pain, irregular bleeding, vaginal discharge, fever.
- signs—abdominal tenderness and guarding; extreme tenderness of the adnexa.

Treatment is by the removal of an IUCD (if present) and the use of broad-spectrum antibiotics.

Ovarian cysts

Ovarian cystic lesions are extremely common. They can be either neoplastic or nonneoplastic. The majority of nonneoplastic cysts arise from developing Graafian follicles; a minority are derived from surface epithelium. They naturally involute in 2–3 months. Persistence however, is a sign of possible neoplasia.

Follicular cysts

These unruptured, enlarged Graafian follicles (>3 cm) are lined by granulosa cells, with an outer coat of thecal cells. These are a common finding during the reproductive years and typically disappear by the resorption of fluid. Most cysts are clinically insignificant though some may secrete oestradiol which can lead to dysfunctional uterine bleeding. Torsion with haemorrhagic infarction is also possible.

Corpus luteum cysts

Are derived from the corpus lutea of pregnancy or menstruation on failure of regression. They are lined by organized luteinized cells and have a cystic haemorrhagic lumen. They can cause irregular menses and can rupture into the peritoneum resulting in an acute abdomen.

Simple cysts

These may represent cysts of follicular origin or epithelial inclusion. The exact classification may not be possible due to a lack of an identifiable lining. They are usually <10 cm and may present as an adnexal mass.

Polycystic ovary syndrome

This is characterized by the classic association of hyperandrogenism, hirsutism, anovulation and infertility and is a metabolic disorder independent of any adrenal or pituitary diseases. Diagnostically at least two out of the following must be present:

1. Polycystic ovaries on ultrasound scan.
2. Clinical (acne, hirsutism) or biochemical hyperandrogenism.
3. Persistent menstrual dysfunction with anovulation.

Patients may also have associated acne and occasional galactorrhoea.

Macroscopically there is bilateral, globular enlargement of the ovaries that demonstrate a linear arrangement of subcapsular follicles (4–8 mm) which contain clear fluid. Microscopically, a thickened capsule covers the cysts, which are at the same stage of development. Prominent follicular atresia and thecal cell hyperplasia are seen.

Complications—polycystic ovary syndrome (PCOS) can manifest with hyperinsulinaemia and hyperlipidaemia, and is compounded by obesity. These can lead to cardiovascular disease and diabetes mellitus. High oestrogen levels may cause endometrial hyperplasia and increase the risk of the development of endometrial carcinoma. Recurrent miscarriage is also well recognized.

Neoplasms of the ovary

Ovarian cancer is responsible for more deaths than any other gynaecological malignancy (7000 cases per year in the United Kingdom, with 4000 deaths), largely because it often presents at an advanced stage. The ovarian tumour marker CA125 is used routinely to monitor for relapse in patients who have undergone treatment. However, it cannot be used as a screening tool as it is has poor sensitivity and specificity.

Primary ovarian cancers account for 4% of all malignancies in women, but only 5%–10% have a direct hereditary component. In these women, mutations are usually found in either the *BRCA1* or *BRCA2* tumour suppressor genes (see Chapter 4). Ninety-five percent of ovarian cancer cases are sporadic and show complex genetic abnormalities, including a high incidence of *p53* mutation (50% of cases) and amplification of the *erbB-2 (HER-2/neu)* oncogene (30% of cases).

There are many types of ovarian tumours and a logical way of classifying them is according to the normal tissue constituents from which they are derived (Fig. 15.4).

Epithelial tumours

Epithelial tumours of the ovary comprise about 70% of all ovarian tumours and about 90% of malignant tumours. They are typically found in adult life.

As with all ovarian tumours, it appears that there is a decreased risk associated with pregnancy and the oral contraceptive pill. This is part of the 'incessant ovulation' hypothesis, whereby continuous monthly repair of the ovarian epithelium has been suggested as one factor in the development of ovarian cancer.

Types—the exact origin of epithelial tumours is unclear and there is now evidence to suggest they arise from the fimbrial end of fallopian tubes. There are at least five recognised types of epithelial tumours:

- Tubal differentiation (serous tumours: high and low grade)
- Endometrial differentiation (endometrial and clear cell tumours)
- Endocervical differentiation (mucinous tumours)
- Transitional differentiation (Brenner tumours).

Microscopically, these tumours are classified into benign, borderline (abnormal tissue architecture with atypical cells but no evidence of invasion) and malignant. The majority

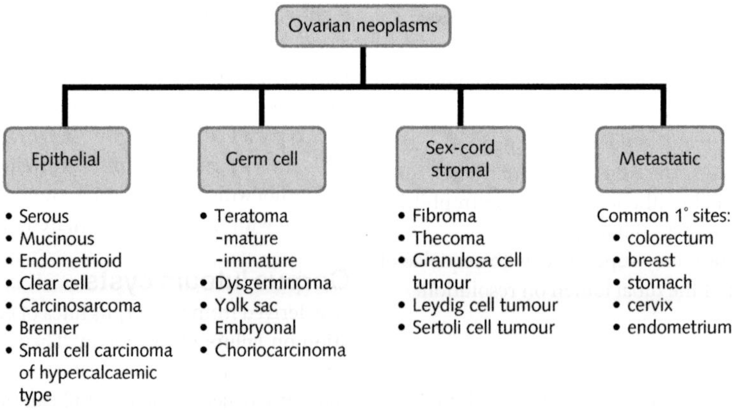

Fig. 15.4 Classification of ovarian neoplasms.

of borderline tumours behave in a benign fashion but some appear capable of low-grade malignancy.

Serous tumours of the ovary

Account for 30%–40% of all ovarian tumours and the majority are benign. A frequent histological finding is concentrically laminated calcified concretions called psammoma bodies.

Benign/borderline: serous cystadenoma—thin-walled, unilocular cystic tumour lined by regular columnar epithelium with or without cilia that may have papillary lesions. They can occur at any age but are most common in the fifth decade. Borderline lesions are characterized by arborizing papillae and nuclear atypia with no frank stromal invasion. They may be multiloculated.

Malignant: Two types of serous ovarian carcinomas are recognized: low grade and high grade. They are considered separate entities and not part of a progressive spectrum as their aetiologies are different.

- ***Low-grade serous carcinoma***—their development is driven by constitutive activation of the MAPK pathway caused by upstream mutations in KRAS, BRAF and erbB-2. They account for the minority of ovarian malignancies (<5%) and follow a stepwise progression from benign → borderline → invasive low grade.
- ***High-grade serous carcinomas***—over 90% have TP53 mutations and are thought to arise from epithelial precursor lesions in the fimbrial end of fallopian tubes: serous tubal intraepithelial carcinomas (STICs). It is thought that these lesions implant onto the ovaries resulting in high-grade carcinoma with no intervening stepwise progression.

Serous carcinomas account for the majority of ovarian malignancies (>70%) and present at an advanced stage with poor outcome. They occur in patients with BRCA mutations.

Endometrioid tumours of the ovary

These ovarian tumours show endometrial differentiation. The vast majority are malignant (endometrioid carcinomas), accounting for 20% of all ovarian carcinomas. They are strongly associated with endometriosis and a synchronous endometrial carcinoma is present in 15–20% of cases. Macroscopically they form cystic, solid masses and contain blood-stained fluid.

Clear cell tumours of the ovary

Clear cell ovarian carcinoma is characterized by the presence of cells with clear cytoplasm that contain abundant glycogen. The nuclei are pleomorphic and bulge into the lumen ('hobnail' appearance). In up to a quarter of cases there is a background atypical endometriotic cyst.

Mucinous tumours of the ovary

These multilocular cystic ovarian tumours of endocervical differentiation contain sticky gelatinous mucin. They are usually unilateral and large, 10–30 cm in diameter.

- Benign (mucinous cystadenoma)—no atypical features or mitoses.
- Borderline mucinous tumours—presence of cellular atypia but with no invasion.
- Malignant (mucinous cystadenocarcinoma)—invasion of the ovarian stroma. Less than 10% of mucinous tumours are malignant. Usually huge with solid areas.

Mucinous tumours can be complicated by pseudomyxoma peritonei if they rupture into the peritoneum (see Chapter 11).

Brenner tumours of the ovary (transitional cell)

Rare tumours that are composed of nests of epithelium resembling transitional cell epithelium of the urinary tract, set within a spindle-cell stroma. The epithelial component may be benign, borderline or malignant. The majority are unilateral and benign and can present with postmenopausal bleeding as the tumour can cause endometrial hyperplasia. In up to 20% of cases there is an associated mucinous cyst adenoma.

Germ cell and sex cord stromal tumours

Germ cell tumours arise from primordial germ cells and represent distorted forms of embryogenesis. They account for 30% of all ovarian tumours and 95% are benign.

The precise origin of sex cord stromal tumours is unknown but they represent steroid-producing ovarian cells and gonadal sex cords and account for 8% of all ovarian tumours. The most common is the mature teratoma (dermoid cyst). Ovarian germ cell and sex cord stromal tumours are summarized in Table 15.4.

Dermoid cyst

These contain a variable number of haphazardly arranged tissues derived from each germ cell layer. Usually they are cystic, containing hair and sebaceous material, although they are infamous for producing teeth. They are also known as teratomas and can be benign or malignant.

Meigs syndrome

This is a triad of ascites, hydrothorax and a benign ovarian tumour. The most common tumours are fibromas and fibrothecomas. The pathogenesis is unknown and symptoms resolve on removal of the tumour.

Metastatic tumours

The ovary is a common site of metastasis, which account for approximately 8% of ovarian tumours. They may be of Müllerian origin (e.g., uterus, fallopian tubes) or from extra-Müllerian sites (typically the breast and gastrointestinal tract).

Krukenberg tumour

This describes bilaterally enlarged ovaries containing metastatic signet ring-cell adenocarcinoma (typically of gastric origin).

Table 15.4 Germ cell and sex cord stromal ovarian tumours[a]

Tumour	% of all ovarian tumours	Age	Appearance	Features	Behaviour
Germ cell tumours					
Mature cystic teratomas (dermoid cyst)	27%–44%	20–40 years, although can be younger	Cyst usually containing hair and sebaceous material plus other tissue, e.g., teeth	Cysts composed of various epithelial types from ectodermal, mesodermal and endodermal origin, e.g., skin, smooth muscle, bowel Fully differentiated	Benign
Immature teratomas	1%	Children and young adults, mean age 18 years	Solid with areas of necrosis and haemorrhage in addition to usual type of dermoid cyst	Similar to mature but contain immature tissue – usually neural	Malignant
Dysgerminoma	1%–2%	Children and young adults, mean age 22 years	• 90% unilateral • Solid, soft and fleshy • White/tan appearance • Polyhedral cells	Similar to seminoma of the testis Raised LDH	Malignant, 1/3 aggressive
Yolk sac tumours	<1%	Mean age 18 years Rare in >40 year olds	• Solid/cystic • Haemorrhagic and necrotic • Microscopic: Schiller–Duval bodies	Secrete α-fetoprotein Raised CA125	Malignant
Embryonal carcinoma	Very rare	Young Mean age 12 years	• Unilateral • Solid • Variegated with haemorrhagic foci • Primitive cells	Can secrete hCG Often found as a component of mixed germ cell tumour	Malignant
Sex cord stromal tumours					
Fibroma	4%	All ages, peak 50–60 years	Unilateral Solid hard, lobulated white/grey masses Composed of fibroblasts with varying amount of thecal differentiation	Unilateral Can be associated with Meigs syndrome	Benign
Thecoma	<1%	Mean 59 years	Unilateral Solid yellow Spindle cells with vacuolated cytoplasm containing lipid	Oestrogen producing, 20% have concurrent endometrial carcinoma	Benign
Granulosa cell tumours	1%–2%	2/3 postmenopausal but any age possible	Unilateral Solid/cystic Yellow/white Oval cells with grooved nuclei Call–Exner bodies	Size ranges from microscopic to macroscopic Oestrogen secreting	Malignant
Sertoli–Leydig cell tumours	<0.5%	Peak second/third decade Mean age 25 years	Unilateral Solid, lobulated and yellow Tubules of Sertoli cells, fibrous stroma and nests of Leydig cells Reinke crystals in Leydig cells	Mixture of cell types usually seen in the testis Commonly masculinization occurs	Benign

[a] *Summary of the key features of ovarian sex cord stromal tumours and germ cell tumours. Oestrogen-secreting tumours induce a relative hyperoestrogenic state that results in a variety of symptoms, e.g., postmenopausal bleeding, irregular bleeding, etc.*
hCG, Human chorionic gonadotrophin; LDH, lactate dehydrogenase.

DISORDERS OF THE PLACENTA AND PREGNANCY

Ectopic pregnancy

This describes any fertilized ovum that is implanted outside the uterine cavity. Ectopic pregnancy occurs in 1 in 300 pregnancies. The fallopian tube (especially in the ampulla) is by far the most common site for this; other sites of abnormal implantation are very rare but include the peritoneal cavity, ovary, cervix and scars.

The aetiology is uncertain but it is possibly the result of some structural abnormality of the fallopian tube, e.g., scarring or adhesions, resulting from previous episodes of salpingitis, endometriosis or previous tubal surgery for contraceptive purposes, i.e., sterilization. However, half of ectopic pregnancies occur without such predisposing factors.

Pathogenesis—following implantation, the proliferating trophoblasts erode the submucosal blood vessels, precipitating severe bleeding into the tubal lumen (haematosalpinx). The muscular wall of the fallopian tube is unable to undergo hypertrophy or distension and so tubal pregnancy is at high risk of rupture.

The types of rupture are:

- into the lumen of the fallopian tube—common in ampullary pregnancy. Mild haemorrhage into the peritoneal cavity occurs, which may collect as a clot in the pouch of Douglas.
- into the peritoneal cavity—occurs most commonly from the isthmus of the tube. Haemorrhage is likely to be severe.
- Retroperitoneal (rare)—rupture occurs into the potential space between the leaves of the broad ligament. Haemorrhage into this site is more likely to be controlled.

RED FLAG

CLINICAL FEATURES OF AN ECTOPIC PREGNANCY

Clinical features of an ectopic rupture are:

- severe lower abdominal pain—usually localized to the side of the ectopic pregnancy with or without referred pain to the shoulder tip.
- vaginal bleeding—occurs after fetal death and is an effect of oestrogen withdrawal.
- signs of anaemia—due to internal blood loss.
- shock, which may occur if haemorrhage is severe and rapid, e.g., due to large vessel erosion. This is the most dangerous and dramatic consequence of tubal pregnancy.

Spontaneous abortion

Many fertilized ova fail to implant successfully. It has been estimated that around 40% of all conceptions fail to convert into recognisable pregnancies. Of those that survive this far, 15% terminate in a clinically recognised spontaneous abortion.

Aetiology—causes of spontaneous abortion differ according to the stage of pregnancy, as shown in Table 15.5.

HINTS AND TIPS

CAUSES OF ABORTION

To remember the causes of abortion at different stages of pregnancy, learn the following rules of thumb:

- First trimester causes—majority are associated with abnormal fetuses.
- Second trimester causes—mainly due to uterine abnormalities.
- Third trimester causes—mainly the result of maternal abnormalities.

Table 15.5 Causes of spontaneous abortion

Time	Cause
First trimester	• Abnormal chromosomal karyotypes, particularly Turner syndrome • Structural developmental abnormalities, e.g., neural tube defects • Maternal systemic lupus erythematosus • Transplacental infection, e.g., *Brucella*, *Listeria*, rubella, *Toxoplasma*, cytomegalovirus and herpes
Second trimester	• Chorioamnionitis • Rupture of membranes • Placental haemorrhages • Structural abnormalities of the uterus, e.g., congenital uterine malformations • Large submucosal leiomyomas • Incompetence of the cervix • Abnormal placentation (but more common in third trimester)
Third trimester	• Uncontrolled hypertension • Eclampsia • Placental abnormalities, e.g., placental haemorrhage, abruption and infarction
At any time	• Endocrine abnormalities: diabetes, hypothyroidism, deficiency of progesterone or luteinizing hormone • Trauma: surgical operation, blow to abdomen, • or hypotensive shock

Nonneoplastic disorders of the placenta

Chorioamnionitis

Inflammation of the fetal membranes (chorion and amnion) characterized by a diffuse neutrophilic infiltrate. The membranes can appear dull and the amniotic fluid cloudy. This is the maternal response to ascending infection from the vagina. A fetal response to the infection (funisitis—inflammation of the umbilical cord) may also be present. The most commonly involved organisms include: group B streptococcus, listeria, *Ureaplasma spp.* and *Gardnerella*. Infection can result in neonatal sepsis, preterm labour and stillbirth.

Placenta accreta, increta and percreta

A spectrum of disorders of abnormal placental implantation whereby the placenta is retained through morbid adherence to the uterine wall. The designation accreta, increta and percreta reflect the degree of placental invasion through the myometrium (Fig. 15.5). They are a cause of second trimester vaginal bleeding and confer a high degree of maternal and fetal morbidity.

Risk factors include previous caesarean section, placenta previa and increased maternal age. The continued rise in incidence directly correlates with the increasing number of caesarean sections performed.

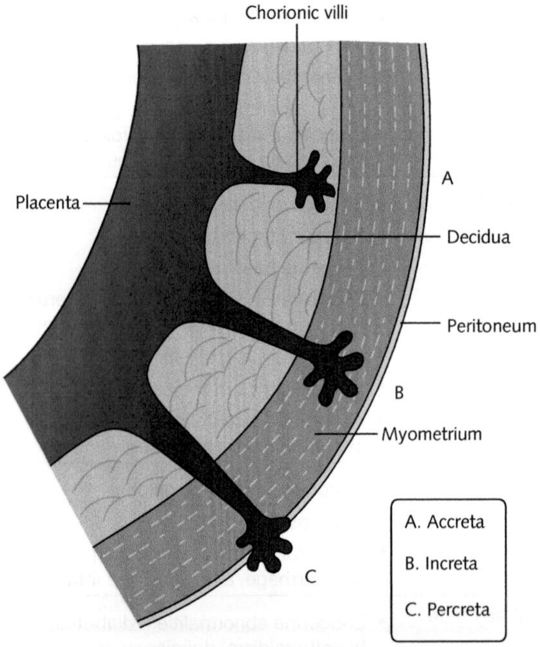

Fig. 15.5 Placenta accreta, increta and percreta. *(A)* Accreta – chorionic villi adherent to myometrium but not invading. *(B)* Increta – chorionic villi invade into the myometrium. *(C)* Percreta – chorionic villi invade through myometrium and into the peritoneum.

Vanishing twin syndrome

This is the apparent disappearance of a fetus in a multigestational pregnancy. Fetal demise is due to chromosomal/developmental abnormalities. The fetus may be reabsorbed, mummified (fetus papyraceus), adherent to the placenta/membranes or may result in a placental anomaly, e.g., a cyst.

Gestational trophoblastic disease

Gestational trophoblastic disease is a group of disorders covering abnormal proliferation of placental tissue and include complete and partial moles, invasive moles, choriocarcinoma and placental site trophoblastic tumour.

Hydatidiform mole

The abnormal development of gestational trophoblast leading to the formation of a benign mass of grape-like clusters of chorionic villi (Fig. 15.6). It occurs in 1 in 2000 pregnancies in the UK and USA, but it is seen more frequently amongst some ethnic groups, such as the Japanese population.

The disease is the result of an error in embryogenesis; the aetiopathogenesis is unknown Table 15.6. There are two types:

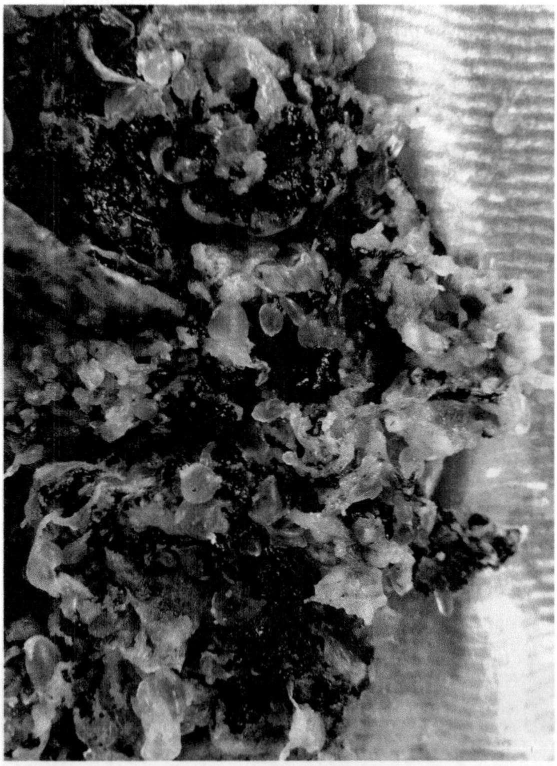

Fig. 15.6 Macroscopic appearance of a complete hydatiform mole. Numerous grape-like clusters of chorionic villi are seen. 'Hydatisa' = a drop of water, 'mola' = false conception.

Table 15.6 Complete and partial hydatiform moles

	Complete mole	Partial mole
Fertilization	One sperm fertilizes a genetically empty egg.	Two sperm fertilize a normal egg.
Genetic material	All paternal	Paternal and maternal
Chromosomal complement	46XX (85%) or 46XY (15%)	Most triploid: 69XXY most common, 69XYY, 69XXX
Embryo present	Not present	Present but usually dies early
Macroscopic appearance	Large clusters of grape-like villi No normal placenta present	Scattered vesicles Placenta present
Microscopic appearance	All chorionic villi abnormal. Large round villi with central cistern formation. Circumferential villous trophoblast hyperplasia	Mixed normal and abnormal chorionic villi Focal cystic swelling of villi with irregular outline Focal trophoblast hyperplasia
Choriocarcinoma	Increased risk 2%–3% Invasive mole 5%–10%	No increased risk

1. ***Complete mole***—entirely of paternal origin (no maternal genetic contribution) and usually forms a bulky mass of grape-like villi that may fill the uterine cavity. There is an excess proliferation of trophoblast and no fetus is present. The risk of subsequent choriocarcinoma is greater than in a partial mole (3% of cases).
2. ***Partial mole***—a partial mole is triploid with most containing one maternal and two paternal haploid sets of chromosomes. Cystic vesicles are found in only a part of the placenta. Fetal parts and some normal placental villi are present along with the abnormal trophoblastic tissue. There is a low risk of subsequent development of choriocarcinoma.

Clinical features:

- Amenorrhoea and other symptoms of pregnancy, followed by continuous or intermittent vaginal bleeding.
- Miscarriage—many molar pregnancies spontaneously miscarry.
- Enlarged soft uterus—often larger than dates would suggest.

Diagnosis is by elevated human chorionic gonadotrophin (hCG) excretion in urine (typically much greater than in normal pregnancies) and by ultrasound for the absence of the fetus. Very high hCG levels may cause extreme morning sickness (hyperemesis gravidarum), promote preeclampsia and can cause hyperthyroidism as hCG has a mild thyroid-stimulating effect.

Treatment is by evacuation of the uterus, with a second aspiration or curettage 2–4 weeks later to ensure complete removal of the mole.

Follow up is by regular hCG levels for at least a year. Detection of hCG may suggest incomplete removal and the persistence of trophoblastic disease. Untreated, this carries a risk of subsequent choriocarcinoma.

Invasive mole

This is a hydatidiform mole that penetrates through the decidua into the myometrium and associated blood vessels. Perforation of the uterus may occur, resulting in invasion of the parametrium. Embolization to other organs, such as lung and vagina, is possible. True malignant transformation is rare.

Choriocarcinoma

This is a malignant tumour of syncytiotrophoblast and cytotrophoblast with absent chorionic villi. It has a propensity for invading vessel walls with blood-borne metastases occurring early to many sites, particularly the lung, brain and liver.

They are rare in the United Kingdom and the United States (at 1 per 50,000 pregnancies) but more common in Asia, South America and Africa.

Aetiology—approximately 70% develop from a hydatidiform mole (majority complete moles), 20% from spontaneous abortion and 10% arise after a normal pregnancy with a variable time lag (months to years).

The prognosis is excellent as the tumours are highly sensitive to cytotoxic chemotherapy (particularly if posttreatment monitoring of hCG levels is carried out).

HINTS AND TIPS

CHORIOCARCINOMA

Choriocarcinoma is not a malignancy exclusive to the placenta. It also occurs in the testis (usually as part of a mixed germ cell tumour) and the ovary.

Placental site trophoblastic tumour

This is a very rare tumour composed of extravillous (intermediate) trophoblast with absent villi arising from the placental implantation site. Trophoblast are seen invading the myometrium but abundant haemorrhage and necrosis are not present, unlike choriocarcinoma. They typically follow nonmolar gestations and are mostly benign, but their behaviour is difficult to predict, i.e., they can be aggressive.

DISORDERS OF THE BREAST

The structure of the normal breast is illustrated in Fig. 15.7.

Nonneoplastic disorders

Acute mastitis and breast abscess

These are uncommon and are usually complications of lactation. The most frequent organism is *Staphylococcus aureus*, which gains access through cracks and fissures of the nipple and areola. An abscess may form if drainage is inadequate.

Mammary duct ectasia

In mammary duct ectasia there is an abnormal progressive dilatation of the large breast ducts, which accumulate inspissated (thickened) secretions. The aetiology is unknown and it affects older women (perimenopausal age range). Patients develop a firm breast lump, but this does not mimic a carcinoma. There may also be a clear or green-coloured nipple discharge.

Fat necrosis

This is usually caused by trauma. Histology shows necrosis with multinucleated giant cells and later fibrosis. It may cause a discrete lump mimicking a carcinoma.

Fibrocystic change

This is a generic term for a number of benign lesions that may occur together, producing lumpiness in the breast tissue. Peak incidence is around the menopause. It is thought that fibrocystic change is caused by hormonal imbalance. Diagnosis is confirmed by needle aspiration of clear fluid (blood-stained aspirate requires further investigation) or biopsy.

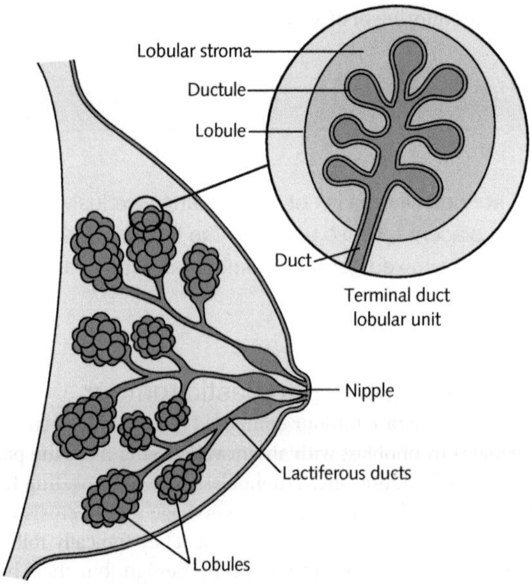

Fig. 15.7 Diagram of the breast.

The histological changes that may be present include:

- cysts—ranging in size from microscopic to palpable lesions 1–2 cm in diameter.
- apocrine metaplasia—epithelial lining of hyperplastic ducts undergoes metaplasia to that of normal apocrine glands.
- fibrosis—replacement of breast tissue by dense fibrous tissue, which can be due to cyst rupture
- sclerosing adenosis—marked proliferation of specialized hormone-responsive stromal tissue and myoepithelial cells, i.e., the number of acini per lobule increases. This forms localized areas of irregular stellate, collagenous sclerosis in which epithelial elements are also present. Occasionally difficult to distinguish from some patterns of invasive carcinoma.

There is no increased risk of a carcinoma unless there is accompanying epithelial hyperplasia (see later).

Epithelial hyperplasia

This describes the proliferation of epithelial cells within ducts or lobules (ductal hyperplasia and lobular hyperplasia respectively). There are two types:

1. Hyperplasia of the usual type—normal cytology and tissue architecture with no signs of malignancy.
2. Hyperplasia of atypical type—biological spectrum between some abnormalities of cytology/architecture and carcinoma in situ.

The risk of subsequent invasive breast carcinoma is increased in individuals with florid usual hyperplasia (1.5–2 fold), and further increased in subjects with atypical hyperplasia (4–5 fold).

Epithelial hyperplasia can only be diagnosed histologically.

> **CLINICAL NOTES**
>
> **TRIPLE ASSESSMENT**
>
> The best form of investigation of a breast mass is so-called 'triple assessment.' This consists of:
>
> - history and examination (of both the lump and regional nodes)
> - imaging (mammography, ultrasound or magnetic resonance imaging)
> - tissue sampling (fine-needle aspiration or core biopsy)

Neoplasms of the breast

Breast lumps are relatively common presentations. Discrete breast lumps or nipple discharge may be a sign of malignancy or a mimic of carcinoma.

DIFFERENTIAL DIAGNOSIS

BENIGN BREAST LUMPS

- Fat necrosis
- Abscess
- Intraductal papilloma
- Fibroadenoma/(benign) phyllodes tumour
- Nodular sclerosing adenosis
- Hamartoma
- Duct ectasia

Fibroadenoma

This is the most common benign tumour of the female breast. There is proliferation of both stroma and epithelium, usually in young women (most frequently the 25–35-year age group). It produces discrete but mobile breast lumps typically 1–4 cm in size, often multiple and bilateral.

Phyllodes tumour

This is a tumour composed of both stroma and epithelium, but the stroma is more cellular than in fibroadenomas. It is less common than fibroadenoma and occurs in the older age group (peak incidence being 45 years of age). Clinically, the tumour presents as a breast lump.

Macroscopically, they are rubbery white lesions consisting of a whorled pattern with slit-like spaces and solid areas.

Microscopically, there is leaf-like architecture. They are classified as benign (90% of cases), borderline (intermediate malignant potential) or malignant.

There is the potential for local recurrence with increasing aggressiveness, and the tumour may eventually metastasize. Phyllodes tumours are therefore excised with a wide margin or, if necessary, are treated by mastectomy.

Papillary lesions

Epithelial proliferation within ducts produces papillary structures. These occur in older women and may produce a blood-stained nipple discharge. Papillomas are usually solitary with no increased risk of a carcinoma. However, a rare condition of multiple intraductal papillomas is premalignant, often showing nuclear atypia and in-situ malignancy.

Carcinoma

Incidence—This comprises 25% of all cancers in women and is the most common cause of death in 35–55-year-old women, increasing with age steeply to 45 years and continuing to increase less steeply thereafter. There are around 55,000 cases each year in the UK; 5-year survival is 86%. There is a 200-fold female preponderance, with the highest rates in America, Western Europe and the Antipodes; the lowest rates are in Africa and Southeast Asia.

Table 15.7 Predisposing factors of breast carcinoma

Predisposing factors for breast carcinoma
Atypical epithelial proliferation (DCIS, LCIS)
First-degree relative with breast cancer (independent of BRCA mutations)
Oestrogen exposure: • Long interval between menarche and menopause • Older age at first pregnancy • Postmenopausal hormone replacement therapy (oestrogen and progesterone) • Contraceptives (oestrogen and progesterone)
Obesity
Alcohol
Ionizing radiation to the chest, e.g., radiotherapy for Hodgkin disease
Increasing age
Increased breast density

DCIS, Ductal carcinoma in situ; LCIS, Lobular carcinoma in situ.

MOLECULAR

BRCA1 AND 2

BRCA 1 (chromosome 17) and *BRCA2* (chromosome 13) are tumour suppressor genes found to be mutated in 20%–25% of hereditary breast cancers and 10% of all breast cancers. Twelve percent of the general population will develop breast cancer, compared with inherited BRCA mutations:

- *BRCA1* mutations: 55%–65% will develop breast cancer.
- *BRCA2* mutation 45% will develop breast cancer.

Predisposing factors of carcinoma

Carcinoma in situ

Ductal carcinoma in situ—Ductal carcinoma in situ (DCIS) refers to neoplastic cells confined to the ducts, with no evidence of invasion through the basement membrane. It may progress to invasive carcinoma, but is highly treatable at the in situ stage. DCIS is more common than lobular carcinoma in situ (LCIS) and can be associated with microcalcifications, which are identifiable on mammography. Treatment is dependent on size and grade, but usually comprises wide local excision and radiotherapy.

Lobular carcinoma in situ—LCIS is more common in younger women and is more likely to affect both breasts. There is an 8–10-fold increased risk of developing invasive carcinoma in either breast.

LCIS is not associated with calcifications on mammography or a mass, and is therefore often an incidental finding on biopsy. The cells are discohesive due to loss of E-cadherin (a cell adhesion protein). Classical (bland morphology) and pleomorphic variants exist.

Paget disease of the nipple

Like extramammary Paget disease in the vulva (see vulva above), the appearance of this intraepithelial neoplasm in the nipple is often an indicator of underlying in-situ or invasive malignancy.

Invasive carcinoma

All breast carcinomas are adenocarcinomas derived from epithelial cells of the terminal ductal lobules. Invasive carcinomas are tumours that have eroded through the basement membrane of their tissue of origin to invade surrounding structures. The most common presentation is a painless palpable mass, excluding those detected early by mammographic screening (see later).

Large masses may cause skin tethering or interfere with lymphatic drainage to produce classic dimpled skin changes (e.g., *peau d'orange*). Nipple retraction can also occur. Axillary lymph nodes may be palpable, reflecting metastasis from the primary site.

RED FLAG

INVASIVE BREAST CANCER

Invasive breast cancer usually presents as a *painless* breast lump or axillary mass.

Investigation is by ultrasound, mammography (less commonly magnetic resonance imaging), core biopsy or fine-needle aspiration cytology. Invasive carcinomas are categorized histologically:

- Invasive ductal (most common 75%)
  - Subtypes: mucinous, tubular, medullary, papillary
- Invasive lobular (E-cadherin negative, increased incidence of bilateral carcinoma)
  - Subtypes: classical, tubulo-lobular, pleomorphic
- Inflammatory carcinoma is characterized by extensive dermal lymphatic invasion.

Macroscopic features—a discrete lump with tethering to the skin or surrounding connective tissue. The macroscopic appearance of the tumour depends on the amount and type of stroma within the carcinoma.

Spread is as follows:

- Direct—skin and muscles of the chest wall
- Lymphatic—axillary lymph nodes (early drainage site), internal mammary lymph nodes
- Haematogenous—lungs, bone, liver, and brain
- Transcoelomic—pleural cavities and pericardium.

Management and prognosis

The mainstay of treatment is surgical excision, often with axillary node clearance. Radiotherapy and chemotherapy are often used after surgery to reduce the risk of relapse.

Prognosis—related to tumour grade and type, size of the tumour, lymph node status and oestrogen/progesterone and *HER-2* receptor status.

Tumour, node, metastasis (TNM) staging for breast carcinoma is used to guide treatment and determine prognosis.

MOLECULAR

ER, PR AND HER2

Hormone receptor (oestrogen (ER) and progesterone receptor (PR)) status of tumours are determined as an indicator of response to tamoxifen therapy. Low-grade tumours tend to have positive receptor status and are more likely to respond to therapy. *C-erbB-2 (HER-2)* is a protooncogene that is found in 15%–20% of breast cancers. It is associated with poorer prognosis, but this may be improved by novel monoclonal antibody therapy (Herceptin).

Screening for breast carcinoma

There is no direct screening method equivalent to the cytology of the uterine cervix. The primary screening modality is mammography, which is more effective in older women with less radiodense breast tissue. Abnormalities seen on mammograms include calcification and soft tissue deformity. In the UK, there is a National Health Service Breast Screening Programme with 3-yearly mammography for all women between 50–70 years. Long-term studies suggest that such screening successfully reduces the mortality from breast carcinoma; it is possible that the age range screened may be extended in the future.

The male breast

Gynaecomastia

This is the benign enlargement of breast tissue.

Aetiology—hormonal influences including increased oestrogen production or receptor sensitivity. It is associated with liver cirrhosis, stilboestrol therapy for prostate carcinoma and drugs, e.g., chlorpromazine.

HINTS AND TIPS

DISCO

Remember the pneumonic 'DISCO' for drugs causing gynaecomastia: ***D***igoxin, ***I***soniazid, ***S***pironolactone, ***C***imetidine, ***O***estrogens.

Carcinoma

Less than 1% of breast carcinomas occur in men. The condition is associated with Klinefelter syndrome and is usually of the ductal type; the lobular type is extremely rare.

DISORDERS OF THE PENIS

Nonneoplastic lesions

Infections

Inflammation of the glans (balanitis) and prepuce (posthitis) can be caused by a variety of bacterial, fungal and viral organisms. Congestion and oedema with exudate on the surface of the glans can cause ulceration and chronic scarring. If untreated, this is a common cause of phimosis. Further discussion is seen in Chapter 5.

Fournier gangrene

Necrotising fasciitis involving the genitalia secondary to bacterial infection along the fascial planes. Pain is severe and extends beyond visual limits of involved skin. A high index of clinical suspicion and rapid diagnosis are needed to prevent high mortality rates. Diagnosis is based on clinical acumen, not histological diagnosis. Early aggressive surgical management is required and involves extensive debridement or amputation to prevent systemic infection and death.

Lichen sclerosus et atrophicus

Clinically known as balanitis xerotica obliterans, it is characterized by a band of lichenoid inflammation and underlying band of sclerosis. It is the commonest cause of phimosis and is associated with squamous cell carcinoma.

Peyronie disease

Superficial fibrosis of fascia results in curvature of the penile shaft and painful erection. May occur secondary to chronic trauma or following infection.

Neoplasms of the penis

Carcinoma in situ

Penile intraepithelial neoplasia (PeIN) is seen in two forms: disease (opaque plaques with shallow ulceration) affecting the shaft and scrotum, and erythroplasia of Queyrat, which is restricted to the glans, presenting with flat, red, glistening plaques. As with VIN, the differentiated subtype is usually preceded by lichen sclerosus. A warty variant is associated with HPV infection (most commonly serotype 16). Penile intraepithelial neoplasia is a precancerous condition and may lead to invasive cancer unless treated vigorously.

Squamous cell carcinoma

This is a well-differentiated, keratinizing, invasive tumour usually seen in elderly men. It occurs most commonly in uncircumcised men and is thought to be associated with previous infection with HPV. It presents as a warty, cauliflower-like growth that bleeds easily. It is typically slow growing but it is often neglected because of patient embarrassment.

DISORDERS OF THE TESTIS AND EPIDIDYMIS

Congenital abnormalities and regression

Cryptorchidism (undescended testis)

This is a condition caused by maldescent of the testes, affecting about 5% at birth, and 1% by the first birthday. In the embryo, the testes develop from the genital ridge high on the posterior abdominal wall. At about 7 months' gestation, the testes migrate down the posterior abdominal wall. They are guided by a cord (the gubernaculum) through the inguinal ring into the scrotum.

Occasionally, migration fails to occur and one (75% of cases) or both (25% of cases) testes become arrested somewhere along the route (Fig. 15.8). There are three common sites of arrest:

1. Abdominal testicle—usually found just inside the internal ring of the inguinal canal.
2. Inguinal testicle—in the inguinal canal, particularly exposed to trauma.
3. Retractile testicle (most common)—either high or low, depending on ability to be manoeuvred into correct position. Usually settles at puberty and does not require surgical correction.

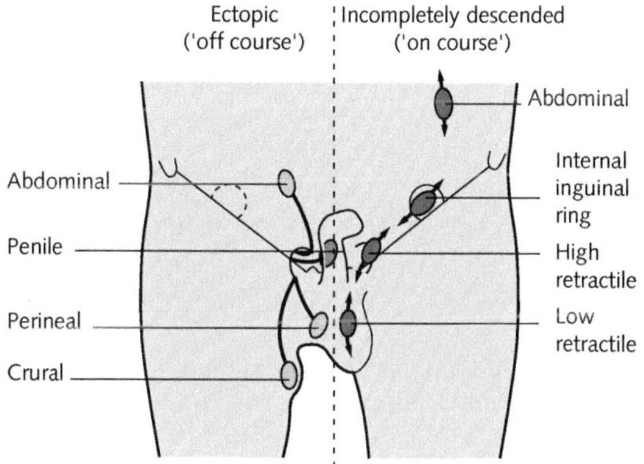

Fig. 15.8 Maldescended testes showing common sites of arrest. (Adapted with permission from Lecture Notes on Urology, 5th edn, by Blandy J, Blackwell Science, 1998.)

Complications

- Infertility—temperature of aberrant locations is higher than in the scrotum and prevents normal germ cell development. The testis remains small and incapable of producing effective spermatozoa.
- Malignancy—more common in an undescended testis; about 1 in 10 of all testicular tumours arise in association with cryptorchidism.
- Inguinal hernia—there is nearly always a patent tunica vaginalis that predisposes to the development of an inguinal hernia.
- Torsion of the testicle (see later).

Management is by detection and correction of testicular maldescent. This is important because of the increased risk of testicular carcinoma. Some restoration of function may be achieved by 'orchidopexy' at an early stage (the testis is surgically pulled down and fixed to the scrotum).

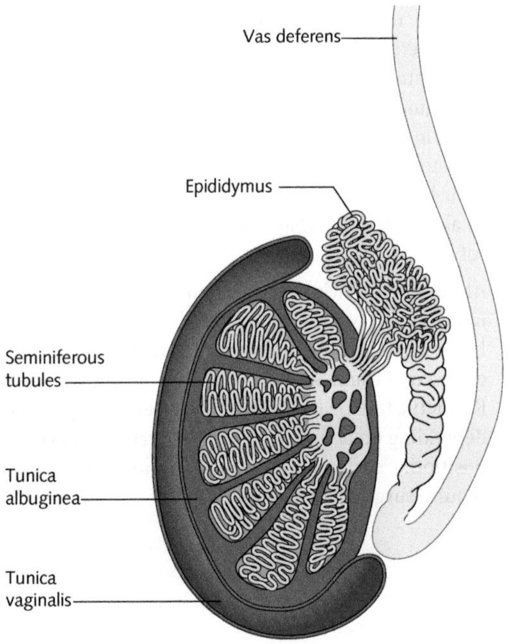

Fig. 15.9 Anatomy of the testis.

Abnormalities of the tunica vaginalis

The tunica vaginalis and tunica albuginea (membrane sheaths surrounding the testes) are invested with mesothelial cells and may be the site of fluid accumulation, inflammation or (uncommonly) tumour formation.

Hydrocele

Fluid which accumulates in the cavity bounded by the tunica vaginalis is termed a hydrocele. This is the most common cause of swelling within the scrotum.

This is often idiopathic, but the aetiology may involve:

- congenital patency of the processus vaginalis, often in continuity with the peritoneal cavity.
- formation secondary to tumours, epididymitis, mumps or acute orchitis.

Haematocele

Blood which accumulates in the cavity bounded by the tunica vaginalis is termed haematocele, and is usually due to trauma or torsion and rarely due to tumour spread.

Chylocele

Chylocele is an accumulation of lymph secondary to obstructed drainage.

Hernias

Indirect inguinal hernias (described in Chapter 11) typically occur as a result of patent processus vaginalis.

Orchitis

Orchitis is inflammation of the testicle, which usually arises following epididymitis. Commonest organisms are *E. coli*, *Chlamydia trachomatis*, *Neisseria gonorrhoeae*, and tuberculosis. Mumps orchitis may occur in unvaccinated children.

Epididymis

Epididymitis

Epididymitis usually arises after a urinary tract infection and can lead to orchitis (see previously).

Spermatocele

Accumulation of nonviable sperm within an epididymal cyst is termed a spermatocele.

Adenomatoid tumours

Adenomatoid tumours are the commonest para-testicular tumour. They are benign and are mesothelial in origin.

Trauma and vascular disturbances

Torsion

This is the twisting of a testicle on its pedicle with obstruction of venous return such that blood continues to enter the testis but cannot leave. The testis is engorged and painful, eventually becoming infarcted (venous infarction). In advanced torsion, the testis is almost black as a result of vascular congestion. Early detection and surgical release are required to preserve testicular viability. Surgical removal is necessary for advanced disease.

Varicocele

This describes variceal dilatation of the veins of the pampiniform plexus of the spermatic cord, and may occur due to compression or valve defect. The appearance is of a 'bag of worms'.

> **HINTS AND TIPS**
>
> **VARICOCELE AND RENAL TUMOUR**
>
> Left-sided varicoceles may indicate a left renal tumour. The left spermatic vein drains indirectly into the inferior vena cava via the left renal vein, whereas the right spermatic vein drains directly. Back pressure from a left renal tumour can therefore result in a varicocele.

Neoplasms of the testis

Tumours of the testis, although relatively uncommon, are important because many occur in young men; they are the most common tumour among 15–35-year-olds. The exact aetiology is unknown but there are links with testicular maldescent and/or dysgenesis, possibly with some genetic susceptibility.

Clinical presentations are:

- painless unilateral enlargement of testis (majority)
- secondary hydrocele
- symptoms of metastases—especially in malignant teratoma, e.g., haemoptysis from lung deposits
- endocrine effects—gynaecomastia, precocious puberty (typically from Leydig or Sertoli cell tumours).

There are two main groups of testicular tumour:

1. Germ cell tumours (97% of cases)—derived from multipotential germ cells of the testis arising mainly as teratomas and seminomas.
2. Nongerm cell tumours (3% of cases)—derived from specialized and nonspecialized support cells of the testis.

Germ cell tumours

Seminoma

This is the most common malignant testicular tumour, accounting for about 50% of all malignant germ cell tumours, with a peak age of onset between 30 and 40 years. Classical seminomas (most common subtype) characteristically show spermatogenic differentiation with delicate fibrous septa and a lymphocytic infiltrate.

Teratoma

This tumour of germ cell origin is composed of three types of tissue representing endoderm, ectoderm and mesoderm. The tumours retain their totipotentiality for differentiation. The peak age of onset is 20–30 years. Most teratomas demonstrate mature, well-differentiated tissue, producing a wide range of organoid structures (e.g., skin, hair, cartilage and bone). Lesions in prepubertal males behave in a benign fashion. Postpubertal teratomas and those with immature elements (e.g., primitive neuroepithelium) are considered malignant.

> **HINTS AND TIPS**
>
> **FEMALE VERSUS MALE TERATOMAS**
>
> The majority of teratomas are benign in women of any age. Teratomas are only benign in prepubertal males.
>
> Teratomas are malignant if occurring in postpubertal males or if they contain immature elements in either sex.

Embryonal carcinoma

Characterised by haemorrhage and necrosis, with high mitotic rate, marked nuclear pleomorphism and in-situ neoplasia within the seminiferous tubules.

Choriocarcinoma

Identical to choriocarcinoma in the placenta (see Placenta above), this highly malignant tumour contains areas of syncytiotrophoblast and cytotrophoblast cells. hCG is a useful marker.

Yolk sac tumour

The pure form is seen in children up to 3 years old and has a good prognosis. The adult (mixed) form is more aggressive. Alpha fetoprotein (AFP) is a useful serological marker.

Combined germ cell tumour

Thirty percent of germ cell tumours consist of a mixture of seminomatous and nonseminomatous germ cell elements. Metastasis can arise from single or multiple elements within the primary tumour.

Prognosis of germ cell tumours

The prognosis of testicular teratomas has improved greatly with the use of adjuvant cytotoxic chemotherapy, and it is related to histological type, as well as to tumour stage. Seminomas are more likely to respond to radiotherapy and adjuvant chemotherapy with carboplatin. In general, germ cell tumours containing trophoblastic, yolk sac and embryonal elements have the worst prognosis.

Nongerm cell tumours

Leydig cell tumour

This rare tumour arises from the Leydig (interstitial) cells of the testis. It may produce androgens, oestrogens or both, causing precocious development of secondary sexual characteristics in childhood or loss of libido/gynaecomastia in adults. Ninety percent are benign.

Sertoli cell tumour

This well-circumscribed tumour is composed of cells resembling normal Sertoli cells of the spermatic tubules. Most lesions are benign.

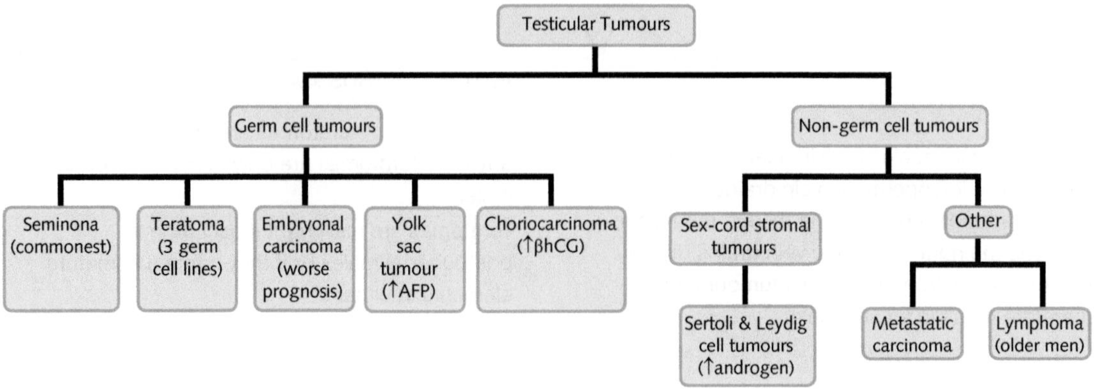

Fig. 15.10 Summary of testicular tumours.

Lymphomas

These comprise approximately 5% of testicular tumours with a peak incidence between 60 and 80 years of age, and are more likely to be bilateral. The commonest type is diffuse large B-cell lymphoma (see Chapter 17).

Metastatic tumours

The spread of other tumours to the testis may occasionally occur, particularly in acute leukaemia.

Fig. 15.10 provides a summary of testicular tumours.

> **HINTS AND TIPS**
>
> **TESTICULAR TUMOUR SEROLOGICAL MARKERS**
>
> Many testicular tumours have useful serological markers:
>
> - Trophoblastic germ cell tumours—↑ hCG
> - Yolk sac tumours—↑ α-fetoprotein
> - Sertoli—↑ androgen

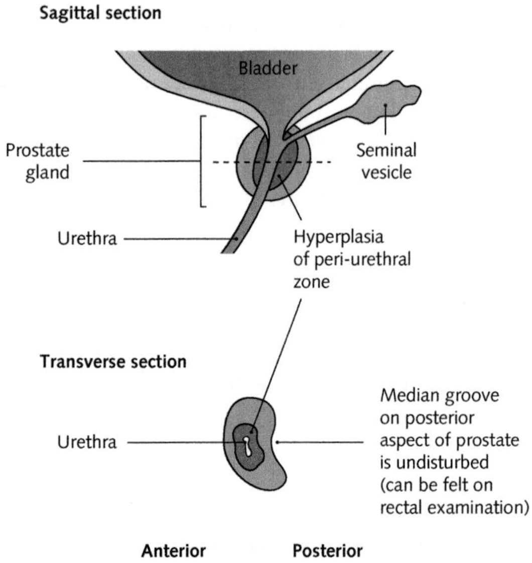

Fig. 15.11 Benign prostatic hyperplasia.

DISORDERS OF THE PROSTATE

Nonneoplastic lesions

Prostatitis

Acute or chronic inflammation of the prostate may be bacterial (most commonly *E. coli*) or granulomatous and may result in a mildly elevated prostate specific antigen (PSA) level.

Benign prostatic hyperplasia

Nonneoplastic enlargement of the prostate is the most common disorder of the prostate, affecting almost all men over the age of 70 years. However, it is found with increasing frequency and severity from about 45 years.

The aetiopathogenesis is uncertain but believed to be a result of androgen–oestrogen imbalance.

Central (periurethral) prostatic glands are hormone sensitive and undergo hyperplasia. Their continuing enlargement compresses peripheral prostatic glands leading to their collapse, leaving only fibrous supporting stroma (Fig. 15.11).

Affected lobes are:

- two lateral lobes (majority of cases)
- posterior lobe (uncommon), causing obstruction of the urinary outflow tract of the internal urinary meatus at the bladder neck.

Histologically:

- There is a nodular pattern of hyperplastic glandular acini separated by fibrous stroma.
- Some nodules are cystically dilated.
- Other nodules contain numerous calcific concretions (corpora amylacea).
- There is often muscular hypertrophy particularly in the region of the bladder neck.

Table 15.8 Complications of benign prostatic hyperplasia

Bladder wall	Hypertrophy of smooth muscle
	Trabeculation: due to prominent bands of thickened smooth muscle
	Diverticula: protrude between trabeculae
Bladder size	Dilation: due to failure of bladder wall compensatory mechanisms
Ureteric changes	Dilation of ureters
Urinary infection (cystitis)	Bladder fails to empty completely after micturition, and residual urine is liable to infection
Kidney disease	Pyelonephritis: from ascending infection
	Impaired renal failure
	Hydronephrosis
	Calculi

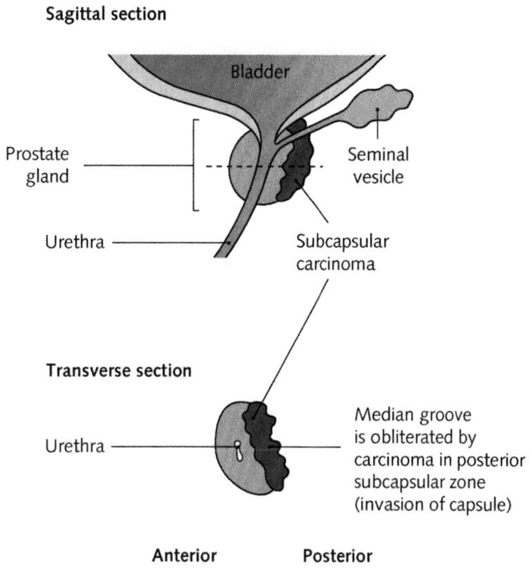

Fig. 15.12 Prostatic carcinoma.

Clinical presentation—compression of the prostatic urethra by the enlarged prostate causes difficulties with micturition, mainly hesitation, poor stream and terminal dribbling.

Complications—prolonged prostatic obstruction can lead to several complications, which are outlined in Table 15.8.

HINTS AND TIPS

CENTRAL VERSUS PERIPHERAL PROSTATE LESIONS

Within the prostate, central lesions are usually benign prostatic hyperplasia (BPH) and peripheral lesions are usually cancer.

Neoplasms of the prostate

Prostatic carcinoma

This is an adenocarcinoma of the prostate and it is shown in Fig. 15.12. It is the second commonest cancer in the UK and is the commonest cancer in males. It is rare before 55 years of age with more than half of cases diagnosed after age 70; 5-year survival is 85%.

Its aetiology is uncertain but there is probably hormonal involvement (reduced androgens).

Unlike benign hyperplasia, carcinoma usually arises in the peripheral zone of the prostate and it is, therefore, often well-established before the development of urinary symptoms. Indeed, some tumours may remain silent even in the presence of widespread metastases.

Types are divided into three groups on the basis of their behaviour:

1. Latent/low grade—small foci of well-differentiated carcinoma, frequently an incidental finding in prostatic glands of elderly men. They remain confined to the prostate for a long period.
2. Invasive/high grade—invade locally and metastasize.
3. Occult/high grade—not clinically apparent in primary site (small tumour) but present as widespread symptomatic metastatic disease.

Macroscopically—there are diffuse areas of firm, white tissue merging into fibromuscular prostatic stromal tissues. Distortion and extension outside the prostatic capsule is common, producing a firm, craggy mass that can be palpated on rectal examination.

Microscopically—the majority have a well-differentiated glandular pattern (good prognosis); a minority have poorly differentiated sheets of cells with no acinar pattern (poor prognosis). Prostate cancer is traditionally graded using the Gleason scale (1–5) and given a Gleason score, but a new system (Gleason grade groups) has been introduced to aid management.

Spread is:

- direct—to the base of the bladder and adjacent tissues. May cause obstruction of the urethra (difficulty in micturition) and may block the ureters, causing hydronephrosis.
- lymphatic—to pelvic and para-aortic nodes.
- haematogenous—most commonly to bone (via the prostatic venous plexus to vertebral veins), but also to the lungs and liver. Bone metastases are typically sclerotic rather than lytic (see Chapter 16).

HINTS AND TIPS

ISOLATED RAISED ALKALINE PHOSPHATASE (ALP)

An isolated raised ALP in an older male patient should always raise clinical suspicion of prostate carcinoma with bone metastases.

Diagnosis:

- Clinical—digital rectal exam.
- Serology—progressively increasing PSA is used as a serum marker for disease, levels being particularly raised when there is metastatic disease. However, raised PSA alone is relatively nonspecific for prostate carcinoma, meaning that screening programmes are likely to have high false-positive rates. (PSA as a screening tool - see Chapter 4.)
- Imaging—ultrasound, X-ray, isotope bone scan (for bony metastases).
- Template mapping core biopsies —histological examination sometimes together with immunohistochemical detection in biopsy material.

CLINICAL NOTES

CLINICAL FEATURES OF PROSTATIC CARCINOMA

The clinical features of prostatic carcinoma:

- Urinary symptoms (hesitancy, poor stream, terminal dribbling)
- Hard, craggy prostate on rectal examination
- Bone metastases: pain (especially back pain), fracture, anaemia

Chapter Summary

- Cervical intraepithelial neoplasia (CIN) and usual-type vulval intraepithelial neoplasia (VIN) are associated with high-risk human papilloma virus (HPV) infection.
- A national cervical cancer screening programme monitors women for CIN and cervical carcinoma.
- The most common gynaecological malignancies are endometrial > ovarian > cervical carcinomas.
- FIGO (International Federation of Gynaecology and Obstetrics) staging system is used in gynaecological malignancies instead of tumour, node, metastasis (TNM).
- Postmenopausal bleeding must always be investigated to exclude a neoplastic process.
- Atypical endometrial hyperplasia is a premalignant condition characterized by increased ratio of architecturally complex glands-to-stromal tissue with nuclear atypia.
- The two main subtypes of endometrial carcinoma (type 1 and 2) have different prognoses and genetic alterations.
- Ovarian cancer is divided into epithelial types, germ cell and sex cord stromal groups with the epithelial type being the most common form of cancer.
- Hydatiform moles are errors in embryogenesis and can be complete or partial. Two to three percent of complete moles can transform into choriocarcinoma.
- Fibroadenomas are the commonest benign tumour of breast.
- *BRCA1* and *BRCA2* mutations predispose to the development of breast carcinoma.
- Ninety-seven percent of testicular neoplasms are germ cell tumours.
- Benign prostatic hyperplasia is the commonest disorder of the prostate.
- Prostate cancer commonly metastasizes to bone via vertebral veins.

Pathology of the musculoskeletal system 16

DISORDERS OF BONE STRUCTURE

Bone pathology requires an understanding of bone structure and function (Fig. 16.1 and Tables 16.1 and 16.2).

Achondroplasia

Achondroplasia is a progressive disorder of enchondral ossification which is the most common cause of nonproportional short stature (dwarfism) worldwide. It occurs in approximately 1 per 15–40,000 births as the result of a

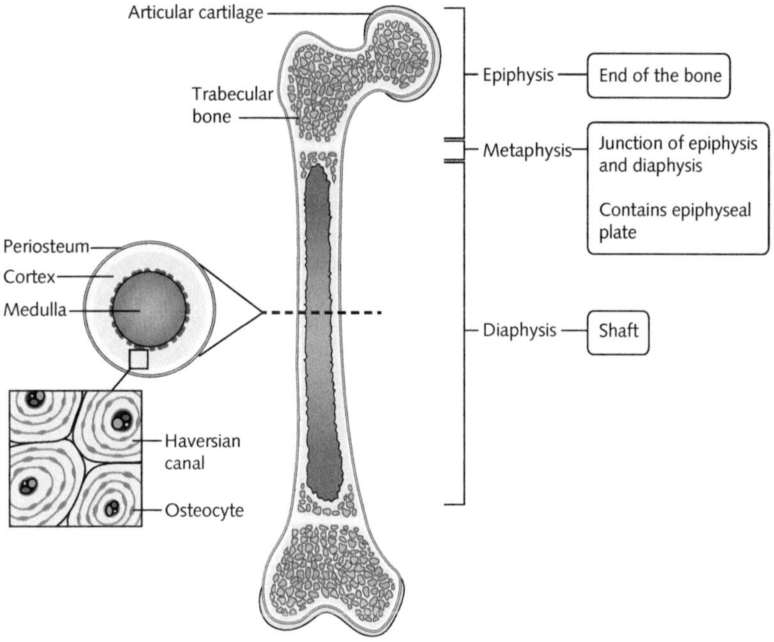

Fig. 16.1 Essential bone anatomy.

Table 16.1 Type and function of bone cells

Cell type	Location	Function
Osteoblast	Surface of new bone	Osteoid/protein synthesis Regulates osteoclast function/bone resorption Become entrapped within osteoid and terminally differentiate to form osteocytes Communicate with other osteocytes via canaliculi
Osteocyte (90% of bone cells)	Lacunae within cortical bone	Bone homeostasis/maintenance Mechano-sensing: response to bone loading/stress
Osteoclast (multinucleated giant cell)	Howship lacunae	Resorbs mineralized bone

Table 16.2 Types of bone

Bone type	Synonyms	Features
Cortical	Compact bone Lamellar	Dense and strong Composed of Haversian canals Concentric parallel lamella—highly organized
Medullary	Spongy bone Trabecular bone Cancellous bone	Formed of struts and trabeculae Contains bone marrow
Woven	Immature bone	Haphazard arrangement of collagen fibres Bulky Associated with states of increased bone turnover, e.g., fractures or neoplastic processes

point mutation in the fibroblast growth receptor 3 protein (FGFR3) on chromosome 4p. In over 80% of cases, the mutation is sporadic (parents are unaffected); the remainder are inherited in an autosomal dominant manner. The FGFR3 mutation results in gain of function causing profound suppression of growth plate chondrocyte proliferation and maturation.

Features:

Achondroplasia is characterized by proximal (rhizomelic) shortening of the limbs, a head that appears large for the body, depressed nasal bridge root and prominent frontal bossing. Other common types of short stature (e.g., pituitary hormone deficiency or malnutrition) are typically proportional, with all bones being equally affected.

Fibrous dysplasia

Fibrous dysplasia is a focal developmental abnormality of bone that affects both children and young adults. Radiologically, the lesions appear as well-demarcated expansile masses which can be cystic, sclerotic, ground glass, monostotic or polyostotic. Soft tissue extension/invasion and periosteal reaction are not seen. The lesions are composed histologically of a mix of fibrous matrix, spindle cells and trabeculae of woven bone. Characteristically, the bony component is curvilinear forming shapes reminiscent of 'Chinese characters'.

The monostotic form is the commonest, with the ribs, face and femur most frequently involved. Presentation is with pain, pathological fracture or entirely asymptomatic.

McCune–Albright syndrome is a hereditary disorder associated with 2%–3% of the polyostotic cases.

Disorders of the bone matrix

Osteogenesis imperfecta (brittle bone disease)

This heterogeneous group of rare congenital disorders is characterized by abnormal collagen formation that results in brittle and fragile bones.

Aetiology—mutation of the genes coding for type I collagen (COL 1A1 and COL 1A2) results in abnormal collagen formation and therefore osteoid production. The pattern of inheritance can be either autosomal dominant or recessive, and it involves mutations on chromosomes 7 and 17.

Appearance—there is a marked variation in severity but widespread weakness of bone results in multiple fractures frequently leading to severe deformity. Lax joint ligaments, blue sclera and hearing loss are also often seen, once more reflecting decreased collagen synthesis.

Osteoporosis

This is a slowly progressive disorder of reduced bone mineral density (T score less than −2.5). Bone biochemistry and overall bony architecture are normal. Osteoporosis is the most common metabolic bone disease and can be primary (idiopathic/age-related) or secondary (occurring due to an identifiable cause, e.g., steroid use), localized or diffuse. Localized osteoporosis may develop in an area of bone secondary to disuse, surrounding inflammation or conditions such as myeloma (see Chapter 17). The risk factors for osteoporosis are summarized in Table 16.3. It is an important

Table 16.3 Type and associated risk factors for osteoporosis.

Type	Risk factors
Idiopathic	Female Early menopause Small stature Thin physique Family history Advanced age Nulliparity
Secondary: generalized[a]	***M***etabolic: low calcium intake, impaired supply of protein (e.g., nephritic syndrome or cirrhosis of liver), scurvy ***A***ssorted endocrine disorders: thyrotoxicosis, panhypopituitarism and Cushing syndrome ***S***teroid therapy ***C***igarette smoking ***A***lcohol abuse ***R***educed physical activities ***A***luminium antacids
Secondary: localized	Disuse atrophy: especially in neurological limb paralysis or post fracture

[a] *The mnemonic 'MASCARA' can be used to help remember the causes of secondary generalized osteoporosis.*

cause of morbidity and even mortality within the elderly, where it is common, as weakened bone predisposes to minimal trauma fractures.

Bone loss in women is accelerated by oestrogen deficiency, making postmenopausal women a high-risk group. Hormone replacement therapy is partly protective.

Radiology—bones appear less dense on X-ray when a loss of 30%–50% has occurred. There is cortical thinning and loss of trabecular bone. Vertebral bodies appear more biconcave giving rise to a 'fish vertebrae' appearance. Diagnosis is by bone scanning at the hip and spine with dual energy X-ray absorptiometry (DEXA) to assess bone density. Osteoporosis is defined by the World Health Organization as a T score of greater than −2.5. Osteopenia is reduced bone density that has not yet reached osteoporotic levels (T score of −1 to −2.5) and normal bone density is a T score of −1 to 1.

Microscopically—Bony trabeculae are thinner, reduced in number and disconnected from each other. This is associated with an amplified osteoclastic activity with increased numbers and depth of resorption pits. Mineralization is not affected and mineral:osteoid ratio is normal.

Complications:

- Bone pain—especially in the back due to crush fractures/wedge fractures of vertebral bodies. This may reduce overall height and cause kyphosis of the spine ('Dowager's hump' if it occurs in the thoracic spine).
- Pathological fractures—following minimal trauma, especially of the femur (hip fracture), proximal humerus and distal radius (Colles fracture).

Osteomalacia and rickets

Osteomalacia and rickets are the same diseases of defective bone mineralization, and are most commonly seen in the developing world. Rickets occurs in children where the metaphyseal growth plates are still open and osteomalacia in adults where the skeleton is mature. They are usually due to a lack of vitamin D, lack of phosphate or disturbances in the metabolism of either (e.g., conversion to active vitamin D via the liver and kidney, familial hypophosphataemia) (Table 16.4). They present with bone pain, tenderness, skeletal deformity (children) and can be associated with proximal muscle weakness.

The ratio of mineral:osteoid is abnormal with an excess of osteoid. Consequently, bone is incompletely calcified, with the development of wide 'seams' of osteoid making the bone weak and prone to fracture.

Radiologically, there is generalized smudgy demineralization and Looser zones (pseudofractures) may be seen. In children, metaphyseal widening, cup-shaped metaphyses and 'frayed and splayed' ends of bones can be appreciated. Rickets also leads to characteristic skeletal changes, e.g., bowing of long bones, bulging costochondral junctions and frontal bossing.

Both disorders are potentially reversible, with early dietary supplementation to correct deficiencies or treatment of underlying disorders.

Table 16.4 Causes of vitamin D and phosphate deficiency[a]

Vitamin D deficiency	
Insufficient exposure to sunlight	Housebound, dark skin pigmentation, full body clothing
Diet	Low intake of calcium, veganism
Malabsorption	Especially conditions causing fat malabsorption, e.g., coeliac disease, gastric surgery, pancreatic insufficiency
Drugs	E.g., phenytoin and barbiturates
Renal failure	Reduced production of bioactive vitamin D
Liver disease	Reduced synthesis and storage of cholecalciferol vitamin D
Genetic	Lack of 1α hydroxylase enzyme in kidney
Phosphate deficiency	
Hypophosphataemia	Genetic: X-linked Acquired: Oncogenic
Fanconi syndrome	Disorder of impaired resorptive function of the proximal renal tubules resulting in phosphaturia, glycosuria, aminoaciduria et al.

[a] *The metabolism and regulation of vitamin D, phosphate and calcium are interlinked. Aberration with one can lead to dysregulation of the others.*

Renal osteodystrophy

Skeletal abnormalities, arising as a result of raised parathyroid hormone (PTH) secondary to chronic renal disease (secondary hyperparathyroidism), are known as renal osteodystrophy.

The pathogenesis of renal osteodystrophy is shown in Fig. 16.2.

Abnormalities vary widely according to the nature of the renal lesion, its duration and the age of the patient, but include:

- osteitis fibrosa cystica (brown tumours)
- rickets or osteomalacia due to reduced activation of vitamin D
- osteosclerosis—increased radiodensity of certain bones, e.g., vertebrae ("rugger-jersey spine")

Symptoms of hypercalcaemia are not a feature of secondary hyperparathyroidism; calcium levels are likely to be decreased as this is driving the compensatory PTH secretion.

Disorders of osteoclast function

Osteopetrosis

This rare, hereditary disorder is characterized by increased density of all cartilaginous bones, especially the vertebrae,

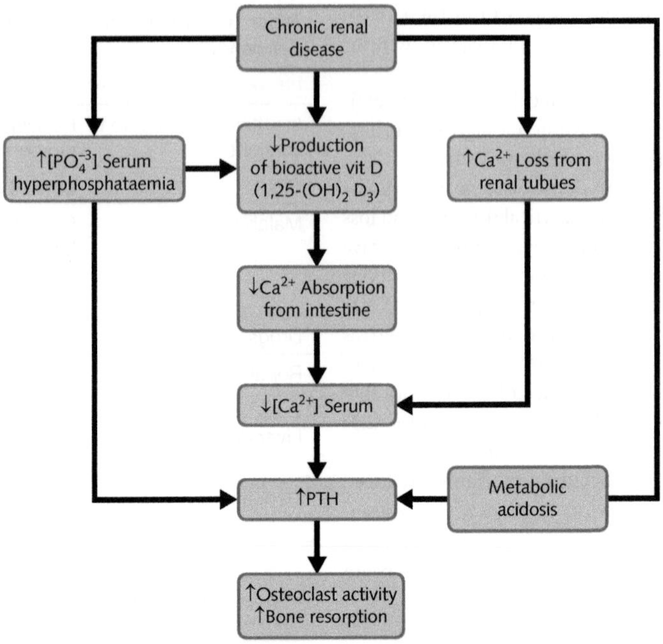

Fig. 16.2 Pathogenesis of renal osteodystrophy. Renal disease causes reduced vitamin D *(vit D)* production, phosphate retention (hyperphosphataemia) and metabolic acidosis. These act directly or indirectly by the action of parathyroid hormone *(PTH)* to cause an increase in osteoclastic activity and bone resorption.

pelvic bones and ribs. It is also known as marble bone and Albers–Schönberg disease.

Pathogenesis—defective resorption of bone by osteoclasts produces diffuse symmetrical skeletal sclerosis.

Appearance—there is no discernible differentiation of cartilaginous bones into cortex and medulla: the cortical compact bone extends into the medulla, which is thus devoid of cancellous bone.

Effect—bones are excessively dense, yet extremely brittle and prone to fracture. The lack of bone marrow function predisposes to infection, extramedullary haematopoiesis and hepatosplenomegaly. Cranial nerve compression can also be seen.

Paget disease of the bone

This is a chronic disease of uncontrolled bone turnover with excessive osteoclastic resorption and haphazard osteoblastic deposition of bone which particularly affects the skull, spine, pelvis and proximal long bones. It is rare before 40 years of age, but increases in incidence with age thereafter. It is relatively common in the United Kingdom, affecting 3% of those over the age of 40, but is rare in Asia, Africa and the Middle East. The aetiology is postulated to be a paramyxovirus or respiratory syncytial viral infection.

Pathogenesis—large, abnormal, multinucleated osteoclasts cause excessive bone erosion with destruction of trabecular and cortical bone. Each wave of bone destruction is followed by a vigorous but uncoordinated osteoblastic response, producing new osteoid to fill the defects left by the osteoclasts. However, both osteoclastic erosion and osteoblastic deposition are random, haphazard and unrelated to functional stresses on the bone, resulting in greatly distorted bone architecture.

Morphology—bone shows a characteristic woven, non-lamellar pattern, indicative of rapid reparative deposition. Well-marked 'cement lines' are often visible, producing the characteristic 'mosaic' or 'crazy-paving' appearance. The bone becomes increasingly sclerotic and brittle, and is therefore prone to fracture. Disruption of bone architecture is followed by progressive increased vascularity in the spaces between the thickened bone trabeculae.

The effects of Paget disease can be widespread (affecting many bones) or localized (15% of cases confined to one area in a single-bone—monostotic Paget disease).

Most patients present with one or both of the following features:

- Bone pain—usually localized to site of most active disease.
- Bone deformity—following extensive disease; most commonly enlargement of the skull, kyphosis or bowing of tibia.

Complications—some patients occasionally present with complications of Paget disease which include:

- Pathological fractures
- Cranial nerve palsies, e.g., CN VIII compression and deafness
- High-output cardiac failure
- Malignant transformation (e.g. osteosarcoma).

Table 16.6 summarises the serum biochemistry of bone disorders

Table 16.6 Serum biochemistry of bone disorders

Condition	Calcium	Phosphate	ALK	PTH	Vitamin D
Osteoporosis	N	N	N	N	N
Osteomalacia/rickets	N or ↓	↓	↑	↑	↓
Hyperparathyroidism	↑	↓	N or ↑	↑↑↑	N
Paget disease	N	N	↑↑↑	N	N
Renal osteodystrophy	N or ↓	↑	↑	↑↑	↓
Metastatic disease	↑	↑	↑	↑	N or ↓

The alterations in serum biochemistry reflect the underlying pathological processes.
ALK, alkaline phosphatase; N, normal; PTH, parathyroid hormone.

INFECTIONS AND TRAUMA

Osteomyelitis

This infection of bone typically affects the cortex, medulla and periosteum, and is most commonly encountered in children under 12 years of age. Adult onset is usually due to compromised host resistance (e.g., severe debilitation, immunosuppression). The most common causative organisms are *Staphylococcus aureus* (over 80% of identified cases), *Mycobacterium tuberculosis, Escherichia coli* (particularly in infants and the elderly) and *Salmonella* species (particularly in patients with sickle cell disease).

Infective organisms gain access to the medullary cavity of the bone by three main routes:

1. Direct implantation through an open wound.
2. Haematogenous spread: following bacteraemia from a focus of sepsis elsewhere.
3. Contiguous Extension from an adjacent site.

Clinical features—abrupt onset of severe pain at the site of bone infection accompanied by fever and malaise. X-rays show areas of lytic destruction with surrounding sclerosis. Subperiosteal abscesses may also be present secondary to infection seeping through the Haversian system.

Sequalae and complications:

- Resolution—with appropriate antibiotic therapy, ideally based on blood cultures or aspiration material.
- Pathological fracture—purulent acute inflammatory exudate formed in closed compartment of marrow cavity causes compression of vessels resulting in necrosis of medullary bone trabeculae and concomitant weakness.
- Adjacent sepsis—destruction of cortical bone may lead to discharge of pus into extraosseous connective tissue, and infection may track through to the skin surface, producing a chronic discharging sinus. Spread may also occur to other bones (malignant osteomyelitis) or neighbouring joints (septic arthritis).
- Limb deformity/length discrepancies – given that osteomyelitis is most common in children, growth disturbance may occur if the metaphyseal plate is damaged.
- Chronic osteomyelitis – cortical bone becomes necrotic (sequestrum) secondary to periosteal elevation resulting in an inadequate blood supply. The infecting organisms may remain viable within the marrow cavity for many years with potential sequestrum providing a nidus. There may be extensive bone destruction, marrow fibrosis and recurrent focal suppuration (Brodie abscess). Reactive new bone formation is seen, particularly around and outside the inflamed periosteum (involucrum), leading to a thickened and abnormally shaped bone.

Diagnosis is by blood culture and isotope scan. Management is by analgesia, antibiotic therapy and potential surgical drainage of abscesses.

Pott disease of the spine:

This is extrapulmonary tuberculosis (TB) infection of the spine. TB infection of the skeleton occurs in 1%–3% of cases of pulmonary TB. The most common site is the spine (Pott disease) followed by the knee and hip. Infection causes progressive destruction of the vertebral bodies with wedge-shaped collapse resulting in thoracic kyphosis. Infection spreads through the intervertebral discs to infect adjacent vertebrae and extends into the soft tissue with abscess formation.

Avascular necrosis

Avascular necrosis (osteonecrosis) is ischaemic death of a segment of bone as a direct result of trauma, or indirectly from other insults/pathologies. These include high steroid administration, alcohol abuse, sickle cell disease and malignancy. It can occur at any age. The commonest sites are the femoral head, scaphoid and talus. This is directly related to the anatomy of their blood supply, some of which is end arterial, which makes them vulnerable to ischaemia.

Perthes disease

This is idiopathic avascular necrosis of the proximal femoral head within the paediatric population (4–8 years old), affecting males five times more frequently than females. Fifteen percent of cases are bilateral. Children present with a painless, atraumatic limp. Pelvic X-rays in the early stages of the disease show blurring of the metaphyseal plate and a smaller, denser epiphyseal head. Later, bone destruction is seen and coxa plana (widening and flattening of the epiphysis) occurs. Treatment is conservative. Hip replacement in adulthood may be required.

Fractures

A fracture is a break in the structural continuity of bone. Note that any break, even if only one cortex is involved, constitutes a fracture. Fractures are the most common abnormality of bone and they are caused by physical trauma.

Types of fracture

Fractures can be classified into two main types according to their relation to surrounding tissues:

1. Closed (simple)—without contact with external environment, i.e., skin or mucous membrane overlying the fracture site is intact. Simple fractures are less likely to become infected.
2. Open (compound)—with direct contact between the fracture and external environment, e.g., a fracture of the tibia in continuity with laceration of overlying skin. Compound factures are more likely to become infected and blood loss can be significant.

Other descriptive terms for fractures are:

- Comminuted—more than two fragments present.
- Complicated—involvement of a nerve, artery or viscus.
- Pathological—fracture occurring in abnormal bone, e.g., in osteoporosis or due to a bone tumour.
- Hairline—slowly developing fracture resulting from repetitive application of force, e.g., a stress fracture.
- Greenstick—usually seen in children. Only one side of a bone is fractured, leaving it bent but intact.
- Crush (compression) - occur in cancellous bone, e.g., vertebral body, heels, when excessive loading force is applied.

Processes of healing

Bone can undergo complete healing by granulation tissue formation with fibrous repair, followed by new bone formation (see Chapter 3 for wound healing of the skin).

The sequence of events in healing of a simple undisplaced fracture are illustrated in Fig. 16.3 and described in Table 16.7.

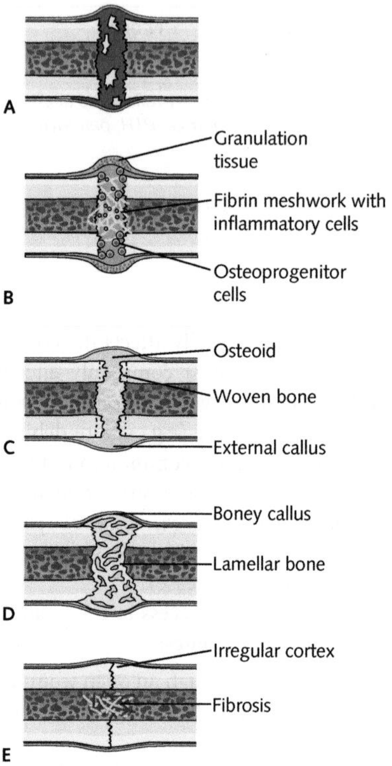

Fig. 16.3 Healing of a simple fracture. (A) Haematoma formation. (B) Organization. (C) Callus formation. (D) Consolidation. (E) Remodelling.

Table 16.7 Stages of fracture repair

Stage of healing	Time course	Events
Haematoma formation	Immediate	Tearing of blood vessels at the site of fracture leads to haematoma formation which fills the fracture gap.
Organization	Within 24 hours	Fibrin mesh allows deposition of platelets and migration of inflammatory cells into the fracture site. These activate osteoprogenitor cells which mature into osteoblasts and osteoclasts. Fibrovascular granulation tissue is formed by fibroblast and capillary proliferation.
Callus formation	1 week	Osteoblasts deposit large quantities of osteoid collagen in a haphazard way producing a woven bone pattern. Fracture is bridged externally by callus (may contain cartilage) and in the medullary cavity by internal callus (rarely contains cartilage). Direct ossification may occur between fractured ends if they are closely apposed.
Consolidation	3 weeks	The callus is well established and has stabilized the fracture site. Endochondral ossification begins to form a bony callus. Remodelling by osteoclastic and osteoblastic activity to replace the bulky woven bone by compact, organized, lamellar bone. This process takes several months.
Remodelling	Months	Formation of new lamellar bone orientated in the direction of loading stress is complete and continuity of the medullary cavity has been restored. Even after reshaping, cortical irregularities and minor marrow space fibrosis persist at the fracture site.

Elements affecting fracture healing

Efficient healing of fractures requires optimal conditions. Factors that prevent efficient healing are:

- poor apposition of fractured bone ends –a fracture is 'reduced' to achieve the best alignment possible
- inadequate immobilization—movement of bone ends at the fracture site
- interposition of foreign bodies or soft tissues between the bone ends
- infection
- corticosteroid therapy
- poor general nutritional status
- poor blood supply

Complications of fractures

The complications of fractures can arise in the immediate/short term as part of the initial injury complex or in the longer term as a result of an aberrant healing process or as a consequence of the initial damage.

Immediate/short-term complications:

- Infection
- Neurological damage—laceration, compression, entrapment of nerves
- Vascular injury and haemorrhage
- Compartment syndrome
- Visceral injury
- Fracture blisters

Longer-term complications:

- Malunion - angulation or rotation of the united fracture leading to deformity.
- Delayed union—when a fracture has not united within the expected time (defined as 25% longer than the average time).
- Nonunion—if union has not occurred within 1 year then the terminology is changed from one of 'delayed union' to one of 'nonunion'. The defect is typically filled with fibrous tissue.
- Joint stiffness/instability.
- Avascular necrosis.
- Myositis ossificans (heterotopic ossification).
- Osteoarthritis (OA).
- Muscle contractures.
- Complex regional pain syndrome.

TUMOURS OF THE BONES

Metastatic disease of the skeleton

The most common tumours in bone are blood-borne metastases from other primary sites, or tumours of the haematopoietic cells located within the marrow spaces of bones, particularly myeloma (see Chapter 17).

Carcinomas

There are five common carcinomas that have a predilection for metastasizing to bone:

1. Breast carcinoma.
2. Bronchial carcinoma.
3. Renal carcinoma.
4. Thyroid carcinoma.
5. Prostate carcinoma.

Metastases are typically multifocal, occurring most commonly in parts of the skeleton that contain vascular marrow, especially vertebral bodies, ribs, pelvis, and the proximal ends of the femur and humerus.

Osteolytic versus osteosclerotic metastases

Most metastatic tumours within bone marrow spaces lead to erosion of bone (osteolytic metastases), through the release of substances that promote osteoclastic resorption (e.g. prostaglandins, parathyroid-hormone-related peptide) (Fig. 16.4). However, prostatic carcinoma (and very rarely breast carcinoma) produce metastatic deposits in which there is osteoblastic stimulation of new bone formation (osteosclerotic metastases) particularly in the lumbosacral vertebrae (Table 16.8).

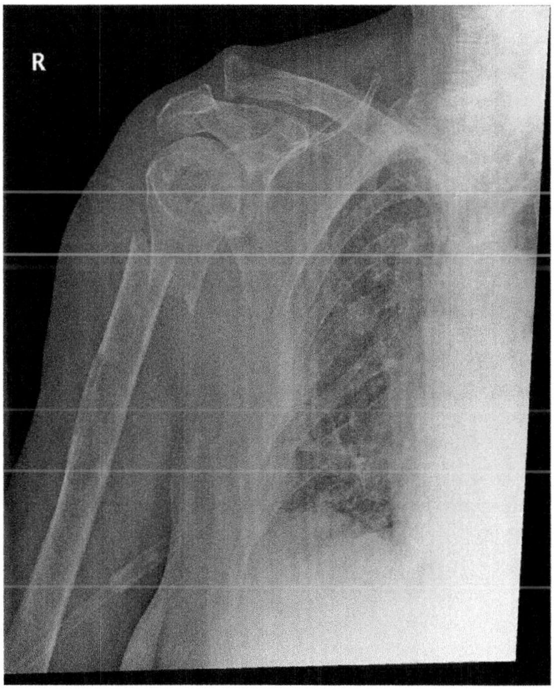

Fig. 16.4 Pathological fracture. X-ray showing a pathological fracture of the right humerus. Numerous osteolytic metastatic deposits can be seen throughout the humeral shaft. The primary cancer was unknown.

Table 16.8 Osteolytic and osteosclerotic metastatic tumours

Osteolytic	Osteosclerotic
Breast (can also be sclerotic)	Prostate carcinoma
Thyroid carcinoma	Urothelial carcinoma (urinary tract)
Renal cell carcinoma	–
Adrenal carcinoma (pheochromocytoma)	–
Ewing sarcoma	–
Wilms tumour	–
Melanoma	–

Osteolytic metastases are more common than sclerotic metastases.

Clinical features:

- bone pain—usually localized to site of deposits;
- pathological fractures—erosion of trabecular bone either directly, or through osteoclast-stimulated bone erosion → bone weakness → fracture;
- leucoerythroblastic anaemia - nucleated red cells and immature myeloid cells in the peripheral blood because of extensive replacement of bone marrow;
- symptoms of hypercalcaemia—caused by the release of calcium from bone by osteolysis.
- nerve and spinal cord compression - spinal metastasis resulting in the protrusion of tumour into the spinal canal causing cord compression (thoracic and cervical vertebrae) or cauda equina syndrome (lumbar vertebrae) as a consequence of canal stenosis.

Haematopoietic malignancies

Haematopoietic malignancies found in bone (e.g., myeloma, lymphomas, leukaemias) are discussed in Chapter 17.

> **HINTS AND TIPS**
>
> Secondary tumours of bone are more common in adults than children, whereas primary tumours of bone are generally more common in children than adults.

Primary bone tumours

Primary bone tumours are rare, accounting for 0.2% of all neoplasms. The majority arise within the second decade with a later peak at over 60 years of age. The commonest sites are the knee and pelvis (Fig. 16.5). They present with progressively worsening pain that is independent of movement and eventually causes nocturnal waking, swelling (late sign), pathological fractures and neurological deficits, or are an incidental finding.

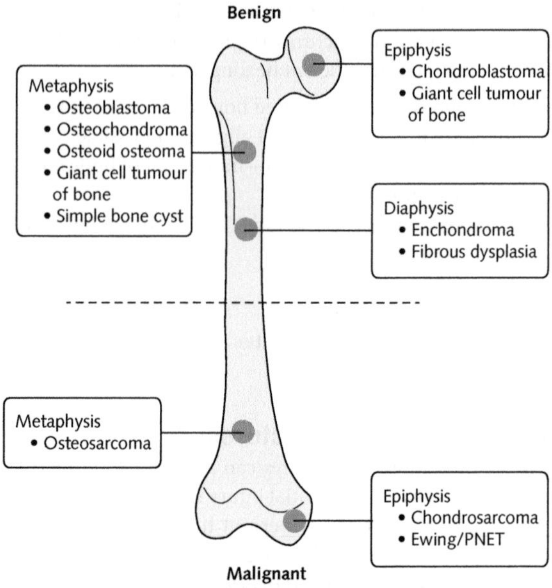

Fig. 16.5 Distribution of primary bone tumours. Primary bone tumours have characteristic sites of predilection within bones. Adapted from World Health Organization Classification of Tumours of Soft Tissue and Bone. 4th ed. Fig. 14.02, p. 245.

Bone-forming tumours

These are rare primary bone tumours, derived from cells involved in bone formation and remodelling.

Osteoma

An osteoma is a benign tumour composed of compact lamellar bone <2 cm in size. It is associated with bones that undergo membranous ossification, chiefly the calvarium, facial bones and jaw. The presentation is usually an incidental finding of a smooth, rounded, sclerotic lesion on X-ray or a visible/palpable, painless swelling. These tumours are slow-growing and do not undergo malignant transformation. The highest incidence is within the 6th decade, with a female preponderance. Patients with Gardner syndrome, a subtype of familial adenomatous polyposis, have multiple osteomas, intestinal polyps and other soft tissue tumours.

Osteoid osteoma and osteoblastoma

These bone-forming tumours are histologically very similar but vary in their size and clinical presentations, as outlined in Table 16.9. Histologically, they are both composed of a central nidus surrounded by haphazard interconnecting trabeculae of osteoid and woven bone set within a fibrovascular stroma.

Table 16.9 Clinical features of osteoid osteoma and osteoblastoma.

	Osteoid osteoma	Osteoblastoma
Frequency	10% of all bone tumours	1%–3% of all bone tumours
Size	<2 cm (average 1.5 cm)	>2 cm (average 3–10 cm)
Age	5–24 years	10–30 years
Location	Long bones—commonest proximal femur>tibia Any bone possible	Spine and sacrum>epiphyses of femur
Pain	Intense pain Intermittent → relentless Worse at night Disproportionate to size of lesion	Dull aching pain Slowly progressive
NSAID effect	Aspirin completely resolves pain	No effect on pain
Behaviour	Indolent, may spontaneously resolve Excision is curative	Locally aggressive—excision is curative

NSAID, Nonsteroidal antiinflammatory drugs.

Radiologically, they are sharply circumscribed lesions characteristically composed of a rim of dense sclerotic bone surrounding a radiolucent nidus.

Osteosarcoma

This is a malignant, high-grade bone-forming tumour of osteoblasts . It occurs most often in adolescent children, with a second peak in the fifth decade of life linked to highly active Paget disease or postradiation exposure. It accounts for 20% of primary bone tumours, being the second commonest. Some cases are associated with familial cancer syndromes, e.g., retinoblastoma syndrome (defect in *RB1*) and the Li-Fraumeni syndrome (defect in *p53)*. The majority originate in the metaphyses around the knee (distal femur or proximal tibia) and a minority in other long bones, e.g., proximal humerus. Symptoms are those of gradually increasing bone pain with tumour growth, with or without a progressively enlarging soft tissue mass. The tumour is often advanced at the time of diagnosis.

Radiologically, osteosarcomas are large ill-defined masses over 5–10 cm with a mixed sclerotic/lytic motheaten appearance. There is cortical and medullary bone destruction with invasion into the soft tissue. Periosteal elevation and reaction (sunburst type) are seen.

Histologically, malignant spindle cells form the tumour bulk, producing osteoid matrix and neoplastic bone associated with adjacent trabecular infiltration/destruction. Necrosis is common.

Tumour growth is rapid and aggressive with replacement of the medullary cavity and metastasis occurring early, with haematogenous spread to the lung.

Prognosis has improved with the adoption of earlier surgical treatment combined with chemotherapy; however 5-year survival is still only 50%. The best prognostic indicator is the extent of tumour necrosis in response to chemotherapy.

Cartilage-forming tumours

Osteochondroma

This is the most common benign tumour of bone comprising of an exophytic protuberant nodule of 'normal' bone capped with hyaline cartilage and an outer layer of perichondrium (also known as 'cartilage-capped exostosis'). Growth ceases with skeletal maturity. It is usually asymptomatic but can present due to fracture through the lesional neck, mechanical effects, or as a hard mass. Lesions arise in the metaphysis of bones formed by enchondral ossification, most commonly the distal femur, upper humerus and proximal tibia and fibula.

Radiologically, osteochondromas are sessile or pedunculated lesions seen projecting from the metaphyseal region away from the joint. Their cortex and medullary cavity are continuous with that of the underlying bone. The cartilage cap is characteristically thin (2–3 mm). They may be solitary or multiple (typically in the autosomal dominant condition multiple hereditary exostoses (MHE)).

Chondrosarcomatous change is rare in solitary lesions but more common in MHE. A cartilage cap of over 1.5 cm is suspicious of malignant transformation.

Enchondroma

This is a benign tumour of hyaline cartilage presenting in 20- to 50-year-olds as an incidental finding or following a pathological fracture. Most commonly located in the short tubular bones of the hands and feet, they may be single (solitary enchondroma) or multiple (enchondromatosis or Ollier disease). Mutation of the *IDH1/IDH2* gene is present in 90% of cases of enchondromatosis. The term 'enchondroma' is used to indicate that the tumour arises and grows within the medullary cavity of bone (compared with osteochondroma, which grows as a nodular exophytic lesion).

Radiologically, enchondromas are well-demarcated, expansive intramedullary masses of over 5 cm, which demonstrate variable radiolucency as they can mineralize over time. Endosteal erosion (<50% of the cortical thickness) can be seen.

Histologically, they are hypocellular lesions formed of chondrocytes set within an avascular hyaline cartilage matrix. Architecturally, multiple nodules or confluent sheets are seen with normal bone marrow interspersed between the nodules. Critically, no surrounding bone entrapment or soft tissue invasion is present.

A solitary enchondroma rarely undergoes malignant change, but occasionally it occurs in multiple enchondromatosis.

Chondrosarcoma

This slow-growing malignant tumour of cartilage often reaches a large size over months to years, eventually breaking through the periosteum into surrounding soft tissue, but usually maintaining a clearly defined border. They occur in those aged over 50 years and have a predilection for the femur, proximal humerus and pelvis. Imaging shows radiolucent lesions with variable amounts of calcification. There is cortical thickening, expansion and deep endosteal scalloping (erosion) of greater than 50%.

Microscopically, the majority are low-grade, well-differentiated tumours resembling enchondromas, but differ by the presence of atypical chondrocytes and permeation into the surrounding bone with bone entrapment. They are locally aggressive and metastasize very late, such that radical local surgery may be curative.

The minority are high-grade, poorly differentiated tumours with marked pleomorphism, high mitotic activity and necrosis. Growth is rapid with early blood-borne metastases.

Other tumours

Ewing sarcoma/PNET

Ewing sarcoma/PNET (primative neuroectodermal tumour) is a highly malignant 'small round blue cell' tumour of bone, probably derived from primitive neuroendocrine cells. This affects children between the ages of 5 and 15 years and usually arises in the metaphysis/diaphyses of long bones, particularly the femur. Severe pain, swelling and tenderness may be associated with fever and leucocytosis (thus tumours are sometimes mistaken for osteomyelitis). Areas of osteolytic bone destruction surrounded by layers of new periosteal bone give the tumour a characteristic 'onion skin' appearance on X-ray. The bulk of the tumour appears as an ill-defined, destructive lytic mass with a motheaten appearance.

It has a characteristic chromosomal translocation—t(11;22) (q24;q12)—that results in the fusion of the *FLI-1* gene from chromosome 11 with the *EWSR1* gene on chromosome 22 to form an oncoprotein. Effective chemotherapy, radiotherapy and surgical excision (often amputation) has increased 5-year survival to 75%.

Giant cell tumour of bone

Also known as osteoclastomas, these are benign but locally aggressive tumours of the mature skeleton occurring more frequently in females aged 20 to 45 years. They arise in the epiphyses of long bones with 50% occurring around the knee; other common sites include the sacrum, vertebrae and distal radius.

The lesion is composed of a mass of round/spindled mononuclear tumour cells and reactive osteoclast like multinucleated giant cells. Mitoses are numerous but morphologically normal. There is gradual expansion of lesions into the metaphysis and erosion of cortical bone. Penetration of the periosteum or articular cartilage may occur with or without soft tissue invasion. Radiologically, these are characterized as sharply defined, eccentric, multilobulated metaphyseal lytic lesions that can be accompanied by a thin, incomplete rim of reactive bone.

Malignant transformation is rare (<1%), however, up to a quarter recur after excision.

Cystic bone lesions

Simple bone cysts

These are unilocular fibrous cysts (also known as solitary/unicameral cysts) containing serous fluid, that arise within the medullary cavity of bones. They generally occur within the metaphyseal areas, the proximal humerus, proximal femur, proximal tibia and calcaneus being the most common sites. Characteristically they appear as well-circumscribed expansive lucencies with symmetrical cortical thinning in the absence of a periosteal bone reaction. The metaphyseal plate is abutted but not crossed. The vast majority occur within the first two decades and 75% are within males. Presentation is typically an incidental finding, but pathological fractures do occur and can result in growth arrest of the limb with subsequent shortening, or avascular necrosis of the femoral head.

Histologically, they are lined by a fibrous membrane which contains variable amounts of hemosiderin and macrophages with cholesterol clefts. Collagen deposition is also seen.

Aneurysmal bone cyst

Aneurysmal bone cysts (ABCs) are rare, locally destructive benign cystic neoplasms composed of multiple blood-filled cysts which lack a cell lining. They normally arise within the metaphyseal regions of long bones, i.e., femur, tibia, humerus or within the pelvis and posterior portions of vertebrae. Normally ABCs appear as eccentric, lytic 'soap bubble' like lesions within bone on X-rays, accompanied by a thin rim of periosteal bone reaction. Soft tissue extension can also occur.

The typical presentation is that of a person over 20 years old with pain and swelling. Neurological deficits can be present if the tumour is located within a vertebral body. Despite treatment, local recurrence can occur.

Upregulation of the ubiquitin specific protease gene *(USP6)* by translocation to a promoter region is the underlying aetiology of this neoplasm. The most common rearrangement is t(16;17)(q22;p13) (Table 16.10).

Table 16.10 Summary of bone tumours

Type	Tumour	Clinical features
Metastatic (secondary)	Carcinoma of bronchus (especially small cell) Adenocarcinomas of the breast, kidney, thyroid, prostate	Metastases occur most commonly to vertebral bodies, ribs, pelvis and proximal ends of femur and humerus
Primary	Bone-forming tumours	Osteoma Osteoid osteoma Osteoblastoma Osteosarcoma
	Cartilage-forming tumours	Osteochondroma Enchondroma Chondroblastoma Chondrosarcoma Chondromyxoid fibroma
	Fibrous and fibroosseous tumour	Fibroma Fibrous dysplasia Fibrosarcoma Pleomorphic undifferentiated sarcoma
	Others	Ewing sarcoma Giant cell tumour of bone Aneurysmal bone cyst

ARTHROPATHIES

Arthropathies are diseases involving the joints. Although there are many ways of classifying arthropathies, the simplest system is by disease process: degenerative, inflammatory (both seropositive and seronegative arthropathies), infectious and crystal-associated (Table 16.11).

Osteoarthritis

Osteoarthritis (OA) is a degenerative disease of articular cartilage. It is associated with secondary changes in underlying bone resulting in pain and impaired function of the affected joint. Although the name suggests that primary OA is an inflammatory process, its main effects on the erosion of cartilage are independent of acute or chronic inflammation, even though inflammatory cells may be present in the affected joint.

Table 16.11 Classification of arthropathies

Disease process	Examples
Degenerative	Osteoarthritis
Inflammatory	Rheumatoid arthritis Ankylosing spondylitis Reactive arthritis Psoriatic arthritis
Infectious	Septic arthritis
Crystal-associated	Gout Pseudogout

It is extremely common—80% of the elderly population show radiographic evidence of OA; only 25% of these are symptomatic.

Females are affected more often than males, except at the hip where both genders are equally prone to OA. It is common over 60 years of age, but may occur in younger age groups following any form of mechanical derangement.

OA affects joints that are constantly exposed to wear and tear, typically large weight-bearing joints (e.g., those of the hip and knee), but also small joints in the hands, particularly the base of the thumb. Although no obvious cause or predisposing factors are seen in the majority of cases, both genetic and environmental factors have been linked to the development of OA. It may arise as a complication of other joint disorders, mainly inflammatory joint disease, congenital joint deformities, trauma to joints, avascular necrosis of bone or as occupational joint disease, e.g., OA of the fingers in typists and of the knee in professional footballers.

Predisposing factors may be fixed or modifiable:

- Fixed—ageing, genetic predisposition, female gender, abnormal joint structure
- Modifiable—abnormal load on joints, repetitive loading, trauma

Pathological changes

Pathological changes involve cartilage, bone, synovium and joint capsule with secondary effects on muscle (Fig. 16.6).

Early stage:

- Erosion and destruction of articular cartilage—degenerate superficial cartilage splits along lines of fibres to produce fronds (fibrillation). Narrowing of the joint space can be seen on radiography.
- Inflammation and thickening of the joint capsule and synovium.

Later stages:

- Sclerosis of subarticular bone—caused by constant friction of naked bone surfaces which now articulate in the absence of cartilage (bone eburnation).
- Osteophytes (irregular outgrowths of bone) form around the periphery of the joint by irregular outgrowth of bone spurs. Some may break off to form loose bodies within the joint (joint mice). In the distal interphalangeal (DIP) joints of the fingers, osteophytes appear as small nodules (Heberden nodes); in the proximal interphalangeal (PIP) joints, they are called Bouchard nodes.

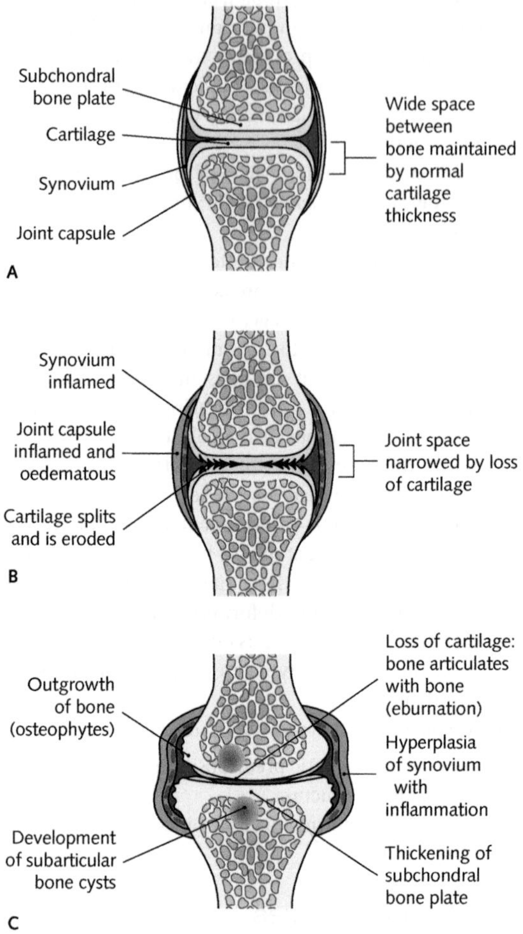

Fig. 16.6 Pathological changes in osteoarthritis (OA). (A) Normal joint. (B) Early stages of OA. (C) Later stages of OA.

- Small subchondral cysts may develop in areas where the bone is not thickened as a result of synovial fluid accumulation in underlying bone.
- Reactive thickening of synovium and joint capsule due to inflammation caused by bone and cartilage debris.
- Disuse atrophy of muscle due to joint immobility.

Clinical features

The main symptoms of OA are pain and limitation in the range of movement of the affected joint, which often leads to functional impairment (e.g., difficulty walking in hip OA). Sometimes OA is associated with visible swelling (usually as an effect of osteophytes).

In OA of the cervical vertebrae (cervical spondylosis), osteophytes compressing emerging spinal nerves are responsible for much of the symptomatology.

CLINICAL NOTES

OSTEOARTHRITIS

Osteoarthritis diagnosis is largely clinical, although there are four classic X-ray signs (of which one or more may be seen):

1. Narrowed joint space
2. Osteophytes (at bone margins)
3. Subchondral bone cysts
4. Subarticular bone sclerosis.

Rheumatoid arthritis

Rheumatoid arthritis (RA) is a chronic inflammatory joint disease caused by a multisystemic connective tissue autoimmune disorder, rheumatoid disease (see later). It affects about 1% of the UK population, females more often than males by a factor of 3:1. Onset is typically between 35 and 45 years of age, but it follows a normal distribution curve and no age group is exempt.

RA mainly affects peripheral synovial joints such as the fingers and wrists, but it can also affect the knees and more proximal joints. The most common presentations are symmetrical.

The aetiology is autoimmune and there is an association with HLA-DR4 haplotype in most ethnic groups. The condition is characterized by autoimmune-mediated activation of CD4+ T cells within affected joints. The antigen for this reaction is unknown, but once it has been triggered, the release of proinflammatory cytokines drives the destruction of the joint.

Eighty percent of RA patients have a circulating autoantibody directed against the Fc portion of native immunoglobulins (rheumatoid factor). The presence of rheumatoid factor (seropositive arthritis) helps to distinguish RA from several other inflammatory joint diseases (seronegative arthritis). However, not all RA patients are rheumatoid factor positive, and not all rheumatoid factor positive patients have RA. The exact role and underlying stimulus of rheumatoid factor is uncertain. However, immunological techniques have demonstrated it in plasma cells located in the synovium of affected joints. The presence of antibodies to anti-cyclic citrullinated peptide (CCP) have also been identified in RA patients and is more specific.

No single criterion is used in the diagnosis of RA, rather a combination of clinical features and serology aid diagnosis, which is based on the American College of Rheumatology 1987 classification criteria. RA is associated with increased mortality, reducing lifespan by an average of 8–15 years.

> **HINTS AND TIPS**
>
> In rheumatoid arthritis, worse prognosis is associated with being female, having metatarsophalangeal joint involvement, systemic involvement, and being positive for both rheumatoid factor and anti-cyclic citrullinated peptide antibodies.

Pathological changes

There are three main pathological changes (Fig. 16.7):

1. Rheumatoid synovitis.
2. Articular cartilage destruction.
3. Focal destruction of bone.

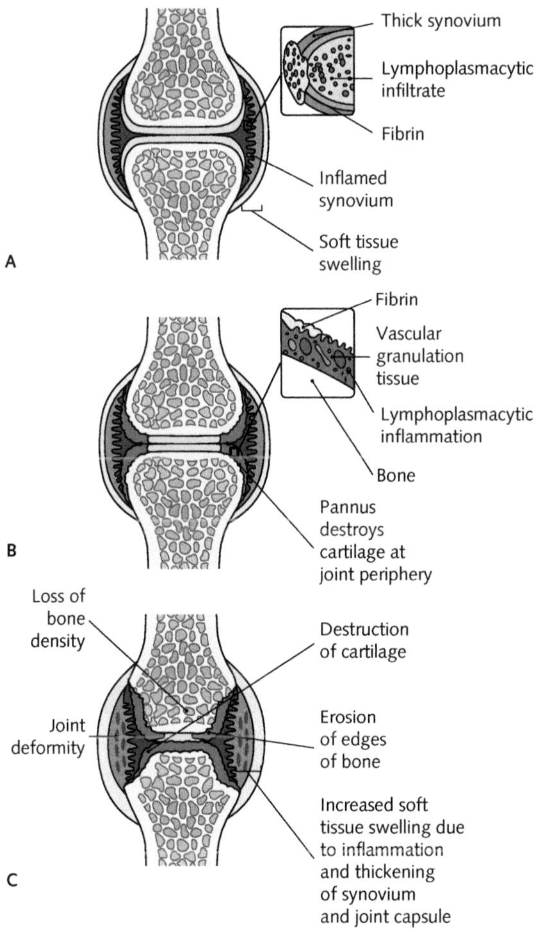

Fig. 16.7 Pathological changes in rheumatoid arthritis. (A) Rheumatoid synovitis. (B) Articular cartilage destruction. (C) Focal destruction of bone.

Rheumatoid synovitis

The synovium becomes swollen and shows a villous pattern. Chronic inflammatory cells (mainly lymphocytes and plasma cells) increase in number within the synovial stroma, often forming an exudate that effuses into the joint space. Fibrin is deposited on the surface of the synovium, which undergoes hypertrophy. Soft tissue swelling from synovial inflammation may be marked. Prolonged inflammation results in ligament laxity and, ultimately, joint deformities.

Articular cartilage destruction

Pannus tissue (macrophages, fibroblasts and granulation tissue) grows across the surface of the cartilage from the joint edges. The articular surface shows loss of cartilage beneath the extending pannus, most marked at joint margins. Pannus formation results in significant morbidity due to destruction of bone and cartilage.

Focal destruction of bone

Osteolytic destruction of bone occurs at the edges of the joint. Bone 'erosions' can be seen on radiography and are associated with joint deformity. There is also increased soft tissue swelling due to inflammation and thickening of the synovium and capsule.

Clinical features

Symmetrical polyarthritis

The insidious onset of arthritis first attacks finger joints (mainly metacarpophalangeal (MCP) and proximal interphalangeal (PIP) joints) followed by metatarsophalangeal joints and joints of the ankles, wrists, knees, shoulders, elbows and hips (in decreasing order of frequency). RA can also affect synovial joints of the spine (particularly cervical). Affected joints become swollen, painful and warm, often with redness of overlying skin. Stiffness tends to be worse in the mornings or following inactivity.

> **HINTS AND TIPS**
>
> In the hands, rheumatoid arthritis tends to affect metacarpophalangeal and proximal interphalangeal (PIP) joints whereas osteoarthritis tends to affect PIP and distal interphalangeal joints.

Joint deformities

As the disease progresses, muscle atrophy and joint destruction result in limitation of joint motion, instability, subluxation and deformities. Subluxation is the partial dislocation of a joint where the bone ends still make contact, but are misaligned. There are also flexion contractures of small joints of the hands and feet, knees, hips and elbows.

Hands:

- Anterior subluxation of the MCP joints with ulnar deviation of the fingers.
- 'Swan neck' deformity—hyperextension of the PIP joint with fixed flexion at DIP joints.
- Boutonnière (buttonhole) deformity—fixed flexion of PIP joint and extension of the terminal interphalangeal joint.
- Z deformity of the thumbs—fixed flexion at MCP joint and hyperextension at interphalangeal joint.

Wrists: There is often a fixed flexion deformity with a prominent, tender ulnar styloid process and pain on pronation/supination.

Knees: Baker cysts (cystic swelling in the popliteal fossa) are seen.

Cervical spine: There is atlantoaxial subluxation.

Deformities are initially correctable but permanent contractures eventually develop such that joints become completely disorganized.

Rheumatoid nodules

Joint changes are often associated with development of subcutaneous rheumatoid nodules, usually over the extensor aspect of the forearm but occasionally found overlying other bony prominences. Nodules are composed of extensive areas of fibrinoid material surrounded by giant cell granulomatous reaction. They occur elsewhere in the body as part of the rheumatoid disease (see later).

Complications

- Secondary OA as a result of loss of articular surface, particularly in weight-bearing joints (e.g., the knee)
- Septic arthritis—infection of the joint secondary to invasion from an ulcerated nodule or infected skin lesion
- Amyloidosis—found in 25%–30% of patients with RA at autopsy
- Carpal tunnel syndrome
- Ruptured extensor tendons of the hand
- Treatment related effects—osteoporosis, peptic ulcer disease and infection secondary to immune suppression are amongst the side effects of steroids, nonsteroidal antiinflammatory drugs and disease-modifying antirheumatic drugs (DMARDs) used to treat RA.

Extraarticular features (rheumatoid disease)

Lungs

Pulmonary involvement causes interstitial pneumonia and fibrosing alveolitis which eventually leads to interstitial pulmonary fibrosis (see Chapter 10). Also, patients may develop lesions similar to subcutaneous rheumatoid nodules, both within the lungs and on pleural surfaces. These rheumatoid nodules are particularly common in patients who already have industrial lung disease caused by inhaling various types of silica; the association of coal-worker's lung with rheumatoid nodules in seropositive miners is called Caplan syndrome. Pleural effusions, bronchitis and bronchiectasis are all more common in rheumatoid patients.

Blood vessels

There may be development of vasculitis which is either:

- acute neutrophilic vasculitis of small to medium size arteries, presenting with purpura and occasional foci of ulceration

or

- lymphocytic vasculitis, producing a more low-key erythematous patchy rash.

Eyes

Secondary Sjögren syndrome (present in 15% of RA patients) and dry eye syndrome (keratoconjunctivitis sicca) caused by lymphocytic inflammation of both lacrimal and mucous glands can occur. Lack of tears leads to secondary inflammation of the cornea. In addition, sight-threatening scleritis may occur because of degeneration of collagenous tissue in the eye.

Haemopoietic and lymphoreticular systems

Anaemia of chronic disease is common in rheumatoid patients and a minority develop hypersplenism or lymphadenopathy. The risk of lymphoma is also increased in long-standing rheumatoid disease. Felty syndrome describes splenomegaly, lymphadenopathy, anaemia and leucopoenia with RA. Sepsis is an important common cause of death in these patients.

Neurological system

Hypertrophied synovium and joint deformities increase the likelihood of peripheral compression neuropathies. Bilateral carpal tunnel syndrome is a relatively common early manifestation of RA. Spinal nerve compression also occurs.

RED FLAG

RHEUMATOID ARTHRITIS

Severe and potentially fatal cord compression can result from atlantoaxial subluxation. Patients must be assessed for joint instability prior to anaesthesia due to neck extension performed during intubation—they are a major anaesthetic risk!

Heart

Approximately one-third of RA patients develop asymptomatic pericarditis, which occasionally becomes complicated by pericardial effusion. Rheumatoid nodules may cause heart block, cardiomyopathy and ischaemia (by coronary artery compression).

Juvenile rheumatoid arthritis

This encompasses many forms and accounts for approximately 15% of cases of juvenile chronic arthritis. By definition, it begins before 16 years of age. Clinical features are similar to those of adults but smaller joints tend to be spared, polyarthritis is less common, rheumatoid nodules are usually absent and rheumatoid factor is often negative (though antinuclear antibodies (ANA) may be positive). Systemic manifestations are more common and prognosis is considered worse than for adults.

Ankylosing spondylitis

This is an example of a seronegative arthritis (rheumatoid factor negative). It is an inflammatory arthritic disorder characterized by a rigid spine due to ossification of the vertebral ligaments. There is typically an insidious onset of recurring episodes of low back pain and stiffness, sometimes radiating to the buttocks or thighs. Symptoms are characteristically worse in early morning and after inactivity. The condition begins in the lumbar vertebral spine and sacroiliac joints, extending upwards to involve thoracic and cervical vertebrae over a period of months or years. There may also be involvement of peripheral joints, mainly the hips and knees.

It affects 0.5% of the population in the United Kingdom, typically presenting in late adolescence and young adults (age 15–30 years of age), and in males more often than females by a factor of 3:1.

The aetiology is unknown but more than 90% of individuals with ankylosing spondylitis have the HLA-B27 antigen (less than 10% of the normal population have this antigen), which suggests an autoimmune disorder. HLA-B27 positivity is a common feature of the seronegative arthritides (Table 16.12).

Morphological changes—chronic inflammation of vertebral ligaments slowly heals by dense fibrosis and ossification ('bony ankylosis') to form a rigid shell that links the periphery of the vertebral bodies. Eventually the vertebral column becomes fused, inflexible and rigid ('bamboo spine' on X-ray).

Systemic manifestations include aortic valve incompetence (secondary to rheumatoid aortitis), anterior uveitis and amyloidosis (rare).

On investigation, erythrocyte sedimentation rate (ESR) and C-reactive protein (CRP) levels are usually raised, serology is negative for rheumatoid factor and X-rays may show sacroiliitis and bridging syndesmophytes between vertebrae.

The disease progresses slowly but unremittingly.

A comparison of common joint diseases is provided (Table 16.13).

Reactive arthritis

This inflammatory syndrome (previously known as Reiter syndrome) is characterized by the triad of arthritis, urethritis and conjunctivitis. It complicates 0.8% of urethral infections in males and 0.2% of cases of dysentery. It occurs in males more often than females by a factor of 15:1 and the

Table 16.13 Comparison of joint diseases

	Osteoarthritis	Rheumatoid disease	Ankylosing spondylitis
Affected age group	Elderly	Any age	Onset usually before 30 years
Sex	Females > males	Females > males	Males > females
HLA association	None known	*HLA-DR4*	*HLA-B27*
Rheumatoid factor	Negative	Positive	Usually negative
Clinical features	Worsening of pain throughout day	Morning stiffness which improves throughout the day	—
Affected joints	Mainly hip, knees and spine Usually asymmetrical	Any Usually symmetrical	Mainly spine
Hands	Heberden nodes (DIP) Bouchard nodes (PIP)	Ulnar deviation Swan neck deformity Boutonnière deformity Z deformity of thumbs Prominent ulnar styloid process	—
Joint pathology	Erosion of cartilage Osteophytes	Destruction of joints Pannus formation	Bony ankyloses
Synovial pathology	Slight synovial hyperplasia	Florid synovial hyperplasia	—
Associated diseases	—	Sjögren syndrome Interstitial lung disease Amyloidosis	Aortic valve incompetence Uveitis Amyloidosis

DIP, Distal interphalangeal; HLA, human leukocyte antigen; MCP, metacarpophalangeal; PIP, proximal interphalangeal.

usual age of onset is 20 to 40 years. More than 80% of patients are *HLA-B27* positive.

The underlying pathological mechanism is unknown but is probably autoimmune, triggered by a prior genitourinary or gastrointestinal infection.

Classification of reactive arthritis is divided into:

- *Genitourinary*—usually follows nonspecific (nongonococcal) urethritis or, less commonly, cystitis or prostatitis.
- *Intestinal or postdysenteric type*—in some parts of the world it may follow dysentery or, occasionally, nonspecific diarrhoea, occurring 10–30 days after intestinal manifestations. Infection is usually with *Salmonella*, *Shigella*, *Yersinia* or *Campylobacter* species.

Clinical features:

- asymmetric arthritis, usually affecting knee or ankle, and developing within weeks of the infectious episode. Clinically and histologically, arthritis resembles RA with chronic inflammatory synovitis.
- dysuria and penile (or vaginal) discharge.
- conjunctivitis (in 30% of cases).

> **HINTS AND TIPS**
>
> REACTIVE ARTHRITIS
>
> Remember: '*Can't see, can't pee, can't climb a tree*' to help remember the conjunctivitis, urethritis and arthritis associated with reactive arthritis.

Prognosis—the first attack typically resolves spontaneously within 6 months. However, 50% of patients relapse and some have continued relapsing chronic arthritis, causing disability but seldom deformity. In a minority of cases, there is development of severe spondylitis and features very similar to those of ankylosing spondylitis.

Psoriatic arthritis

Five to seven percent of psoriasis patients develop arthropathy, which takes one of four forms:

1. Distal arthritis—the most common form. Affects the DIP joints of the hands and feet, causing 'sausage-like' swelling of the digits.
2. Rheumatoid-like arthritis—polyarthropathy similar to rheumatoid disease, usually symmetrical but negative for rheumatoid factor (seronegative arthritis). More common in women.
3. Arthritis mutilans—progressive deformity of the hands and feet caused by erosion of the small bones. Often associated with severe psoriasis.
4. Ankylosing spondylitis/sacroiliitis—in *HLA-B27*-positive patients.

Others

Inflammatory bowel disease-associated arthritis

Enteropathic arthritis is seen at some stage in up to 20% of patients with ulcerative colitis and Crohn disease. Typically, it involves knee joints, but occasionally ankles, elbows and digital joints. Sacroiliitis and ankylosing spondylitis are also more frequent in patients with inflammatory bowel disease.

Neuropathic (Charcot) joint disease

A Charcot joint is the degeneration, bone destruction and ultimate deformity of a weight-bearing joint. This joint disease occurs secondary to the loss of position sense within the joint, which although swollen and deformed, is painless. Possible causes of loss of joint sensation include diabetic neuropathy, tabes dorsalis, syringomyelia, leprosy and cauda equina lesions (e.g., myelomeningocele).

Sarcoid arthritis

Arthritis occurs in 10% of patients with sarcoidosis, with onset typically in the first year of the disease. It may be of two types:

1. Early acute transient type—polyarticular, symmetrical arthritis typically affecting knees and ankles, and usually associated with erythema nodosum. Arthritis is typically self-limiting.
2. Chronic persistent type—polyarticular, associated with chronic sarcoidosis.

Crystal arthropathies

These diseases are characterized by deposition of crystals in joints and soft tissues. Affected patients usually present with an episode of acute arthritis, inflammation being caused by the deposition of crystals. There are two main types of crystal arthropathies: monosodium urate gout ('true gout' or simply 'gout') and calcium pyrophosphate gout ('pseudogout'). A comparison of the two types is shown in Table 16.14.

Gout

This acute inflammatory crystal arthropathy is caused by the deposition of urate crystal in joints and soft tissues as a result of hyperuricaemia. Prevalence is about 1% of the UK population and it is largely confined to men (90%), although some women develop the condition postmenopausally. It can present at any time over the age of 20.

Aetiology—uric acid is normally derived from the breakdown of purines and is excreted in urine. Increased concentrations of serum uric acid (hyperuricaemia) can result in gout (Table 16.15).

However, it should be noted that the majority of patients who have a raised blood uric acid level will never develop

Table 16.14 Comparison of gout and pseudogout

	True gout	Pseudogout
Commonest location	Big toe	Knee
Crystal type	Monosodium urate	Calcium pyrophosphate
Underlying process	Hyperuricaemia	Chondrocalcinosis
Joints affected	Small	Large
Pain	Severe (because of crystal shape)	Moderate
Crystal shape	Needle	Rhomboid
Polarization	Negative birefringence	Positive birefringence

Table 16.15 Causes of hyperuricaemia

Reduced excretion of uric acid	Commonest Uncertain origin Associated with hyperlipidaemia, renal failure, lactic and thiazide diuretics
Overproduction of uric acid	Less common Associated with high cell turnover (e.g., leukaemia, chemotherapy, severe psoriasis) Rarely due to congenital enzyme defects of purine metabolism

gout or any of its complications. The condition has a familial tendency, and it is believed to be polygenically inherited.

Pathogenesis

Gout affects the joints, soft tissues and kidney, as discussed further.

Joints—supersaturation of urate in synovial fluid results in the precipitation of needle-shaped urate crystals in certain joints, forming white powdery deposits on the surface of articular cartilage, beneath which degenerative changes can be seen. Crystal release into the synovial fluid stimulates an acute inflammatory reaction leading to excruciating pain (due to the shape of the crystals), oedema and the redness seen in acutely inflamed joints. Microscopically, neutrophil polymorphs can be seen to phagocytose urate crystal in joint fluid. Tophi (large aggregations of urate crystals surrounded by inflammation) are pathognomonic of chronic gout.

Soft tissues—uric acid crystals are also deposited in the soft tissues around joints, where their presence excites a foreign body, giant cell reaction. These soft tissue masses may also enlarge to produce tophi, especially around the pinna of the ear.

Kidney—in 10% of patients, urate crystals deposited in the kidney may lead to an interstitial nephritis and to renal calculi composed of uric acid. Crystals may also cause urinary obstruction, increasing the likelihood of complications such as pyelonephritis.

Clinical features

Characteristics of gout are:

- intermittent attacks of excruciating pain, oedema and redness (acute gouty arthritis)
- monoarthropathy (90%); polyarthropathy (two or more affected joints) 10%
- metatarsophalangeal joint of the big toe is most commonly affected (podagra, 75% of cases), but gout occasionally affects the ankle and, less commonly, the knee and hip.

Recurrent attacks affecting the same joint eventually lead to articular cartilage destruction, chronic synovial thickening and secondary OA—chronic gouty arthritis.

Diagnosis:

- Clinical features (as described previously)
- Raised serum urate level
- Presence of crystals of monosodium urate in aspirated synovial fluid from joint (detected with polarizing light)

Prognosis—some patients have only a single attack or suffer another only after an interval of many years. More often there is a tendency towards recurrent attacks that increase in frequency and duration so that, eventually, attacks merge and the patient remains in a prolonged state of subacute gout.

Chronic tophaceous gout

Repeated acute attacks of gout cause tophi formation with inflammation, fibrosis and hyperplasia of the synovial lining of the joint and eventually produces chronic arthritis.

Pseudogout

This acute inflammatory crystal arthropathy (also known as calcium pyrophosphate deposition disease, CPPD) is caused by deposition of calcium pyrophosphate crystals in articular cartilage of joints (chondrocalcinosis). CPPD is most common in the elderly and affects males more often than females.

The aetiology can be sporadic, metabolic or familial:

- *Sporadic*—in the vast majority of cases, the cause of pyrophosphate deposition is unknown but it is probably an age-related phenomenon.
- *Metabolic*—in patients under the age of 60 years, the disease is often associated with hyperparathyroidism, haemochromatosis or other less common metabolic or endocrine disorders.
- *Familial*—in a minority of patients, the disease is inherited as an autosomal dominant disorder.

Pathogenesis

Chondrocalcinosis is often asymptomatic. However, if crystals are shed into the joint space, patients develop an acute arthritis similar to that seen in urate gout. This shedding of crystals may be precipitated by trauma or intercurrent illness, or it may be spontaneous.

With time, damage to cartilage leads to the development of secondary OA.

Clinical features

As with gout, the affected joint becomes suddenly painful, warm, swollen and tender. The most commonly affected joint is the knee (>50% of cases), followed by the wrist, shoulder and ankle. The duration of the attack can vary from days to weeks and recurrent attacks are uncommon. ***Diagnosis*** – is by X-ray—cartilaginous calcification is usually obvious on X-ray—and by the presence of calcium pyrophosphate dihydrate crystals in aspirated synovial fluid (detected with polarizing light).

Intraarticular aspiration and corticosteroids are the most effective treatment for acute pseudogout (antiinflammatory drugs and colchicine also work but are often avoided in the elderly).

Septic arthritis

This acute inflammation of a joint is caused by infection—typically bacterial. This may affect any age group but children and young adults are most commonly affected. It is a medical emergency, with a mortality rate of 10%. In older adults, most cases are associated with penetrating injury. Males are affected more often than females by a factor of 2:1. The knee and hip are the most common sites.

Aetiology—a wide range of bacteria may be responsible, but *S. aureus*, streptococci, *Haemophilus* and *Salmonella* species are the most important. Patients who have developed septic arthritis always have bacteraemia.

Risk factors are diabetes, RA, joint puncture, surgery and immunosuppressed states.

Bacteria gain access to a joint via:

- local trauma—well-recognized complication of penetrating injury such as open fractures, insertion of surgical prosthesis and nonsterile, intraarticular injection of steroids for established autoimmune arthritis.
- spread from adjacent infective foci—especially in neonates with epiphyseal osteomyelitis.
- haematogenous spread—most common route, usually from the skin or upper respiratory tract. Intravenous drug users are particularly likely to develop septic arthritis associated with Gram-negative bacteraemia. Patients with sickle cell disease are prone to Salmonella septic arthritis.

Clinical features—there is an abrupt onset of severe pain, tenderness, swelling and erythema. The majority of cases affect a single joint only, but some cases of gonococcal arthritis and arthritis in intravenous drug abusers may affect more joints.

RED FLAG

Acute onset of a painful, stiff, hot and swollen joint requires immediate aspiration (arthrocentesis) to exclude septic arthritis.

DIFFERENTIAL DIAGNOSIS

CAUSES OF AN ACUTE MONOARTHRITIS

Common causes	Gout
	Pseudogout
	Septic arthritis
	Osteomyelitis
	Trauma
	Avascular necrosis of the femoral head
	OA
	Haemarthrosis
Less common causes	Malignancy
	RA
	Haemoglobinopathy
	Reactive arthritis

Complications—untreated, it proceeds rapidly to joint destruction often with osteomyelitis, sinus formation, ankylosis and dislocation of joints.

CLINICAL NOTES

Fluid cytology is performed on swollen and inflamed joints to aid diagnosis. Synovial fluid is aspirated from the diseased joint, and a wet preparation (unstained fluid placed directly onto a slide and covered) is viewed under the microscope and polarized. This particularly aids in diagnosis of crystals.

DISORDERS OF THE NEUROMUSCULAR JUNCTION

Overview

Several diseases of muscle have been shown to result from disorders affecting transmission at the neuromuscular junction (NMJ).

Clinical presentation of NMJ dysfunction:

- Fatigability—primarily affecting proximal limb muscles, extraocular muscles (causing ptosis or diplopia) and muscles of mastication, speech and facial expression.
- Periodic paralysis—sudden reversible attacks of paralysis and flaccidity.

Disorders can be classified into two types, presynaptic and postsynaptic abnormalities, depending on which of the synaptic membranes is affected.

Presynaptic abnormalities

Botulism

This rare form of food poisoning is caused by ingestion of a toxin produced by the bacterium *Clostridium botulinum*, found in imperfectly treated tinned food or preserved fish contaminated with the microbe.

Pathogenesis—the toxin binds irreversibly to the presynaptic nerve terminals of axons whose neurotransmission is acetylcholine (ACh) mediated. These include the NMJ, autonomic ganglia and parasympathetic nerve terminals. Binding of the toxin prevents fusion of ACh vesicles with the neuronal membrane, thereby preventing ACh release and neurotransmission.

Clinical symptoms are chiefly vomiting and paresis of skeletal, ocular, pharyngeal and respiratory muscles. Antitoxin is available, but it has no effect once the toxin is bound. Recovery of transmission is achieved by terminal axonal sprouting and the formation of new synaptic contacts. Mortality can be high.

Lambert–Eaton myasthenic syndrome

This rare autoimmune disorder is characterized by proximal muscle weakness and absent reflexes that both improve with exercise. Autoantibodies are thought to bind to presynaptic voltage-gated calcium channels at the NMJ. This causes the reduced release of ACh in response to nerve stimulation. Forty percent of cases are associated with lung carcinoma, usually small cell subtype, when it is considered a paraneoplastic syndrome. Small cell lung carcinoma cells express calcium channels, suggesting that cross-reactive autoantibody production is triggered by these tumour antigens.

Postsynaptic abnormalities

Myasthenia gravis

This autoimmune disease is characterized by a progressive failure to sustain maintained or repetitive contractions of striated muscle. Prevalence is about 1 in 30,000. The disease usually appears between the ages of 15 and 50 years, and females are more often affected than males.

Aetiology—autoantibodies against the postsynaptic acetylcholine receptor (AChR) are produced by B lymphocytes that are defectively controlled by T lymphocytes as a result of a disorder of the thymus gland. Antibody binding to AChRs causes accelerated receptor degradation, damage to the postsynaptic membrane via a complement reaction and blocking of acetylcholine binding resulting in severely impaired neurotransmission.

Thymus pathology coexists in 75% of cases of myasthenia gravis; 15% of cases have a thymoma (see Chapter 17) and 65% have thymic gland hyperplasia. There is a strong link to other autoimmune diseases, including thyrotoxicosis (Graves disease), diabetes mellitus, RA, and systemic lupus erythematosus (SLE). There is linkage with various human leucocyte antigens (HLA), such as B8 and DRw3.

Presentation:

- Early symptoms—intermittent ptosis or diplopia, weakness when chewing, swallowing, speaking or of moving the limbs. Movement is initially strong, but it rapidly weakens by the end of the day or after exercise. Reflexes are normal.
- Later symptoms—respiratory muscles may be involved and respiratory failure is not an uncommon cause of death. Asphyxia occurs readily as the cough may be too weak to clear foreign bodies from the airways. Muscle atrophy may occur in long-standing cases.

The disease runs a relapsing/remitting course, and relapses may be precipitated by emotional disturbances, infections, pregnancy or severe muscular effort.

Most patients with appropriate treatment have a relatively normal lifespan (mortality 3%–4%). Onset at age over 40 years and thymoma are key risk factors for a poorer prognosis.

MYOPATHIES

Introduction

Skeletal muscle is composed of bundles of muscle fibres which are individual muscle cells. In cross-section, muscle fibres are polygonal, of similar size, with peripherally located nuclei, and are surrounded by a thin fibrous sheath called the endomysium. Fat is not normally present.

Two types of muscle fibres are recognized based on their contractile and metabolic characteristics. Slow twitch (type I) muscle fibres have aerobic metabolism and are used during sustained periods of activity. Fast twitch (type II) muscle fibres use anaerobic metabolism and are recruited in explosive events such as sprinting as they are efficient at rapid energy generation and powerful shortening.

Definition

Myopathy is any condition that primarily affects muscle physiology, structure or biochemistry.

Muscular dystrophy

X-linked muscular dystrophy

Muscular dystrophy is the term used to describe inherited degenerative muscle diseases.

X-linked muscular dystrophy is characterized by the progressive degeneration of single muscle cells over a prolonged period of time. It results in muscle fibre destruction with the development of fibrosis.

Duchenne muscular dystrophy

Duchenne muscular dystrophy (DMD) affects 1 in 3500 male births and is the most common form of muscular dystrophy in childhood. The disorder is due to a mutation of the gene coding for dystrophin, a protein that normally anchors the actin cytoskeleton of muscle fibres to the basement membrane via a membrane glycoprotein complex (Fig. 16.8). Dystrophin helps to transmit the forces of contraction, meaning that muscle fibres in patients with DMD are liable to tearing with repeated contraction leading to permanent loss.

A spectrum of clinical severity exists in DMD as a result of different mutations within the dystrophin gene:

- Severe DMD—complete failure to produce dystrophin due to frameshift mutations.
- Moderate to severe forms of DMD—dystrophin is produced but anchorage is inefficient because of mutations in binding sites for either membrane glycoprotein complex or actin cytoskeleton.
- Mild form of DMD (Becker muscular dystrophy (BMD)) - in-frame deletion mutations produce a truncated but functional dystrophin protein which is still capable of anchoring muscle to basement membrane. BMD has a later onset than DMD.

Morphological features - there is loss of the total number of muscle fibres with a resultant increase in endomysial thickness and perimysial fat infiltration. The remaining muscle fibres show variability in size and include small rounded forms, large hypercontracted fibres and necrotic fibres.

Clinical features—childhood onset of proximal muscle weakness is associated with a high serum creatine phosphokinase level (caused by muscle necrosis) and calf pseudohypertrophy due to fat and fibrous tissue replacement of muscle. Cardiac muscle is also affected leading to cardiomyopathy (see Chapter 9).

The prognosis depends on the degree of severity. For severe DMD it is very poor; most affected individuals are wheelchair-dependent in their early teens and die in their early twenties from cardiac complications or respiratory insufficiency (Table 16.16).

Table 16.16 Features of Duchenne and Becker muscular dystrophy

	Duchenne muscular dystrophy	Becker muscular dystrophy
Incidence	1/3500	1/20,000
Age of onset	3–5 years	≥11 years
Life expectancy	20 years	40 years
Mobility	Wheelchair bound by age 11 years	Walking or wheelchair bound in later life >35 years
Dystrophin mutation	Out-of-frame deletions, duplications or nonsense	In-frame deletions
Dystrophin protein	Complete loss or nonfunctional	Truncated and partially functional

Myotonic disorders

Myotonic disorders are diseases in which there is a continuing contraction of muscle after voluntary contraction has ceased.

Myotonic muscular dystrophy

This autosomal dominant disorder is characterized by progressive distal muscle weakness, myotonia (inability to relax muscles) and several nonmuscle features including cataracts, frontal baldness in males, gonadal atrophy, cardiomyopathy and (in some cases) dementia.

This is the most common inherited muscle disease of adults, affecting 1 in 8000.

The genetic abnormality is an unstable CTG repeat sequence in a cyclic adenosine monophosphate (cAMP)-dependent protein kinase located on chromosome 19. The disease shows anticipation, meaning that it appears at a younger age in each succeeding generation. The mechanism by which this mutation causes myotonia is unknown.

Microscopically, affected muscles show abnormalities of fibre size with fibre necrosis, abundant internal nuclei and replacement by fibrofatty tissue.

The disorder usually becomes apparent in adolescence or early adulthood with facial weakness and disturbed gait.

Prognosis—death is commonly due to involvement of respiratory muscles in middle age.

Acquired myopathies

Idiopathic inflammatory myopathies

This is primary inflammation of muscle with resulting fibre necrosis. The inflammatory infiltrate is mainly composed of CD8 + T lymphocytes and monocytes as part of an abnormal immune response. There are three main types of inflammatory myopathies, any of which may occur as part of an immune-mediated systemic disease such as systemic sclerosis.

Polymyositis

This is the most common inflammatory muscle disorder, though still relatively rare, occurring most frequently in adults, with females affected more often than males by a factor of 3:1. It is characterized by symmetrical weakness and pain of the proximal limb muscles.

Aetiology—cytotoxic T cells and other lymphoid cells are found within the endomysium and are seen invading non-necrotic muscle fibres suggesting an autoimmune response to myocytes, but the mechanism of sensitization is unknown.

Associations:

- Increased predisposition in people with *HLA-B8/DR3*.
- Connective tissue diseases such as SLE, RA or systemic sclerosis.
- Autoimmune diseases: Hashimoto thyroiditis and myasthenia gravis.
- Interstitial lung disease and myocarditis.
- Dermatomyositis—see later.
- Malignancy—10% of patients will develop or have a malignancy at the time of presentation. Most common associated malignancies are breast and ovarian cancers in women and lung and prostate cancers in men.

Clinical features—an insidious onset in the third to fifth decade of life, with symmetrical proximal muscle weakness initially affecting the lower limbs and neck flexors. Progression is typically slow, over weeks to months, but it may eventually involve pharyngeal, laryngeal and respiratory muscles leading to dysphagia, dysphonia and respiratory failure. Blood tests show elevated muscle enzymes (creatine kinase, aspartate aminotransferase, lactate dehydrogenase) and tests for rheumatoid factor and ANA are often positive (anti-Jo-1 antibodies present in 20%). Inflammatory markers (ESR and CRP) can be mildly raised or normal. Muscle biopsy is the gold standard for diagnosis.

Dermatomyositis

This can present on its own or as part of an overlap syndrome with other connective tissue diseases. It has the muscle components of polymyositis accompanied by characteristic skin lesions:

- Heliotrope rash—purple rash on upper eyelids with associated periorbital oedema
- Gottron papules—erythematous scaling patches over the knuckles
- Shawl/'V' sign—erythematous, scaling photosensitive rash on neck, back and sometimes anterior chest
- Mechanics hands—cracked and thickened skin on the ventral surface of the hands
- Nail bed changes—dilated capillary loops, irregular cuticles and periungual telangiectasia.

Twenty-five percent of dermatomyositis cases will have an associated malignancy.

Inclusion body myositis

This slowly progressive inflammatory muscle disorder is similar to polymyositis, but typically affects both proximal and distal muscles in an asymmetric pattern. It also occurs mainly in the elderly with a male preponderance. By light microscopy, histological features appear similar to polymyositis, but with electron microscopy vacuoles containing filamentous inclusion bodies can be seen within fibres.

Other myopathies

Weakness and wasting of muscles are not exclusive to inflammatory myopathies and occur in other conditions/disease processes. The main causes are:

- corticosteroid-induced myopathy—either therapeutic or in Cushing disease. Corticosteroids are associated with type II muscle fibre atrophy.
- myopathies of thyroid dysfunction—associated with both hyperthyroidism and hypothyroidism.
- myopathy of osteomalacia—painful myopathy often without much wasting or weakness.
- alcoholic myopathy.
- drug induced myopathy, e.g., chloroquine, statins, D-penicillamine, corticosteroids.

Changes are usually reversible with appropriate therapy.

Chapter summary

- Primary bone tumours are rare, metastatic tumours are more common.
- Primary bone tumours have characteristic sites, age ranges and X-ray appearances. The majority occur around the knee.
- The commonest malignant bone tumours are osteosarcoma, chondrosarcoma and Ewing sarcoma/primitive neuroectodermal tumour (PNET).
- Benign bone lesions include enchondroma, osteoid osteoma and osteochondroma.
- Bone disease can be intrinsic to the bone matrix resulting in increased turnover, demineralization and loss of substance in varying proportions.
- Arthropathies can be due to degeneration, inflammation, infection or crystals.
- Osteoarthritis is the commonest arthropathy.
- Inflammatory arthropathies may be seropositive or seronegative for rheumatoid factor, and may be associated with systemic disease.
- Septic arthritis is a clinical emergency.
- Crystal arthropathies should be diagnosed on fluid cytology.
- Myositis is an acquired symmetrical weakness with pain affecting proximal limb muscles; it usually occurs in adults.
- X-linked muscular dystrophies present in children and cause progressive proximal weakness without pain.

Pathology of the blood and immune system 17

AUTOIMMUNE DISEASE

Systemic autoimmune disease

Autoimmune diseases that cause damage in many tissues and organs are termed 'multisystemic' or 'systemic' autoimmune diseases and are associated with a variety of autoantibodies (Table 17.1). They can occur in isolation or as part of overlap syndromes where features of more than one disease are present.

Table 17.1 Autoimmune diseases and associated antibodies[a]

Condition	Antibodies involved
SLE	ANA (speckled pattern) Anti-dsDNA (specific) Anti-histone (drug induced) Anti-RNP Anti-Smith (specific, predicts renal disease) Anti-La Anti-Ro Rheumatoid factor positive
Antiphospholipid syndrome	Antiphospholipid Anticardiolipin Lupus anticoagulant
Systemic sclerosis • Diffuse systemic • Limited cutaneous (CREST syndrome)	Anti-Scl-70 (more severe clinical course and visceral involvement. In females, confers increased risk of malignancy.) Anti-Jo-1 Anti-RNA pol-1 ANA positive
	Anti-centromere
Sjögren syndrome	Rheumatoid factor positive Anti-La Anti-Ro (crosses placenta causing fetal heart block) ANA positive
Polymyositis	Anti-Jo-1 (can be positive in dermatomyositis)
Rheumatoid disease	Rheumatoid factor positive Anti-CCP
Vasculitides	ANCA positive

[a] *No one antibody is 100% specific however, some are more specific than others for certain conditions and confer additional clinical phenotypes. Antibody positivity is variable from patient to patient. Anti-La and -Ro can be present in SLE but are more commonly associated with Sjögren syndrome.*
ANCA, Antineutrophil cytoplasmic antibody; ANA, antinuclear antibody; CREST, calcinosis, Raynauds phenomenon, esophageal dysmotility, sclerodactyly, telangiectasia; dsDNA, double stranded DNA; SLE, systemic lupus erythematosus; RNP, ribonucleoprotein.

Systemic lupus erythematosus

This inflammatory disorder of connective tissue is associated with autoantibodies to a wide variety of autoantigens. Many tissues are affected but synovial joints, skin, kidneys and the brain are the major target organs. It affects 30 per 100,000 of the UK population with a female to male ratio of 9:1. Presentation is commonly in the young and middle-aged with a peak incidence at 20 to 30 years old. The aetiology is unknown, but there is a strong familial association and drugs (hydralazine, procainamide, minocycline), chemicals and unidentified viral infections have been implicated.

Pathogenesis: Systemic lupus erythematosus (SLE) appears to be a disorder of immune intolerance to 'self', as a wide array of autoantibodies are seen (Table 17.1). None of these antibodies are specific for SLE and most have been detected in other connective tissue disorders or in diseases with an immunological basis.

Clinical features: The disease is a great mimicker, indolent to fulminant, and can affect almost every organ system. Presentation is commonly in a young woman, with fever, joint pain and a rash. Other symptoms include malaise, weight loss and marked musculoskeletal symptoms. Specific diagnostic criteria are outlined in Table 17.2 and diagnosis is made on a combination of clinical features and laboratory investigations. The disorder follows a protracted course of relapses and remissions. Renal, central nervous system (CNS) and cardiac lesions are the most important prognostically.

Microscopically: the appearance is highly variable, depending on severity and organ system involved. The underlying pathology is that of immune complex deposition. Within small blood vessels, this leads to an acute necrotizing vasculitis with fibrinoid necrosis of the vessel walls and deposition of fibrinoid material within the surrounding tissues.

Immunofluorescent stains are used to visualize the location and type of immune complex deposition. Characteristically there is 'full house' positivity in SLE for all of the antibody stains.

Rheumatoid disease

Rheumatoid disease is a common and important multisystemic autoimmune disease. It is covered in detail in Chapter 16.

Antiphospholipid syndrome

This is a prothrombotic autoimmune disease with autoantibodies against phospholipids. The two major antiphospholipid antibodies are: lupus anticoagulant and anticardiolipin antibody. Coombs test can be positive and β_2 microglobulin antibodies can be present; antineutrophil cytoplasmic antibody (ANCA) is negative. *Note:* positive anticardiolipin antibodies give a false-positive test for syphilis.

> **HINTS AND TIPS**
>
> ANCA AND ANA
>
> **ANCA**—antineutrophil cytoplasmic antibody. Antibodies against elements found in the cytoplasm of neutrophils. Two types:
> - pANCA—perinuclear—antibodies against proteinase 3.
> - cANCA—cytoplasmic- antibodies against myeloperoxidase (MPO).
>
> Positive in various autoimmune diseases but most strongly associated with vasculitis.
>
> **ANA**—antinuclear antibody.
>
> Antibodies against elements found in the nucleus. These include Ro and La, anti-centromere, Jo-1, histones, topoisomerase (Scl70). The pattern of ANA positivity can also be described, i.e., speckled, centromeric, nucleolar.

Presentation is in the young to middle-aged, with patients at risk of deep vein thrombosis, stroke, myocardial infarction, renal disease and miscarriage. Most cases are primary, but it can occur as part of an overlap syndrome with SLE.

> **HINTS AND TIPS**
>
> CLOT
>
> Features of antiphospholipid syndrome can be remembered by 'CLOT'
>
> ***C***oagulation defect—arterial/venous thrombosis
> ***L***ivedo reticularis
> ***O***bstetric—recurrent miscarriages
> ***T***hrombocytopenia

Scleroderma disorders

This is the term for a group of disorders characterized by chronic inflammation of connective tissues followed by progressive fibrosis. It affects 3.7 people per million, with a 4:1 female bias in people aged 30–65 years. The commonest symptom is bilateral skin thickening of the fingers and hands which, if it extends proximally to the metacarpophalangeal joints, is sufficient for a diagnosis of 'scleroderma'. Other symptoms are variable and include Raynaud phenomenon, oesophageal reflux, lethargy and musculoskeletal pain.

> **CLINICAL NOTES**
>
> CREST
>
> ***C***alcinosis
> ***R***aynaud disease
> *(O)**E***sophageal dysmotility
> ***S***clerodactyly
> ***T***elangiectasia
> and
> Primary pulmonary hypertension

The classification of the sclerodermal disorders determines the course and prognosis of the disease (Table 17.3). In general, limited cutaneous disease (CREST) is associated

Table 17.3 Classification of scleroderma diseases[a]

Classification	Features
Localized	
• Linear scleroderma	A long narrow plaque of sclerosis found on the skin
• Generalized morphea	Four or more plaques affecting two or more body regions
Systemic	
• Limited cutaneous systemic sclerosis (limited scleroderma/ CREST syndrome)	Still has organ involvement Increased risk of pulmonary hypertension Associated anticentromere antibodies
• Diffuse cutaneous (diffuse scleroderma)	Lung fibrosis, PAH, renal disease, cardiac disease, small bowel malabsorption, constipation/overflow diarrhoea, erectile dysfunction Anti-Scl-70 antibodies
• Systemic sclerosis sine scleroderma	Rare—visceral but no cutaneous involvement.
Overlap syndromes—account for 20%	For example, with polymyositis, Sjögren syndrome and rheumatoid disease

[a] Limited cutaneous systemic sclerosis is more common than diffuse cutaneous systemic sclerosis.
PAH, Pulmonary artery hypertension.

with a better survival rate compared with diffuse disease with extensive organ involvement.

Pathology: Increased deposition of collagen (types I, II, IV and VII), glycosaminoglycans and fibronectin within the connective tissues and walls of small blood vessels results in collagenous fibrosis. Vasculopathy is also present with intimal proliferation and leaking of red blood cells into the interstitium.

Sjögren syndrome

A disease characterized by dry eyes (keratoconjunctivitis sicca) and dry mouth (xerostomia) owing to autoantibodies against exocrine glands, most notably lacrimal and salivary. This results in lymphocytic infiltration, fibrosis and destruction of the glands. Onset is around 30 to 40 years of age, with a 9:1 female predominance. Other symptoms include parotid swelling, polyarthritis and lethargy.

Serologically, antinuclear antibody (ANA) is positive with or without positivity for Ro and La antibodies. This is important as Ro can cross the placenta and cause fetal heart block. Histologically, diagnosis is by lip biopsy to assess the minor salivary glands.

Sjögren syndrome can be primary, associated with HLA-B8, DR3 and DQA1, or secondary as part of an overlap syndrome.

Organ-specific disease

Autoimmune diseases involving a single organ or cell type are known as organ-specific autoimmune diseases. Table 17.4 provides an overview of these conditions, providing page references to detailed discussions of each elsewhere.

> **HINTS AND TIPS**
>
> **ORGAN-SPECIFIC AUTOIMMUNE DISEASE**
>
> Although organ-specific autoimmune diseases specifically affect one organ, they frequently occur together, e.g., Addison disease is often associated with autoimmune gastritis.

Hashimoto thyroiditis

This causes hypothyroidism secondary to antibody-mediated destruction of the thyroid gland (see Chapter 14).

Graves disease

Thyrotoxicosis due to overstimulation of thyroid-stimulating hormone receptors by autoantibodies (see Chapter 14).

Type 1 diabetes mellitus

Type 1 (insulin-dependent) diabetes mellitus results from antibody-mediated destruction of β-cells within the pancreatic islets of Langerhans, which produce insulin. It is characterized by hyperglycaemia responsive to insulin (see Chapter 14).

Addison disease

This is adrenal insufficiency caused by the autoimmune-mediated destruction of the adrenal cortex (80%) or by infection (20%) (see Chapter 14).

Autoimmune gastritis

This is chronic inflammation of the gastric mucosa mediated by gastric parietal cell antibodies with or without intrinsic factor autoantibodies, and may lead to pernicious anaemia (see Chapter 11).

Vitiligo

In this multifactorial condition there is patchy depigmentation of skin caused in part by autoimmune destruction of melanocytes (see Chapter 18).

Myasthenia gravis

This is the autoimmune antibody-mediated destruction of acetylcholine receptors within the neuromuscular junction (see Chapter 16).

Table 17.4 Organ-specific autoimmune diseases

Disease	Associated autoantibody	Clinical features
Graves disease	Anti-TSH receptor antibody	Hyperthyroidism
Hashimoto disease	Anti-TPO and/or anti-Tg antibodies	Hypothyroidism
Type I diabetes mellitus	Anti-islet β-cell antibody	Insulin-responsive hyperglycaemia
Addison disease	Anti-21 hydroxylase antibodies/ adrenal antibodies	Adrenal insufficiency
Autoimmune gastritis	Anti-parietal cell and/or anti-intrinsic factor antibodies	Pernicious anaemia
Vitiligo	Abs against melanocytes /tyrosine	Hypopigmentation
Myasthenia gravis	Anti-AChR	Muscle fatigue

Ab, Antibody; AChR, acetylcholine receptor antibody; Tg, thyroglobulin; TPO, thyroid peroxidase; TSH, thyroid-stimulating hormone.

DISEASES OF IMMUNODEFICIENCY

Immunodeficiency is an impairment of the body's immune response mechanisms, resulting in a predisposition to acquiring infections and certain malignancies. They can be congenital or acquired:

- ***Primary immunodeficiencies:*** a rare group of congenital diseases that usually result from genetic defects in one or more of the effector components of the immune system. Symptoms commonly develop in infancy, after the initial protection of maternally derived IgG antibodies starts to decline between 3 and 6 months of age (Fig. 17.1). More than 95 inherited immunodeficiency disorders have now been identified.
- ***Secondary immunodeficiencies***: acquired disorders from extrinsic/environmental causes that are common compared to primary causes.

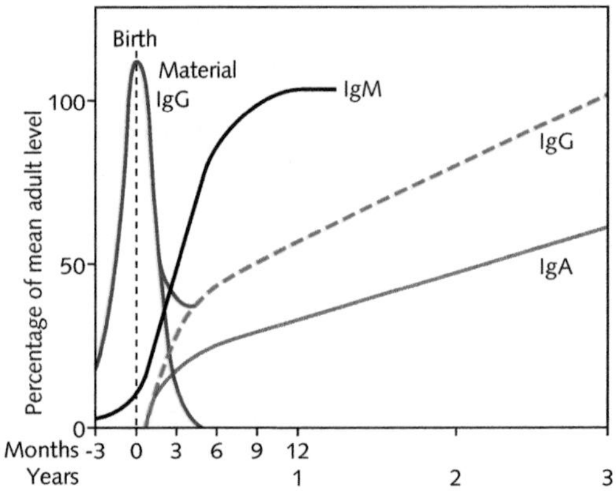

Fig. 17.1 Serum immunoglobulin levels in the neonate. (Adapted with permission from Newell S, Lecture Notes in Paediatrics, 8th ed. Blackwell Publishing, London, 2008.)

HINTS AND TIPS

INFECTIONS LINKED WITH B AND T CELL DEFICIENCIES

The type of infection associated with diseases of immune deficiency depends on the category of immune disorder:

- B-cell deficiencies (defective antibody response)—increased susceptibility to opportunistic infections caused by extracellular organisms.
- T-cell deficiencies (defective cell-mediated immunity)—increased susceptibility to opportunistic infections caused by intracellular organisms (fungi/viruses).
- Mixed B- and T-cell deficiencies (defective antibody response and cell-mediated immunity)—increased susceptibility to most infections.

Primary immunodeficiencies

B-cell deficiencies

X-linked agammaglobulinemia of Bruton

This is an X-linked recessive disorder of B-cell maturation and differentiation failure affecting males. It is caused by a lack of Bruton tyrosine kinase (BTK) enzyme on chromosome Xq22, which is normally involved in light chain rearrangements.

The disease is characterized by:

- deficiency of B cells and plasma cells
- negligible levels of circulating immunoglobulins
- small lymph nodes with no germinal centres
- absent tonsils.

T-cell numbers and functions are normal and infections are, therefore, primarily bacterial. Recurrent bacterial infections of the upper respiratory tract (e.g., by *Streptococcus pneumoniae)* are a common first presentation.

Selective IgA deficiency

The commonest form of immunodeficiency, selective IgA deficiency affects 1 in 600 whites. Circulating B cells bearing surface IgA are immature and fail to differentiate into IgA-secreting plasma cells. Most are asymptomatic; however, others present with recurrent ear, sinus and respiratory tract infections and bowel colonization with *Giardia*, *Salmonella* and other enteric pathogens.

Common variable immunodeficiency

Common variable immunodeficiency (CVID) is a heterogeneous group of conditions, both inherited and acquired. The common feature is agammaglobulinemia, characterized by an increased susceptibility to bacterial infections presenting from infancy into adulthood. Both sexes are equally affected.

The bone marrow contains normal numbers of immature B cells but there is a failure of differentiation of B cells into plasma cells, resulting in low levels of all classes of immunoglobulins.

CVID is more common and more variable than the X-linked form (hence the name); however, the pattern of infections are similar, chiefly the lungs, sinuses and gastrointestinal (GI) tract. There is increased risk of developing malignancies, autoimmune and granulomatous diseases.

Table 17.5 Summary of immunodeficiencies

Category	Deficiency	Example
Primary	B cell (antibody deficiency)	Transient hypogammaglobulinemia of infancy X-linked agammaglobulinemia Acquired common variable immunodeficiency Hypogammaglobulinemia Selective IgA or IgG subclass deficiencies
	T cell	Thymic hypoplasia (DiGeorge syndrome)
	Mixed B and T cell	Severe combined immune deficiency
Secondary	B cell (antibody deficiency)	Myeloma Protein deficiency
	T cell	AIDS Hodgkin disease Non-Hodgkin lymphoma Drugs, e.g., steroids, ciclosporin, azathioprine
	Mixed B and T cell	Chronic lymphocytic leukaemia Post bone marrow transplantation Post chemotherapy/radiotherapy Chronic renal failure Splenectomy

T-cell deficiencies

22q11 Deletion syndrome (DiGeorge syndrome)

This is a rare group of phenotypically overlapping disorders, including DiGeorge syndrome, which are caused by a microdeletion in chromosomal band 22q11.2. This results in developmental failure of the third and fourth pharyngeal pouches with variable consequences, one of which is hypoplasia/complete absence of the thymus and parathyroid glands. Patients have characteristic facies and a spectrum of embryological sequelae, e.g., tetralogy of Fallot, tracheooesophageal fistulae and craniofacial malformations, as well as behavioural and psychiatric problems. Infantile hypocalcaemia can occur.

Affected individuals have a mild immunodeficiency with decreased numbers of circulating T cells, and with normal or reduced immunoglobulin levels. They are susceptible to recurrent infections, especially systemic viral and fungal infections. Less than 1% have a severe immunodeficiency.

Mixed T- and B-cell deficiencies

Severe combined immunodeficiency

This inherited deficiency of lymphocytic stem cells is characterized by:

- deficiency in the number and function of T and B cells
- negligible circulating immunoglobulins
- greatly reduced cell-mediated immunity
- hypoplastic thymus.

There is always a T-cell deficiency in severe combined immunodeficiency (SCID) with variable loss of B cells (30%) and NK cells, caused by a variety of mutations. The most frequent is in the common γ chain of the interleukin receptor, which is shared by IL2, 4, 7, 9 and 15 located on the X chromosome (X-linked SCID). Autosomal recessive SCID presents with deficiencies in a variety of immune-related proteins such as major histocompatibility complex (MHC) class II (bare lymphocyte syndrome).

SCID presents during the first few months of life with a failure to thrive, persistent/recurrent infections that are typically more severe, more frequent and require longer courses of antibiotics, chronic diarrhoea and dermatitis. Death usually occurs within the first 2 years of life from multiple infections, although bone marrow transplant can effect a cure in some cases.

Wiskott–Aldrich syndrome

An X-linked combined immunodeficiency disorder secondary to mutations in the WAS gene. Wiskott–Aldrich syndrome accounts for 3% of all primary immunodeficiencies. It is described by the classic triad of microthrombocytopenia, recurrent bacterial infections and eczema in males. Presentation is in infancy, commonly with chronic bloody diarrhoea, purpura and recurrent sinopulmonary/ear infections. Characteristically, normal levels of IgG, reduced IgM and raised IgA and IgE are seen.

Autoimmune disease is common and there is an increased risk of haematopoietic malignancies.

Secondary immunodeficiencies

Secondary immunodeficiencies are those that result from extrinsic or environmental causes (Table 17.6).

Table 17.6 Causes of secondary immunodeficiencies

Cause	Examples
Physiological	Pregnancy, age: senescence or prematurity
Infection	HIV, measles
Iatrogenic	Immunosuppressants, corticosteroids, radiation
Malignancy	
Biochemical/nutritional	Diabetes mellitus, malnutrition
Other	Burns, hyposplenism

AMYLOIDOSIS

Amyloidosis is the pathological deposition of the abnormal extracellular fibrillary protein, amyloid, in different tissues. Amyloid is composed of a meshwork of rigid, straight fibrils created from precursor peptides (Table 17.7) forming a cross-β-pleated sheet. The β-pleated sheet structure is important because enzymes are incapable of digesting such large molecules in this form.

- ***Macroscopically:*** involved organs may have a waxy, pale appearance and are often firm and heavy.
- ***Microscopically:*** amyloid appears as an extracellular amorphous, hyaline, pale eosinophilic material deposited within blood vessel walls and interstitial tissues. Electron microscopic studies reveal the fibrillary nature.

Congo-red dye stains amyloid brick red and imparts apple-green birefringence under polarized light.

Amyloid formation

Greater than fifteen distinct forms of amyloid have been described, but three predominate:

- AA (amyloid associated)
- AL (amyloid light chain)
- Aβ amyloid.

Amyloid formation occurs due to the production of:

- abnormal amounts of normal precursor peptide (common), e.g., immunoglobulin light chains in multiple myeloma or serum amyloid A protein in acute phase response. It may be a result of overproduction, reduced degradation or reduced excretion of protein or

Table 17.7 Types of amyloid and their clinical association

Amyloid subtype	Precursor protein	Clinical association	Clinical features
AL	Ig light chain—predominantly λ type.	Plasma cell dyscrasias, e.g., myeloma, Waldenström macroglobulinemia	'Glove and stocking' neuropathy Macroglossia Restrictive cardiomyopathy Carpal tunnel syndrome Nephrotic syndrome Skin thickening
AA	SAA Acute phase reactant synthesized by the liver undergoes proteolysis into smaller 'AA' proteins	Chronic inflammation (secondary amyloid), e.g., rheumatoid arthritis, tuberculosis, inflammatory bowel disease Also associated with intravenous heroin addicts	Splenomegaly Hepatomegaly Nephrotic syndrome Renal vein thrombosis
Aβ	β amyloid precursor protein which is a transmembrane glycoprotein	Alzheimer disease.	Found at the core of cerebral plaques and blood vessels in Alzheimer disease
Aβ_2 microglobulin	β_2 microglobulin. Component of MHC class I molecules	Long-term haemodialysis	Carpal tunnel syndrome Joint arthropathy
ATTR	TTR: transport protein for thyroxine and retinol	Familial amyloid polyneuropathies (mutated TTR)	Amyloid deposition in peripheral and autonomic nerves
		Senile systemic amyloidosis (normal TTR)	Occurs in elderly Heart deposition: restrictive cardiomyopathy, arrhythmias

AA, Amyloid associated; Aβ, amyloid; AL, amyloid light chain; ATTR, amyloid transthyretin; Ig, immunoglobulin; MHC, major histocompatibility complex; SAA, serum amyloid-associated protein; TTR, transthyretin.

- normal amounts of abnormal protein (rare), e.g., mutations in transthyretin, which make these proteins more prone to misfolding and aggregation.

Normally, misfolded proteins would be degraded by proteasomes intracellularly or by macrophages extracellularly; however, in amyloidosis, degradation fails and the misfolded proteins form extracellular aggregates.

HINTS AND TIPS

AMYLOID PROTEIN

It is the physical arrangement of the constituent amino acids that make a protein an amyloid rather than any specific amino acid sequence.

There are many different types of amyloid, each being formed from different precursor amino acids with the precursors themselves often being fragments of larger proteins.

Classification of amyloidosis

Clinically, amyloidosis is inherited or acquired and can be:

- systemic—involving many tissues owing to a predilection for deposition in blood vessel walls and basement membranes. Usually fatal, with death generally occurring from renal or cardiac disease.
- localized—affecting only one organ or tissue, e.g., Alzheimer disease. The skin, lungs and urinary tract are the most frequent sites.

In both cases, the progressive accumulation of amyloid leads to cellular dysfunction by preventing the normal processes of diffusion through extracellular tissues and by physical compression of functioning parenchymal cells.

DISORDERS OF WHITE BLOOD CELLS

Leucopenia

Leucopenia is defined as a reduction in circulating leucocytes. The classification of leucocytes is shown in Fig. 17.2.

Neutropenia

Neutropenia, a deficiency of polymorph neutrophils, is the most important form of leucopenia. A 2.5×10^9/L neutrophil count is the lower limit of normal (except in Afro-Caribbean races and in the Middle East, where it is 1.5×10^9/L). Levels less than these values are classified as neutropenia.

Neutropenia may be selective or part of a general pancytopenia. Clinical features depend on the degree of neutropenia:

- Mild—usually asymptomatic.
- Moderate to severe ($<0.5 \times 10^9$/L)—associated with a progressive increase in risk and severity of infection, and increase in recurrent infections.
- Levels $<0.2 \times 10^9$/L are associated with a high mortality from overwhelming infection.

Severe neutropenia (agranulocytosis) can result in predominantly bacterial infections which are usually opportunistic, most commonly Gram-positive skin organisms (e.g., *Staphylococcus* and *Streptococcus* species) or gram-negative gut bacteria (e.g., *Pseudomonas, Escherichia coli*, etc.).

They can be either localized (e.g., mouth, throat, skin or anus) or generalized (neutropenic sepsis). The latter may be rapidly fatal.

Treatment is of the underlying cause and with antimicrobial therapy.

Leucocytosis

Leucocytosis is defined as an increase in numbers of circulating white blood cells.

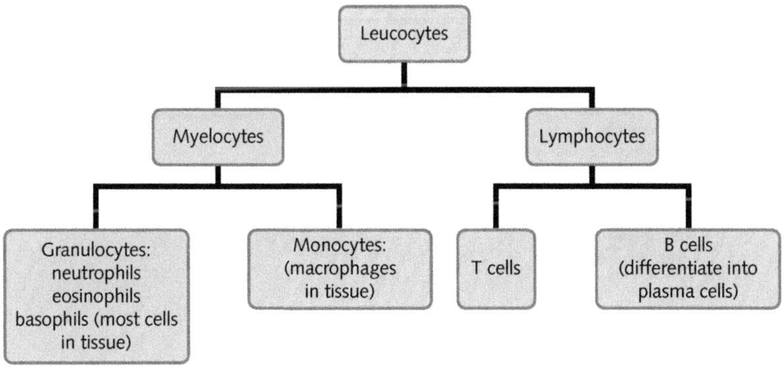

Fig. 17.2 Classification of leucocytes.

Types of leucocytosis

Each type of leucocyte (see Fig. 17.2) may be increased in number (neutrophilia, eosinophilia, etc.). Monocytosis and lymphocytosis are the terms used for increases in monocytes and lymphocytes, respectively.

Neutrophilia is the most common cause of leucocytosis, produced by common events such as acute bacterial infection or acute inflammation.

Leucocytosis can be:

- Primary—caused by bone marrow disease, e.g., leukaemias, lymphomas (described later).
- Secondary—reactive leucocytosis caused by the normal response of bone marrow to abnormal conditions, e.g., infection.

Lymphomas

Lymphomas are clonal, neoplastic proliferations of lymphoid cells in solid organs, and can be classified by cell type (B cells or T cells), tumour architecture (e.g., diffuse or follicular), or subdivided into Hodgkin lymphomas or non-Hodgkin lymphomas (Fig. 17.3).

Hodgkin lymphoma

Hodgkin lymphoma affects 4 per 100,000 in the UK, with a male predominance. It can occur at any age but there is a bimodal distribution of incidence: one in young adults (15–25 years old) and the other in late middle-age (40–60 years old).

Clinically, it is characterized by the painless enlargement of one or more groups of superficial lymph nodes, most often in the neck (e.g., cervical nodes). The disease is initially localized to a single peripheral lymph node region, but it spreads in a fairly consistent pattern to adjacent nodes via the lymphatics, then to the spleen and other organs via the bloodstream.

One-third of patients have systemic symptoms (so-called 'B symptoms'), notably weight loss, pyrexia (including episodic Pel–Ebstein fevers) and night sweats.

Diagnosis of Hodgkin lymphoma is made on examination of aspirated or biopsied lymph nodes:

- Macroscopically—affected lymph nodes are enlarged, with a smooth surface and thickened capsule.
- Microscopically—subdivided into classical Hodgkin lymphoma (characterized by the presence of large binucleate Reed–Sternberg (RS) cells), and nodular lymphocyte-predominant Hodgkin lymphoma (characterized by popcorn cells). Classical Hodgkin lymphoma has four recognized subtypes according to the Rye classification system (Fig. 17.4).

The aetiology of Hodgkin lymphoma is obscure, as is the origin of the malignant RS cells. Although no causal link has been established with Epstein–Barr virus (EBV), Hodgkin lymphoma sufferers are three times more likely to have had glandular fever in the past.

CLINICAL NOTES

STAGING AND TREATMENT OF HODGKIN LYMPHOMA

The stage (extent of spread) of Hodgkin lymphoma is determined by the Ann Arbor staging system. A clinical addition is the presence of 'B symptoms'—systemic features associated with poorer prognosis. Treatment (with radiotherapy or chemotherapy) depends on the stage. Ten-year survival is 80%, but long-term survivors of chemotherapy and/or radiotherapy are at increased risk of secondary cancers.

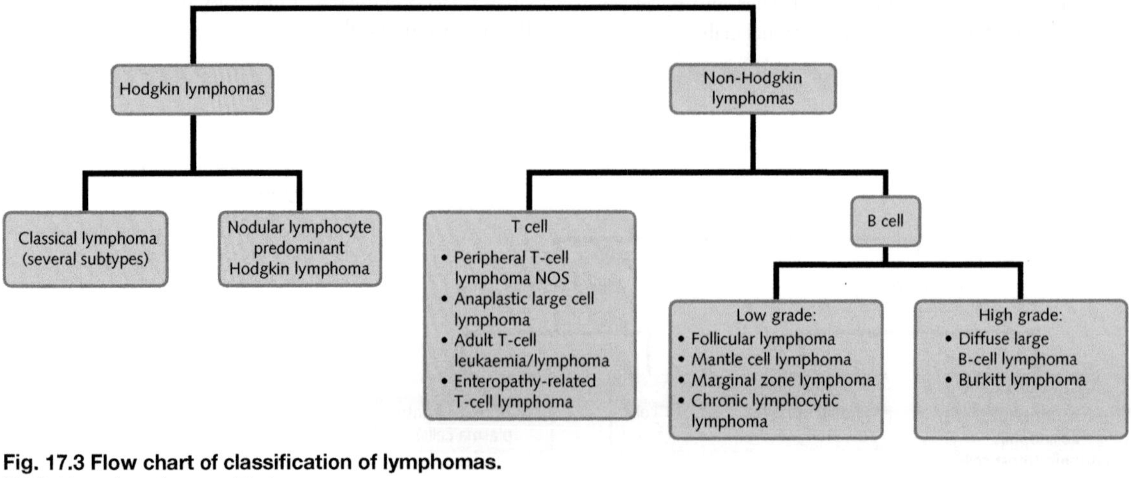

Fig. 17.3 Flow chart of classification of lymphomas. *NOS*, Not otherwise specified.

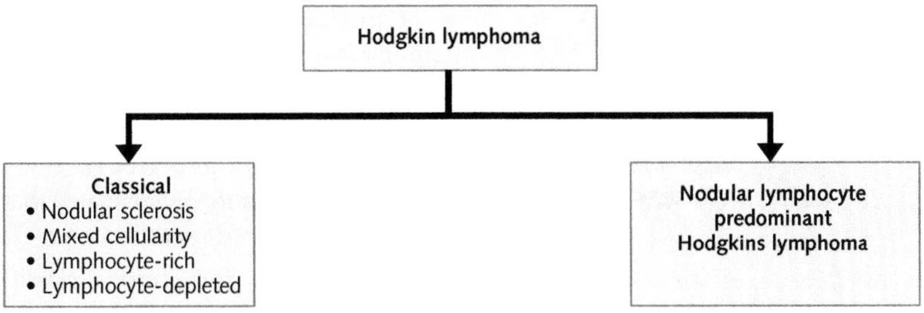

Fig. 17.4 Rye classification of Hodgkin disease. (Adapted with permission from medicshandbook.com, 2011.)

Non-Hodgkin lymphomas

Non-Hodgkin lymphomas (NHLs) include all lymphomas other than Hodgkin lymphoma and are subdivided by cell type and grade (Fig. 17.3). They are predominantly diseases of middle and later life, with males slightly more affected than females.

The aetiology of NHLs is poorly understood but several factors have been implicated:

- Immunosuppression—increased incidence in primary immunosuppressive diseases, e.g., X-linked agammaglobulinaemia and in secondary immunosuppression, e.g., drug induced after transplantation and immune senescence.
- Viral infection—with lymphotropic viruses, e.g., EBV, human T-lymphotropic virus (HTLV-1) and HIV.
- Bacterial infection—*Helicobacter pylori* infection linked to gastric lymphoma.
- Radiation.

Chromosomal translocations are a feature of many types of lymphoma.

> **MOLECULAR**
>
> **COMMON LYMPHOMA TRANSLOCATIONS**
>
> - Burkitt lymphoma—t(8;14), *c-myc* translocation
> - Follicular lymphoma—t(14;18)
> - Mantle cell lymphoma—t(11;14).

These translocations cause a neoplastic transformation as a result of the transfer of an oncogene or oncogene-regulatory gene to an abnormal site. This causes the increased expression of these oncogenes, e.g., *bcl-2* in follicular lymphoma, which inhibits apoptotic cell death.

The majority (70%) of NHLs are B-cell lymphomas, which are derived from follicle centre cells. These tumours have either follicular or diffuse architecture.

> **HINTS AND TIPS**
>
> **UNDERSTANDING THE LYMPH NODE**
>
> Recognizing the normal development of lymphocytes (Fig. 17.6) and normal lymph node architecture (Fig. 17.5) is essential to understanding lymphomas and other neoplastic proliferations of white blood cells.

Clinical features

The clinical manifestations of NHLs are similar to those of Hodgkin disease but they are more varied because of their heterogeneous nature. The majority of cases present with asymmetric, painless lymphadenopathy in one or more peripheral lymph node regions. However, extranodal presentation is more frequent than in Hodgkin lymphoma, with 20% of all NHLs originating within extranodal sites.

Systemic symptoms are often prominent in extensive disease, along with hepatosplenomegaly.

Management and prognosis

Treatment is by single or combination chemotherapy or biological therapy, with which some patients show long-term remission, if not cure.

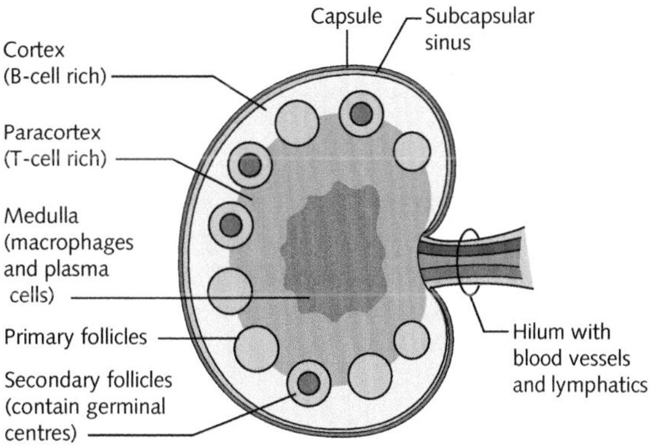

Fig. 17.5 Normal lymph node architecture.

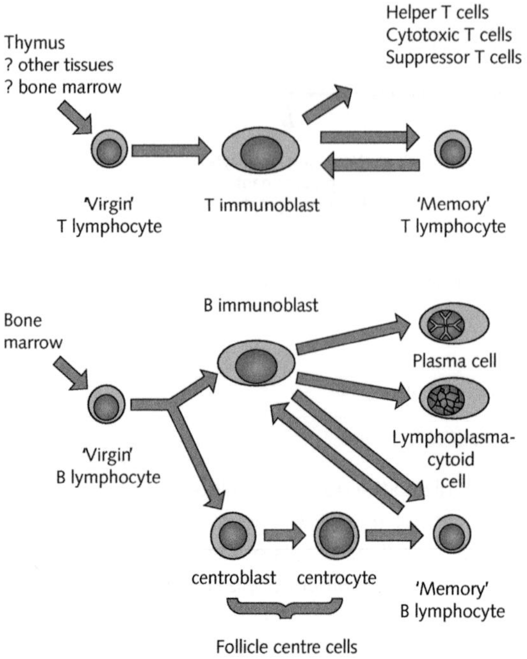

Fig. 17.6 Normal lymphocyte development. (Adapted with permission from Hoffbrand V, Pettit J, Essential Hematology, 5th ed. Wiley-Blackwell, 2005.)

The prognosis depends on the type of lymphoma and varies widely from highly proliferative and rapidly fatal diseases (e.g., immunoblastic lymphoma) to indolent and well-tolerated malignancies (e.g., chronic lymphocytic leukaemia [CLL]).

> **HINTS AND TIPS**
>
> **RICHTER TRANSFORMATION**
>
> Occasionally, low-grade lymphomas (usually chronic lymphocytic leukaemia) undergo transformation into high-grade lymphomas. Approximately 5% transform into diffuse large B-cell lymphoma, and <1% to Hodgkin lymphoma. This is known as Richter transformation.

T-cell lymphomas

T-cell lymphomas are less common than their B-cell counterparts. They are almost always of high grade and tend to have poor prognoses. Cutaneous forms (including mycosis fungoides) can occur.

Leukaemias

Leukaemias are neoplastic proliferations of white blood cell precursors in the bone marrow and peripheral blood.

Classification—leukaemias are classified into acute or chronic, based on clinical progression:

- Acute—characterized by numerous immature 'blast' cells (leucocyte precursors) and rapid disease progression.
- Chronic—characterized by large numbers of precursor cells that are more differentiated than blast cells and associated with slower disease progression.

These groups are then further classified into two main groups depending on their lineage:

- Myeloid leukaemia (cells of granulocytic series).
- Lymphocytic leukaemia (cells of the lymphoid series).

Aetiology—in the majority of cases, the cause of leukaemia is unknown. However, certain factors are known to initiate leukaemic transformation:

- Genetics—slight familial tendency (high concordance in monozygotic twins); chromosome abnormalities (both quantitative and qualitative) are present in about 50% of patients; increased incidence in Down syndrome.
- Ionizing radiation—excessive exposure in therapy, e.g., for malignant disease; nuclear explosions/accidents, e.g., Hiroshima and Chernobyl.
- Drugs—prolonged chemotherapy, e.g., with alkylating agents (cause myeloid leukaemia).
- Immune status—increased incidence in immunosuppressed individuals.
- Viruses—e.g., HTLV-1 causes adult T-cell leukaemia/lymphoma.
- Industrial benzene exposure.

Common features of leukaemias

The common features of leukaemias are bone marrow failure, gout and metastasis.

Bone marrow failure

Overproduction of leucocyte precursor cells causes the suppression of normal blood cell production, thus:

- deficiency of red cell production → anaemia
- deficiency of platelet production → thrombocytopenia (risk of haemorrhage)
- deficiency of normal leucocyte production → leucopenia (failure to control infection).

Gout

Increased cell turnover leads to increased uric acid synthesis, which may result in gout.

Metastasis

There is infiltration of organs such as the liver, spleen, and less commonly lymph nodes, meninges and gonads by the leukaemic cells.

Acute leukaemia

Acute leukaemia is a malignant disorder in which haemopoietic blast cells constitute >20% of bone marrow cells.

There are two main types: acute lymphoblastic leukaemia (ALL) and acute myeloblastic leukaemia (AML). These

Table 17.8 Features of acute lymphoblastic and acute myeloblastic leukaemia

Type	Acute lymphoblastic leukaemia	Acute myeloblastic leukaemia
Epidemiology	Mainly (>90%) affects children of less than 14 years, with highest incidence at 3–4 years Second increase in incidence occurs around middle-age	Occurs at all ages and is the commonest form of acute leukaemia in adults
Proliferating-cell type	Neoplastic lymphoblasts (lymphocyte precursor cells)	Neoplastic myeloblast (granulocyte/ monocyte precursor cell)
Degree of differentiation	Blast cells show no differentiation	Blast cells usually show some evidence of differentiation to granulocytes
Prognosis	Children aged 2–9 years: 50%–75% cure rate Adults: 35% cure rate with chemotherapy; 50% with allogeneic bone marrow transplant	20%–25% cure rate with standard chemotherapy 50% with allogeneic bone marrow transplant

are further subclassified according to cytological features of the blast cells. ALL is further subclassified according to B- and T-cell lineages. Table 17.8 outlines the features of ALL and AML.

The clinical features of both AML and ALL are similar. They commonly present with symptoms of anaemia (e.g., tiredness, malaise, breathlessness, angina) and their course is typified by a series of overwhelming infections and mucosal haemorrhage.

Onset is frequently rapid and progression to death from anaemia, haemorrhage or infection occurs within weeks if no treatment is given.

The clinical course is less catastrophic in childhood ALL.

Haematological investigations reveal:

- anaemia—normocytic, normochromic.
- leucocytosis—although leucopenia may be an occasional feature, despite massive marrow infiltration with blast cells.
- neutropenia—susceptibility to overt infections.
- thrombocytopenia—petechiae, purpura, epistaxis, bleeding gums, GI haemorrhage, cerebral haemorrhage.
- blood film—this shows blast cells and can be diagnostic.
- bone marrow biopsy—this shows a hypercellular marrow with normal elements replaced by blast cells.
- involvement of other organs:
  - skeleton (bone pain, especially in children)—probably caused by osteolytic lesions
  - lymphadenopathy
  - symptoms and signs secondary to CNS infiltration.

Cytogenetics and immunological staining can help diagnosis. For prognosis see Table 17.8.

Chronic leukaemias

Chronic lymphocytic leukaemia

This chronic low-grade lymphoproliferative disorder is characterized by the proliferation of an abnormal lymphoid clone of leucocyte precursors in the bone marrow. It is the most common leukaemia of adults, comprising about 30% of all leukaemias, with males affected more often than females by a factor of 2:1. It is a disease predominantly of the elderly, with peak incidence at 65 years old.

This disease is much less aggressive than other leukaemias, following an indolent course over a period of years.

Haematological changes are:

- leucocytosis—small, nonfunctional lymphocytes of B-cell origin
- anaemia and thrombocytopenia—late developments
- secondary autoimmune haemolytic anaemia—develops in 10% of cases.

The lymph nodes, liver and spleen are characteristically involved, and their normal architecture may become completely effaced by the infiltrating cells.

Survival for more than 10 years from diagnosis is common, and where CLL affects the elderly, death is often from an unrelated cause. CLL in younger individuals tends to be more aggressive.

Chronic myeloid leukaemia (CML) is discussed later.

Myeloproliferative disorders

These are autonomous proliferations of one or more myeloid cell lineages (erythroid, granulocytic, megakaryocytic) with differentiation to mature forms (Table 17.9). The main types of myeloproliferative disorders are CML, polycythaemia rubra vera, essential thrombocytosis and myelofibrosis. Progression from one disorder to another within the group is common.

Chronic myeloid leukaemia

CML is a clonal proliferative disorder of neoplastic myeloid precursor cells within the bone marrow. About 90% of cases are characterized by the presence of a specific karyotypic abnormality—the Philadelphia chromosome—within the haemopoietic stem cells. This involves reciprocal translocation of part of the long arm (q) of chromosome *22* with the long arm of chromosome 9. This creates a chimeric gene *(BCR-abl)*, which produces a tyrosine kinase thought to be involved in the pathogenesis of CML.

Table 17.9 Myeloproliferative disorders and their basic features

Disorder	Principal proliferations	Bone marrow morphology	Clinical features
Polycythaemia rubra vera	Erythroblasts	Increased cellularity, especially erythroid	Erythrocytosis with increased Hb and PCV Often neutrophilia and thrombocytosis Pruritus (relating to basophilia) Thrombosis or haemorrhage Splenomegaly
Myelofibrosis	Fibroblasts	Increased deposition of collagen/reticulin; bone marrow difficult to aspirate	Leucoerythroblastic blood picture Anaemia with teardrop poikilocytes Hepatosplenomegaly
Chronic myeloid leukaemia	Myeloblasts	Increased cellularity, especially myeloid	Leucoerythroblastic blood picture Anaemia, neutrophilia, basophilia Splenomegaly
Essential thrombocythaemia	Megakaryoblasts	Increased megakaryocytes	Thrombocytosis Thrombosis or haemorrhage Occasional splenomegaly

Hb, Haemoglobin; PCV, packed cell volume.

MOLECULAR

PHILADELPHIA CHROMOSOME

Treatment of Philadelphia-chromosome-positive chronic myeloid leukaemia has been transformed by the drug imatinib, a tyrosine kinase inhibitor which offers long-term remission as long as the patient remains on the drug.

CML occurs in all age groups, but most frequently between the ages of 40 and 60 years. The disease has three recognized stages:

1. Chronic phase—characterized by anaemia and splenomegaly; responsive to chemotherapy.
2. Accelerated phase—owing to the emergence and dominance of a more malignant clone of myeloid cell, the disease becomes harder to control.
3. Blast crisis phase—transformation to an acute leukaemia (usually AML), often rapidly fatal. Progression from chronic phase is unpredictable and may occur at any time.

Haematological investigation reveals leucocytosis and normocytic anaemia. Note that in contrast to acute leukaemias, neutropenia, lymphopenia and thrombocytopenia are not common in the chronic phase and that infection and bleeding are not typical.

There is sometimes massive splenomegaly, and often hepatomegaly.

Polycythaemia

Polycythaemia (erythrocytosis) is essentially the opposite of anaemia, defined as a sustained increase in red cell numbers, usually with a corresponding increase in haemoglobin concentration and haematocrit.

Relative polycythaemia

This occurs when the haematocrit reading is raised due to a decrease in plasma volume, usually as a result of fluid loss (haemoconcentration). This is not 'true' (absolute) polycythaemia.

Absolute polycythaemia

Primary

Primary polycythaemia occurs in a rare condition termed polycythaemia rubra vera, which is one of the myeloproliferative disorders.

Secondary

Most cases of polycythaemia are secondary to conditions resulting in:

- chronic hypoxia (common)—physiological polycythaemia, e.g., high altitude, cyanotic heart disease, respiratory disease (such as chronic bronchitis, emphysema), smoking, haemoglobinopathies (resulting in defective release of O_2 to tissues).
- renal tumours and ischaemia (rare)—pathological polycythaemia, e.g., renal carcinomas or cysts, renal artery stenosis.

Both chronic hypoxia and renal tumours/ischaemia result in increased erythropoietin hormone production, which stimulates bone marrow production of red cells (Table 17.10).

Treatment is by venesection or myelosuppression using chemotherapy or radioactive phosphorous-32. Treated patients have a mean survival of about 13 years, with increased morbidity and mortality from coronary and cerebral disease related to the raised haematocrit.

Polycythaemia rubra vera

This idiopathic condition is characterized by an increase in red cell concentration, usually with concomitant increases in haemoglobin concentration and haematocrit. Red cell mass is greatly increased.

The disorder has a prevalence of 2 per 100,000 in the UK. It typically affects middle-aged people, with males affected more often than females.

Progression of this disease is chronic, but some cases evolve into myelofibrosis or acute leukaemia.

Onset is usually insidious and nonspecific, e.g., malaise, fatigue, headache, dizziness and itching after a bath. Symptoms are caused by vascular engorgement, increased haematocrit and thrombosis, with or without haemorrhage. Diagnosis requires raised red cell mass without another cause and palpable splenomegaly.

Essential thrombocythaemia

This condition is characterized by increased platelet production due to a clonal proliferation of megakaryocytes without a systemic cause. It is most commonly seen in patients over 50 years of age and is often associated with a *JAK2* mutation. Its features are:

- large, atypical platelets with increased platelet count, often $>600 \times 10^9$/L
- combined pathological haemorrhages and thromboembolic episodes
- spleen enlargement, but it is usually normal or reduced in size because of thromboembolic infarction.

Treatment with chemotherapy and antiplatelet drugs (e.g., aspirin) is effective and median survival with treatment is 8–10 years.

Table 17.10 Comparison of main features of primary and secondary polycythaemia

	Primary	Secondary
Prevalence	Rare	Common
Cause	Unknown	Hypoxia Renal tumours/ ischaemia
Erythropoietin	Normal or decreased	Increased
Blood film	↑RBCs (may be hypochromic) ↑Leucocytes ↑Megakaryocytes	↑RBCs (normochromic)
Splenomegaly	Common	None

RBC, Red blood cell

Myelofibrosis

This condition is characterized by a proliferation of fibroblasts in the bone marrow and obliterative marrow fibrosis, with a corresponding massive extramedullary haematopoiesis in the liver and spleen.

The condition is a chronic disorder of late and middle-age. It may arise de novo (with unknown aetiology) or as an end stage of other myeloproliferative disorders. Like essential thrombocythaemia, myelofibrosis is associated with *JAK2* mutations.

The disease is usually slowly progressive, with a median survival of a few years. Acute leukaemic transformation sometimes occurs.

Clinical features are:

- blood film—typically leucoerythroblastic; erythropoiesis is ineffective leading to anaemia with marked anisocytosis and teardrop poikilocytes
- splenomegaly
- hepatomegaly.

Symptoms are usually caused by anaemia and massive splenomegaly. Systemic symptoms (e.g., fever, weight loss) are usually late features. Bone marrow aspirates typically produce a 'dry tap', therefore bone marrow trephine is usually needed for diagnosis.

Myelodysplastic syndromes

This group of acquired neoplastic disorders of the bone marrow is characterized by increasing bone marrow failure with quantitative and qualitative abnormalities of at least one myeloid cell line (red cells, granulocytes and platelets) due to a defect of stem cells.

In most cases, the disease arises de novo and the aetiology is likely to be as for the leukaemias. Approximately one-third of patients progress to AML, often after many years. In a significant proportion of cases, the disease is secondary to treatment with chemotherapy or radiotherapy for a previous neoplastic disease.

The hallmark of the disease is ineffective haematopoiesis resulting in pancytopenia despite a marrow of either normal or increased cellularity.

Bone marrow contains morphologically abnormal cells including ring sideroblasts and hypogranular white cells, often with abnormal chromosomes.

Clinical features—more than half the patients are over 70 years old and more than 75% are over 50; males are affected more often than females. Symptoms are generally sequelae of the variable cytopenias.

Treatment is via stem cell transplant or supportive, by blood transfusion and treatment of infection.

Morbidity and deaths are largely attributable to the refractory cytopenias, either directly (e.g., from haemorrhage) or indirectly (e.g., from transfusion-related haemosiderosis).

COMMON PITFALLS

MPN VERSUS MDS

Myelofibrosis, myeloproliferative neoplasia (MPN) and myelodysplastic syndrome (MDS) are overlapping entities that are commonly confused. Do not panic—remember the clue is in the name:

Myelo: relates to the bone marrow and *myeloid* cell lineage which encompasses red cells, megakaryocytes (produce platelets) and granulocytes (eosinophils, neutrophils, etc).

MPN = myelo + proliferative.

Proliferative = increase in number: *dysregulated proliferation* of ≥1 cell line with maturation. The proliferation is clonal (cells are all the same) with abnormal clones replacing normal polyclonal cells with various degrees of reactive fibrosis.

Includes:

Chronic myeloid leukaemia (CML), megakaryocytes: essential thrombocythaemia (ET), red blood cells: polycythaemia vera (PV), and myelofibrosis.

Myelofibrosis = myelo + fibrosis.

Fibrosis = generation of excess fibrous connective tissue replacing normal tissue. This is a type of MPN which can be primary or develop after progression of CML, ET or PV.

MDS = myelo + dysplastic

Dysplastic = abnormal growth: *ineffective proliferation and differentiation* of ≥1 myeloid cell line; confusingly, it may occur in conjunction with MPN. (NB: leukaemia = proliferation with no change in differentiation.)

Hairy cell leukaemia

This rare B-cell leukaemia is characterized by variable numbers of 'hairy' cells in the blood, bone marrow, liver and other organs. Hairy cells are so named because of their characteristic irregular outline caused by cytoplasmic projections or 'hairs' typically seen on blood film.

The disease has a peak incidence at 40 to 60 years old, affecting males more often than females by a factor of 6:1.

It is characterized clinically by features of pancytopenia (mainly recurrent infections) and splenomegaly.

The disorder typically runs a chronic course and remission is common with chemotherapy, immunotherapy or splenectomy.

Plasma cell dyscrasias

This describes the malignant, monoclonal proliferation of plasma cells in the bone marrow. Subclassification is based on the number of sites involved (multiple sites = multiple myeloma, solitary site = plasmacytoma) and the percentage of abnormal plasma cells.

Monoclonal gammopathy of uncertain significance (MGUS)

This is an abnormal plasma cell proliferation amounting to less than 10% of nucleated bone marrow cells. It is characterized by paraproteinaemia in the absence of associated organ-specific effects.

Plasmacytoma

This rare disease is characterized by a discrete solitary tumour of proliferating monoclonal plasma cells, usually in the bone.

Proliferation does not occur in parts of the skeleton beyond the primary lesion and marrow aspirates distant from the primary tumour are usually normal.

The associated M component (paraprotein) usually disappears following radiotherapy to the primary lesion. However, a minority of cases progress to multiple myeloma.

Multiple myeloma

This typically affects the elderly, with almost all cases occurring after the age of 40. There is a male predominance.

Pathogenesis—normal plasma cells produce polyclonal immunoglobulins. In myeloma, only monoclonal immunoglobulins or light chains are produced; these are referred to as the 'M component' or paraprotein.

The M component is usually IgG (>60%), but may be IgA (20%) or just the immunoglobulin light chain (κ (kappa) being more frequent than λ (lambda)). IgM-producing plasma cells are a feature of Waldenström macroglobulinaemia.

Serum protein electrophoresis, shows increased levels of β_2-microglobulin and a dramatic increase in the levels of gamma globulins (Fig. 17.7).

Diagnosis of myeloma requires two out of the following three findings:

- bone marrow plasmacytosis
- serum or urinary paraprotein (M component)
- skeletal lesions (see later).

Renal impairment

In two-thirds of cases of IgG and IgA myeloma, monoclonal free light chains are also produced, which are small enough to enter the urine, where they are called Bence–Jones proteins.

During passage through the tubules, the protein precipitates as 'casts', causing damage to the tubular epithelial cells.

Light chains that pass through capillaries are converted into amyloid (systemic amyloidosis); causing damage to many organs including the kidneys.

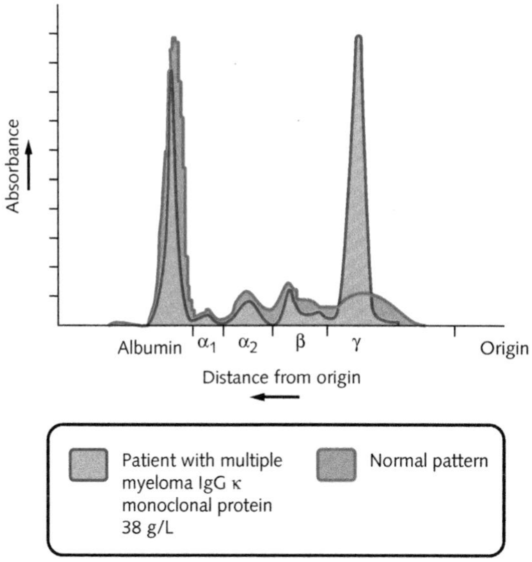

Fig. 17.7 Serum electrophoresis showing characteristic gamma band of multiple myeloma. (Adapted with permission from Hoffbrand V, Pettit J, Essential Hematology, 5th ed. Wiley-Blackwell, 2006.)

Raised blood uric acid (from increased cell turnover) worsens renal impairment (urate nephropathy), as does increased blood calcium from bone osteolysis (hypercalcaemia).

Bone changes

These are characteristic of myeloma:

- Hypercellular bone marrow with a large proportion of malignant plasma cells, especially in the skull, ribs, vertebrae and pelvis.
- Osteolysis of medullary and cortical bone due to increased numbers of bone-resorbing osteoclasts: thought to be stimulated by interleukin 1 (IL1) produced by the malignant plasma cells.
- Osteolytic lesions are seen as 'punched out' defects in the bones, the skull showing this appearance particularly well ('pepper-pot skull').
- Pathological fractures may occur, especially in the vertebrae, causing spinal cord compression.

Haematological findings

These are as follows:

- Anaemia—usually normochromic, normocytic
- Marked rouleaux formation—red cells adhere forming cylinders with a 'stack of coins' appearance
- Raised blood viscosity—depending on the type of immunoglobulin
- Reduced concentration of unaffected immunoglobulins—'immune paresis'
- Abnormal plasma cells—occasionally seen in peripheral blood, but most are in the bone marrow
- Neutropenia and thrombocytopenia—common features of bone marrow failure in late stages.

HINTS AND TIPS

CLINICAL FEATURES OF MYELOMA 'CRAB'

The mnemonic 'CRAB' can aid in remembering the clinical features of myeloma:

- *C*alcium—hypercalcemia.
- *R*enal failure and recurrent infections (due to deficient antibody levels and bone marrow failure).
- *A*naemia (lethargy, breathlessness, tachycardia) and abnormal bleeding tendency (M component may interfere with platelet function and coagulation factors; thrombocytopenia in advanced disease).
- *B*one pain—especially backache and pathological fractures.

Treatment involves chemotherapy and radiotherapy but median survival is only 3 years with treatment. Allogeneic bone marrow transplant may benefit some patients.

Note: acute and chronic graft versus host disease (where donor graft cells attack recipient host cells) may occur secondary to transplant.

DISORDERS OF THE SPLEEN AND THYMUS

Splenomegaly

The spleen serves as the site of filtration and phagocytosis of the following:

- Effete cells and cell debris, especially red cells
- Microorganisms
- Abnormal or excess material derived from metabolic processes.

HINTS AND TIPS

FIVE CAUSES OF MASSIVE SPLENOMEGALY

The main causes of massive splenomegaly are:

- malaria
- visceral leishmaniasis (kala-azar)
- marginal zone lymphoma
- chronic myeloid leukaemia
- myelofibrosis.

Splenomegaly (enlargement of the spleen) is a common physical sign. It can have many causes, the main types of which are summarized in Table 17.11.

A palpable spleen is at least twice its normal size and is vulnerable to traumatic rupture.

Effects of splenomegaly

Irrespective of the cause, enlargement of the spleen may result in the development of hypersplenism, i.e., a decrease in the circulating numbers of erythrocytes, leucocytes and platelets (pancytopenia), resulting from the destruction or pooling of these cells by the enlarged spleen.

Hypersplenism is often accompanied by a compensatory response—hyperplasia of the bone marrow.

Splenectomy leads to clinical and haematological improvement.

Congestive splenomegaly

This is enlargement of the spleen caused by any condition that leads to a persistent elevation of splenic venous blood pressure.

Morphological features—sinusoids of the spleen are initially distended with red cells. Fibrosis of both the spleen and capsule eventually occurs and sinusoids then appear ectatic and empty.

The cut surface of the spleen has a purple-red colour with an inconspicuous white pulp and it is often flecked with firm, brown nodules (called Gamna–Gandy nodules) that represent foci of fibrosis and phagocytosed minerals.

Foci of extramedullary haemopoiesis are an occasional feature and are thought to be secondary to dysfunctional erythropoiesis.

Splenic infarcts

Splenic infarction follows occlusion of the splenic artery or its branches and it may be caused by:

- emboli that arise in the heart (most common). These may be septic if associated with infective endocarditis.
- local thrombosis, e.g., in sickle cell diseases, myeloproliferative disorders and malignant infiltrates. Patients with sickle cell usually undergo autosplenectomy by age 8 years, making them prone to infection by encapsulated micro organisms.

Infarcts may be single or multiple and are generally wedge shaped and pale.

Trauma

Splenosis

This is the autotransplantation (seeding) of the spleen after trauma; its appearance may be concerning on imaging. The deposits of splenic tissue can be numerous and derive their

Table 17.11 Causes of splenomegaly

Cause	Comments
Infections	Bacterial, e.g., typhoid, tuberculosis, brucellosis, infective endocarditis Viral: infectious mononucleosis Protozoal: malaria, leishmaniasis, trypanosomiasis, toxoplasmosis
Congestion	Owing to persistent elevation of splenic venous blood pressure, the cause of which may be: • Prehepatic: thrombosis of hepatic, splenic or portal vein • Hepatic: long-standing portal hypertension associated with cirrhosis • Posthepatic: raised venous pressure of inferior vena cava, e.g., due to right-sided heart failure, which is transmitted to the spleen via the portal system
Storage disease	Heritable enzyme deficiencies, which result in storage of material in splenic macrophagic cells, e.g., Gaucher disease, Niemann–Pick disease and Tay–Sachs disease
Neoplasia	Primary: rare Secondary: • Lymphomas: Hodgkin disease and non-Hodgkin lymphomas • Leukaemias: especially chronic leukaemias • Metastases: splenic metastases from solid tumours, e.g., carcinomas or sarcomas, are rare • Extramedullary haemopoiesis, e.g., in myeloproliferative diseases and diseases with diffuse marrow replacement by tumour
Haematological disorders	Haematological anaemias, e.g., hereditary spherocytosis, β-thalassaemia, autoimmune haemolysis Autoimmune thrombocytopenia: destruction of antibody-coated platelets in spleen results in accumulation of foamy histiocytes in sinuses
Immune disorders	Felty syndrome: follicular hyperplasia in spleen associated with hypersplenism and rheumatoid disease Sarcoidosis: spleen infiltrated by granulomas Amyloidosis: spleen infiltrated with amyloid

blood supply from surrounding tissues. In contrast, an accessory spleen (splenunculus) is supplied by the splenic artery.

Disorders of the thymus

This is a primary lymphoid organ composed of lymphoid cells and specialized epithelial cells. The function of the thymus is the differentiation, maturation and selection of T cells.

Thymic activity is maximal in the fetus and in childhood; regression is rapid after puberty.

Developmental disorders

Thymic hypoplasia and aplasia

These occur due to the developmental failure of either:

- epithelial tissue—thymus is completely absent or is represented by a fibrous streak, e.g., DiGeorge syndrome or
- lymphoid tissue—severe combined immunodeficiency syndromes, ataxia telangiectasia and reticular dysgenesis.

Both types of developmental disorder result in T-cell deficiency associated with a disordered, cell-mediated immune response.

Thymic hyperplasia

This is a rare condition in which lymphoid follicles composed of B cells develop in the thymic medulla. It is often accompanied by an increase in the size of the thymus and is associated with autoimmune disease, especially myasthenia gravis. In some cases, autoantibodies are thought to be produced by the lymphoid tissue.

Thymomas

These rare tumours are derived from thymic epithelial cells; they can be benign or malignant.

Histologically thymomas are composed of uniform epithelial or spindle cells variably mixed with reactive lymphoid cells.

Benign thymomas

The majority (80%–90%) of thymomas are benign, well-circumscribed, encapsulated, lobulated tumours. Most are asymptomatic, but some present with local disease caused by the compression of adjacent mediastinal structures:

- Respiratory tract—dyspnoea and cough
- Oesophagus—dysphagia
- Great veins—cyanosis and suffusion of the face.

The remainder present with autoimmune disease—15% of patients with myasthenia gravis have a thymoma. Complete surgical excision is curative.

Malignant thymomas

Around 10% to 20% of thymomas are malignant (thymic carcinoma) and are staged based on the extent of invasion into adjacent structures.

DIFFERENTIAL DIAGNOSIS

MEDIASTINAL MASSES

Anterior mediastinal masses (remember the 'Ts'): ***T***hymoma, ***T***eratoma, ***T***hyroid tumour, and ***T***errible lymphoma

Posterior mediastinal masses: lymphoma, neurogenic tumours, foregut cysts.

DISORDERS OF RED BLOOD CELLS

Abnormalities of red cell size and shape

Many haematological and systemic disorders are associated with specific abnormalities of red cell size (anisocytosis) and/or abnormal red cell shape (poikilocytosis) (Fig. 17.8).

Anaemia classifications

Anaemia can be defined as a total reduction in the circulating red cell mass with reduced oxygen carrying capacity of the blood. This is recognized by a haemoglobin concentration that is below the normal range for the patient's age and sex. The normal haemoglobin range in males is 13.0–18.0 g/dL (130–180 g/L) and in females is 11.5–16.5 g/dL (115–165 g/L).

Anaemia can be classified by the underlying mechanism for reduced haemoglobin, as shown in Table 17.12.

It is worth noting that, in clinical practice, anaemia is usually classified by the mean corpuscular volume (MCV) of red cells—this can be increased (macrocytic anaemia), normal (normocytic) or reduced (microcytic).

HINTS AND TIPS

RULE OF THUMB ANAEMIA TYPES

Rules of thumb for different types of anaemia by size:

- Macrocytic—megaloblastic anaemia (vitamin B_{12} or folate deficiency) or haemolytic anaemia (new immature red blood cells—reticulocytes—are large in size).
- Normocytic—anaemia of chronic disease or hypoplastic anaemias (bone marrow suppression).
- Microcytic—iron-deficiency anaemia or thalassaemia.

Fig. 17.8 Diagrammatic representation of anisocytosis and poikilocytosis. Anisocytosis refers to abnormalities in red cell size, and poikilocytosis refers to abnormalities in red cell shape. (Adapted from Underwood, 2009.) *Hb,* Haemoglobin; *MAHA*, microangiopathic haemolytic anaemia; *HUS*, haemolytic uraemic syndrome.

Anisocytosis		
Morphology	**Features**	**Clinical association**
 Microcyte	• <6 µm	• Iron deficiency • Thalassaemia
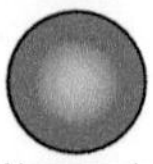 Normocyte	• Biconcave disc • Central area of pallor • 6–8 µm	• Normal red blood cell
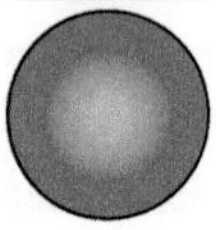 Macrocyte	• >8 µm	• Liver disease • Alcohol abuse • Hypothyroidism • Pregnancy • Megaloblastic anaemia
Poikilocytosis		
 Spherocyte	• Spherical - loss of concave shape • Uniformly dense • Small	• Hereditary spherocytosis • Autoimmune haemolytic anaemia • Burns
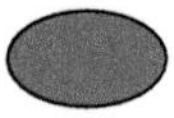 Elliptocyte	• Oval shaped • Rounded edges • Central pallor • Longer than a normocyte	• Hereditary elliptocytosis • Severe iron deficiency anaemia
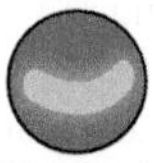 Stomatocyte	• Elliptical central area of pallor • Looks like a mouth	• Liver disease • Hereditary stomatocytosis
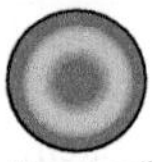 Target cell	• Central disc of Hb-dense staining • Rim of pallor • Peripheral rim of Hb	• Iron deficiency • Haemoglobinapathies • Liver disease • Hyposplenism
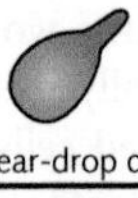 Tear-drop cell	• Pear shaped	• Myelofibrosis • Marrow infiltration
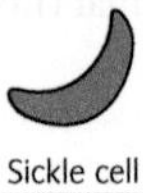 Sickle cell	• Crescent shaped • Elongated with pointed ends	• Sickle cell disease
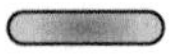 Pencil cell	• Cigar shaped • Long axis ×5 length of short axis • Hypochromic variant of elliptocytes	• Iron deficiency
 Acanthocyte	• 2–10 spicules • Irregular shape and thickness • Broad base • Irregularly distributed	• Liver disease • Abetalipoproteinaemia • Renal failure
 Echinocyte	• 10–30 spicules • Equal size and shape • Regularly distributed	• Liver disease • Ureamia • Post splenectomy • Storage artifact
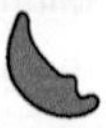 Schistocyte	• Fragmented rbc • Smaller than normal erythrocyte • Irregular shape	• MAHA • HUS • Mechanical cardiac valves • Burns

Table 17.12 Causes of anaemia[a]

Mechanism	Causes
Increased red cell loss, lysis or pooling	Blood loss Haemolysis: • Intrinsic abnormalities of red cells: hereditary (membrane defects, enzyme defects, haemoglobinopathies) and acquired (paroxysmal nocturnal haemoglobinuria) • Extrinsic abnormalities of red cells: antibody-mediated red cell destruction and mechanical trauma to red cells Hypersplenism
Impaired red cell production	Deficiency of haematinics: • Megaloblastic anaemias: lack of vitamin B_{12} or folate • Iron-deficiency anaemia Dyserythropoiesis (production of defective red blood cells): • Anaemia of chronic disorders • Myelodysplasia • Sideroblastic anaemia Hypoplasia of marrow (failure to produce cells): • Aplastic anaemia • Red cell aplasia Invasion of marrow by malignant cells: • Leukaemias • Myeloproliferative diseases • Non-haematological malignancies

[a] *Anaemia is the result of an imbalance between the rate of loss and rate of production of red blood cells.*

The colour of a red cell (representing the quantity of haemoglobin) is also described with the terms hypochromic (low), normochromic (normal) and hyperchromic (high).

The sections that follow describe the mechanisms that cause these anaemias.

COMMON PITFALLS

ANAEMIA IS NOT A DIAGNOSIS

'Anaemia' is not a diagnosis. It must be qualified and the underlying cause must be identified, e.g., 'The patient has a macrocytic anaemia secondary to B_{12} deficiency'.

Anaemia from blood loss

Acute blood loss

Following acute blood loss, a state of cardiovascular collapse may occur. On cessation of haemorrhage, the plasma volume begins to be restored from the interstitial fluid compartment; this results in haemodilution and anaemia becomes apparent.

The blood picture shows:

- normocytic and normochromic anaemia
- increased reticulocytes (immature red blood cells), reflecting increased haemopoiesis
- transient leucocytosis and thrombocytosis.

The plasma proteins and other biochemical constituents are restored rapidly (in 2–3 days). Full red cell restoration may take up to 6 weeks (Table 17.13).

Table 17.13 Lifespan of blood cells

Cell	Lifespan
Red blood cells	120 days
Neutrophils	8 hours–3 days
Lymphocytes	3 days Memory T and B cells: years
Eosinophils	In blood: 8 hours; In tissue: 6 days
Basophils	Hours to days
Monocytes/macrophages	Monocytes: 3 days Macrophages: 6–16 days
Platelets	10 days

Chronic blood loss

Chronic blood loss is the most common cause of iron-deficiency anaemia, characterized by a microcytic hypochromic blood film. The main causes of chronic haemorrhage are:

- diseases of the GI tract—particularly peptic ulceration and carcinoma (colorectal, stomach)
- menorrhagia.

Patients with unexplained iron-deficiency anaemia require careful screening for an occult cause of blood loss.

Haemolytic anaemias

The basic pathological change in all haemolytic anaemias is a reduction in the lifespan of the red cell due to an increased rate of destruction; this is termed haemolysis. The effects of increased haemolysis are:

- anaemia—commonly macrocytic due to increased reticulocytes in the blood, but may be normocytic.
- bone marrow erythroid hyperplasia.
- splenomegaly (see page 317).
- unconjugated hyperbilirubinaemia due to red cell breakdown, which may lead to the development jaundice, pigmented gallstones and kernicterus in neonates.
- haemoglobinuria—leading to acute tubular necrosis in the kidney.

Aetiology

The aetiology of haemolytic anaemias can be broadly classified into:

- congenital abnormalities of red cells—hereditary defects (intrinsic to the cell)
- acquired abnormalities of red cells—(extrinsic to the cell).

Fig. 17.9 outlines the further subdivisions of causes of haemolytic anaemia.

Membranopathies

These are disorders affecting the red cell membrane.

Hereditary spherocytosis

Hereditary spherocytosis is the most common cause of hereditary haemolytic anaemia in the UK. It is usually an autosomal dominant condition, presenting at any age, caused by an abnormality in one of the cytoskeletal-associated membrane proteins: ankyrin, spectrin or band 4.2 protein.

The cells are spherical due to defective vertical interactions between the cytoskeleton and membrane. Their deformability is reduced and they are abnormally fragile.

Reduced deformability causes their retention in the splenic microcirculation where they undergo metabolic stress caused by a lack of glucose and acidosis. Increased fragility of metabolically stressed cells causes spontaneous lysis or premature phagocytosis by the splenic macrophages.

Blood film shows:

- increased microspherocytes, which are more deeply stained with loss of the central pallor of normal erythrocytes.
- polychromasia and reticulocytes.

The general clinical features are anaemia, splenomegaly (splenectomy usually performed) and fluctuating jaundice.

Hereditary elliptocytosis

Hereditary elliptocytosis is similar to spherocytosis but the red cells are elliptical. This is caused by abnormalities of horizontal interactions of spectrin heterodimers. This condition is autosomal dominant but not as severe as hereditary spherocytosis and does not usually cause anaemia or jaundice.

Enzymopathies

Enzyme deficiencies

In erythrocytes, 90% of glucose is metabolized anaerobically to lactate via the Embden–Meyerhof glycolytic pathway (similar to regular glycolysis except that the end product is lactate, not pyruvate). Ten percent of glucose is used in the hexose monophosphate shunt (pentose phosphate pathway) to increase the levels of reduced nicotinamide-adenine dinucleotide phosphate (NADPH) to those required for the reduction of glutathione. Reduced glutathione is essential for maintaining haemoglobin (Hb) in the reduced (ferrous) state (Fig. 17.10).

The most common enzymopathies are glucose-6-phosphate dehydrogenase (G6PD) deficiency, glutathione synthetase deficiency and pyruvate kinase deficiency. Many other enzymopathies of glycolytic enzymes exist but they are extremely rare, e.g., deficiencies of hexokinase, glucose phosphate isomerase and phosphofructokinase. The effects are similar to pyruvate kinase deficiency.

G6PD deficiency

G6PD deficiency is an X-linked recessive condition that is especially common among Afro-Caribbean people. It results in

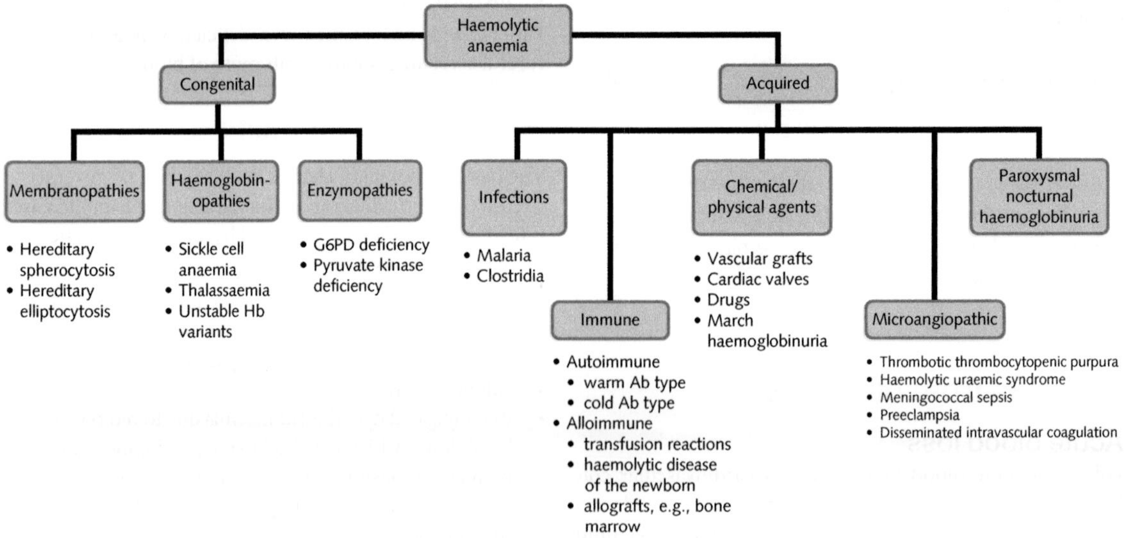

Fig. 17.9 Causes of haemolytic anaemia. *Hb*, Haemoglobin.

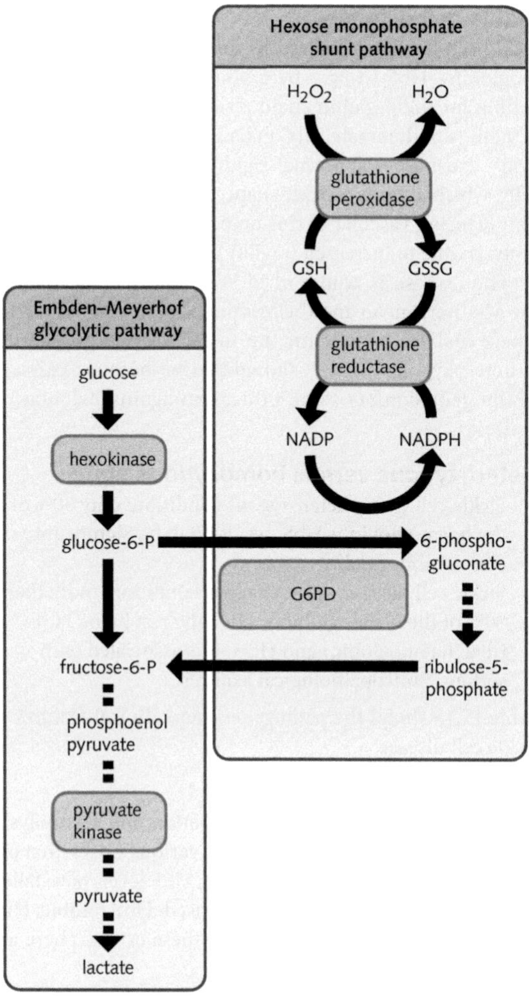

Fig. 17.10 Metabolic pathways of the red cell. *Fructose-6-P,* Fructose-6-phosphate; *glucose-6-P,* glucose-6-phosphate; *G6PD,* glucose 6 phosphate dehydrogenase; *GSH,* reduced glutathione; *GSSG,* oxidized glutathione; *H_2O_2,* hydrogen peroxide; *NADP,* oxidized nicotinamide-adenine dinucleotide phosphate; *NADPH,* reduced nicotinamide-adenine dinucleotide phosphate.

a decreased ratio of NADPH:NADP. Glutathione protects the cell from oxidative stress and NADPH is required for glutathione reduction, therefore with decreased availability of glutathione, the cell has increased susceptibility to oxidative stress.

Spontaneous anaemia is rare but episodic acute haemolytic crises are frequently precipitated by infections, certain foods (e.g., fava (broad) beans) or drugs (quinine, naphthalene (moth balls), ciprofloxacin).

Blood films during haemolytic crises show increased poikilocytosis with bite-shaped defects ('bite' cells) or surface blebs ('blister' cells) and Heinz bodies (red cells containing oxidized, denatured haemoglobin). The blood film is normal between haemolytic episodes.

Female heterozygotes have the advantage of being resistant to falciparum malaria.

A deficiency of glutathione synthetase leads to defective synthesis of glutathione causing a similar syndrome to G6PD deficiency.

Pyruvate kinase deficiency

Pyruvate kinase deficiency is a rare, autosomal recessive defect that results in congenital chronic haemolytic anaemia. Red cells become rigid due to reduced adenosine triphosphate formation and failure of membrane ion pumps. The cells become dehydrated, distorted and removed by the spleen.

This is characterized by mild anaemia, jaundice and gallstones. The blood film shows poikilocytosis and distorted 'prickle cells'.

Haemoglobinopathies

Haemoglobinopathies are caused by either:

- decreased α- or β-globin synthesis—the α- and β-thalassaemias
  or
- synthesis of abnormal haemoglobin—e.g., sickle cell disease, other unstable haemoglobins.

Anaemias are usually a combination of both dyshaematopoiesis and haemolysis.

Thalassaemias

Normal adult haemoglobin (HbA) is composed of two α-globin chains and two β-globin chains ($\alpha_2\beta_2$). In thalassemia there is absent or reduced synthesis of one of the globin chains. This results in a microcytic, hypochromic anaemia, with excessive production of the non-affected haemoglobin chain often producing insoluble red cell inclusions. This can impair erythropoiesis and cause premature cell death (haemolysis).

The disease is inherited; many different causative mutations have been identified. It is common in the Mediterranean, Middle and Far East and South-East Asia, where carrier rates of 10%–15% are found.

α-Thalassaemia

This is mainly caused by deletion (rather than mutation) of parts of the α-globin genes. Normal individuals have four copies of the α-globin gene, two on each chromosome 16. There are, therefore, four possible degrees of α-thalassaemia, depending on how many genes are affected (Fig. 17.11). Haemolysis is less severe than in β-thalassaemia.

β-Thalassaemia

This is caused by a mutation of the β-globin gene (β) leading to either reduced (β^+) or absent (β0) synthesis of the β-globin chain. Normal individuals have two copies of each β-globin gene (one on each chromosome 11). There are, therefore, two possible degrees of β-thalassaemia (Table 17.14):

1. Thalassaemia minor—heterozygous trait associated with mild anaemia (β^+ β) or (β0 β) and is usually clinically silent.
2. Thalassaemia major—homozygous syndrome associated with severe haemolytic anaemia ($\beta^+ \beta^+$) (β0 β0). This requires blood transfusions for survival.

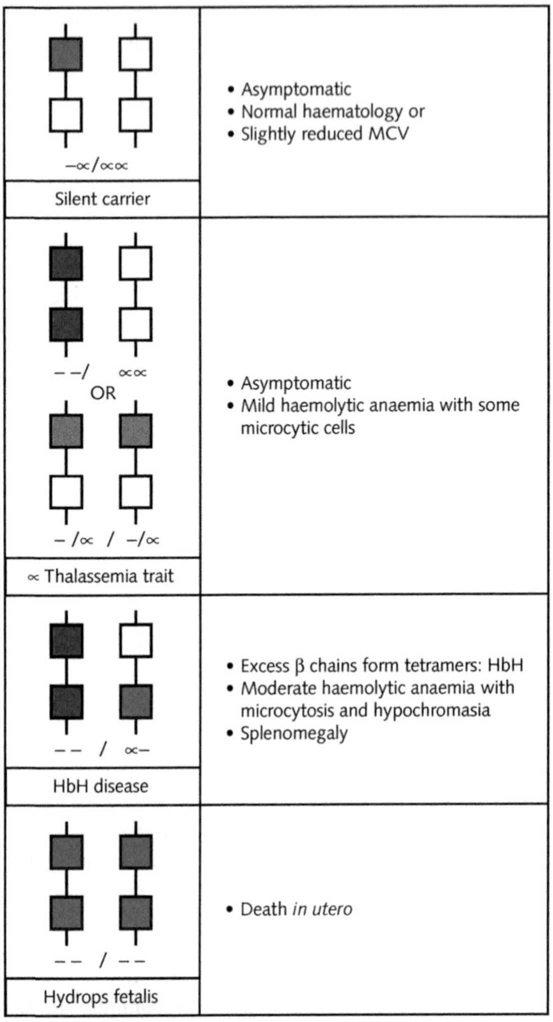
−∝/∝∝
Silent carrier
• Asymptomatic
• Normal haematology or
• Slightly reduced MCV
− −/ ∝∝
OR
− /∝ / −/∝
∝ Thalassemia trait
• Asymptomatic
• Mild haemolytic anaemia with some microcytic cells
− − / ∝−
HbH disease
• Excess β chains form tetramers: HbH
• Moderate haemolytic anaemia with microcytosis and hypochromasia
• Splenomegaly
− − / − −
Hydrops fetalis
• Death *in utero*

Fig. 17.11 Alpha thalassemia mutations. *HbH,* haemoglobin H; *MCV,* mean corpuscular volume.

Sickle cell disease

Sickle cell disease is caused by an abnormal form of haemoglobin—HbS ($\alpha_2\beta_2^S$)—by a point mutation in the gene coding for the β-globin chain resulting in the substitution of valine for glutamate. HbS polymerises at low oxygen tensions, causing an abnormal rigidity and deformity of red cells, which assume a sickle shape. These undergo aggregation (causing vascular occlusion of small vessels) and haemolysis (due to increased fragility).

The disease is common in West and Central Africa, the Mediterranean and the Middle East. In areas of Africa where malaria is endemic, up to 30% of the population is heterozygous. This is thought to be because carriage of the gene confers some protection against falciparum malaria.

Heterozygous versus homozygous state

- Sickle cell trait—heterozygous condition: only 30% of the haemoglobin is HbS, resulting in no significant clinical abnormality.
- Sickle cell disease—homozygous condition: more than 80% of the haemoglobin is HbS, the rest being HbF (fetal haemoglobin) and HbA. It is associated with serious clinicopathological features.

Table 17.15 shows the pathogenesis and clinical features of sickle cell disease.

'Crises' of sickle cell disease

In addition to the effects of aggregation and haemolysis, sickle cell disease is characterized by various 'crises' that occur after the age of 1 or 2 years, when HbF levels have fallen and the proportion of HbS has increased. HbF inhibits HbS polymerization, initially preventing these crises. There are three main patterns:

1. Sequestration crises—sudden pooling of red cells in the spleen and/or liver, which can lead to death from a rapid fall in haemoglobin.

Table 17.14 β-Thalassaemia disorders

	Globin chains present	Clinicopathological features
Thalassaemia minor	Heterozygous $\beta^0\beta$	Moderate reduction in HbA
	Heterozygous $\beta^+\beta$	Compensatory increase in $HbA_2(\alpha_2\ \delta_2)$
		Mild anaemia with hypochromic cells
Thalassaemia major	Homozygous $\beta^0\ \beta^0$	Hypochromic microcytic anaemia
	Homozygous $\beta^+\ \beta^+$	Severe haemolysis with hepatosplenomegaly
	occasionally$\beta^+\ \beta^0$	Marrow hyperplasia causing skeletal deformities
		Iron overload from repeated transfusions

HbA, *Adult haemoglobin.*

Table 17.15 Pathogenesis and clinical features of sickle cell disease

Pathogenesis	Clinical features
Vascular occlusion	• Cerebral infarction • Retinopathy → blindness • Pulmonary infarction → acute respiratory distress • Cor pulmonale • Haematuria and polyuria • Splenic atrophy → hyposplenism → infections • Bone necrosis → osteomyelitis • Leg ulcers
Chronic haemolysis	• Anaemia • Jaundice and gallstones • Haemochromatosis (caused by iron overload in transfused patients)

2. Infarctive crises—blood vessel occlusion in bone, causing the 'painful crises' (especially femoral head), spleen (leading to splenic atrophy) and skin (leg ulcers).
3. Aplastic crises—infection with parvovirus B19, which targets erythroblasts and lyses them, causing an aplastic crisis with rapid fall in blood haemoglobin.

Treatment of sickle cell disease includes the avoidance of factors known to precipitate crises, especially hypoxia. Hydroxyurea chemotherapy raises the HbF percentage in red cells. Mean survival figures are variable, reflecting differing standards of medical care. However, the death rate in infancy and childhood is higher in underdeveloped countries.

Acquired defects of the red cell

Paroxysmal nocturnal haemoglobinuria

This rare disorder of young adults is caused by a non-malignant clonal expansion of abnormal erythrocytes, which are sensitive to complement mediated lysis. The cells lack the enzyme required for the synthesis of glycosyl-phosphatidyl inositol, which anchors several complement regulating proteins to the cell membrane. Chronic intravascular haemolysis occurs with urine characteristically appearing dark in the morning due to concentrated haemoglobinuria. Clinically there is a triad of:

- haemolytic anaemia
- pancytopenia (from bone marrow failure)
- venous thrombosis.

Venous thrombosis is a frequent complication involving large calibre vessels, commonly the hepatic, portal, cerebral and pulmonary veins, with half of patients dying from thrombotic complications. There is also progressive chronic renal failure.

Alloimmune antibody-mediated haemolytic anaemia

Incompatible ABO blood transfusion

This classic example of red cell haemolysis is caused by alloantibodies (Table 17.16).

For example, if donor blood is group A (cells contain A antigen) and recipient blood is group O (plasma contains anti-A and anti-B antibodies), then anti-A antibodies of the recipient will cause agglutination and haemolysis of donor red blood cells.

CLINICAL NOTES

CLINICAL EFFECTS OF ABO INCOMPATIBILITY

The clinical effects of an ABO incompatible transfusion are:

- Massive intravascular haemolysis leading to collapse, hypotension and lumbar pain.
- Haemoglobinuria is common and renal failure may ensue.
- Disseminated intravascular coagulation may be triggered by red cell lysis.

The effects may be precipitated with only a few millilitres of incompatible red cells.

Transfusion-induced haemolysis due to incompatibility of the rhesus system is generally milder, since antibodies to the rhesus system are not complement fixing.

Haemolytic disease of the newborn

This haemolysis of red blood cells in rhesus (Rh)-positive fetuses is caused by the placental passage of maternal anti-rhesus IgG antibodies from rhesus-negative mothers. It is particularly associated with D antigen of the rhesus blood group. The pathogenesis is as follows:

Table 17.16 ABO blood group system

Genotype	Phenotype	Serum antibodies	Frequency of phenotype in UK
OO	O	Anti-A, Anti-B	Most common
AA or AO	A	Anti-B	Common
BB or BO	B	Anti-A	Rare
AB	AB	None	Rarest

- First pregnancy—Rh-positive fetus in Rh-negative mother with no antibodies: healthy baby. However, fetal red blood cells enter maternal circulation during birth (or miscarriage) causing maternal isoimmunization with subsequent production of anti-Rh antibodies.
- Subsequent pregnancies—maternal anti-Rh antibodies acquired during a previous pregnancy cause haemolysis in Rh-positive fetuses: haemolytic disease of the newborn (HDN).

Incidence of HDN is now reduced by prophylactic anti-RhD injection in Rh-negative mothers, removing RhD^+ fetal cells before isoimmunization can occur.

Autoimmune haemolytic anaemia

This is the most common type of haemolytic anaemia, caused by the immune destruction of red blood cells by the patient's own antibodies. It may be idiopathic, secondary to other diseases or drug related.

It is divided into two main groups according to the temperature at which the haemolytic reactions occur.

1. 'Warm' antibody type

The autoantibody is IgG and is most reactive at 37 °C. It is the more common form leading to chronic anaemia with microspherocytosis. Red cell destruction occurs in the spleen.

Clinical features are those of haemolytic anaemia: pallor, jaundice, and splenomegaly.

2. 'Cold' antibody type

The autoantibody is IgM and is most reactive at 4 °C but can still bind complement and agglutinate red cells at 30 °C; the temperature of peripheral tissues (hands, feet, nose and ears). There is destruction of red cells by Kupffer cells of the liver.

Clinical features are those of anaemia with blue and cold extremities, occasionally progressing to ischaemia and ulceration. The disorder is chronic and usually mild.

Table 17.17 summarizes the antibody-mediated haemolytic anaemias.

Table 17.17 Summary of antibody-mediated haemolytic anaemias

Isoimmune	Transfusion reactions Haemolytic disease of the newborn
Autoimmune	
• ***'Warm' antibody type (auto antibody is IgG class)***	Primary: idiopathic (50%) Secondary: • chronic lymphocytic leukaemia • lymphoma related • systemic lupus erythematosus and other autoimmune disorders • viral infections • drug related, e.g., methyl-dopa, penicillin, quinidine
• ***'Cold' antibody type (auto antibody is IgM class)***	Primary: idiopathic Secondary: • lymphoma related • infectious mononucleosis • *Mycoplasma pneumoniae* • mumps • malaria

Mechanical trauma to red cells

Mechanical damage to red cells may lead to reduced lifespan and haemolysis.

There are several groups of mechanical haemolysis, as described below.

Microangiopathic haemolytic anaemia (MAHA)

Intravascular haemolysis secondary to physical trauma of erythrocytes occurring within small blood vessels. This is caused by fibrin mesh formation due to increased activation of the coagulation system. It is commonly present in:

- disseminated intravascular coagulation (see later)
- haemolytic uraemic syndrome
- thrombotic thrombocytopenic purpura (TTP)
- SLE
- malignancy

Blood film shows the presence of schistocytes (especially triangular cells).

Macroangiopathic haemolytic anaemia

This is intravascular haemolysis secondary to physical trauma of erythrocytes occurring within large blood vessels, caused by prosthetic (usually mechanical) heart valves or conditions and resulting in turbulent blood flow such as coarctation of the aorta.

CLINICAL NOTES

MARCH HAEMATURIA

Repetitive and prolonged foot striking, e.g., soldiers marching and marathon running, can uncommonly lead to the passage of free haemoglobin in the urine, resulting in russet-coloured urine post exercise. This is a result of mechanical trauma to red blood cells and resolves spontaneously.

Malaria

Haemolysis is common in malaria. *Plasmodium* species enter erythrocytes where they multiply and mature to form schizonts, which are released by erythrocyte rupture. Massive splenomegaly is often present (see Chapter 5).

Table 17.18 Causes of macrocytic anaemia

Macrocytic anaemia
Alcohol
Liver disease
Haemorrhage
Hypothyroidism
B_{12}/folate deficiency (megaloblastic anaemia)
Pregnancy
Drugs, e.g., azathioprine
Myelodysplasia
Haemolytic anaemia
Aplastic anaemia

Macrocytic anaemia

This is an anaemia where the MCV is >95 fL, for which there are many causes (Table 17.18). Alcohol is the commonest cause of a raised MCV with or without anaemia.

Megaloblastic anaemia

This is a cause of macrocytic anaemia resulting from impaired DNA synthesis in bone marrow precursor cells secondary to vitamin B_{12} or folic acid (folate) deficiency. This causes asynchronous maturation of the cell's nucleus and cytoplasm with the formation of abnormally large red cell precursors (megaloblasts) which develop into abnormally large red cells (macrocytes). The causes and effects of vitamin B_{12} and folate deficiency are outlined in Table 17.19.

Microcytic anaemia

In this condition, the MCV of an erythrocyte is <80 fL, for which there are many causes; iron deficiency is the most common (Table 17.20).

Iron-deficiency anaemia

Iron is abundant in meat, vegetables, eggs and dairy foods.

Requirements are:

- men and postmenopausal women—9 mg per day
- menstruating women—15 mg per day
- pregnancy—27 mg per day
- children—9mg per day.

Absorption of iron is via the duodenum and upper jejunum in the ferrous (Fe^{2+}) form.

Table 17.19 Comparison of vitamin B_{12} and folate deficiency

	Vitamin B_{12} deficiency	Folate deficiency
Source	Animal produce – meat, eggs	Most foods—especially green vegetables, fruit, cereals meat and eggs.
Requirements	1 µg/day (heat stable, liver stores = several years)	Minimally, 200 µg/day (heat labile, liver stores = 50–100 days)
Nutritional deficiency	Uncommon (only in vegans)	Common—malnutrition from anorexia, alcoholism, poor diet, etc.
Time of onset	Slow (years)	Over several weeks
Area of absorption	Absorbed in terminal ileum and requires intrinsic factor	Absorbed in jejunum (and duodenum)
Disease causing deficiency	Reduced absorption: • Reduced intrinsic factor ◦ Pernicious anaemia ◦ Gastrectomy • Inadequate uptake ◦ Diseases of terminal ileum e.g., Crohn disease ◦ Surgical removal of terminal ileum Inadequate intake: • Rare, occasionally seen in veganism • Bacterial overgrowth	Reduced absorption: • Drugs—especially anticonvulsants • Jejunal disease Inadequate intake Increased requirements • Pregnancy and lactation • Haemolysis
Drug involvement	No	May be drug related (anticonvulsants or antimetabolites)
Deficiency state	Megaloblastic anaemia – associated with neutropenia and thrombocytopenia	Megaloblastic anaemia – associated with neutropenia and thrombocytopenia
Neurological involvement	Neurological lesions frequent: subacute combined degeneration of the cord, peripheral neuropathy, optic neuropathy	Linked to fetal neural tube defects. No adult involvement.

Table 17.20 Causes of microcytic anaemia

Microcytic anaemia

Iron deficiency
• Increased loss
  ○ Bleeding
• Increased utilization
  ○ Growth
  ○ Pregnancy
• Inadequate intake
  ○ Dietary deficiency, e.g., vegan/vegetarian
• Malabsorption, e.g., coeliac disease

Anaemia of chronic disease • Chronic infections, e.g., tuberculosis, HIV • Chronic inflammation e.g., inflammatory bowel disease, rheumatoid arthritis, systemic lupus erythematosus • Malignancy (independent of bone marrow infiltration)
Thalassemia

The causes of iron deficiency are:

- chronic blood loss—most common cause e.g., diseases of the GI tract, menorrhagia, lesions of the urinary tract
- increased requirements, e.g., in childhood and pregnancy
- malabsorption due to gastrectomy, coeliac disease
- inadequate intake, i.e., dietary deficiency.

Blood film:

- hypochromic microcytic erythrocytes
- low numbers of reticulocytes for the degree of anaemia
- poikilocytosis (especially 'pencil' and 'target' cells)
- anisocytosis.

Laboratory findings: reduced total serum iron, reduced serum ferritin (iron storage protein), reduced transferrin saturation (iron-carrying protein) and largely increased total iron-binding capacity.

Treatment is of the underlying cause and iron supplementation (ferrous sulphate).

Dyserythropoiesis

This group of disorders is characterized by the production of defective red cells.

Anaemia of chronic disease

This is a common cause of anaemia, second only to iron deficiency. There are no other obvious causes for the anaemia other than that the patient has a chronic disease such as:

- autoimmune disease (non-organ-specific), e.g., rheumatoid disease, SLE, inflammatory bowel disease.
- chronic infective disease, e.g., tuberculosis, malaria and schistosomiasis.
- neoplasia: lymphoma and some carcinomas.

Iron stores are replete; however, the flow of iron is blocked by the effect of cytokines (IL1 and tumour necrosis factor) inhibiting the release of iron from macrophages to plasma to erythrocytes. Erythropoiesis is reduced as the normal response of erythropoietin (Epo, the hormone that stimulates erythropoiesis) to anaemia is suppressed. Iron therapy therefore does not correct the anaemia; however, exogenous Epo administration may be beneficial. The anaemia improves with treatment of the underlying chronic condition.

Blood film: mainly normocytic and normochromic or mild hypochromasia and microcytosis.

Laboratory findings: a reduced serum iron and reduced serum iron-binding capacity (as iron is plentiful), but the iron stores (ferritin) are normal or increased (Table 17.22).

Table 17.21 Causes of a normocytic anaemia

Anaemia of chronic disease
Chronic renal failure
Acute blood loss
Haemolytic conditions
Hypothyroidism
Mild iron-deficiency anaemia
Myelodysplasia

HINTS AND TIPS

FERRITIN AS AN ACUTE PHASE REACTANT

Ferritin is an acute phase reactant and will therefore be elevated if the patient is unwell. Be careful interpreting it in this situation.

Sideroblastic anaemia

Ultimately, this is caused by defective haem synthesis, resulting in the accumulation of excess cytoplasmic iron

Table 17.22 Serology of microcytic anaemia

Indices	Iron-deficiency anaemia	Anaemia of chronic disease	Thalassaemia
Hb	Low	Low	Normal or low
MCV	Low	Low	Low
Serum iron	Low	Low	Normal
TIBC	High	Normal or low	Normal
Ferritin	Low	Normal or increased	Normal
Transferrin saturation	Low	Normal	Normal
BM iron stores	Absent	Increased	Normal or increased

BM, Bone marrow; Hb, haemoglobin; MCV, mean corpuscular volume; TIBC, total iron binding capacity.

(haemosiderin) around the nucleus of erythrocyte progenitors within the bone marrow. These cells are called ring sideroblasts. Peripheral erythrocytes are hypochromatic.

The disease can be:

1. Hereditary sideroblastic anaemia—various mutations.
2. Acquired:
   a. Primary sideroblastic anaemia—subtype of the myelodysplastic syndromes
   b. Secondary sideroblastic anaemia
      - neoplastic diseases of the bone marrow, e.g., myeloma
      - drug/toxin related, e.g., alcohol, lead, isoniazid.

Bone marrow hypoplasia

This is a descriptive term for conditions where there are a reduced number of haematopoietic cells within the bone marrow.

Aplastic anaemia

This is a pancytopenia resulting from aplasia of all three stem cell lineages within the bone marrow. Microscopically, the marrow is hypocellular with extensive fat replacement. Anaemia is usually normocytic but a mild macrocytosis can be seen.

Aetiology:

- Primary
  - Congenital, e.g., Fanconi anaemia, a rare autosomal recessive disorder of DNA repair.
  - Idiopathic
- Secondary
  - Ionizing whole body irradiation—therapeutically (e.g., haematological neoplasms) or in nuclear accidents (e.g., Chernobyl).
  - Drugs—chloramphenicol, phenylbutazone.
  - Toxins—benzene, insecticides, dichloro-diphenyl trichloroethane.
  - Viruses—parvovirus B19, EBV, viral heptitides.

Pure red cell aplasia

This normocytic anaemia is caused by the maturation arrest of erythroblasts only. In contrast to aplastic anaemia, leucocytes and platelets are not affected. There are three main forms:

1. Acute/transient form—occurs after parvovirus infection or exposure to certain toxins.
2. Chronic acquired red cell aplasia—autoimmune, can be associated with thymomas, haematological malignancies.
3. Congenital red cell aplasia—Diamond-Blackfan anaemia

Bone marrow infiltration

The normal haematopoietic elements of the bone marrow may be extensively replaced/obliterated by infiltrating neoplastic cells or fibrotic processes:

- leukaemias
- lymphomas with bone marrow involvement
- myelofibrosis
- disseminated malignancies.

Patients develop leucoerythroblastic anaemia characterized by circulating erythroblasts and primitive white cells. Extramedullary haematopoiesis commonly develops.

DISORDERS OF HAEMOSTASIS

Definitions of clinical lesions

Petechiae

Individual small purple spots of a nonblanching rash are called petechiae.

Purpura

This skin rash results from bleeding into the skin from capillaries. It is caused either by defects in capillaries or by defects or deficiencies of platelets.

Ecchymosis

This is a bruise larger than 1 cm, presenting as a bluish-black mark on the skin resulting from the release of blood into the tissues either through injury or through spontaneous leaking of blood from vessels.

Abnormalities of the vessel walls

This heterogeneous group of conditions (the 'nonthrombocytopenic purpuras') is characterized by easy bruising and spontaneous bleeding from small vessels. The underlying lesions are of two main types:

1. Abnormal perivascular connective tissue which leads to inadequate vessel support.
2. Intrinsically abnormal or damaged vessel wall.

Haemorrhages are mainly in the skin, causing petechiae, ecchymoses or both. In some disorders, there is also bleeding from the mucous membranes. Bleeding is not usually serious.

Infections

Some bacterial and viral infections cause purpura as a result of either vascular damage (vasculitis) by the organism or through disseminated intravascular coagulation (DIC), e.g., measles, meningococcal septicaemia.

Scurvy and Ehlers–Danlos syndrome

Vitamin C is required for the hydroxylation of proline as a step in collagen synthesis. In both Ehlers–Danlos syndrome (an inherited disorder of collagen synthesis) and scurvy (vitamin C deficiency), capillaries are fragile because of defective collagen synthesis.

Perifollicular petechiae, bruising and mucosal haemorrhages are common.

Steroid purpura

Cushing syndrome arises from long-term steroid therapy and results in purpura (amongst other symptoms) caused by loss of vascular supportive tissue.

Henoch–Schönlein purpura

This immune complex hypersensitivity reaction (type III) is usually found in children and often follows an acute infection. It is characterized by red wheals and a purple rash on the buttocks and extensor surfaces of the lower legs caused by bleeding into the skin from inflamed capillaries and venules.

Arthritis, acute glomerulonephritis, haematuria and GI symptoms may also occur.

It is a self-limiting condition but occasionally patients develop renal failure.

Reduced platelet count (thrombocytopenia)

The normal platelet count is 150–450 × 10^9/L. The causes of thrombocytopenia are discussed below.

Decreased platelet production

This is the most common cause of thrombocytopenia.

Generalized disease of bone marrow

This is seen in aplastic anaemia and neoplastic bone marrow infiltration that obliterates normal haemopoietic elements.

Ineffective megakaryopoiesis

- Megaloblastic anaemia (folate or vitamin B_{12} deficiency)—is characterized by decreased numbers of platelets.
- Paroxysmal nocturnal haemoglobinuria—may cause ineffective megakaryopoiesis.

Decreased platelet survival

Immune destruction: idiopathic thrombocytopenic purpura (ITP)

The autoimmune destruction of antibody-coated platelets by the reticuloendothelial system, especially the spleen, increases the likelihood of haemorrhage within the:

- Skin—petechiae and ecchymoses.
- Mucous membranes—e.g., epistaxis, bleeding gums, menorrhagia, haematuria, melaena.
- CNS—possibly fatal intracranial haemorrhage.

There is often associated anaemia secondary to blood loss.

Clinical types are:

- acute—often in children and usually self-limiting with spontaneous resolution. May be postinfective, e.g., measles.
- chronic—over 6 months duration, usually in adults, mainly idiopathic but occasionally related to other autoimmune diseases, CLL or drug induced—e.g., quinine, heparin, sulphonamides.

Non-immune destruction

This is mainly through thrombotic thrombocytopenic purpura (TTP) and haemolytic uraemic syndrome (HUS).

HUS and TTP are thought to represent the same disease process but with different distributions of thrombotic lesions.

Thrombocytopenia occurs due to abnormal platelet activation and consumption. Platelets adhere to the endothelium of capillaries and precapillary arterioles where they undergo aggregation, with fibrin deposition, which results in microvascular occlusive platelet plugs and microangiopathic haemolytic anaemia.

Aetiology—the underlying cause of the disorder is obscure but the following pathogenic factors have been implicated:

- Immune-mediated vessel damage.
- Platelet hyperaggregation due to deficiency of an IgG. inhibitor of platelet-agglutinating factor in normal plasma.
- Diminished production of prostaglandin by vessel walls.
- Excess of high-molecular-weight multimers of von Willebrand factor, which interact with platelet agglutinating factor, causing platelet adhesion to vascular endothelium.

In TTP, occlusive plugs lead to widespread ischaemic organ damage, especially of the brain and kidney, resulting in neurological abnormalities and progressive renal impairment. In HUS, organ damage is limited to the kidney. Children tend to develop HUS rather than TTP.

DIC can also cause widespread consumption of platelets, resulting in simultaneous thrombosis and haemorrhage.

Dilutional thrombocytopenia

Platelets are unstable at 4 °C so blood transfusions contain few viable platelets. Therefore, transfusion with massive amounts of stored blood may cause thrombocytopenia. The effect can be minimized by replacement with specific products, e.g., fresh frozen plasma and platelet concentrates.

Defects of platelet function

Congenital

Defective adhesion (Bernard–Soulier syndrome)

This rare disease causes life-threatening haemorrhages. The platelets are deficient in glycoprotein receptors (glycoprotein Ib/IX complex), which are essential for the binding of von Willebrand factor. The platelets are larger than normal with defective adherence to exposed subendothelial connective tissues and defective platelet aggregation. There is also a variable degree of thrombocytopenia.

Defective aggregation: thrombasthenia (Glanzmann disease)

This failure of primary platelet aggregation is due to a deficiency of membrane receptors (glycoprotein IIb–IIIa complex) for fibrinogen binding.

Defective secretion (storage pool disease)

A common, mild defect of platelet function. It causes easy bruising and bleeding after trauma. It is caused by a deficiency of 'dense granules' within the platelets, which normally store adenosine diphosphate (ADP). The decreased storage pool of ADP prevents complex platelet functions such as thromboxane release.

Acquired

Aspirin

Aspirin therapy is the most common cause of defective platelet function, and it produces an abnormal bleeding time.

Aspirin irreversibly inhibits cyclooxygenase, causing impairment in thromboxane A_2 synthesis, which is necessary for platelet release and aggregation. After a single dose, the effects last 7–10 days.

Bleeding tendency is mild, with increased skin bruising and bleeding after surgery. The use of aspirin may contribute to GI haemorrhage associated with acute mucosal erosions. It can be life threatening.

Uraemia

In uraemia, defects may be caused by an abnormal arachidonate metabolism with reduced synthesis of thromboxane. Platelet interactions with the subendothelium are abnormal and bleeding may be severe.

Clotting factor abnormalities

Hereditary factor abnormalities

Von Willebrand disease

This is the most common of the hereditary coagulation disorders. It is usually an autosomal dominant disorder of abnormal platelet adhesion associated with low factor VIII activity. The primary defect is the reduced production of von Willebrand factor, a protein synthesized by platelets and endothelial cells which has two main functions:

1. The promotion of platelet adhesion.
2. As a carrier molecule for factor VIII, protecting it from premature destruction.

The disease is characterized by operative and posttraumatic haemorrhage, mucous membrane bleeding (e.g., epistaxis, menorrhagia) and excessive blood loss from superficial cuts and abrasions.

Severe bleeding episodes are treated with factor VIII concentrates that contain both von Willebrand factor and factor VIII.

Haemophilia A (factor VIII deficiency)

A common hereditary disorder of blood coagulation. It is characterized by the absence or low levels of plasma factor VIII.

Inheritance is X-linked but 33% of patients have no family history and the disorder presumably results from spontaneous mutation.

Blood clotting time is prolonged and, in severe disease, the blood is incoagulable. Bleeding into muscles, joints, retroperitoneal tissue, the urinary tract and epistaxis may occur. Operative and posttraumatic haemorrhage is life threatening, both in severely and mildly affected patients.

Mild, moderate and severe forms of the disease are recognized, depending on the residual clotting factor activity. Haemophilia A 'breeds true' in that the same severity of disease is seen in all affected members of a family.

Haemophilia B (factor IX deficiency/Christmas disease)

Inheritance, clinical features and treatment principles of factor IX deficiency are identical to those of haemophilia A. However, factor IX deficiency is less common, the incidence being only about one-fifth of that of haemophilia A.

The features of the most common hereditary clotting factor deficiencies are summarized in Table 17.23 and Fig. 17.12.

Acquired factor abnormalities

Acquired disorders of coagulation are far more common than the inherited disorders, and multiple clotting factor deficiencies are usual.

Table 17.23 Common hereditary clotting factor abnormalities

	Haemophilia A	Haemophilia B	Von Willebrand disease
Deficiency	Factor VIII	Factor IX	Von Willebrand factor→ factor VIII deficiency
Inheritance	X-linked	X-linked	Dominant
Prevalence in the UK	1 in 10,000	1 in 50,000	1 in 5000
Main sites of haemorrhage	Muscle, joints: after trauma or postsurgical	Muscle, joints: after trauma or postsurgical	Mucous membranes: after trauma and postsurgical

Vitamin K deficiency

Vitamin K is essential for γ-carboxylation and hence activation of factors II, VII, IX and X, as well as proteins C and S (inhibitors). The deficiency is associated with decreased activity of these proteins, leading to coagulopathies. This may present in the neonatal period or in later life.

Vitamin K is obtained from green vegetables and bacterial synthesis in the gut. It is a fat-soluble vitamin and requires bile for its absorption.

Causes of vitamin K deficiency:

- inadequate diet
- malabsorption—e.g., obstructive jaundice (reduced bile), coeliac disease
- drugs—warfarin (a vitamin K antagonist).

In emergency life-threatening bleeds, vitamin K and prothrombin complex concentrates are used.

Neonates are particularly susceptible to vitamin K deficiency because of their lack of gut bacteria and low concentrations of the vitamin in breast milk. Vitamin K can be prophylactically supplemented at birth.

Liver disease

This is commonly associated with coagulation defects owing to:

- impaired absorption of vitamin K caused by biliary obstruction, producing decreased activation of vitamin K-dependent factors (II, VII, IX and X, proteins C and S)
- reduced synthesis of clotting factors and fibrinogen
- increased amounts of plasminogen activator in severe hepatocellular disease and cirrhosis
- thrombocytopenia from hypersplenism associated with portal hypertension
- dysfibrinogenemia: functional abnormality of fibrinogen found in many patients with liver disease
- qualitative platelet disorders.

Disseminated intravascular coagulation

DIC is characterized by increased coagulation, which leads not only to widespread thrombosis but also to haemorrhage owing to consumption of platelets and coagulation factors. Thus (paradoxically) both thrombosis and haemorrhage are features of this disorder.

The disorder may cause a severe haemorrhagic syndrome with high mortality or may run a milder, more chronic course.

Aetiology—this is shown in Table 17.24.

Pathogenesis—the causes listed in Table 17.24 activate the coagulation system in small vessels throughout the body via:

- release of procoagulant material into the circulation
- widespread endothelial damage and platelet aggregation (some bacteria, viruses and immune complexes may have a direct effect on platelets).

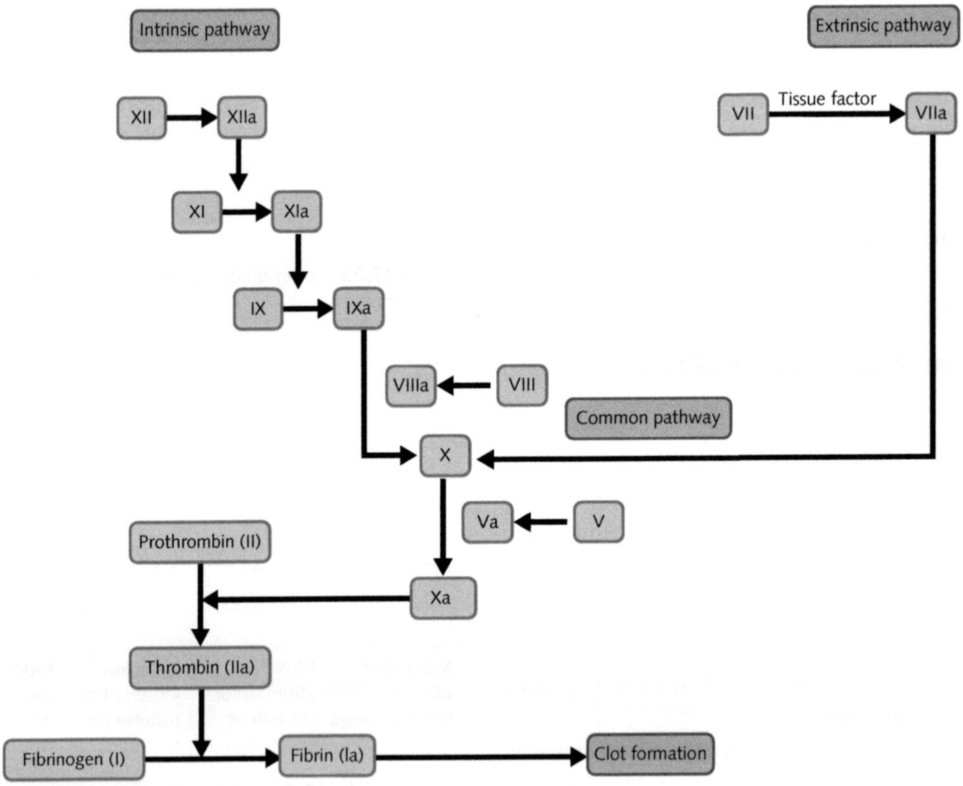

Fig. 17.12 Clotting cascade.

Table 17.24 Causes of disseminated intravascular coagulation

Causes	Examples
Infections	Septicaemia, viral infections (purpura fulminans), malaria
Malignancy	Carcinomas of pancreas, lung and prostate Acute promyelocytic leukaemia
Obstetric complications	Amniotic fluid embolism, placental abruption, retained dead fetus
Hypersensitivity reactions	Anaphylaxis, incompatible blood transfusion
Widespread tissue damage	Burns, major accidental trauma, major surgery, shock, intravascular haemolysis, dissecting aortic aneurysm
Liver disease	Various causes

The main effects of DIC are:

- thrombosis—ischaemic organ damage
- microangiopathic haemolysis
- haemorrhage—consumption of platelets, clotting factors and fibrinogen.

HINTS AND TIPS

DIC, THROMBOSIS AND HAEMORRHAGE

- Disseminated intravascular coagulation (DIC) is a very important condition.
- Remember that it causes both thrombosis and haemorrhage. It may be triggered by a wide variety of conditions (Table 17.24) and can be rapidly fatal if not recognized quickly.

Activation of fibrinolytic system results in increased fibrin degradation products (e.g., D-dimer, which is measurable). These products may themselves have anticoagulant effects causing further haemorrhage.

Treatment is of the underlying cause, with clotting factor and platelet replacement.

Thrombosis

Thrombosis can affect both arteries and veins and is considered in detail in Chapter 9.

PORPHYRIA

Porphyria comprises a group of seven rare metabolic disorders related to enzyme deficiencies in the haem biosynthetic pathway (Table 17.25). There is an accumulation of toxic porphyrin precursor products (aminolevulinic acid and porphobilinogen) that precipitate acute neurovisceral attacks (acute porphyria) or cutaneous disease (cutaneous porphyria).

Within the UK, acute intermittent porphyria (AIP) is the commonest and most severe type of porphyria, whereas porphyria cutanea tarda (PCT) is the commonest worldwide. Presentation is usually between 20 and 40 years of age and symptoms are dependent on the type of porphyria, i.e., acute versus cutaneous:

Acute (neurovisceral) symptoms: attacks of severe abdominal or back pain, muscle pain, paraesthesia, numbness, dark reddish-purple urine, hallucinations, seizures, tachycardia, hypertension and absent reflexes.

Cutaneous symptoms: photosensitivity causing pruritus, swelling, pigmentation, hypertrichosis, vesicular/bullous eruptions with scarring and dark reddish-purple urine.

Pathophysiology: Eighty-five percent of haem is synthesized within red blood cells, the remainder within the liver; therefore, the principal sites of enzyme deficiency can be erythroid or hepatic. The types of

Table 17.25 Types of porphyria

Type of porphyria	Inheritance	Enzyme deficiency
Neurovisceral		
Porphyria cutanea tarda	Autosomal dominant	Uroporphyrinogen III decarboxylase
Congenital erythropoietic porphyria	Autosomal recessive	Uroporphyrinogen III synthase
Erythropoietic porphyria	Autosomal dominant	Ferrochelatase
Cutaneous porphyria		
Acute intermittent porphyria	Autosomal dominant	Hydroxymethylbilane synthase
ALA dehydratase deficiency	Autosomal recessive	ALA dehydratase
Neurovisceral and cutaneous		
Variegate porphyria	Autosomal dominant	Protoporphyrinogen
Hereditary coproporphyria	Autosomal dominant	Coprophyrinogen oxidase

ALA, δ-aminolevulinic acid.

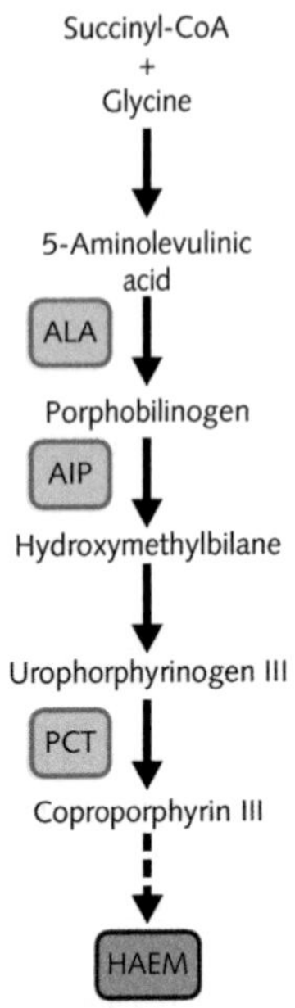

Fig. 17.13 Simplified haem biosynthetic pathway. Simplified biosynthetic pathway of haem showing the enzymatic defects of the major types of porphyria. Eighty-five percent of haem is synthesized within red blood cells, the remainder within the liver. *AIP,* Acute intermittent porphyria; *ALA,* δ-aminolevulinic acid dehydratase deficiency; *PCT,* porphyria cutanea tarda.

porphyria arise due to defects in different enzymes along the haem synthetic pathway (Fig. 17.13).

Porphyria cutanea tarda

This is the most common type of porphyria, with cutaneous symptoms of vesicular and bullous eruptions on sun-exposed skin, skin fragility and milia. Most patients will have underling hepatic damage secondary to uroporphyrinogen III decarboxylase deficiency in the liver causing iron overload. There is an associated increased risk of hepatocellular carcinoma.

There are two types of PCT:

Type 1: sporadic (80%)—precipitated by excess alcohol, oestrogens, iron overload (any cause) and viral hepatitis, which drive increased porphyrin production in the liver.

Type 2: familial (20%)—autosomal dominant with low penetrance.

Acute intermittent porphyria

AIP is an autosomal dominant neurovisceral porphyria with no cutaneous involvement. The most common symptoms are abdominal pain, vomiting and constipation with motor polyneuropathy, possible depression and psychosis. It is caused by deficiency in hydroxymethylbilane synthase. Attacks are precipitated by fat-soluble drugs, e.g., barbiturates, steroids, anticonvulsants, alcohol and physiological stress.

Chapter Summary

- Antiphospholipid syndrome is associated with recurrent miscarriages.
- ANA is positive in systemic lupus erythematosus, Sjögren syndrome, dermato/polymyositis and scleroderma.
- Rheumatoid factor is positive in rheumatoid arthritis, Sjögren syndrome, primary biliary cholangitis and mixed essential cryoglobulinemia.
- ANCA is useful in the diagnosis of vasculitides.
- Scleroderma is a generic term for a group of diseases with different presentations and prognosis. It can be limited or systemic.
- Porphyria is a group of disorders caused by enzymatic defects in the haem synthetic pathway.
- Immunodeficiencies can be primary or secondary, and involve T cells, B cells or both, as well as defects in the innate immune system.
- Recurrent infections, persistent, unusual sites, unusual organisms, resistance to usual antibiotics should raise the possibility of a primary immunodeficiency.
- 'Amyloid' is an umbrella term that refers to aggregations of normal proteins transformed into insoluble fibrils that cannot be degraded by macrophages and that accumulate within tissues.
- Anaemia is a total reduction in the circulating red cell mass with reduced oxygen-carrying capacity of the blood. It can be classified into micro-, normo- or macrocytic anaemia.
- Classical Hodgkin lymphoma has a bimodal age distribution and often presents as unilateral neck lymphadenopathy.
- Non-Hodgkin lymphomas are subdivided into low-grade and high-grade lymphomas; low-grade lymphomas can transform into high-grade forms.

- Acute leukaemias are more common and have better prognoses in children.
- Plasma cell dyscrasias are a spectrum of diseases with monoclonal plasma cell proliferations.
- Determining location of a mass within the mediastinum is useful in forming differential diagnoses at this site.
- Warfarin and liver dysfunction are common causes of coagulation defects of the vitamin K-dependent factors (II, VII, IX and X and proteins C and S).
- Disseminated intravascular coagulation causes both haemorrhage and thrombosis.

Pathology of the skin 18

NORMAL SKIN

The skin is the largest organ in the body. It is composed of three layers—epidermis, dermis and subcutis—which are further subdivided histologically (Figs 18.1 and 18.2). Understanding the distribution and features of skin lesions, in combination with clinical presentation, aids in the diagnosis of skin conditions.

TERMINOLOGY OF SKIN PATHOLOGY

Macroscopic appearances

Macule

This localised (<1 cm), flat area of discoloration can be hyperpigmented, e.g., a freckle, hypopigmented, e.g., vitiligo, or erythematous, e.g., a capillary haemangioma.

Papule

This is a small, raised, solid lesion of the skin, <1 cm in diameter.

Nodule

This is similar to a papule but >1 cm in diameter. It is solid and can involve any layer of the skin.

Patch

A patch is a flat lesion like a macule, but >1 cm.

Plaque

A plaque is a >1 cm raised lesion that forms a plateau-like elevation of skin.

Wheal

This is similar to a papule or plaque but is transitory and compressible. It is caused by dermal oedema, is red or white in colour and usually signifies urticaria.

Blister

This fluid-filled space within the skin is caused by the separation of cells and the leakage of plasma into the space. This term encompasses vesicles and bulla.

Vesicle

This small blister (<5 mm in diameter) contains clear fluid within or below the epidermis.

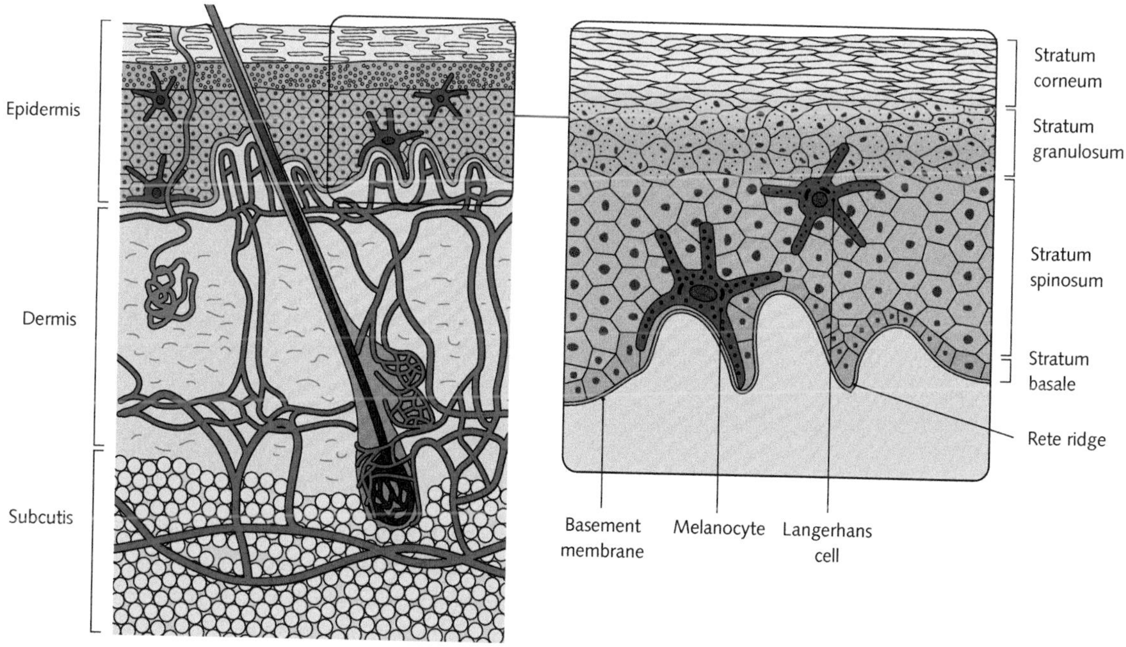

Fig. 18.1 Normal skin and epidermis.

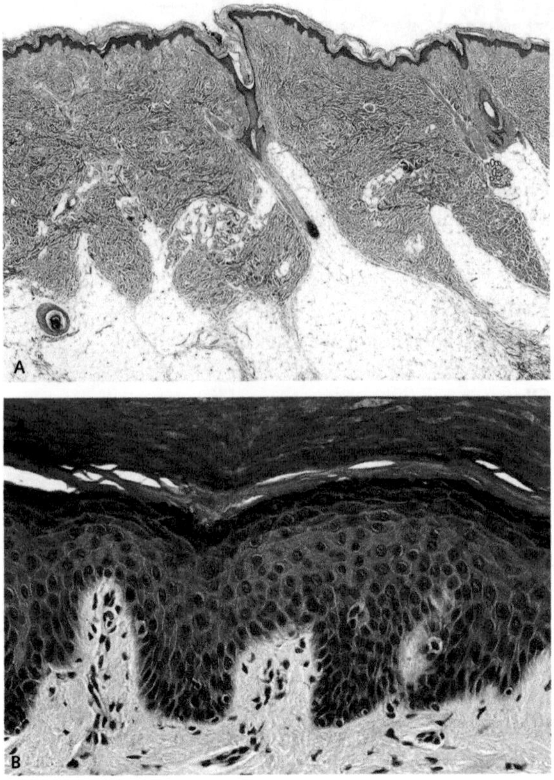

Fig. 18.2 **Histology of normal skin.** (A) Microscopic appearance of the skin. (B) Microscopic appearance of the epidermis. (From: The structure and function of skin. McKee's Pathology of the Skin. McGrath, JA. Published January 1, 2012. Pages 1-31. © 2012. Fig. 1.1 and 1.2)

Bulla

This is similar to a vesicle but >5 mm in diameter.

Pustule

This is a small (<1 cm), pus-containing blister, commonly indicating infection.

Scale

Scaling is excess keratin accumulation, usually indicating inflammation of the epidermis.

Lichenification

There is a thickening of the epidermis with exaggeration of the normal skin creases caused by scratching or rubbing of skin.

Excoriation

This is caused by the destruction or removal of the surface of the skin, usually by scratching, but also by chemical application or other traumatic means.

Onycholysis

This is the separation of part or all of a nail from its bed. It may occur in psoriasis and in fungal infections of the skin and nail bed, and is more common in women.

Microscopic definitions

Hyperkeratosis

Hyperkeratosis is thickening of the outer horny layer of the skin (stratum corneum).

Acanthosis

This diffuse thickening of the epidermis is caused by an increased number of cells in the strata spinosum and basale (prickle and basal layers).

Dyskeratosis

With dyskeratosis, there are abnormal immature cells in the strata spinosum and basale.

Acantholysis

This refers to the loss of cellular cohesion and separation of epidermal keratinocytes caused by the rupture of intercellular bridges. Bulla formation often results.

Vacuolization

This is the formation of intracellular, fluid-filled spaces (vacuoles).

Papilloma

This is a benign lesion in which hyperplastic epidermis forms frond-like lesions with central fibrovascular cores.

Lentiginous

This describes skin where there is linear proliferation of cells along the basal layer.

Erosion

This is the loss of part of the epidermis. It does not extend into the dermis and it heals without scarring.

Ulceration

Ulceration is a full-thickness defect of the epidermis; sometimes there is also loss of the dermis.

HINTS AND TIPS

VOCABULARY OF DERMATOLOGY

The vocabulary of dermatology is quite distinct from that of other specialities.
Learning the common dermatological terms is essential to correctly describe different skin disorders.

INFLAMMATION AND SKIN ERUPTIONS

Psoriasis

Definition

Psoriasis is a chronic, noninfectious, waxing and waning inflammatory disease of the skin characterized by erythematous plaques covered with thick, silvery scales (Fig. 18.3).

It affects about 2% of the population in the United Kingdom and it can start at any age, but the peak onset is in the second and third decades of life.

The aetiology of psoriasis is unclear; however, many patients show a family history. It is associated with HLA haplotypes Cw6, B13 and B17.

Environmental factors are thought to trigger the disease in genetically susceptible individuals.

Pathogenesis:

- Hyperproliferation of normal keratinocytes.
- Increased skin turnover, resulting in absent granular layer—accumulation of abnormal keratin results in a scale.

Histological features:

- Uniform elongation of the rete ridges separated by papillary dermis in which there are large numbers of dilated capillaries.
- Scale—composed of flakes of thickened surface keratin, which contain remnants of nuclei (parakeratosis).
- Neutrophil polymorphs that migrate through the epidermis and may be trapped beneath the thickened horny layer forming small aggregates (Munro microabscesses).

Precipitating factors: a number of factors have been identified that can precipitate psoriasis:

- Köebner phenomenon: lesions at sites of trauma.
- Infection: β-haemolytic streptococcal throat infection may precipitate guttate psoriasis.
- Drugs: β-blockers, lithium and antimalarials can precipitate or worsen psoriasis.

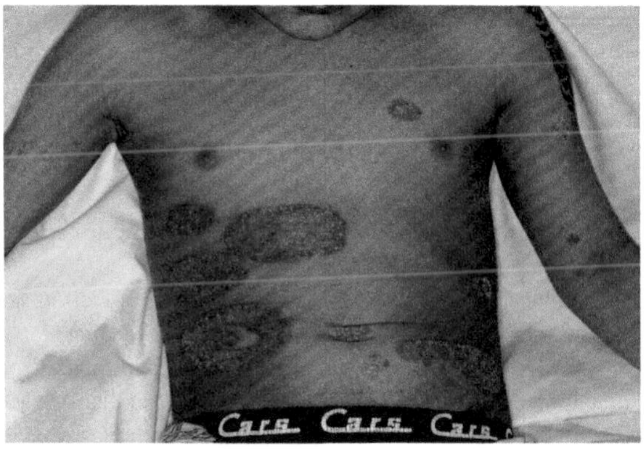

Fig. 18.3 Psoriasis.

Table 18.1 Types of psoriasis

Type	Features
Plaque	Most common type. Disc shaped, erythematous plaques covered with white silvery scale.
Guttate	Symmetrical 'drop-like' lesions. May be associated with streptococcal infection in the young.
Flexural	Smooth erythematous plaques, often glazed.
Localized	Scalp, palmoplantar pustulosis, napkin (nappy area in infants) and acrodermatitis of Hallopeau (nails) types.
Generalized	Rare, but potentially life threatening.

Psoriasis most commonly affects the extensor surfaces of the knees and elbows, the trunk and the scalp. Nail involvement is frequent and may present as a salmon patch on the nail bed, under the nail. Nail pitting and subungual hyperkeratosis may be followed by onycholysis.

Several types of psoriasis exist, which are of variable appearance and behaviour (Table 18.1).

Many types of arthropathies can occur in psoriasis. These are discussed in detail in Chapter 16.

Eczema and dermatitis

Definitions

Eczema and dermatitis are synonymous terms for noninfective inflammatory conditions of the skin. They are not diseases but reactive conditions occurring in response to certain stimuli, many of which are unknown. They can be acute or chronic.

Acute and chronic forms

Acute eczema/dermatitis

Acute eczema/dermatitis is characterized by:

- erythema—caused by an inflammatory cell infiltrate (lymphocytes) around dilated vessels in the upper dermis
- fluid-filled vesicles—caused by epidermal oedema with separation of keratinocytes (known as spongiosis)
- lesions—these are itchy (histamine release), erythematous and vesicles may weep and crust.

Chronic eczema/dermatitis

Prolonged scratching of the itchy, acute-stage lesions causes secondary changes, which result in the chronic form of the condition. It is characterized by:

- thickening of the prickle cell layer (acanthosis)
- thickening of the stratum corneum (hyperkeratosis)
- elongation of the rete ridges and dermal collagenization

- dilation of dermal vessels and infiltration of the dermis with inflammatory cells.

Characteristic thickening, which occurs as a result of scratching, is termed lichenification.

> **HINTS AND TIPS**
>
> **DERMATITIS VERSUS ECZEMA**
>
> The terms 'dermatitis' and 'eczema' essentially describe the same reactive condition, i.e., they are histopathologically identical. Although the terms are often used interchangeably, eczema is sometimes used to describe the reaction that occurs in response to an endogenous stimulus, whereas dermatitis is used to describe the reaction that occurs in response to an exogenous stimulus.

Atopic eczema

This chronic form of eczema is often associated with a strong family history of other atopic diseases such as asthma and hay fever. Although 10%–15% of the population are atopic, only about 5% of these individuals will develop atopic eczema. The condition follows a relapsing/remitting course. It is more common in children than in adults.

> **HINTS AND TIPS**
>
> **ATOPIC TRIAD**
>
> The atopic triad comprises: eczema (atopic dermatitis), allergic rhinitis (hay fever) and asthma. Patients with one are likely to have the others.

The aetiology of atopic eczema and other atopic diseases is not well understood. However, there is a genetic predisposition.

Pathogenesis:

- Individuals prone to atopy have higher circulating levels of immunoglobulin E (IgE) antibodies than nonatopic individuals.
- On exposure to certain allergens, IgE-mediated, type 1 hypersensitivity reactions are triggered, causing mast cell degranulation with the release of histamine and other inflammatory mediators. Uncontrollable itching is common.
- In the skin, this type of hypersensitivity reaction results in the histological changes of acute eczema, which on scratching becomes chronic eczema.

Atopic eczema presents at an early age, with 85% presenting before 1 year and 95% by 5 years.

The appearance of atopic eczema varies between different age groups:

- Infancy—babies develop the typical acute form of eczema on the face and hands, often with secondary infection.
- Childhood—progression from acute to chronic condition. Usually involves flexural areas such as the antecubital and popliteal fossae, neck, wrists and ankles
- Adults—chronic condition with lichenified (and sometimes nodular) lesions. The hands are most commonly affected but a few adults also develop the chronic, severe form of generalized atopic eczema, which is often precipitated by stressful situations.

The complications of eczema are:

- bacterial infection—typically with *Staphylococcus aureus*.
- viral infection—increased susceptibility to the development of viral warts, molluscum contagiosum and widespread eruption following secondary infection with herpes simplex (eczema herpeticum).
- sleep disturbance (itchiness)—potentially causing behavioural or developmental difficulties.

Contact dermatitis

Contact dermatitis is a form of dermatitis precipitated by exogenous agents. It can be classified into:

- irritant contact dermatitis—the most common form. Caused by contact of the skin with abrasives, acids, alkalis, solvents or detergents
- allergic contact dermatitis—caused by a type 4 (delayed-type) hypersensitivity reaction to allergens such as nickel (e.g., under a watch, earrings).

Lesions are localized to the site of contact, and they are most common on the hands and face.

Other forms

Seborrhoeic dermatitis

This is a common, chronic inflammatory condition in which the skin is reddened and covered by a thick, waxy or white scale. The eruption often occurs in the sebaceous gland areas of the scalp and face, although other regions may also be involved.

The aetiology is unknown but genetic factors and overgrowth of the commensal yeast *Pityrosporum ovale* (*Malasezzia furfur*) have been implicated.

There are two main types:

1. Infantile type: usually involves the scalp ('cradle cap') or groin ('napkin rash').
2. Adult type: may involve the scalp and face (affecting the sides of the nose, scalp margin, eyebrows and ears), the back (erythematous follicular eruption with papules or pustules) or flexural sites (e.g., axillae, groin and submammary areas) and are often secondarily colonized by *Candida albicans*.

Discoid eczema

A condition of unknown aetiology, this is characterized by 'coin-shaped', symmetrical, eczematous lesions, which typically affect the limbs of elderly men, and young men who drink alcohol excessively. Secondary bacterial infection is common.

Asteatotic eczema (eczema craquelé; winter eczema)

This dry eczema with cracking of the skin appears as a fine, 'crazy-paving' pattern of fissuring, commonly affecting the limbs and trunk of the elderly. Causes are excessive washing of patients in institutions, a dry winter climate, hypothyroidism and the use of diuretics.

Stasis dermatitis

This is erythematous, scaly and dry skin secondary to chronic venous stasis, usually seen on the legs.

Lichen planus

Lichen planus is a papular rash affecting flexural sites, mucous membranes and the glans penis; it is self-limiting, though may last years. It may exhibit the Köebner phenomenon (lesions occurring at sites of trauma).

CLINICAL NOTES

KÖEBNER PHENOMENON

Köebner phenomenon is the occurrence of lesions within areas of cutaneous trauma, e.g., bites, lacerations, burns. The lesions follow the route of injury. Conditions which classically display this phenomenon include:

- Psoriasis
- Lichen planus
- Vitiligo

BLISTERING DISORDERS

Bullae are large blisters within the skin caused by the separation of two tissue layers and the leakage of plasma into the space. The contents of bullae vary and may include inflammatory cells, fibrin and blood, which are important diagnostically. There are many causes of blisters and bullae apart from primary skin disorders, e.g., skin infections, drug reactions and insect bites.

Blistering skin conditions can be grouped according to the level within the skin that the tissue split occurs (Fig. 18.4).

Pemphigus

This rare but potentially fatal group of autoimmune disorders is marked by successive outbreaks of blisters on the skin and mucous membranes.

Aetiopathogenesis—Immunoglobulin G (IgG) autoantibodies bind to desmoglein 3 present in desmosomes forming the intercellular junctions between keratinocytes. Binding of IgG activates complement, releasing proteolytic enzymes and resulting in loss of cellular adhesion (acantholysis) and splitting of the epidermis. Variants of pemphigus occur depending on the level of the split, the most common is pemphigus vulgaris.

Direct immunofluorescence staining is positive for IgG that is distributed around keratinocytes.

Clinical presentation—pemphigus vulgaris typically affects those 50–60 years of age and is characterized by flaccid, thin-walled, superficial blisters over the scalp, face, back, chest and flexures (Fig. 18.5). These rupture, resulting in painful erosions. Oral erosions are present in 50% of cases and are often the presenting symptom. If left untreated, the blistering is progressive and ultimately fatal. Treatment is with systemic steroids and immunosuppressive agents.

Organ-specific autoimmune disorders, e.g., myasthenia gravis, are also associated with pemphigus.

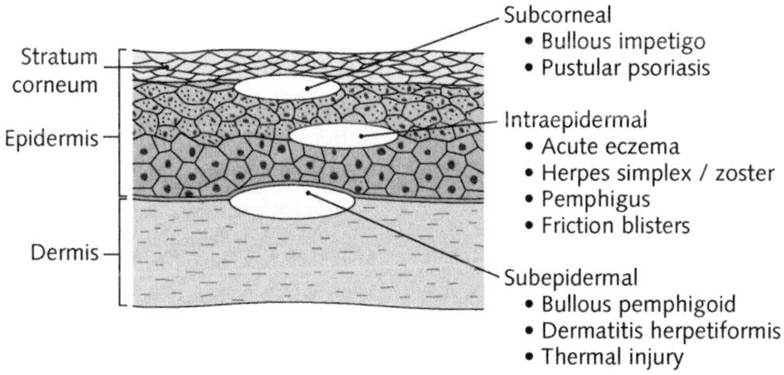

Fig. 18.4 Location of blisters within the skin. Blisters/bullae form owing to loss of cohesion between cells within the skin. They can form at different levels within the skin dependent on the disease process. Subcorneal blisters form beneath the stratum cornea, intraepidermal blisters form between the keratinocytes within the epidermis and subepidermal blisters between the basal layer of epidermis and dermis.

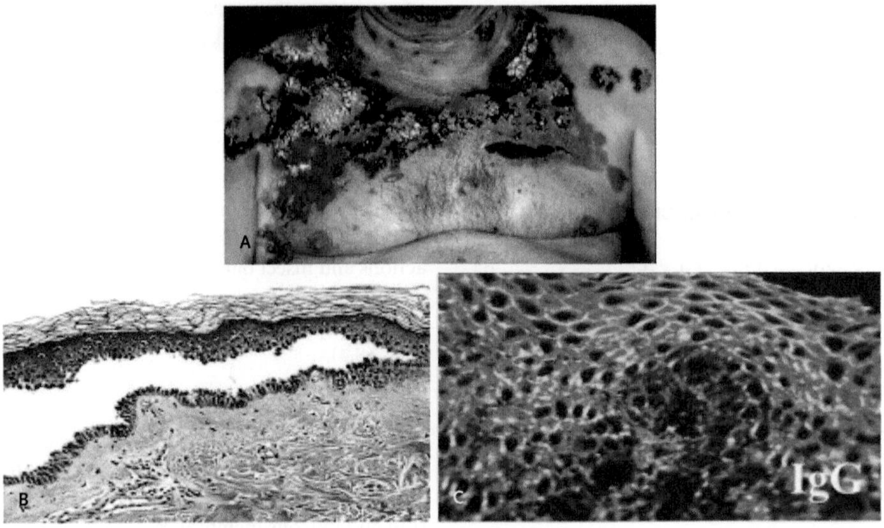

Fig. 18.5 Pemphigus vulgaris. (A) Macroscopic appearance of flaccid blisters and erosions. (B) Microscopic picture showing epidermal detachment caused by a split within the epidermis splitting, in this case suprabasal i.e., above the basal layer of keratinocytes. (C) Immunofluorescent staining showing localization of IgG around the epidermal keratinocytes.

HINTS AND TIPS

BLISTERS GO BUST

Remember:

In pemphig***US*** the blisters go b***US***t and are ***SU***perficial (i.e., intraepidermal).

In pemphigoi***D*** the blisters are ***D***eep (i.e., subepidermal).

CLINICAL NOTES

IMMUNOFLUORESCENCE

Immunofluorescent stains are used for diagnosis to detect the presence and distribution of antibodies/complement in blistering skin disorders. Unlike other histological specimens, skin biopsies must be submitted in saline for immunofluorescent analysis, *not* formalin.

Bullous pemphigoid

This is a chronic, itchy blistering disorder of the elderly.

Aetiopathogenesis—an autoimmune disorder, in which IgG with or without IgE autoantibodies to collagen XVII are deposited at the basement membrane of the epidermis.

Complement is activated and neutrophils are recruited to the site, releasing proteolytic enzymes which results in subepidermal bullae formation. The bullae contain a mix of fibrin and inflammatory cells, including large numbers of eosinophils.

Clinical presentation—large, tense, dome-shaped blisters commonly appear on the limbs, abdomen and flexures, but are occasionally localized to one site, often the lower leg. Unlike pemphigus, the bullae in pemphigoid tend to remain intact and oral lesions only occur in 10% of cases. An urticarial eruption may precede the onset of blistering (Fig. 18.6).

The disease is self-limiting in about 50% of cases.

Dermatitis herpetiformis

This is a rare symmetrical eruption of intensely itchy blisters on extensor surfaces.

Aetiopathogenesis—Greater than 90% of patients with dermatitis herpetiformis have coeliac disease (see Chapter 11). Subepidermal blisters form because of the granular deposition of immunoglobulin A (IgA) at the dermal papillae, which is directed against epidermal transglutaminase (eTG).

Clinical presentation—groups of small, intensely itchy vesicles or papules are seen on the knees, elbows, scalp, buttocks and shoulders. They may appear as crusts because of scratching. Onset is usually in the third or fourth decade of life, with males affected more often than females by a factor of 2:1.

A summary of blistering disorders is given in Table 18.2.

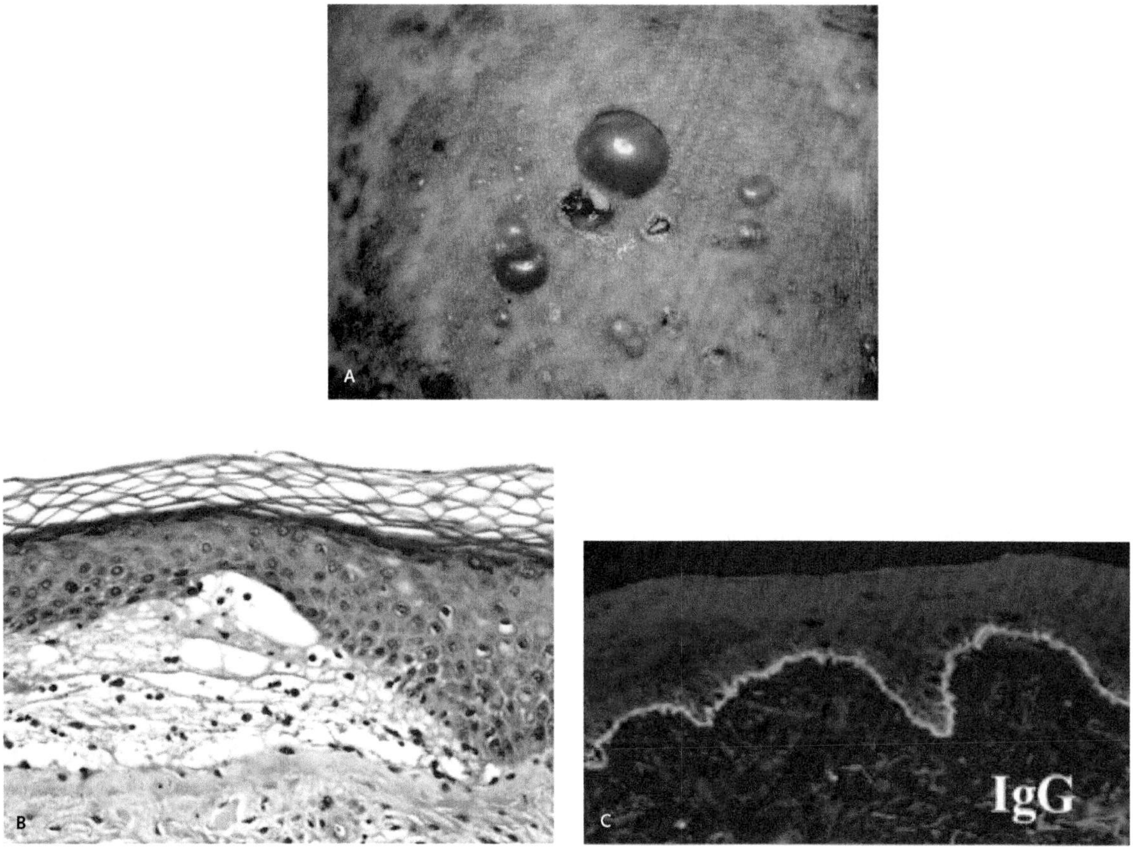

Fig. 18.6 Bullous pemphigoid. (A) Macroscopic appearance of tense, dome shaped blisters. (B) Microscopic picture showing epidermal detachment caused by subepidermal splitting of the epidermis and dermis. (C) Immunofluorescent staining showing localization of IgG to the basement membrane of the epidermis.

Table 18.2 Summary of blistering disorders

Disorder	Type of bullae	Autoimmunity	Clinical features
Pemphigus vulgaris	Intraepidermal	IgG deposited on intercellular junctions of keratinocytes	Flaccid, superficial bullae that rupture to form erosions More common in the middle-aged High mortality
Bullous pemphigoid	Subepidermal	IgG ± deposited on the basement membrane	Large, tense bullae More common in the elderly Self-limiting in about 50% of cases
Dermatitis herpetiformis	Subepidermal	IgA deposited on dermal papillae	Groups of small, itchy vesicles Usually presents in the third or fourth decade Males > females Associated with coeliac disease

Steven–Johnson syndrome/toxic epidermal necrolysis

These very rare conditions are a spectrum of severe cutaneous drug reactions. Many drugs are implicated; however, the most commonly involved are:

- antibiotics: sulphonamides, erythromycin, penicillins, ciprofloxacin
- anticonvulsants: carbamazepine, lamotrigine, phenytoin, phenobarbital
- nonsteroidal antiinflammatory drugs: oxicams, indomethacin, oxybutazone.

Patients can present within a week or up to 2 months following drug commencement. A flu-like prodrome occurs before a painful, erythematous spreading rash appears. It consists of coalescing macules with flaccid blisters evolving over hours to days. Severe skin loss results as the blisters merge causing sheets of skin to detach exposing the underlying dermis. Mucosal membranes are also involved, including the eyes, lungs and gastrointestinal (GI) system.

A high degree of morbidity and mortality is associated with these conditions, with 10%–30% dying. Death results from bacterial infection, sepsis, dehydration, multiple organ failure, acute respiratory distress syndrome or disseminated intravascular coagulation.

INFECTIONS AND INFESTATIONS

Bacterial infections

Normal skin microflora

The skin is colonized by numerous microorganisms known as microflora or the microbiome. The majority are Gram positive bacteria which colonize the superficial layers of the dermis and hair follicles. Examples include:

- *Staphylococcus epidermidis*
- *Micrococcus*
- *Corynebacterium*
- *Propionibacterium*
- *Bacteroides*
- *Pseudomonas aeruginosa*
- *Malasezzia*
- *Candida.*

Microflora are an important defence against disease as they prevent colonization by pathogens, deprive pathogens of nutrients and help to stimulate the immune system.

Staphylococcal infections

Impetigo

This highly contagious superficial skin infection is caused by either *S. aureus* or *S. pyogenes*, or both. It typically affects children and there is a predilection for the face and hands; however, it may occur anywhere on the body.

It may be bullous or nonbullous and is characterized by areas of yellow 'honey-coloured' crusted exudate which arise from vesicles or bullae. Satellite lesions of impetigo occur caused by autoinfection from the primary site. Impetigo can form punched-out full-thickness ulcers (ecthyma) that scar on healing; *Streptococcus pyogenes* is the causative agent.

Common differential diagnoses are herpes simplex or fungal infections.

Folliculitis

This is inflammation of hair follicles, which can be caused by infection *(S. aureus)*, irritation from regrowing hairs (e.g., after shaving), drugs or inflammatory skin disorders such as lichen planus.

Clinically, folliculitis is characterized by the production of tiny pustules located in the necks of hair follicles (superficial folliculitis). The inflammation can also occur deep within the follicle.

A furuncle (boil) is when there is deep infection of the follicle by *S. aureus*. An inflammatory nodule develops containing an expanding collection of pus that destroys the follicle and extends into the surrounding dermis.

A carbuncle is a deep infection of a group of adjacent follicles by *S. aureus*. The result is a painful suppurating mass that has multiple drainage channels.

Staphylococcal scalded skin syndrome

This acute toxic illness, usually of infants and children younger than 5 years old, is characterized by the shedding of sheets of skin following a widespread, confluent blistering rash. It is accompanied by fever and irritability. The denuded erythematous areas that result resemble 'scalded skin' and are treated as if they were burns.

It is caused by potent exotoxins (epidermolytic toxin A and B) produced by a specific strain of *S. aureus* and it may follow impetigo. The exotoxins disrupt the epidermis at the granular cell layer.

Streptococcal infections

Cellulitis

This is an infection of deep dermis and subcutaneous tissues, caused mostly by streptococci. It may be primary or complicate a wound or other skin condition. Limbs are usually affected and the distribution is unilateral.

The appearance of cellulitis is preceded by systemic flu-like symptoms of fever and rigours. The affected limb then appears red, warm, swollen, tender and painful. Blistering, ulceration and abscess formation may also occur.

> **COMMON PITFALLS**
>
> **BILATERAL CELLULITIS**
>
> 'Bilateral cellulitis' is a diagnosis often made but seldom correct. Cellulitis is usually unilateral. Conditions which mimic cellulitis include chronic lipodermatosclerosis, stasis dermatitis and lymphoedema. The commonest scenario is that of an elderly/debilitated person, with or without comorbidities,(e.g., heart failure or diabetes), who has stasis/venous dermatitis. A helpful tip is to enquire as to whether the appearance of their legs has changed recently.

Erysipelas

This is a superficial cellulitis caused by *S. pyogenes*. The presentation is as an acute, erythematous, well-demarcated lesion that is often oedematous and tender. It usually affects the face or the lower leg.

Mycobacterial infections

Cutaneous tuberculosis

Cutaneous extrapulmonary tuberculosis (TB) is an uncommon form of TB, but it is occasionally seen in the elderly and in recent immigrants from endemic TB areas.

Cutaneous manifestations of TB include:

- **Lupus vulgaris**—a slowly progressive chronic skin lesion characterized by well-demarcated reddish-brown plaques. It usually occurs following reactivation of preexisting disease, typically affecting the head and neck. If untreated it leads to scarring. It is the most common form of cutaneous TB.
- **Scrofuloderma**—cutaneous involvement from direct spread from an underlying focus, usually a lymph node (commonly cervical). Fistulae and scarring may occur.
- **Tuberculosis verrucosa cutis**—inoculation of the skin in an individual with immunity from a previous infection results in a warty plaque. Typically, it affects the hands, knees or buttocks and is the most common form of cutaneous TB in developing countries.

All types of cutaneous TB are characterized by giant cell, necrotizing granulomatous inflammation in the dermis leading to the destruction of dermal collagen and skin appendages. Scarring is common and sometimes destruction of deeper tissues such as cartilage occurs.

> COMMON PITFALLS
>
> LUPUS VULGARIS, LUPUS PERNIO
>
> Be aware! These conditions have nothing to do with systemic lupus erythematosus:
>
> - **Lupus pernio**: this is cutaneous sarcoidosis
> - **Lupus vulgaris**: this is progressive and persistent cutaneous tuberculosis.

Leprosy (Hansen disease)

This is a chronic granulomatous disease caused by *Mycobacterium leprae. M. leprae* is an obligate intracellular organism preferring temperatures of <37°C. It preferentially infects the skin, nerves and mucous membranes, especially the nasal mucosa.

Leprosy is rare in the United Kingdom but is common in Africa (Democratic Republic of Congo, Nigeria), Asia (India, Bangladesh) and Brazil. The number of new cases worldwide is approximately 500,000–700,000 per year. Transmission is person to person and although the exact mechanism is unclear, it is thought to be by nasal droplet inhalation. Leprosy has a low infectivity so prolonged close contact (months) with a person with untreated leprosy is required to contract it, i.e., you cannot catch leprosy from shaking hands!

The clinicopathological features of leprosy depend on the degree of cell-mediated immunity instigated by the host against the infection. This varies on a spectrum from strong (tuberculoid leprosy) to weak (lepromatous leprosy). Incubation times vary from months to years and disease progression is extremely slow (decades) with affected people dying with, rather than from, the disease.

Tuberculoid form: There is a vigorous T cell-mediated response to the organism, resulting in well-formed nonnecrotizing granulomas containing minimal bacteria (paucibacillary). Lesions are focal.

Lepromatous form: There is a minimal or absent immune response to the organism resulting in numerous bacteria (multibacillary). Skin lesions are diffuse with or without organ involvement.

Clinical presentation—Table 18.3 outlines the clinical features of lepromatous and tuberculoid forms of leprosy. Intermediate forms on this spectrum are also seen, e.g., where the lesions are tuberculoid in form but numerous.

Spirochaetal infections

Spirochaetes are Gram-negative slender, corkscrew-shaped bacteria with double membranes. Three genera are pathogenic to humans: *Treponema*, *Borrelia* and *Leptospira*. They cannot be cultured and require silver stains (e.g., Warthin–Starry) to be visualized, as they are too small to be identified by Gram staining.

Syphilis

Syphilis is a chronic infectious venereal disease caused by the spirochaete *Treponema pallidum*, which is usually transmitted by sexual intercourse (Chapter 5). There are three clinical stages, with skin manifestations present during the secondary stage.

Clinical features of secondary syphilis:

- Presentation is ~4–12 weeks after the onset of the primary chancre (primary syphilis). The spirochaetes spread and proliferate within the skin and mucous membranes.
- Nonitchy, nonpainful red or copper-coloured papular/macular eruption on the trunk, palms and soles of the feet.
- Often accompanied by lymphadenopathy, general malaise and weight loss.
- Greyish-white warty papules (condylomata lata) in moist areas, e.g., the anogenital area, axilla, under the breasts and inner thighs.
- Mucosal patches appearing raw and red, e.g., mouth and genital area.

Untreated, the eruption resolves in 1–3 months; however, a third of untreated patients progress to tertiary syphilis after ~5 years.

Lyme disease

Also known as borelliosis, this cutaneous and systemic infection is caused by the spirochaete *Borrelia burgdorferi* and spread by *Ixodes* ticks from deer and wild animals. The

Table 18.3 Presentation of lepromatous and tuberculoid leprosy

	Tuberculoid leprosy	Lepromatous leprosy
Bacteraemia	Bacteraemia rare	Bacteraemia with spread to peripheral sites
Number of skin lesions	One or a few (1–5)	Multiple skin lesions (>5) with extensive cutaneous involvement
Symmetry	Asymmetrical	Symmetrical
Distribution	Often affects the face, buttocks, extensor surfaces	Typically involves arms, legs, buttocks, face, ears, wrists, elbows and knees
Type of skin lesion	Single, raised, red patch with elevated borders or a hypopigmented spot Sensation is impaired within the plaque.	Variety of lesions: macules, papules, plaques and nodules Poorly defined, raised, red and indurated centres Sensation may be lost
Peripheral nerves	Palpable thickened nerves supply the lesion and may be painful	Nerves palpable but degree not as severe as tuberculoid form Remain functional early on in disease so sensation is maintained
Disfigurement	Progression is slow; combined effect of extensive destruction of tissue by immune response and repeated trauma to desensitized areas results in severe disfigurement, especially to hands and feet	Progression causes a thickened, furrowed appearance of face (leonine facies) with eyebrow loss, earlobe thickening, teeth loss Reabsorption of digits owing to sensory loss and repeated trauma
Other organs	Not a feature	Testes—sterility because of atrophy Gynaecomastia Eyes—corneal ulcers, photophobia Nose—saddle deformity owing to collapse of nasal bridge, nasal congestion, epistaxis Larynx—hoarse voice

initial infection is characterized by *erythema chronicum migrans*, which is a targetoid rash centred on the tick bite that slowly extends outwards as the spirochaetes spread within the dermis (Fig. 18.7). This may be accompanied by intermittent systemic symptoms, e.g., fever and lymphadenopathy. For further discussion see Chapter 7.

Other bacterial infections

Anthrax

This rare infection, caused by *Bacillus anthracis*, is associated with farm animals, particularly cattle. It can cause cutaneous, intestinal or pulmonary disease depending on the route of entry. There is no human-to-human spread.

Cutaneous form: Infection is via a break in the skin and direct inoculation of the bacteria. Those at risk include taxidermists, vets and farmers. After inoculation, a boil forms which enlarges and ulcerates over 7–10 days to form a black eschar that heals with scarring. If treated, the mortality risk is ~1%.

Intestinal disease: Infection is via the ingestion of contaminated meat products. Symptoms develop after 2–5 days with abdominal pain, nausea, vomiting and haemateme-

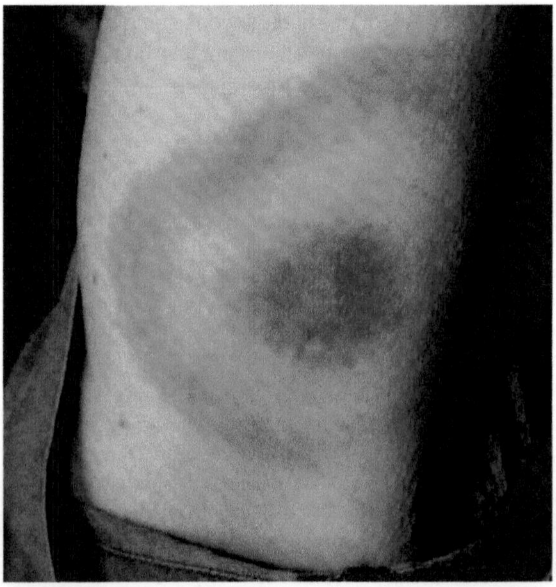

Fig. 18.7 Erythema chronicum migrans. Targetoid rash with migrating erythematous border characteristic of Lyme disease.

Table 18.4 Summary of bacterial skin infections

Causative bacteria	Associated skin disease
Staphylococci	Impetigo, ecthyma, folliculitis, scalded skin syndrome
Streptococci	Erysipelas, impetigo, necrotizing fasciitis
Mycobacteria	TB (lupus vulgaris, scrofuloderma, warty TB), leprosy
Spirochaetes	Secondary syphilis, yaws/bejel/pinta, Lyme disease
Others	Anthrax, Gram-negative infections

TB, Tuberculosis.

sis. Extensive ulceration is present throughout the GI tract. Even if treated, mortality is 20%–60%.

Pulmonary disease: Infection occurs via the inhalation of spores or aerosolized material. The symptoms develop over 1–3 days with progression to high grade fever, shortness of breath, haemoptysis, chest pain and haemorrhagic mediastinitis. Mortality is nearly 100% regardless of treatment.

Table 18.4 provides a summary of bacterial skin infections.

Viral infections

Viral warts

These common, benign, hyperkeratotic, papillomatous growths on the skin are caused by infection with human papillomavirus (HPV), of which there are many strains.

The virus infects the keratinocytes in the stratum granulosum (granular layer) and produce vacuolated cells with viral inclusions.

Common warts

Firm, dome-shaped, horny papules (1–10 mm in diameter), are usually multiple. They are found mainly on the hands, but can also affect the feet, face and genitalia.

Plantar warts

Commonly known as verrucae, these occur on the soles of the feet and are often covered by callus (hyperkeratosis). Removal of the callus reveals the presence of thrombosed capillaries which appear as black dots. Continual pressure causes inward growth, which results in tenderness. They may be single, multiple or confluent (mosaic warts).

Plane warts

These are flat, skin-coloured papules usually found on the hands and face. They are usually multiple. They resist treatment but eventually resolve spontaneously.

Genital warts

These affect the genitalia and the perianal region, and certain subtypes (HPV 16 and 18) are linked to increased risk of cervical cancer (see Chapters 4 and 15).

Molluscum contagiosum

These lesions are caused by a DNA poxvirus. They appear as discrete, umbilicated pearly pink papules in groups.

Clinical presentation—mainly affects children or young adults. The most commonly affected areas are the face, neck and trunk, but it can affect the upper thighs when sexually acquired.

The virus is transmitted by contact, including sexual transmission, or on towels.

Untreated, the papules disappear in 6–9 months. Fig. 18.8

Herpes simplex

A common, acute vesicular eruption of the skin or mucous membranes, this is caused by infection with herpes simplex virus (HSV).

Pathology:

- HSV are double-stranded DNA viruses which infect fibroblasts and epithelial cells.
- There are two types: HSV1 and HSV2.
- Infection causes the formation of infectious vesicles containing viral particles.
- Latent infection follows primary infection with the virus lying dormant within the dorsal root ganglia.
- Reactivation at various intervals, which can be years later, occurs.

Clinical presentation:

1. HSV type 1—primary infection usually occurs in childhood, causing a cold sore present on or around the lips. Epithelial infection may be accompanied by fever, malaise or local lymphadenopathy and lasts for about 2 weeks
2. HSV type 2—primary infection usually occurs in adulthood and is mainly associated with genital herpes. It presents as a vesicular rash on the penis, vulva, thigh or buttock. It is sexually transmitted (see Chapter 5).

Note both HSV type 1 and 2 viruses can cause genital herpes and cold sores, depending on the site of the initial infection.

Complications:

- Secondary bacterial superinfection—usually staphylococcal.
- Eczema herpeticum—atopic eczema may be complicated by herpes simplex infection. Rarely, eczema herpeticum can be fatal.
- Herpetic keratitis—Corneal ulceration that threaten sight.
- Disseminated herpes simplex—occasionally occurs in the newborn or in immunosuppressed patients. Active HSV is transmissible from mother to child at birth and is an indication for elective caesarean section
- Chronic herpes simplex—common in HIV patients.
- Herpes encephalitis—serious complication of HSV infection.
- Erythema multiforme—immune-mediated disease characterized by erythematous lesions on the hands and feet.

Herpes zoster (shingles)

This acute, vesicular eruption occurs in a dermatomal distribution. It is caused by the reactivation of latent varicella zoster virus (VZV).

Following an attack of chickenpox, VZV becomes dormant in the dorsal root ganglion of the spinal cord. On reactivation (the causes of which are unknown), the virus migrates down the sensory nerve to affect one or more dermatomes on the skin (Fig. 18.9).

CLINICAL NOTES

CLINICAL PRESENTATION OF SHINGLES

Shingles clinical presentation:

- Densely grouped vesicles and erythema in the distribution of one dermatome.
- Usually thoracic dermatomes, except in the elderly (in whom the ophthalmic division of the trigeminal nerve is more common).
- Pain, tenderness and paraesthesia may precede vesicular eruption.
- Vesicles become pustular and form crusts, which resolve after 2–3 weeks and may leave scarring.
- Vesicular blisters contain virus, which when shed, may cause chickenpox in varicella zoster virus-naïve contacts.
- Local lymphadenopathy is common.

Complications:

- Secondary bacterial infections
- Postherpetic neuralgia—occurs in one-third of those over 60 years old, but infrequently in patients under 40 years old. Pain usually subsides within 6 months.

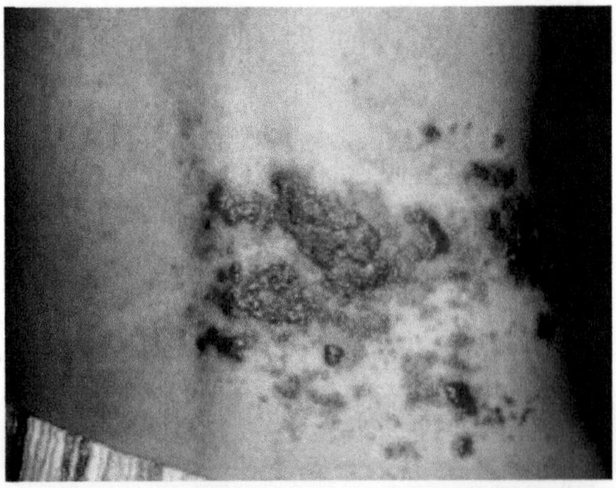

Fig. 18.9 Herpes zoster infection. A strip-like eruption of densely packed vesicles on a background of erythema. This demonstrates the dermatomal distribution of shingles.

- Ophthalmic scarring—corneal ulcers and scarring may occur following shingles of the ophthalmic division of the trigeminal nerve.
- Motor palsy—rare; viral involvement may spread from the posterior horn of the spinal cord to the anterior horn where it infects motor nerves, resulting in palsies or paralysis of individual muscles or muscle groups.
- Disseminated herpes zoster—may occur in the immunosuppressed leading to potentially fatal varicella pneumonia or encephalitis.

Superficial fungal infections

Superficial fungal infections (mycoses) affect any keratinized or external mucosal surface. Infections are caused by dermatophytes, a group of related filamentous (hyphal) fungi, or nondermatophytes which are unrelated fungi, e.g., yeasts and moulds.

Dermatophyte infections

Dermatophytes reproduce by spore formation and inhabit the keratin of the skin, hair and nails. They are collectively termed 'ringworm' but comprise three genera:

1. Microsporum
2. Trichophyton
3. Epidermophyton.

Table 18.5 outlines the common dermatophyte infections.

Yeast infections

Candida albicans

Candida albicans is a yeast-type fungus. It is a commensal organism of the vagina and alimentary canal and commonly produces opportunistic infections. Predisposing factors may be humidity, diabetes, broad-spectrum antibiotic therapy, immunodeficiency, preexisting skin conditions and extremes of age.

Clinical presentation: in infection, hyphal forms of *C. albicans* are seen, and the infection is termed candidiasis, which can present in numerous patterns.

- ***Genital:*** vulvovaginal ('thrush') where white-yellowish plaques on inflamed mucous membranes produce itching and discomfort, and sometimes a white curd-like vaginal discharge.
- ***Oral:*** adherent white plaques to the gums, tongue or inside the cheeks. They leave a sore red base on removal.
- ***Intertrigo:*** An inflammatory rash between two skin surfaces that are in contact (e.g., within the groin or under the breasts). It can be caused by or aggravated by *C. albicans* infection.

Malassezia

There are several different species of *Malassezia*, which can result in a variety of skin infections, including pityriasis versicolor, folliculitis and seborrhoeic dermatitis. Causative species include *M. furfur* and *M. globose*, amongst others.

Table 18.5 Dermatophyte infections and their clinical effects[a]

Affected area	Most common organism	Clinical presentation
Tinea corporis (trunk and limbs)	*Trichophyton verrucosum* *Microsporum canis* *Trichophyton rubrum*	Oval erythematous scaling patches with central healing over time to form a ring lesion Single or multiple lesions Itchy Usually asymmetrical
Tinea pedis (athlete's foot)	*Trichophyton rubrum* *Trichophyton interdigitale* *Epidermophyton floccosum*	Most common form of dermatophyte infection in the UK Common in young men Redness, erosion and scaling which is often interdigital, but diffuse involvement of skin also occurs
Tinea capitis (scalp/hair)	*Microsporum canis* *Trichophyton tonsurans* *Microsporum distortum*	Usually affects children Hair loss and scaling Yellow crust with matted hair Kerion
Tinea cruris (groin)	*Trichophyton rubrum* *Epidermophyton floccosum* *Trichophyton interdigitale*	Commonly affects adult men ('jock itch') Often spread from foot infection by towels Red, scaly, itchy rash with brown patches Starts on groin flexures and spreads to thighs
Tinea barbae (beard)	*Trichophyton verrucosum*	Affects beard and moustache area of adult males Inflamed and bumpy areas From contact with infected animals

[a] *Different parts of the world have slightly different causative species.*

Infestations

Insect bites and stings

These are a cutaneous inflammatory reaction to insect parts (nonvenomous) or to injected foreign substances (venomous). Common culprits include garden insects (wasps, bees, ticks), insects of household pets (fleas, mites) and bedbugs.

Bites are usually grouped on a limb and lesions vary from itchy wheals to quite large bullae, depending on the insect and the type of immune response elicited.

Secondary bacterial infection of excoriated insect bites is common.

Scabies

Scabies is caused by the burrowing of the female mite *Sarcoptes scabiei* through the stratum corneum, where she lays her eggs. After a few days, the eggs hatch into larvae, which moult and mature in the epidermis. The new mites mate, the male dies, and the fertilized female burrows into the skin and continues the cycle. Transmission is by direct skin-to-skin contact.

Clinical presentation—intensely itchy, raised lesions, often red and scaling, typically arise on the sides of fingers, palms, nipples and genitalia. The head and neck are usually spared. Itchiness is worse at night and linear tracks (burrows) ~1 cm long, are often seen within the web spaces of the fingers or wrists. The mites can be seen at the end of the burrows on dermatoscopy.

Itching causes excoriation that can result in secondary bacterial infection. Untreated, the condition becomes chronic.

CLINICAL NOTES

SKIN SCRAPING

Rapid diagnosis of fungal infections can be made with potassium hydroxide (KOH) wet mount preparations. KOH removes the associated tissues of a specimen leaving the fungal elements visible under a microscope. Uses include dermatophyte detection in hair and nails, aspergillus in sputum.

Tropical skin infections and infestations

Leishmaniasis

Leishmaniasis is caused by the protozoan *Leishmania*, which is transmitted by female sand flies. It is a common disease in the tropics and subtropics occurring as one of three forms and caused by different species of *Leishmania* (Table 18.6).

Cutaneous larva migrans

Also known as 'creeping eruption', this is a parasitic skin infection caused by the hookworm larvae of dogs or cats. The larvae burrow through the skin (most commonly the feet, toe web spaces, hands and knees), leaving intensely itchy red tracks in their wake. Humans are an accidental host and the larvae cannot complete their life cycle so die within 8 weeks.

Table 18.6 Different types of leishmaniasis[a]

Type of leishmaniasis	Endemic areas	Clinical presentation
Visceral (kala azar)	Asia, Africa and South America	Affects the spleen, liver and bone marrow, causing a pentad of fever, weight loss, hepatosplenomegaly, pancytopenia and hypergammaglobulinaemia. Increased pigmentation/darkening of the skin.
Cutaneous	Mediterranean coast, Middle East and Asia	Characterized by 'tropical sore', a red-brown nodule that appears at site of inoculation and develops over months, either ulcerating or spreading slowly to form a crusty plaque. Usually painless with variable lymphadenopathy.
Mucocutaneous	Central and South America	Characterized by a skin lesion similar to that of 'tropical sore' as parasites spread from skin to the mucous membranes. It is followed by necrotic ulcers and destruction of the midface structures including nasal septal perforation. Nose, mouth and oropharynx affected.

[a] *There are over 20 species of Leishmania that infect humans, examples include L. donovani, L. brasiliensis and L. tropica. The type of infection caused is determined by species, environmental conditions and host factors.*

Deep mycoses

These are infections of the dermis/subcutis by organisms found in the soil occurring by implantation, e.g., stepping on a thorn. They are rare in the UK and most prevalent within the tropics. Infections include:

- Mycetoma—commonly occurs on the foot (Madura foot) and is caused by several fungi including *Madurella* spp and *Actinomadura madurae*. Infection can persist for years and presents as a nodule with numerous discharging sinuses.
- Sporotrichosis—a rare disease caused by the *Sporothrix schenckii* fungus which enters the skin through a penetrating injury with contaminated/rotting plant material. Infection presents as a small enlarging pink or purple nodule on hands or fingers. It causes a suppurative chronic granulomatous skin infection and spreads via the lymphatic channels.

Onchocerciasis

This endemic disease of Africa and Central America is caused by the nematode worm *Onchocerca volvulus*, transmitted by blackfly (*Simulium* spp) bites. The adult worms cause an itchy papular eruption on the skin, which progresses to form fibrous nodules. Larvae (microfilariae) are produced by the adults inciting an intense inflammatory skin eruption upon death. Microfilariae migrate to and invade the eye, resulting in total or partial blindness (called 'river blindness' in Africa as blackflies live near rivers).

DISORDERS OF SPECIFIC SKIN STRUCTURES

Epidermis

Epidermal naevi

These are congenital lesions that are present from birth or develop in childhood. They are formed from an overgrowth of the epidermis and occur along the lines of Blashko, therefore appearing linear, and are commonly on the trunk and limbs. Initially the naevi are tan/brown macules which become thickened, warty and enlarge with time. Most are a few centimetres long but they can be extensive.

Epidermal and pilar cysts

These are benign, keratin-filled, firm, skin-coloured cysts, normally 1–3 cm in diameter.

Epidermal cysts are derived from the epidermis and pilar cysts are derived from the outer root sheath of the hair follicle. These are often incorrectly grouped together as 'sebaceous cysts'.

Seborrhoeic wart/keratosis

This common, benign tumour of basal keratinocytes typically occurs on the trunk, face and arms of the elderly and is of unknown aetiology. They are also known as senile keratoses.

The lesions are usually multiple and increase in number over time, being rare under the age of 35. They are often greasy looking (hence seborrhoeic), but they are not associated with seborrhoea nor with sebaceous glands. They have a 'stuck on' appearance akin to a barnacle, with well-defined edges and a range in colour from light tan to darkly pigmented.

Microscopically, lesions show basal cell proliferation, hyperkeratosis, pseudohorn cyst formation and a variable degree of pigmentation.

Dermis

Hypertrophic scar and keloid

These are both forms of excessive scar tissue formation following an injury.

Keloid

Scar tissue formation extends beyond the margin of the original injury and appears as firm, smooth nodules of various shapes. They occur mainly over the upper back, chest or

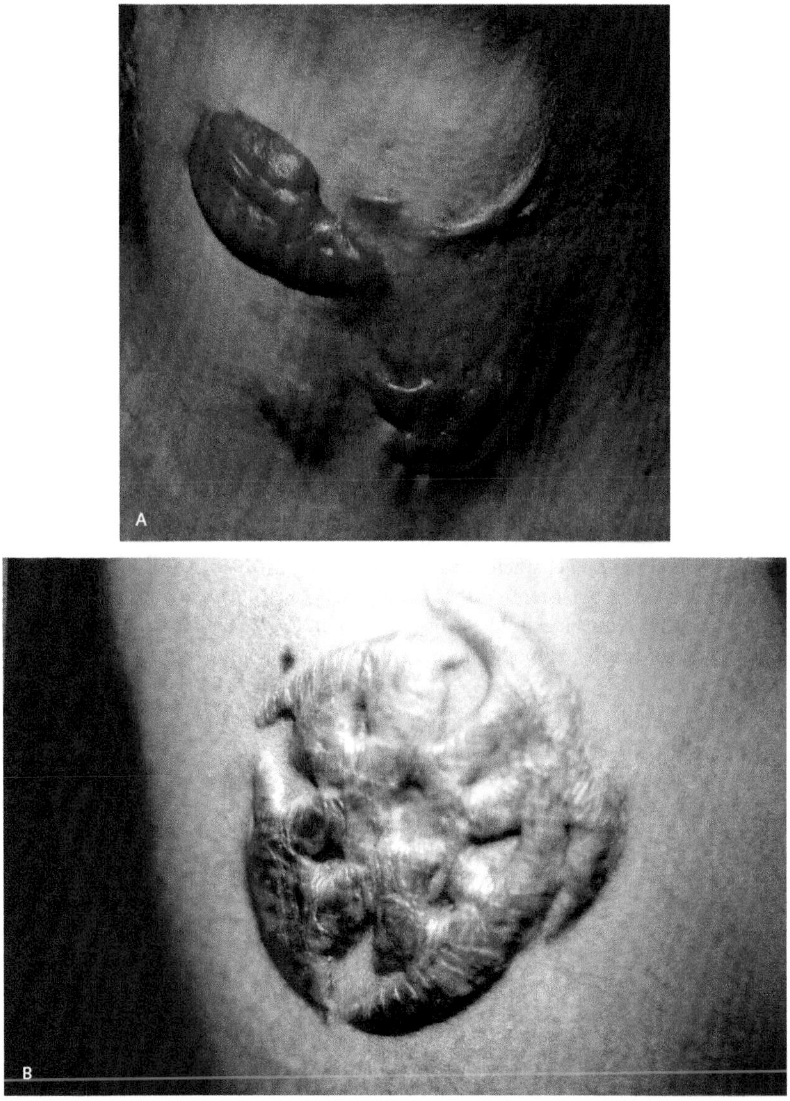

Fig. 18.10 **Keloid scar.** Examples of keloid scars. Scar tissue can be seen overgrowing the margins of the original wound (A) Keloids on a neck. (B) Keloid formation in response to a tattoo.

ear lobes, evolve over time, and are more common in black people (Fig. 18.10).

Hypertrophic scar

Scars that may be raised above the skin, pink or red but do not extend beyond the margins of the initial wound. They may spontaneously regress.

Morphoea

Morphoea is a form of localized scleroderma of which there are many variants. It is important to note that morphoea is not systemic sclerosis (see Chapter 17). Classical presentation is a thickened, ivory-white sclerotic plaque with a violaceous border. These may be multiple. Histologically, the mid to deep dermis is replaced with dense sclerosis obliterating normal adnexal structures such as hair follicles and sweat glands.

Dermatofibroma (histiocytoma)

These firm, reddish-brown nodules are common in young adults, occurring in females more often than males, and usually appear on the lower legs. Histologically, they consist of whorled bundles of spindle cells and fibroblasts with hyperplasia and hyperpigmentation of overlying epidermis. Dermatofibroma can be mistaken for a melanocytic naevus or malignant melanoma.

Sweat and the sebaceous structures

Acne vulgaris

This inflammatory disorder of the pilosebaceous apparatus is characterized by open and closed comedones (blackheads and whiteheads), papules, pustules, nodules, cysts and scars that affects the face, back and shoulders. It is extremely common in adolescents, the peak age being 18 years.

Aetiopathogenesis: The cause is multifactorial and includes a combination of:

- increased sebum excretion
- hyperkeratosis and reduced desquamation of the follicles
- blockage of pilosebaceous units with excess keratin and sebum, causing microcomedo formation
- release of inflammatory mediators
- colonization of ducts with the commensal bacteria *Propionibacterium acnes.*

P. acnes causes the evolution of comedones into inflammatory papules, nodules or cysts, which often form scars on healing. This may persist until the early twenties and even into the fifth decade of life in a few patients, especially women.

Rosacea

This chronic inflammatory disease of the face typically affects the middle-aged or elderly and is characterized by intermittent facial flushing on top of persistent erythema, telangiectasia and pustules. There are no blackheads, whiteheads or nodules and the trunk and limbs are rarely affected.

Rosacea is often complicated by:

- rhinophyma—sebaceous gland hyperplasia and fibrous thickening of the nose
- eye involvement—blepharitis (inflammation of the eyelids)
- sunlight and topical steroids—which exacerbate the condition.

The aetiology is unknown.

Hair disorders

Alopecia

This is hair loss. It is commonly classified into three main types: diffuse non-scarring, localized non-scarring and scarring (cicatricial). A brief summary of the various causes of alopecia is presented in Table 18.7.

In the assessment of alopecia, biopsies from an active area of alopecia are taken. These are meticulously examined histologically to evaluate the number and types of hair present, follicle density, scarring and any concomitant conditions such as lupus or fungal infections.

Diffuse non-scarring

There is diffuse reduction in hair density. The patient usually notices excessive numbers of hairs on the pillow, brush or comb.

The causes of diffuse nonscarring alopecia are numerous but common causes include:

- androgenic alopecia (male/female pattern)—inherited, androgen-dependent hair loss. Extremely common in men but it also occurs in women, becoming more pronounced after menopause.
- telogen effluvium—an increased number of hair follicles enter telogen (rest phase) and become synchronized. The cause is usually physiological stress, e.g., high fever, childbirth, surgery or drugs. The hairs are then shed in unison 3 months later.
- drugs—e.g., cytotoxics, heparin, warfarin, carbimazole, colchicine, vitamin A, β blockers and valproic acid.

Localized non-scarring

There is patchy hair loss. The causes are:

- alopecia areata—an autoimmune common condition characterized by round bald patches, usually on the scalp, mediated by $CD8^+$ T-cells attacking the hair follicles. It is associated with autoimmune disorders, atopic eczema and Down syndrome.
- infections—e.g., with scalp ringworm (tinea capitis) or secondary syphilis.
- traction—very common, especially in black people, from prolonged tightly braided hair styles/weaves/ponytails.

Scarring (cicatricial) alopecia

This is caused by scarring of the scalp with the destruction of hair follicles and permanent hair loss. The condition can be primary or secondary, diffuse or localized. Primary causes include:

- central centrifugal cicatricial alopecia—the most common form of scarring hair loss in black women. It begins at the vertex and extends outwards leaving a shiny appearing scalp. Histologically, there is lymphocytic inflammation of the hair bulb, fibrosis and desquamation of the root sheath. The progression can be halted but hair loss is permanent in fibrosed areas.
- lichen planopilaris—this is lichen planus of the scalp.

Secondary causes include trauma (chemical/thermal), infection, e.g., shingles, and other skin conditions, e.g., sarcoidosis, systemic sclerosis.

Excess hair

Hirsutism

This is the growth of coarse, pigmented hair with an androgenic distribution in a female.

Table 18.8 outlines the aetiology of hirsutism.

Table 18.8 Aetiology of hirsutism

Idiopathic	Most common form; probably because of increased hypersensitivity of end organs to androgens
Lactogenic	Exogenous androgens, progestogens
Virilizing tumours	Ovarian tumours (Sertoli–Leydig cell) Adrenal tumours (androgen producing)
Endocrine disorders	Congenital adrenal hyperplasia Cushing syndrome Acromegaly Polycystic ovary syndrome

Hypertrichosis

This is excessive growth of hair in a non-androgenic distribution. It is less common than hirsutism and can be:

- localized—as a feature of some naevi (e.g., vascular, congenital melanocytic) or following topical steroid application.
- generalized—fine terminal hairs appear on the face, limbs and trunk. Mostly drug-induced (e.g., ciclosporin, androgenic steroids and phenytoin) but can also be caused by malnutrition (e.g., anorexia nervosa), porphyria cutanea tarda or underlying malignancy.

Fat disorders

Panniculitis

This is a generic term used to encompass a group of conditions characterized by inflammation of the subcutaneous fat. Clinically, the appearances are similar, presenting as nodules or plaques which are thick and firm and usually associated with overlying erythema, pain/tenderness.

Diagnosis is made on microscopic features seen on biopsy. Histologically, an inflammatory infiltrate is present, either involving the septae between fat lobules, the lobules themselves or a mixture of both. The type of inflammatory infiltrate and presence of vasculitis also help to diagnose the type of panniculitis. Examples of panniculitis include erythema nodosum, necrobiosis lipoidica, rheumatoid nodules and drug reactions.

Erythema nodosum

This is the most common form of panniculitis. It usually affects the shins but may occur on the forearms or elsewhere. Typically young adults are affected, with a female bias.

Clinically, there is an acute presentation of multiple, bilateral subcutaneous tender/painful red nodules which are hot to touch. These are initially bright red and then fade like a bruise over time.

Histologically, septal panniculitis is seen with a mixed inflammatory infiltrate in the absence of vasculitis.

> **HINTS AND TIPS**
>
> **CONDITIONS ASSOCIATED WITH ERYTHEMA NODOSUM**
>
> Erythema nodosum is an important rash to identify as it is often associated with systemic pathology. Important associations include:
>
> - inflammatory bowel disease
> - infections—e.g., throat
> - sarcoidosis
> - tuberculosis
> - pregnancy
> - drug reactions—e.g., sulphonamides.

Lipoma

This is a soft, subcutaneous tumour of mature adipocytes. They can be solitary or multiple and mostly found on the trunk, neck and upper extremities in adulthood.

Liposarcoma

These are the most common malignant soft tissue tumours and, unlike lipomas, rarely arise within the skin. Instead they are deep seated, usually occurring in the thigh or retroperitoneally. They often reach a large size as they grow silently until they impinge on adjacent structures, producing symptoms.

Vascular lesions

Vascular naevi

Vascular naevi are composed of malformations of dilated blood vessels within the skin. They are always present at birth, becoming more visible as the infant grows. They are categorized by the type and size of vessel present. The most common are capillary vascular malformations:

Salmon patch—these are small, poorly defined patches of pink skin, caused by capillary malformation. This lesion (present in ~50% of neonates) is typically located on the neck or eyelids. If on the neck they are commonly referred to as 'stork bites'. Most resolve within the first year of life.

Port wine stain naevus—these are large, well-defined patches of red/purple skin which are also caused by capillary malformations. They are less common (<1% of neonates) and often affect one side of the face. They evolve to become bumpy with time and they do not spontaneously regress.

Angiomas

These are benign tumours of blood vessels caused by endothelial cell proliferation, unlike vascular naevi, which are malformations. There are many different types that present at various ages.

Capillary haemangioma (strawberry naevus)—these are superficial infantile haemangiomas and form in the upper dermis developing within the first few weeks of life. They appear as red, nodular lesions which grow and reach their maximum size in the first 12 months and then involute. Most cases have regressed by 5–7 years of age and the majority are located on the head and neck (Fig. 18.11).

Cavernous haemangioma—these are infantile haemangiomas which form in the deep dermis/subcutis. They present as soft blue/red nodular swellings.

Campbell de Morgan spots (cherry angioma)—these are very common capillary tumours of middle-aged to elderly patients. Characteristically they are small, bright-red papules (1–2 mm diameter) that commonly arise on the trunk but can occur anywhere. They may also appear blue or nearly black and their numbers increase over time.

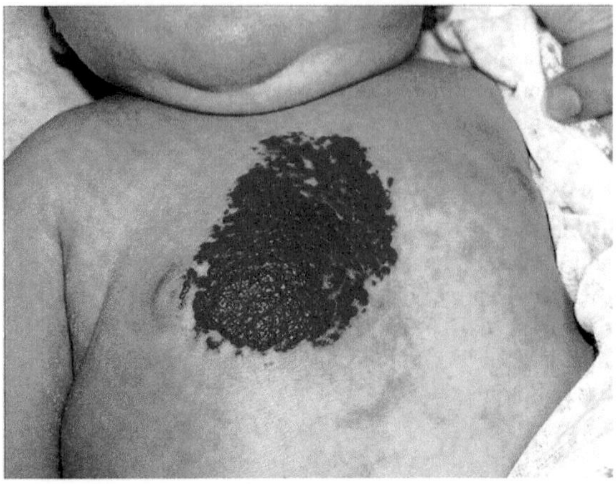

Fig. 18.11 Capillary haemangioma.

Pyogenic granuloma (lobular capillary haemangioma)

This is a benign, rapidly growing, bright-red shiny nodule arising mainly on the fingers, face (lips) and neck, most commonly in young adults and children. It is neither pyogenic nor granulomatous; instead, it is a well-circumscribed dermal lesion of lobules of proliferating capillaries. They can cause concern owing to their appearance and rapid growth.

Glomus tumour

These tumours arise from the glomus body, which is normally involved in the regulation of temperature by controlling blood flow to the skin. They occur as red/blue solitary lesions on the palms or fingers, 1–2 cm in size. They are characteristically painful. Histologically, a well-circumscribed dermal proliferation of sheets of glomus cells and small blood vessels is seen.

Kaposi sarcoma

This malignant disorder is characterized by bluish-brown plaques or nodules formed from a proliferation of small blood vessels and spindle cells in the dermis. It is caused by infection with the Kaposi sarcoma herpes virus (human herpes virus 8—HHV8). It commonly occurs in association with AIDS but is also endemic in certain African regions.

The lesions are multicentric, affecting the skin and mucous membranes, often beginning on the feet. They may disseminate widely to involve internal organs. Slit-like spaces dissecting collagen and extravasated red blood cells are seen histologically.

HINTS AND TIPS

VASCULAR NAEVI AND OTHER CONGENITAL SYNDROMES

The presence of vascular naevi should raise the question of whether other developmental malformations are also present:

Sturge–Weber syndrome: a port wine stain naevus within the distribution of the trigeminal nerve can be associated with underlying meningeal angiomas causing epilepsy, visual field defects and glaucoma.

Nail disorders

Trauma

Traumatic conditions are as follows:

- Subungual haematoma—bleeding under the nail following trapping of a fingernail or toenail.
- Splinter haemorrhages—seen with infective endocarditis, vasculitis and trauma.
- Onychogryphosis—thickened rams-horn-like big toenails, usually in response to trauma, ageing or psoriasis.
- Brittle nails (onychoschizia)—usually caused by repeated exposure to detergents and water.

Infections

Infections include:

- tinea unguium—fungal infection of the nails (Table 18.9).
- acute paronychia—infection of the soft tissue adjacent to nails which occurs and presents quickly. It is commonly caused by *S. aureus* and HSV.
- chronic paronychia—infection of the soft tissue adjacent to nails with a slow onset and long course (weeks), commonly caused by *C. albicans* or pseudomonas.

Lesions around the nails

These include:

- viral warts—common around the nail fold
- periungual fibroma—associated with tuberous sclerosis
- melanoma—subungual melanoma, which produces a pigmented longitudinal streak in a nail and may cause its destruction
- myxoid cyst—found over distal toes and finger interphalangeal joints, it contains mucin
- pyogenic granuloma—see vascular lesions above.

DISORDERS OF PIGMENTATION

Hypopigmentation

Albinism

This is a rare (1 in 17,000) autosomal recessive disease characterized by lack of pigmentation in the skin, hair and eyes. Melanocyte numbers are normal but melanin production fails because of a deficiency or defect in the enzyme tyrosinase.

Table 18.9 Nail changes and their possible causes

Nail change	Description	Possible causes
Nail plate surface		
Beau lines	Transverse ridges Affects all nails	Severe systemic illnesses that stop nail growth
Ridging	Transverse	Beau lines, eczema, psoriasis, chronic paronychia
	Longitudinal	Secondary to trauma
Pitting	Small holes/pits in nail bed	Psoriasis, eczema, alopecia areata, lichen planus
Discoloration		
Colour change	Blue	Haematoma, cyanosis, antimalarials
	Blue-green	*Pseudomonas* infection
	Brown	Fungal infection, cigarette stains, chemotherapy, decorative henna
	Brown longitudinal streak	Melanocytic naevus, malignant melanoma, Addison disease
	Red-brown streaks (splinter haemorrhages)	Infective endocarditis, vasculitis, trauma
	White spots/lines	Trauma to nail matrix (not calcium deficiency)
	White (leuconychia)	Hypoalbuminaemia, chronic renal failure, congenital
	Yellow	Psoriasis, tinea unguium, jaundice, tetracycline
	Yellow nail syndrome	Rare disorder of yellow thickened nails associated with lymphoedema, pleural effusions and possible bronchiectasis
Nail shape		
Koilonychia	Concave (spoon-shaped) nails	Iron deficiency anaemia Repeated exposure to detergents
Cuticle and nail fold		
Clubbing	Swelling of nail bed with loss of the angle between the nail fold and nail plates.	Respiratory: bronchiectasis, lung cancer, empyema, fibrosing alveolitis; lung abscess Cardiovascular: infective endocarditis, congenital heart disease Gastrointestinal tract: Crohn disease, ulcerative colitis, cirrhosis
Nail-fold telangiectasia	Reddened nail folds caused by dilated capillaries	Inflammatory connective tissue disorders including systemic sclerosis and dermatomyositis
Onycholysis	Separation of part or all of nail from its bed	Psoriasis, tinea unguium, trauma, thyrotoxicosis, tetracyclines

It is associated with poor sight, photophobia and nystagmus. People with albinism have an increased risk of skin tumours on exposure to ultraviolet (UV) light. Prenatal diagnosis is possible.

Vitiligo

This common disorder (1% of the population) is characterized by the appearance of symmetrical white or pale macules on the skin, which are caused by focal melanocyte loss.

Aetiopathogenesis—it has been suggested that vitiligo is an autoimmune disease of melanocytes, as it is often associated with other autoimmune diseases, such as pernicious anaemia, thyroid disease and Addison disease.

The exact aetiology is unknown, but about 30% of patients have a family history.

Clinical presentation—vitiligo affects all races, but is more conspicuous in dark-skinned individuals.

Onset is usually between 10 and 30 years of age. It commonly affects the hands, wrists, knees, neck and areas around orifices (e.g., mouth). It has an unpredictable course, ranging from progression to repigmentation (rarely).

Phenylketonuria

Phenylketonuria (PKU) is an autosomal recessive inborn error of metabolism caused by a deficiency of phenylalanine hydroxylase, which normally converts phenylalanine to tyrosine. The prevalence of PKU is 1 per 25,000 and it is detected by routine screening tests.

Patients have fair hair and skin because of impaired melanin synthesis (phenylalanine and tyrosine are precursors of melanin). The concentration of phenylalanine and its metabolites is increased and damages the neonatal brain. Untreated, mental retardation and choreoathetosis develop, although a low phenylalanine diet can prevent neurological damage.

Hyperpigmentation

Freckles and lentigines

Freckles (ephelides)

Freckles are small, light-brown, well-demarcated macules that darken on exposure to sunlight. They contain normal numbers of melanocytes but melanin production is increased. They are common in childhood, especially in fair-skinned children.

Lentigines

Lentigines (also known as lentigos) are similar in appearance to freckles but they are more scattered and they do not darken in the sun. Their outline may be more irregular than freckles. They contain increased numbers of melanocytes. They may develop in childhood, but are more common in the elderly. They usually occur in sun-exposed skin (solar lentigos).

Drug-induced pigmentation

This can be caused by stimulation of melanogenesis or by drug deposition in the skin. Drugs commonly responsible include amiodarone, bleomycin, psoralens, chlorpromazine and minocycline.

Other causes

Addison disease

This is characterized by hypoadrenalism, with overproduction of adrenocorticotrophic hormone (ACTH) by the pituitary gland. ACTH stimulates melanogenesis, resulting in hyperpigmentation of mucosae and skin creases.

Addisonian-like pigmentation is also seen in Cushing syndrome, hyperthyroidism and acromegaly.

Peutz–Jeghers syndrome

This rare, autosomal dominant disorder is characterized by perioral lentigines and intestinal polyps.

Postinflammation

Hyperpigmentation occurring after resolution of a dermatosis (e.g., eczema or lichen planus) may be seen. It is caused by deposition of melanin pigment from the epidermis into the dermis. This pigmentation tends to be more pronounced in darker skin.

A summary of the causes of hypopigmentation and hyperpigmentation is given in Table 18.10.

TUMOURS OF THE SKIN

Skin tumours may be benign or malignant, and may be subclassified based on their cell of origin. Table 18.11 summarizes some of the main skin tumours and their precursor lesions. It should be noted that many skin tumours arise from skin adnexa (e.g., sweat gland tumours), but this is beyond the scope of this book.

MELANOCYTIC LESIONS

Naevi

Definition

Naevi are benign, pigmented lesions on the skin formed from a proliferation of one or more of the normal constituent cells of the skin. Although often congenital (birthmarks), they may be acquired.

Table 18.10 Cause of hypopigmentation and hyperpigmentation

	Causes of hypopigmentation	Causes of hyperpigmentation
Genetic	Albinism and PKU	—
Chemical	Phenols, hydroquinone	—
Drugs	—	Oestrogens, amiodarone, bleomycin, psoralens, chlorpromazine, minocycline
Endocrine	Hypopituitarism (↓ACTH and ↓MSH)	Addison disease, chronic renal failure, Cushing syndrome, hyperthyroidism, acromegaly, melisma
Infective	Leprosy, yaws, pityriasis versicolor	—
Metabolic	—	Haemochromatosis, jaundice, porphyria
Nutritional	—	Carotenaemia (orange discoloration), pellagra, malabsorption/malnutrition
Postinflammatory	Cryotherapy, eczema, morphoea	Eczema, lichen planus, systemic sclerosis
Other	Vitiligo, lichen sclerosis, halo naevi	Acanthosis nigricans, melanoma, naevi

ACTH, Adrenocorticotrophic hormone; MSH, melanin-stimulating hormone; PKU, phenylketonuria.

Table 18.11 Summary of lesions of the skin

Cell of origin	Benign	Premalignant	Malignant
Melanocyte	Benign melanocytic naevi: junctional, compound and intradermal	–	Melanoma
Keratinocyte	Solar lentigo	• Actinic keratosis • Bowen disease	• Squamous cell carcinoma • Basal cell carcinoma
Lymphocyte	–	–	Mycosis fungoides
Neuroendocrine cell	–	–	Merkel cell carcinoma
Myofibroblast	Dermatofibroma	–	Dermatofibrosarcoma protuberans

Melanocytic naevi

These consist of localized benign proliferations of melanocytic cells and are the most common type of naevus (also known as 'moles'). They present in most white people, but are less prevalent in those with Down syndrome; they are also less common in black people.

The aetiology of naevi development is unknown but it seems to be an inherited trait in many families:

- About 1% of naevi are congenital.
- The majority develop during childhood or adolescence; numbers reach a peak at puberty and they have a tendency to decline during adult life.
- A few new naevi develop during the third and fourth decade of life, especially if provoked by excessive sun exposure or pregnancy.

Naevi can be classified according to the position of the naevus cells within the skin as follows:

- Junctional naevi—flat circular macules consisting of rounded nests of melanocytes in the lower epidermis at the dermo-epidermal junction.
- Compound naevi—papules or nodules with an irregular surface, which consist of junctional nests of melanocytes combined with an intradermal mass of melanocytic cells.
- Intradermal naevi—dome-shaped papules or nodules composed entirely of melanocytic cell clusters within the upper dermis (no junctional component present).

These different types of naevi are thought to arise by progression from junctional to intradermal (Fig. 18.12).

Other variants are:

- congenital naevi—usually over 1 cm in diameter; they may be protuberant or hairy and have a small risk of malignant change.
- blue naevi—usually a solitary intradermal naevus, most commonly found on the extremities; it appears blue owing to abundant deep dermal pigment.
- halo naevi—white halo of depigmentation surrounds the naevi. Represents involution of naevus following immune response against naevus cells. Mainly seen in children and adolescents.
- familial dysplastic naevus syndrome—familial condition characterized by large numbers of benign and atypical (or 'dysplastic') naevi. Affected individuals have a greatly increased risk of developing malignant melanoma.

Clinically, malignant naevi appear larger than normal and have an irregular edge, surface and pigmentation. They are also more likely to be itchy and to bleed. Junctional components of junctional or compound naevi carry the highest risk for malignancy. Invasion is preceded by nuclear pleomorphism with increased mitoses and cellular atypia.

Melanoma

This malignant tumour of melanocytes usually arises in the skin, and is the fifth most common cancer in the UK. Incidence is 4% and rising steadily. Five-year and 10-year survival is 90%.

It occurs in all races but it is more common in whites. Incidence is proportional to geographical latitude, which suggests an effect of UV radiation. The most common site in males is on the back but in females it is the lower leg.

The aetiology is unknown but repeated exposure to UV radiation is thought to play an important role.

Major risk factors for the development of melanoma (with decreasing risk) are:

- familial dysplastic naevus syndrome—rare but lifetime risk of melanoma is over 50%
- congenital naevus
- previous melanoma
- immunosuppression
- fair skin—melanin pigmentation appears protective.

MOLECULAR

BRAF AND MELANOMA

Several tumours, including melanomas, can demonstrate a mutation in the BRAF gene (V600E). If present, patients with this mutation may be treated with targeted BRAF inhibitor drugs, and therefore have a better prognosis.

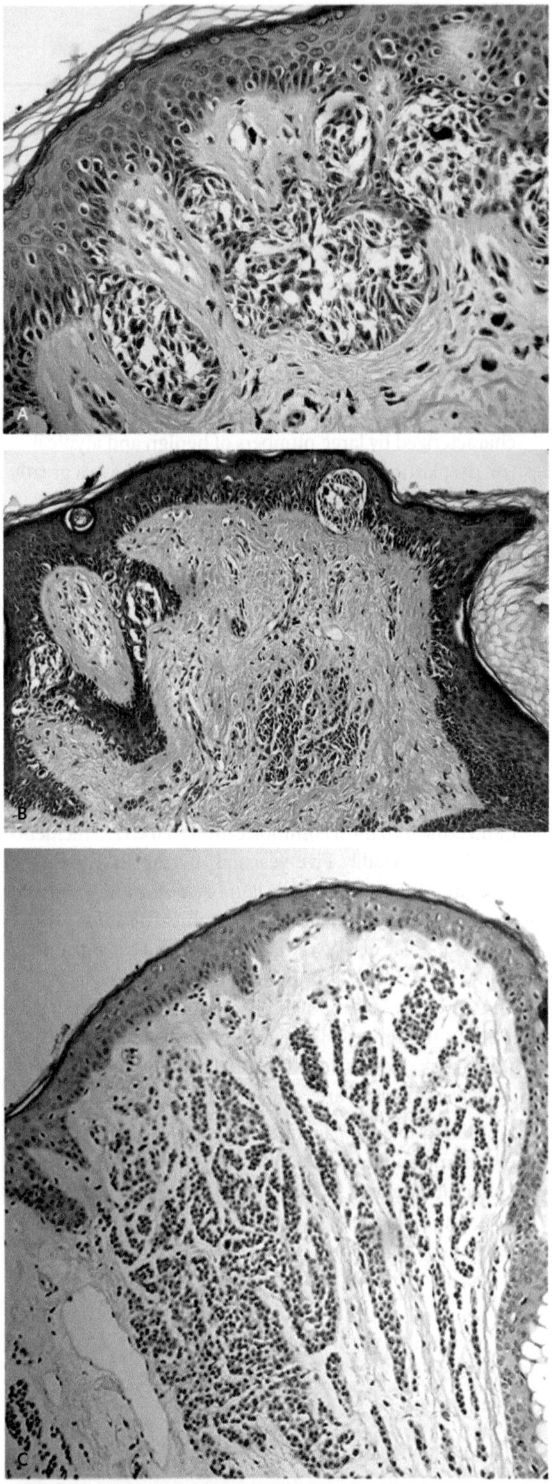

Fig. 18.12 Microscopic pictures of junctional, compound and intradermal naevi.
(A) Junctional naevus: melanocytes form nests within the epidermis and are limited to the epidermis. (B) Compound naevus: melanocytes are within the epidermis and dermis. (C) Intradermal naevus: melanocytes are within the dermis only.

Diagnosis—one or more of the following changes observed or reported in a naevus or pigmented lesion may suggest melanoma:

- Size—usually increased
- Shape—irregular outline
- Colour—irregular pigmentation
- Inflammation—at the edge of lesion
- Crusting—oozing or bleeding lesion
- Itchiness—a common symptom.

HINTS AND TIPS

THE ABCS OF MELANOMA

Remember your ABCs for the malignant changes in a melanocytic naevus:
*A*symmetry—an asymmetrical lesion
*B*order—irregular edges
*C*olour—changes in pigmentation
*D*iameter—growth of the lesion
*E*volution—the patient has noted a change over time

Classification

Four main types of malignant melanoma are recognized.

Superficial spreading melanoma

A flat tumour with variable pigmentation and irregular edges. This is the most common type.

Lentigo maligna melanoma

A nodular lesion arising in a preexisting lentigo maligna. This typically occurs in sun-damaged skin of the face in elderly patients. Lentigo maligna is similar to a benign lentigine but it is generally larger (>2 cm) and has atypical melanocytes.

Acral lentiginous melanoma

This resembles lentigo maligna melanoma but it affects the palms, soles and nail beds (subungual melanoma). It is the most common form of melanoma in Asian and Afro-Caribbean people, suggesting it develops independently of UV radiation exposure. It is often diagnosed late and consequently has poor survival figures.

Nodular malignant melanoma

An aggressive pigmented nodule that may grow rapidly and ulcerate. It is the second commonest subtype and typically arises on the legs and trunk.

Staging and prognosis of malignant melanoma

The most important criteria in determining prognosis for a melanoma is the presence of ulceration, the mitotic rate and the thickness of the tumour. Depth of invasion is assessed using the Breslow method (Fig. 18.13). The Breslow thick-

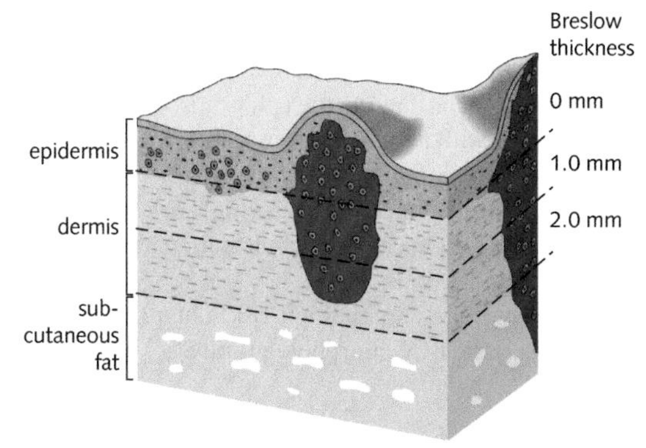

Fig. 18.13 Breslow thickness.

Table 18.12 Five and ten-year survival rates based on Breslow thickness

Breslow thickness (mm)	5-year survival rate (%)	10-year survival rate (%)
<1.00	97	92
1.01–2.00	91	80
2.01–4.00	79	63
>4.00	71	50

ness is the measured thickness in millimetres (on a histological section) from the granular layer of the epidermis to the deepest identifiable melanoma cell.

The Breslow thickness is directly related to the risk of metastasis and therefore prognosis. (Table. 18.12).

NEOPLASTIC LESIONS OF THE EPIDERMIS

Squamous lesions

Solar elastosis

This is accumulation of elastin in the dermis of sun-damaged skin.

Actinic keratosis

These present as roughened, scaly brownish to red lesions, usually <1 cm across, which may bleed when rubbed. They typically arise on sun-exposed areas (also known as solar keratosis), especially the face, scalp and hands of the middle aged and elderly.

Histologically, they show hyperkeratosis and parakeratosis, abnormal basal keratinocytes with loss of maturation, and a mild to moderate degree of pleomorphism and mitotic figures.

The lesions are considered premalignant, with up to 10% evolving into squamous cell carcinoma (SCC).

Bowen disease

This carcinoma in-situ typically occurs on skin which has not been exposed to sun; it is associated with previous exposure to arsenicals. It is characterized by:

- slowly extending, pink or lightly pigmented, scaly plaques up to several centimetres in size. Can look like psoriatic plaques.
- full-thickness dysplasia with prominent nuclear pleomorphism and large numbers of mitoses (Fig. 18.14).

Carcinomas usually remain in situ for many years but have the capacity to transform into SCCs.

Keratoacanthoma

This is a well-circumscribed squamous cell tumour that typically arises on the face of elderly white males. It grows very rapidly, changing from a small, red papule to a large, domed nodule with raised edges and a central mass of keratin within a few weeks. The base of the tumour is not infiltrative and it rarely metastasizes. The majority spontaneously regress within a few months. Some schools of thought classify keratoacanthomas as a low-grade SCC. However, owing to its ability to regress, lack of infiltration and lack of metastasis, other schools consider it a benign lesion.

Squamous cell carcinoma

This malignant tumour is derived from keratinocytes of the upper layers of the epidermis. It is typically seen on the face in elderly or middle-aged individuals. Tumours are locally invasive and they may also metastasize.

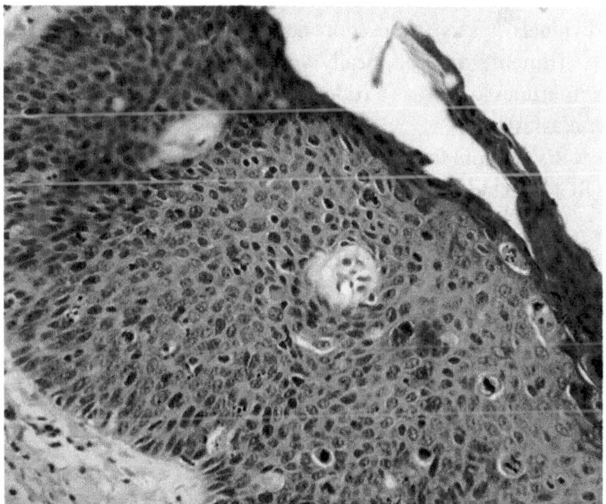

Fig. 18.14 Histology of Bowen disease. Microscopic appearance of Bowen disease with the epidermis showing full-thickness dysplasia with abnormal mitoses, lack of cellular maturation from top to bottom and pleomorphic keratinocytes. There is no invasion into the dermis as the basement membrane is intact. This is a good example of carcinoma in-situ.

The aetiology of SCC is related to:

- chronic UV exposure
- chemical carcinogens (e.g., tar, arsenic and machine oil)
- X-ray radiation
- chronic ulceration and scarring
- smoking (lip lesions—aggressive, frequently metastasize)
- common wart virus (HPV) in immunosuppressed individuals
- genetic (e.g., xeroderma pigmentosum).

Histologically, tumours consist of disorganised keratinocytes with typical malignant cytology, which destroy the dermoepidermal junction and form invading strands of malignant squamous cells into the dermis. Foci of keratinization are seen within well-differentiated tumours.

Clinical presentation:

- Dome-shaped nodules, which usually arise in sun-exposed sites such as the face, neck, forearm or hand.
- Nodules typically develop into roughened keratotic areas, ulcers or horns.
- Often difficult to distinguish from keratoacanthomas (see previous section).
- Less aggressive forms may arise within actinic keratosis as a small papule, which progress to ulceration and then crust over.
- More aggressive forms may arise at the edge of chronic skin ulcers (e.g., a Marjolin ulcer), but this is rare.

Basal cell carcinoma

This is a malignant tumour that arises from the basal keratinocytes of the epidermis. It is the most common form of human cancer, typically seen on the face of elderly or middle-aged individuals. It is five times more common than SCC.

Tumours may be locally very invasive (hence they are sometimes known as a rodent ulcer), but they almost never metastasize.

Risk factors for the development of basal cell carcinoma (BCC) include:

- repeated UV exposure
- light-skinned races
- X-ray irradiation
- chronic scarring
- genetic predisposition (Gorlin syndrome).

Tumours are typically composed of basophilic cells that invade the dermis. They appear as well-defined islands with peripheral palisading of cells.

Clinical presentation—they typically occur on sun-exposed sites, commonly around the nose, inner canthus of the eyelids and the temple. They may have a glistening pearly edge and show numerous telangiectatic vessels on the surface. Tumours grow slowly but relentlessly. Some subtypes may destroy underlying cartilage, bone and soft tissue structures. These often have central ulceration with an adherent crust.

There are four main types of BCC:

1. Nodular—circumscribed dermal tumours.
2. Superficial—confined to the epidermis, often multifocal, with a high recurrence rate; these are often given topical therapy.
3. Infiltrative/morphoeic—this is a high-risk subtype which may have focal areas of ulceration and often perineural invasion.
4. Basosquamous—another high-risk subtype, it shows areas of classic BCC morphology and SCC morphology.

CLINICAL NOTES

MOHS

Management of basal cell carcinomas of the face is usually via a procedure known as Mohs surgery (named after Dr Frederic Mohs).

Procedure—the tumour is narrowly excised, and an on-site pathologist reviews frozen sections of the tumour margins. If negative, the surgery is considered complete; if positive, more thin margin sections are taken and reviewed by the pathologist until the tumour is completely, but narrowly excised. This method preserves cosmesis.

Other tumours of the skin

Mycosis fungoides (cutaneous T-cell lymphoma)

This is the commonest primary cutaneous T-cell lymphoma. It is a slowly progressive (years), indolent tumour of $CD4^+$ (T helper) lymphocytes in the skin.

There are three stages:

1. Patch stage—erythematous eczematous lesions, usually on the trunk or legs. They may persist for 10 or more years. They have atypical lymphocytes with cerebriform nuclei in the basal layer of the epidermis.
2. Plaque stage—erythematous plaques develop, typically affecting the trunk. Atypical lymphocytes infiltrate the full thickness of the epidermis and form Pautrier microabcesses. This stage may last for years.
3. Tumour stage—tumour nodules or ulcers develop within the plaques. A dermal infiltrate is seen microscopically. Mean survival time is 2.5 years.

Dermatofibrosarcoma protuberans

Dermatofibrosarcoma protuberans (DFSP) is a locally invasive dermal tumour of proliferating myofibroblasts with low-grade malignancy. DFSP is similar in appearance to dermatofibromas, but is locally invasive. It entraps fat, giving it a classic lace-like appearance. It does not metastasize but often recurs following excision.

Merkel cell carcinoma

This is a malignant neuroendocrine tumour of the skin which arises in Merkel cells (of neural crest origin). It has the morphological appearance of small cell carcinoma of the lung. It is highly aggressive and has a poor prognosis.

Metastatic lesions

Metastases to the skin are uncommon. The commonest metastatic entities to skin are breast, lung, colon and kidney carcinomas.

Chapter Summary

- Psoriasis is a chronic noninfective inflammatory disease; it presents as silver scales over extensor surfaces.
- Eczema encompasses numerous dermatoses with characteristic spongiotic inflammation.
- Blistering disorders arise from splitting of the skin and accumulation of plasma. They are characterized by the level of the split and the contents of the blister.
- Skin infections can be bacterial, viral or fungal.
- Leishmaniasis and onchocerciasis are examples of parasitic tropical skin infections.
- Leprosy and tuberculosis are examples of mycobacterial skin infections.
- Syphilis and Lyme disease are examples of spirochaetal skin infections.
- Tumours, benign and malignant, may arise from any structure/cell type within the skin. Common examples include lipomas, haemangiomas and dermatofibromas.
- Nail changes can reflect primary disease of the nails, systemic disease or involvement by dermatoses.
- Alopecia can be scarring or non-scarring, diffuse or focal.
- Hypopigmentation and hyperpigmentation are the result of either changes in melanocyte proliferation, or the amount of melanin produced by melanocytes.
- Melanocytic naevi are pigmented proliferations of melanocytes.
- Ulceration, Breslow thickness and mitotic rate are key prognostic factors in melanoma.
- Squamous cell carcinomas, basal cell carcinomas and melanomas are all associated with chronic sun exposure.
- Mycosis fungoides is a slowly progressive primary cutaneous T-cell lymphoma.

SELF-ASSESSMENT

Single best answer (SBA) questions

Chapter 2 Postmortem pathology

1. A terminally ill patient falls in her nursing home and presents to A&E. She dies 3 hours later. The foundation year doctor is told to refer the case to the coroner. Which of the following is *not* an indication for coronial referral?
   A. Unknown cause of death.
   B. The patient had an operation 3 months ago.
   C. The patient has not seen a doctor within 2 weeks.
   D. The patient had a morphine overdose.
   E. There is a suspicion of neglect in her nursing home.

2. A foundation year doctor is confused about when she is allowed to write a death certificate. Which of the following instances prevents her from writing a death certificate?
   A. She has not treated the patient in the last 14 days.
   B. She was not present at time of death.
   C. She has not been paid for writing a medical certificate of cause of death.
   D. She has not seen the body after death.
   E. She was not the doctor pronouncing death.

Chapter 3 Inflammation, repair and cell death

1. A 12-year-old boy with a 1-day history of sore throat was seen by his GP. On physical examination, the most prominent finding was a purulent pharyngeal exudate. He most likely has an acute inflammation. In acute inflammation, which of the following is true?
   A. The predominant cell type is the neutrophil.
   B. The inflammation is usually initiated by cell-mediated immunity.
   C. The duration may be for months.
   D. Plasma cells are frequently present.
   E. Lymphocytes are present at the start of the process.

2. The histopathology report for a tissue biopsy shows that there is acute inflammation. Which of the following features are seen in tissue with acute inflammation?
   A. Vasoconstriction.
   B. Increased blood flow.
   C. Histamine sequestration.
   D. Diuresis.
   E. Nitrate release.

3. Which of the following statements about necrosis is correct?
   A. It is a reversible cellular injury.
   B. It maintains plasma membrane integrity.
   C. It is caused by oxygen free radicals.
   D. It does not result in an inflammatory response.
   E. It is an energy-dependent process.

4. Apoptotic cells usually exhibit distinctive morphological features. Which of the following is true of pure apoptosis?
   A. It is initiated by Golgi body disintegration.
   B. It occurs in groups of cells.
   C. It results in cell shrinkage and fragmentation.
   D. DNA is cleaved by proteases.
   E. It results in an inflammatory response.

5. Trauma to the breast can result in which type of necrosis?
   A. Liquefactive necrosis.
   B. Coagulative necrosis.
   C. Caseous necrosis.
   D. Fat necrosis.
   E. Fibrinoid necrosis.

Chapter 4 Cancer

1. During an oncology department multidisciplinary team meeting, the oncologist mentions some medical terminology. Which of the following definitions is correct?
   A. Dysplasia is a change from one type of differentiated epithelium to another.
   B. Anaplasia is an almost complete lack of differentiation
   C. Carcinoma is a benign tumour of epithelial derivation.
   D. Metaplasia is the disordered development of cells with loss of organization.
   E. Carcinoma in situ is a carcinoma with stromal invasion.

2. Which of the following statements regarding cancers is correct?
   A. Tumours arise from single cells.
   B. Lymphomas are benign tumours of lymphoid cells.
   C. Cells in a tumour are genetically identical.
   D. Transcoelomic spread occurs through the lymphatic system.
   E. Melanomas are benign skin tumours; malignant melanomas are malignant skin tumours.

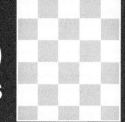

3. You are reading a histopathology report which describes the excised tumour as malignant. Which of the following is not a common histological feature of malignant tumours?
   A. Pleomorphism.
   B. Nuclear hyperchromasia.
   C. Anisonucleosis.
   D. Abnormal and increased mitoses.
   E. Inconspicuous nucleoli.

4. Which of the following statements about tumour suppressor genes is correct?
   A. Tumour suppressor genes encode proteins that positively regulate cell growth.
   B. DNA mismatch repair genes are mutated in familial adenomatous polyposis.
   C. Gain of function of tumour suppressor genes results in neoplastic growth.
   D. Viral proteins cannot deregulate tumour suppressor function.
   E. *p53* triggers apoptosis and cell-cycle arrest.

5. Which of the following carcinogenic agents is associated with increased risk of gastric mucosa-associated lymphoid tissue (MALT) lymphomas?
   A. Benzene.
   B. Epstein–Barr virus (EBV).
   C. *Helicobacter pylori.*
   D. Human papilloma virus (HPV).
   E. Ultraviolet (UV) radiation.

Chapter 5 Infectious disease

1. Which of the following is true of viruses?
   A. They are prokaryotes.
   B. They only possess RNA.
   C. If of the non-enveloped type, may release new particles by budding.
   D. They are obligate extracellular parasites.
   E. They may cause cell lysis.

2. A 34-year-old man who presented with infection with a resistant species of enterobacteria was commenced on oral ciprofloxacin. Which of the following is true of bacterial antibiotic resistance?
   A. It is uncommon.
   B. It is conferred via extrachromosomal RNA.
   C. It cannot be directly transferred between bacteria.
   D. It may occur through the alteration of the target site for an antibiotic.
   E. Methicillin-resistant *Staphylococcus aureus* (MRSA) is virtually impossible to treat.

3. A 39-year-old man with untreated HIV presents with shortness of breath worsening on exertion and a nonproductive cough. Blood tests showed CD4 count to be <200 cells/mm^3. Chest X-ray showed bilateral fluffy hilar opacities. Bronchial washings showed proteinaceous, foamy-appearing alveolar casts in which silver stain showed round, cup-shaped organisms. What is the likely infectious agent?
   A. Aspergillus.
   B. *Cryptococcus neoformans.*
   C. *Pneumocystis jirovecii.*
   D. *Mycobacterium tuberculosis.*
   E. *Mycobacterium avium intracellulare.*

Chapter 6 Molecular pathology

1. Which of the following is true of the polymerase chain reaction (PCR)?
   A. Is not temperature-dependent.
   B. Occurs on a gel.
   C. Amplifies DNA.
   D. Sequences DNA.
   E. Involves restriction enzymes.

2. Which of the following is true about the RAS protein?
   A. RAS directly activates mitogen-activated protein kinase (MAPK).
   B. Numerous anticancer drugs directly inhibit RAS.
   C. RAS is adenosine triphosphate (ATP)-dependent.
   D. RAS is part of an intracellular signalling cascade.
   E. K and B forms exist.

Chapter 7 Pathology of the nervous system

1. A 65-year-old woman presented with headache, vomiting, nausea, and papilloedema. Upon admission to hospital, the patient was noticed to have gait instability, urinary incontinence and focal neurological signs. A diagnosis of hydrocephalus was made. Which of the following is true of hydrocephalus?
   A. It is a decrease in the volume of cerebrospinal fluid (CSF) within the brain.
   B. It results in the constriction of the cerebral ventricles.
   C. Increased absorption of CSF at the arachnoid villi is the commonest form.
   D. A ventricular shunt can be used in the management.
   E. All causes of hydrocephalus are acquired.

2. A 34-year-old woman was hit in the head by a cricket ball. After she was hit, she managed to walk off the field without any symptoms. By the time she reached hospital, she had died. Upon autopsy, a diagnosis of extradural haemorrhage (EDH) was made. Which of the following is true of extradural haemorrhage?
   A. Occurs between the dura and outer surface of the arachnoid membrane.
   B. It is not usually associated with a skull fracture.

C. It is due to bleeding from the cortical bridging veins.
D. It may be associated with a posttraumatic lucid period.
E. It is not a surgical emergency.

3. An 82-year-old man dies after an episode of pneumonia. Upon autopsy, an incidental finding of Alzheimer disease is made. Which of the following is true of Alzheimer disease?
A. It is usually familial.
B. It is characterized by cerebral oedema.
C. Neurofibrillary tangles occur within neurones.
D. Affects half of all people over the age of 80 years.
E. It is not usually associated with memory disturbance.

4. A patient with a cerebral hemisphere mass was informed by the neurosurgeon that it is a tumour. Which of the following is true about neoplasms of the central nervous system (CNS)?
A. Gliomas are the least common primary CNS tumour.
B. Astrocytomas rarely affect children.
C. Oligodendrogliomas are slow-growing tumours.
D. Meningiomas commonly invade deep CNS tissue.
E. Prostatic carcinoma often causes brain metastases.

5. A secretary presents to her general practitioner with pain and tingling in both her hands which has been progressively getting worse over the last month. This is maximal first thing in the morning and it is preventing her from typing at work. Which of the following is true of carpal tunnel syndrome?
A. Pollicis brevis is wasted.
B. Trousseau sign is positive.
C. The cuboid bone is part of the carpal tunnel.
D. Sensory loss occurs over the medial 2.5 fingers.
E. Causes wrist drop.

Chapter 8 Pathology of the head and neck

1. A 45-year-old man who recently moved to the UK from Hong Kong presents with a history of nasal obstruction and epistaxis. A diagnosis of nasopharyngeal carcinoma is made. Which of the following is true of nasopharyngeal carcinoma?
A. It commonly presents with axillary lymphadenopathy.
B. It is associated with Epstein–Barr virus.
C. It is common in southern Africa.
D. It commonly causes destruction of the surrounding bone.
E. There is abundant lymphoid tissue with necrotizing granulomatous inflammation.

2. Which of the following is true of squamous cell carcinoma of the oral cavity?
A. It occurs least commonly on the lips.
B. It is more common in women than men.
C. It has a positive association with cigarette smoking.
D. It has a positive association with moderate alcohol intake.
E. It has a 5-year survival of about 10%.

3. A 75-year-old man presents with a lateral neck lump that is nontender and increasing in size. He is a heavy smoker. What is the most likely diagnosis?
A. Carotid body tumour.
B. Tonsillitis.
C. Lymphoma.
D. Epidermoid cyst.
E. Laryngeal carcinoma.

4. Which is true of laryngeal tumours?
A. Papillomas occur bilaterally on the vocal cords.
B. Persistent hoarse voice is a worrying symptom.
C. Lymphoma is the commonest tumour of the larynx.
D. Lymphoma is the commonest tumour of the tonsils.
E. Subglottic laryngeal carcinomas have the best prognosis.

Chapter 9 Pathology of the cardiovascular system

1. A 24-year-old man was found to have a ventricular septal defect upon echocardiogram. Which of the following is true of ventricular septal defect?
A. It usually produces a right-to-left shunt of blood.
B. It is not associated with Eisenmenger syndrome.
C. It produces a diastolic murmur.
D. It may be of a membranous or muscular location.
E. It is the least common congenital cardiac abnormality.

2. Coarctation of the aorta was diagnosed in a 4-year-old child. Which of the following is true of coarctation of the aorta?
A. It is more common in females.
B. It causes hypertension distal to the narrowing.
C. It is often associated with a bicuspid mitral valve.
D. It can cause right-ventricular failure.
E. It is associated with weak and delayed femoral pulsations.

3. Upon autopsy an incidental finding of atherosclerosis was made. Which of the following is true of atherosclerosis?
A. It is characterized by the accumulation of protein-rich material in the intima of arteries.

B. It is common in the pulmonary arteries.
C. It is associated with hypocholesterolaemia.
D. It may be seen as a pathological response to endothelial injury.
E. It is characterized by neutrophil lipid uptake to form foam cells.

4. During a routine checkup at the GP, a 34-year-old man had consistently high blood pressure of 149 mmHg systolic. Benign hypertension is characterized by:
A. Fibrinoid necrosis of arterioles.
B. Hypotrophy of the muscular media of the arteries.
C. Fibroelastic thinning of the intima.
D. Hyaline change in arteriole walls.
E. Sudden and severe increase in blood pressure.

5. A 56-year-old man has arrived in hospital complaining of chest pain which radiated to his left hand, and upon investigation had ECG changes concurrent with acute myocardial infarction (MI). Which of the following is true of MI?
A. It results in necrosis of the myocardium following severe ischaemia.
B. It induces chronic inflammatory changes.
C. The infarcted tissue is replaced by new cardiac muscle.
D. Occlusion of the left anterior descending coronary artery results in an inferior MI.
E. Dressler syndrome is an acute complication which may occur within a few days of MI.

6. A 67-year-old man presents to the general practitioner with breathlessness upon exertion, orthopnoea and oedema of legs, feet and ankles. Which of the following of heart failure is true?
A. It is when the heart is unable to maintain cardiac output.
B. Right-sided heart failure is more common than left-sided failure.
C. Left-sided heart failure may commonly develop as a result of right-sided failure.
D. It is not a complication of myocardial infarction.
E. It is not associated with valve disease.

7. After a 12-hour plane flight, a 53-year-old female flight attendant noticed a heavy ache over her right calf, with associated swelling and tenderness. Which of the following is true of thrombosis?
A. A thrombus is the pathological term for a clot.
B. It is predisposed by both blood stasis and turbulence.
C. Antiphospholipid antibody decreases risk of arterial and venous thrombosis.
D. The most common site of venous thrombosis is the portal vein.
E. Factor V Leiden mutation is protective against thrombosis.

8. A 26-year-old athletic Italian man presents reporting symptoms of dyspnoea on exertion and palpitations. He has also felt lightheaded and dizzy. What is the most likely diagnosis?
A. Hypertrophic cardiomyopathy.
B. Dilated cardiomyopathy.
C. Restrictive cardiomyopathy.
D. Arrhythmogenic right-ventricular cardiomyopathy (ARVC).
E. Takotsubo cardiomyopathy.

9. A 50-year-old female presents with a thromboembolic stroke causing right-sided hemiplegia. Which of the following is the most likely source of emboli?
A. Right carotid artery stenosis.
B. Left deep vein thrombosis (DVT).
C. Abdominal aortic aneurysm.
D. Atrial fibrillation (AF).
E. Berry aneurysm.

Chapter 10 Pathology of the respiratory system

1. A 56-year-old man who is a chronic smoker presented to hospital with an acute exacerbation of chronic obstructive pulmonary disease (COPD). Which of the following is true of chronic obstructive pulmonary disease?
A. It is characterized by chronic bronchitis, emphysema and bronchiolitis.
B. The obstructive lung disease can be completely reversed with bronchodilators.
C. It causes hypoinflated lungs.
D. It is exclusively a disease of smokers.
E. Lung fibrosis is a feature of emphysema.

2. Which of the following is true of chronic bronchitis?
A. It is defined as a productive cough on most days for 1 month of the year for at least 2 successive years.
B. Most cases are due to cigarette smoking.
C. Hypersecretion of mucus is associated with hypotrophy of the bronchial mucus-secreting glands.
D. It is characterized by an acute inflammation of the bronchioles.
E. Lung function tests show a restrictive pattern.

3. A 12-year-old boy presents to his GP with coughing, wheezing and shortness of breath. The GP

subsequently diagnosed him with asthma. Which of the following is true of asthma?
A. Causes irreversible airway narrowing.
B. May be caused by a type II hypersensitivity reaction.
C. Bronchospasm, oedema and mucus plugging are commonly seen.
D. It is sometimes associated with α-1-antitrypsin deficiency.
E. Hypotrophy of bronchial smooth muscle may occur.

4. Which of the following is true of cystic fibrosis (CF)?
A. It is associated with infections with *Pseudomonas spp.*
B. It is the most common autosomal dominant condition in Europe.
C. It is due to defective transport of potassium ions.
D. It is not associated with malabsorption.
E. It is due to a mutation in a gene on chromosome 9.

5. A 67-year-old man is admitted to hospital with bronchial breathing at the right lung base, associated crackles and pyrexia. A clinical diagnosis of pneumonia was made. Which of the following is true of pneumonia?
A. Pneumonia is most commonly caused by viral infections.
B. Most cases of bacterial community-acquired pneumonia are due to Gram-negative organisms.
C. Empyema is a type of pneumonia.
D. Red hepatization is a pathological stage in bronchopneumonia.
E. Lobar pneumonia is more commonly seen in those without an underlying lung condition.

6. A 29-year-old woman with cervical lymphadenopathy is seen in a surgical outpatient clinic. An excision biopsy was performed and sent for histopathology. Which of the following is true of pulmonary tuberculosis?
A. It is most commonly due to *Mycobacterium avium intracellulare.*
B. It is caused by direct cytopathic effects of the infecting organism.
C. It is not associated with chronic lung disease.
D. It is a common cause of death in AIDS.
E. It is not characterized histologically by granulomas.

7. A 78-year-old smoker complaining of a persistent dry cough had a chest X-ray which showed a 2 cm mass lesion in the right upper zone. Biopsies were sent for histological examination. Which of the following is true of lung carcinomas?
A. Adenocarcinomas are the commonest type.
B. They are not associated with cigarette smoking.
C. They are not associated with asbestos.
D. They are rarely metastatic at the time of presentation.
E. They do not cause pleural effusions.

8. Which of the following is true of idiopathic pulmonary fibrosis?
A. It is an infectious condition.
B. It causes interstitial atrophy.
C. It is an obstructive lung disease.
D. It causes peripheral lung honeycombing.
E. It is not a cause of finger clubbing.

9. Which of the following is an example of a restrictive lung disease?
A. Emphysema.
B. Idiopathic pulmonary fibrosis.
C. Bronchiectasis.
D. Asthma.
E. Chronic bronchitis.

10. A 48-year-old man has suddenly developed acute onset of chest pain, cough, dyspnoea, tachypnoea and marked anxiety. He underwent an operation 2 days ago. Which of the following is true of a pulmonary embolism (PE)?
A. A positive D-dimer confirms the diagnosis of a PE.
B. It may be precipitated by mural thrombus in the left ventricle.
C. It does not cause ventilation and perfusion mismatching.
D. It is the shape of the vessel in which it originated.
E. It is usually caused by thromboembolism from arm veins.

11. Which of the following is true of mesothelioma?
A. It develops rapidly after exposure to asbestos.
B. It mainly spreads via the bloodstream.
C. It is slowly progressive with a long life expectancy.
D. It has been decreasing in incidence.
E. It is associated with recurrent pleural effusions.

Chapter 11 Pathology of the gastrointestinal system

1. A 78-year-old man with a 3-month history of weight loss and dysphagia is diagnosed with oesophageal carcinoma. Which of the following is true of oesophageal carcinoma?
A. It is most commonly adenocarcinoma.
B. It may develop into Barrett metaplasia.
C. Adenocarcinoma is the most likely pattern in heavy smokers or drinkers.
D. It accounts for 20% of cancers in the UK each year.
E. It causes dysphagia for solids more than liquids.

2. A 54-year-old woman with a history of chronic alcohol use presents with coffee-ground haematemesis which quickly turns to frank blood. Which of the following is true of oesophageal varices?
   A. They are dilated submucosal veins in the oesophagus.
   B. They are not associated with cirrhosis of the liver.
   C. Rupture causes slight bleeding.
   D. They are associated with portal vein hypotension.
   E. Variceal banding is not used in the management.

3. A 25-year-old woman presents to her GP with intermittent nausea and vague abdominal pain for the past 18 months. A *Campylobacter*-like organism (CLO) test at the time of endoscopy is positive for *Helicobacter pylori*. Which of the following is true of *H. pylori*-associated gastritis?
   A. It is an example of an acute gastritis.
   B. *H. pylori* colonizes the epithelium above a layer of mucus.
   C. Epithelial damage is caused by the immune response against *H. pylori.*
   D. It is most commonly seen at the pyloric fundus.
   E. It is usually a transient infection.

4. A 32-year-old man presents with malaise and unintentional weight loss of 10 kg over the past 2 months. He is investigated and is noted to be anaemic. Imaging shows a mass in his stomach. Endoscopy with biopsy is performed and he is diagnosed with gastric carcinoma. Which of the following is true of gastric carcinoma?
   A. It is usually of squamous cell type.
   B. It is more common in females than males.
   C. It occurs most commonly in the body of the stomach.
   D. It is commoner in Europe than Japan.
   E. It has a positive association with *Helicobacter pylori* infection.

5. A 45-year-old man has developed iron-deficiency anaemia secondary to chronic bloody diarrhoea. A colonic biopsy showed the presence of ulcerative colitis. Which of the following is true of ulcerative colitis?
   A. It is characterized by transmural inflammation.
   B. It has a positive association with cigarette smoking.
   C. It is characterized by granulomatous inflammation.
   D. It is commonly complicated by fistulae.
   E. It is characterized by continuous disease distribution in the colon.

6. A 24-year-old woman presents with weight loss and vague abdominal discomfort for 2 years. Endoscopy with duodenal biopsy suggests coeliac disease, which is confirmed by serological tests. Which of the following is true of coeliac disease?
   A. It is caused by a normal immune response to gluten.
   B. It is associated with intestinal villous hypertrophy.
   C. It most commonly affects the large intestine.
   D. Anti-endomysial antibodies are a useful blood test to aid diagnosis.
   E. It is associated with HLA-B27.

7. A 67-year-old man has a positive faecal occult blood test. He is referred for colonoscopy which identifies three polyps in his sigmoid colon. These are biopsied—two show high-grade dysplasia and the third shows a well-differentiated adenocarcinoma. Which of the following is true of colorectal carcinoma?
   A. It is often a progression from adenoma.
   B. Familial adenomatous polyposis patients rarely develop colorectal cancer if untreated.
   C. It is staged by the Breslow system.
   D. It usually presents earlier if affecting the right (ascending) colon.
   E. It most commonly develops in the caecum.

8. A 32-year-old man presents to A&E alarmed as he passed bright red blood after defaecation. It was painless and he only became aware when he saw it in the toilet. He reports no other symptoms. What is the most likely diagnosis?
   A. Anal fissure.
   B. Haemorrhoids.
   C. Rectal carcinoma.
   D. Perianal haematoma.
   E. Proctalgia fugax.

Chapter 12 Pathology of the hepatopancreaticobiliary system

1. Which of the following is true of liver cirrhosis?
   A. It is a reversible condition in which the liver's normal architecture is diffusely replaced by nodules.
   B. A rare cause of cirrhosis is alcoholic liver disease.
   C. A common cause of cirrhosis is chronic autoimmune hepatitis.
   D. The normal architecture is replaced by fibrosis and nodules of regenerating hepatocytes.
   E. Prothrombin time is reduced.

2. Which of the following is true of Wilson disease?
   A. It is an autosomal dominant condition.
   B. It results from a mutation in a gene for the iron transporter protein.
   C. Free copper overspills into the blood and deposits in the cornea and the brain.
   D. There are no psychiatric symptoms.
   E. The liver is not affected.

3. Which of the following is true of hepatitis B?
   A. It is an RNA virus.
   B. It may be transmitted by drinking infected water.
   C. Initial infection is chronic in the majority of cases.
   D. Vaccination utilizes the hepatitis B surface antigen (HbsAg).
   E. Cirrhosis and hepatocellular carcinoma (HCC) are not complications of chronic infection.

4. A 54-year-old woman presented with increasing abdominal distension. Physical examination revealed an enlarged liver. Her serum α-fetoprotein is 40 times the upper limit of normal. Which of the following is true of HCC?
   A. It is the most common malignant tumour of the liver.
   B. It has a positive association with hepatitis A.
   C. It is more common in males than females.
   D. There is a median survival of 3 years following diagnosis.
   E. It arises from bile duct epithelium.

5. A 43-year-old woman is noted to have mild jaundice and some weight loss. Her alkaline phosphatase level is elevated, and she has a positive antimitochondrial antibody. She was subsequently diagnosed with primary biliary cholangitis (PBC). Which of the following is true of PBC?
   A. It is more common in males.
   B. It is not associated with autoimmune diseases.
   C. It rarely results in liver transplantation.
   D. It is strongly associated with ulcerative colitis.
   E. It progresses to cirrhosis.

6. A man presents with painless obstructive jaundice and weight loss. Imaging shows a mass in the head of the pancreas and a diagnosis of ductal adenocarcinoma is made. Which of the following is true of ductal adenocarcinoma of the pancreas?
   A. It is not associated with excess alcohol ingestion.
   B. It is more common in women than men.
   C. It commonly occurs in the tail of the pancreas.
   D. It is normally squamous in origin.
   E. It usually occurs in subjects older than 60 years of age.

Chapter 13 Pathology of the kidney and urinary tract

1. Which of the following is true of adult polycystic kidney disease?
   A. Only one kidney is affected.
   B. It is an inherited autosomal recessive disease.
   C. There are no vascular associations.
   D. Enlarging cysts replace and compress functioning renal parenchyma.
   E. There are no liver associations.

2. Which of the following is true in glomerular disease?
   A. Nephrotic syndrome in an adult is strongly suggestive of minimal change nephropathy.
   B. Most cases of membranous glomerulonephritis have an identifiable cause.
   C. Minimal change disease rapidly progresses to renal failure in children.
   D. A proliferative glomerulonephritis with autoantibodies against type III collagen is indicative of Goodpasture syndrome.
   E. Streptococcal sore throat may be a cause of glomerulonephritis.

3. Which of the following is true of renal cell carcinoma (RCC)?
   A. It invades the renal artery.
   B. Polycythaemia can occur as a paraneoplastic syndrome.
   C. Proteinuria is a common presenting feature.
   D. It appears brown with a central scar.
   E. The most common type is papillary RCC.

4. A 67-year-old man presents with painless haematuria. Urine cytology shows single atypical cells with hyperchromatic nuclei. Cystoscopy is performed and shows a papillary lesion. This is biopsied and a diagnosis of papillary urothelial carcinoma is made. Which of the following is true of bladder cancer?
   A. It is largely a disease of women.
   B. It is usually a squamous cell carcinoma.
   C. It does not cause urinary obstruction.
   D. It most commonly arises at the base of the trigone and around the ureteric orifices.
   E. It is not linked to exposure to environmental carcinogens.

Chapter 14 Pathology of the endocrine system

1. Which of the following is true of Graves disease?
   A. It is equally common in males and females.
   B. A minority of individuals are positive for thyroid-stimulating hormone (TSH)-receptor antibodies in their serum.
   C. It causes no change in the thyroid gland.
   D. Only a minority of individuals show signs of exophthalmos.
   E. It causes the same change in thyroid hormone levels as Hashimoto thyroiditis.

2. Which of the following is true of malignant thyroid tumours?
   A. They include toxic adenomas.
   B. They may be caused by childhood radiation exposure.

C. Papillary carcinomas tend to be found in elderly patients.
D. Medullary carcinoma is derived from thyroxine-secreting cells.
E. Anaplastic carcinoma is not associated with a history of multinodular goitre.

3. Which of the following are causes of Cushing syndrome:
   A. Addison disease
   B. Corticosteroid administration
   C. Sheehan syndrome
   D. Phaeochromocytomas
   E. Waterhouse–Friderichsen syndrome

4. Which of the following is true of type 1 diabetes mellitus?
   A. It is not an autoimmune-induced disorder.
   B. It has no genetic predisposition.
   C. It is a disease of middle-aged/elderly onset.
   D. It shows destruction of insulin-secreting cells of the islets of Langerhans.
   E. It shows plasma insulin levels that are raised or normal.

5. Which of the following is true of type 2 diabetes mellitus (DM)?
   A. It is a disease most commonly of children
   B. It is thought to develop from tissue insulin resistance
   C. It is commonly treated with insulin in the first instance
   D. It may be complicated by diabetic ketoacidosis
   E. It is not associated with vascular complications

6. A 40-year-old presents with attacks of sweating and is found to be hypertensive. Abdominal imaging shows a solitary lesion in the adrenal gland. A diagnosis of phaeochromocytoma is made. Which statement is true regarding phaeochromocytomas?
   A. 10% are familial.
   B. The majority are malignant.
   C. They are a type of paraganglioma.
   D. They can be associated with multiple endocrine neoplasia (MEN) type 1 syndrome.
   E. They arise from adrenal cortex

Chapter 15 Pathology of the reproductive system

1. A 42-year-old woman from a developing country moves to the United Kingdom and has a Pap smear as part of the screening programme. She is diagnosed with carcinoma of the uterine cervix. Which of the following is true? Carcinoma of the uterine cervix:
   A. Is usually of adenomatous differentiation.
   B. Is preceded by cervical intraepithelial neoplasia (CIN).
   C. Is associated with serotypes 6 and 11 of human papilloma virus (HPV).
   D. Has no association with cigarette smoking.
   E. Has no association with HIV infection.

2. A 26-year-old woman is diagnosed with endometriosis. Which of the following statements regarding endometriosis is correct? Endometriosis:
   A. Is defined as endometrial glands or stroma occurring outside of the uterus.
   B. Rarely affects the ovaries.
   C. Is not caused by retrograde menstruation.
   D. Worsens after the menopause.
   E. Is progesterone driven.

3. A 24-year-old woman presents to her general practitioner with lower abdominal pain and vaginal discharge. She is diagnosed with pelvic inflammatory disease (PID). Which of the following is true?
   A. PID is a combined inflammatory disorder of the fallopian tubes, ovaries and peritoneum.
   B. Intrauterine contraceptive device is not a predisposing factor.
   C. *Pseudomonas* is a common aetiological agent.
   D. PID reduces the risk of ectopic pregnancies.
   E. PID is not linked to infertility.

4. Which of the following is true of breast carcinoma?
   A. It is the most common cause of death in women aged over 60 years of age.
   B. Predisposing factors include mutation of *BRCA1* and *BRCA2* genes.
   C. Screening is not carried out in the United Kingdom.
   D. Tamoxifen can be used if oestrogen-receptor negative.
   E. Ductal carcinoma is the rarest type.

5. A 76-year-old man presents with urinary retention. He had a digital rectal examination which revealed an enlarged prostate with a craggy nodular feel. Biopsy confirmed malignancy. Which of the following is true of prostate carcinoma?
   A. It is a squamous cell carcinoma.
   B. It affects the central zone of prostate.
   C. It is more likely to cause urinary symptoms than benign prostatic hyperplasia.
   D. It rarely metastases.
   E. The majority have a well-differentiated glandular pattern.

6. A 45-year-old female presents with bloating, indigestion and weight loss. On examination, bilateral adnexal masses are felt. Ultrasound scan shows large,

bilateral solid ovarian masses with a small volume of ascitic fluid. The stomach was noted to be thickened. What is the most likely diagnosis?
A. Meigs syndrome.
B. Mucinous adenocarcinoma of the ovaries.
C. Endometriosis.
D. Krukenberg tumour.
E. Polycystic ovarian syndrome.

7. A 72-year-old female presented with postmenopausal bleeding (PMB) for 2 months. On examination, she was slim and no abdominal or pelvic masses were palpable. Hysteroscopy showed a thickened and bulky endometrium. Further work-up showed her to have omental cake; histology showed a high-grade carcinoma. What is the most likely diagnosis?
A. Endometrioid endometrial adenocarcinoma.
B. Endometriosis.
C. Serous endometrial adenocarcinoma.
D. Leiomyoma.
E. Pseudomyxoma peritonei.

Chapter 16 Pathology of the musculoskeletal system

1. Which of the following is true of osteoporosis?
A. It is an uncommon bone disorder
B. It is not a cause of pathological fractures
C. Microscopically, bone trabeculae are thickened
D. Diagnosis is by X-ray
E. Bones appear less dense on X-ray/DEXA scan T score of –2.5

2. A 56-year-old woman is on long-term corticosteroid therapy for severe rheumatoid arthritis. Which of the following is true of rheumatoid arthritis?
A. It affects 10% of the population
B. The likelihood of onset increases with age, therefore peaking in the elderly
C. All patients have circulating rheumatoid factor
D. It causes the development of a pannus with joint destruction
E. There are no extraarticular features

3. The mother of a 6-year-old boy notices he is 'walking funny' one day. He denies being in any pain. On examination he has a limp, but his range of motion is maintained. There is no history of trauma or fever. What is the most likely diagnosis?
A. Slipped upper femoral epiphysis (SUFE)
B. Perthes disease
C. Septic arthritis
D. Still disease
E. Osgood–Schlatter disease

4. Which arthropathy is associated with HLA-DR4 haplotype?
A. Ankylosing spondylitis
B. Rheumatoid arthritis
C. Psoriatic arthritis
D. Osteoarthritis
E. Reactive arthritis

5. A 68-year-old man presents to the accident and emergency department 'off legs' with back pain and general malaise. On further questioning he admits to difficulty passing urine and numbness on his buttocks. Blood tests show an isolated raised alkaline phosphatase (ALP). What is the most likely diagnosis?
A. Decompensated liver disease
B. Benign prostatic hyperplasia (BPH)
C. Metastatic prostate carcinoma
D. Alcoholism
E. Urinary tract infection (UTI)

6. Synovial fluid was aspirated from a swollen joint and sent to the cytology department where rhomboid-shaped crystals with weak positive birefringence under polarized light were found. What joint disease is this an indicator of?
A. Pseudogout
B. Gout
C. Rheumatoid arthritis
D. Osteoarthritis
E. Septic arthritis

7. A 68-year-old woman presents with long-standing pain in her right thigh which is persistent and dull in nature and relieved by ibuprofen. X-ray shows focal distortion of the normal boney architecture. Serum markers show normal calcium, phosphate and parathyroid hormone (PTH) with a raised alkaline phosphatase. What is the most likely diagnosis?
A. Osteomalacia
B. Paget disease
C. Metastatic tumour
D. Osteoid osteoma
E. Osteoporosis

Chapter 17 Pathology of the blood and immune system

1. Which of the following is true of amyloidosis?
A. Amyloid is a structureless polypeptide.
B. Amyloid is negative with Congo red staining.
C. It has no systemic effects.
D. The most common amyloid in reactive systemic amyloidosis is the AL type.
E. It may follow long-term haemodialysis.

2. Which of the following is true of leucopenia and leucocytosis?
   A. Agranulocytosis is used to describe severe thrombocytopenia.
   B. Neutropenia forms part of Kostmann syndrome.
   C. Leucocytosis is most commonly caused by an increase in lymphocytes.
   D. Leucocytosis always indicates infection.
   E. Basophilia is commonly seen in allergic reactions.

3. A lymph node biopsy was performed on a 45-year-old man who presented with a low-grade fever, night sweats and generalized malaise for a couple of months. He was found to have cervical lymphadenopathy. A diagnosis of Hodgkin disease was confirmed upon biopsy. Which of the following is true of Hodgkin disease?
   A. It is characterized histologically by Reed–Sternberg cells.
   B. It is more common in females than males.
   C. It is currently staged using the Rye classification.
   D. It has a better prognosis if B symptoms are present.
   E. The mixed cellularity type has the most favourable prognosis.

4. Which of the following is true of non-Hodgkin lymphoma (NHL)?
   A. It is not linked to immunosuppression.
   B. Gastric lymphoma has been linked to *Escherichia coli* gastroenteritis.
   C. The majority of cases are derived from T cells.
   D. Point mutations of susceptibility genes are commonly associated.
   E. Extranodal presentation is more common in NHL than in Hodgkin lymphoma.

5. A 67-year-old man was found to have numerous small, mature lymphocytes. A diagnosis of chronic lymphocytic leukaemia (CLL) was made. Which of the following statements is correct regarding chronic lymphocytic leukaemia?
   A. It is characterized cytogenetically by the Philadelphia chromosome.
   B. It is the least common leukaemia in adults.
   C. It has a median survival of 9 months.
   D. It is more common in females than males.
   E. It may affect lymph nodes.

6. Which of the following is true of sickle cell disease?
   A. It is caused by a point mutation in the DNA coding for the α-globin chain.
   B. It is more common in Europe than Africa.
   C. It is associated with gallstones.
   D. It is associated with hypersplenism.
   E. It does not confer resistance to malarial infection.

7. Which of the following is true of haemolytic anaemia?
   A. It can occur in rhesus-negative fetuses.
   B. It does not cause brain damage in neonates.
   C. When autoimmune, 'warm' type results in macrospherocytosis.
   D. When autoimmune, 'cold' type results in red cell agglutination.
   E. It is not associated with lymphoma.

8. Which of the following is true of microcytic anaemia?
   A. It is commonly seen in pregnancy.
   B. It is commonly seen in liver disease.
   C. It is a feature of renal failure.
   D. It is a characteristic of acute blood loss.
   E. It is commonly caused by iron deficiency.

Chapter 18 **Pathology of the skin**

1. Which of the following definitions are correct regarding skin pathology?
   A. A nodule is a raised lesion <1 cm across.
   B. A vesicle is a blister greater than 5 mm across.
   C. A macule describes a raised lesion of altered skin colour.
   D. A pustule is a blister containing clear fluid.
   E. Spongiosis means epidermal oedema.

2. A 25-year-old man present presents with oval plaques on his elbows and head. On examination, they are red with a silvery adherent scale. Which of the following is true of psoriasis?
   A. It is an infective condition.
   B. It is characterized by a reduced turnover of epithelial cells.
   C. It may be precipitated by lithium administration.
   D. It commonly affects skin at the antecubital fossa.
   E. It is not associated with pitting of the nails.

3. A 7-year-old girl with history of asthma and hay fever is brought to the general practioner, as she has been scratching her elbow and wrist as they are 'really itchy'. There is an inflamed, erythematous area, which is weeping. She is diagnosed with atopic eczema. Which of the following is true of atopic eczema?
   A. It is decreasing in incidence.
   B. It is less common where there is a strong family history.
   C. It is a type 2 hypersensitivity reaction.
   D. It increases in incidence with increasing age through childhood.
   E. It increases the likelihood of skin infection.

4. Which of the following is true of blistering disorders?
   A. Pemphigoid describes subcorneal separation of skin tissue.
   B. Pemphigus is associated with erosions.
   C. Pemphigoid has a higher untreated mortality than pemphigus.
   D. Pemphigus is associated with coeliac disease.
   E. Dermatitis herpetiformis involves granular IgG deposition at the dermal papillae of normal-looking skin.

5. A worried mother brings her 2-month-old baby to see the general practioner (GP) as she has noticed a red lump growing on his nose. The GP diagnoses a strawberry naevus. Which of the following is true of strawberry naevi?
   A. They are a type of capillary vascular malformation.
   B. They require prompt surgical excision.
   C. They are an early sign of immunodeficiency.
   D. They are benign and spontaneously regress.
   E. They are a common example of angiosarcoma.

6. Which of the following is true of melanoma?
   A. It arises from epidermal keratinocytes.
   B. It is associated with repeated intense ultraviolet (UV) light exposure.
   C. It has no increase in incidence with familial dysplastic naevus syndrome.
   D. It has a good prognosis with a depth of invasion of 3.5 mm.
   E. It never arises within lentigo maligna.

Extended-matching questions (EMQs)

Each answer can be used once, more than once or not at all.

Chapter 3 Inflammation, repair and cell death

Chemical mediators of inflammation

A. Bradykinin
B. C-reactive protein
C. Histamine
D. Interferon
E. Interleukin (IL)-1
F. IL-2
G. IL-4
H. IL-6
I. IL-10
J. IL-12
K. Nitric oxide
L. Platelet activating factor
M. Serotonin
N. Thromboxane
O. Tumour necrosis factor

For each scenario below, choose the most likely corresponding option from the list given above.

1. Released from platelets causing platelet aggregation and vasoconstriction.
2. Is a pyrogen in the acute inflammatory response.
3. Is a potent vasodilator derived from endothelial cells.
4. Key in macrophage activation.
5. Causes the terminal differentiation of B-cells to plasma cells.

Chapter 5 Infectious disease

Sexually transmitted infections (STIs)

A. *Burkholderia cepacia*
B. *Chlamydia trachomatis*
C. *Haemophilis ducreyi*
D. Herpes simplex virus
E. HIV
F. Human papillomavirus
G. *Neisseria gonorrhoeae*
H. *Plasmodium ovale*
I. *Treponema pallidum*
J. Trichomonas
K. *Trypanosoma brucei*

For each scenario below, choose the most likely corresponding option from the list given above.

1. A 28-year-old female with a history of pelvic inflammatory disease (PID) is trying to conceive. She has been pregnant once but unfortunately it was an ectopic pregnancy. Her past sexual history includes multiple sexual partners. The oral contraceptive pill is the only previous contraceptive method she has used. A routine vaginal swab as part of her initial investigations tests positive.
2. A 60-year-old woman is brought to the GP by her daughter who is concerned that 'mum is losing her marbles' and that 'she seems very vague about things and forgetful, which is not like her'. On questioning, the woman reports dizziness and blurred vision. On examination, she has multiple, nontender nodules over her skin and her daughter thinks that it might be the return of a rash she had many years ago. This was extensive with brown lumps on her palms, soles and chest.
3. A 55-year-old woman complains of an itchy vulva. On examination a white area is observed on her vulva, which is biopsied. The report is that of a high-grade dysplastic lesion with no evidence of invasive squamous cell carcinoma.
4. A 37-year-old African man presents to his GP with a painful ulcer on his foreskin. He has recently returned from visiting Africa and reports that the ulcer started as a red lump, which he thought was a spot as it contained pus, but it is now not healing. On examination, he has bilateral inguinal lymphadenopathy, which is firm and tender. His GP prescribes antibiotics and suggests an HIV test.
5. A 40-year-old man presents with rectal pain, passing blood with his stool and faecal urgency. On examination, he has tender inguinal lymph nodes and sigmoidoscopy shows proctitis. On further questioning he admits to having sexual intercourse with men.

Chapter 6 Molecular pathology

Genetic techniques

A. Chromosomal in-situ hydridization (CISH)
B. Fluorescent in-situ hybridization (FISH)
C. Flow cytometry
D. Immunohistochemistry
E. Karyotype analysis

F. Microarray
G. Nanopore technology
H. Next-generation sequencing
I. Polymerase chain reaction (PCR)
J. Pyrosequencing
K. Sanger sequencing

For each scenario below, choose the most likely corresponding option from the list given above.

1. Massively parallel sequencing technology.
2. Labelled antibodies hybridized to tissue sections.
3. Best method for detecting chromosomal abnormalities using fusion or break-apart probes.
4. Thermocycling reaction using deoxynucleoside triphosphates (dNTPs) and DNA polymerase which forms the basis of many genetic tests.
5. Technique by which most of the human genome was sequenced.

Clinically relevant mutations

A. *BCR-ABL*
B. *BRCA*
C. *C-KIT*
D. *EGFR*
E. *ER/PR*
F. *EWSR-FLI1*
G. *HER2*
H. *MLH2*
I. *p53*
J. *RAS*

For each scenario below, choose the most likely corresponding option from the list given above.

1. Mutation involved in Lynch syndrome.
2. Mutation present in 95% of gastrointestinal stromal tumours (GIST).
3. Disease-defining mutation in chronic myeloid leukaemia (CML).
4. If mutated, precludes antiepidermal growth factor receptor (anti-EGFR) therapy.
5. Can be mutated in breast and gastric carcinoma.

Chapter 7 Pathology of the nervous system

Neural pathology

A. Acute bacterial meningitis
B. Alzheimer disease
C. Extradural haemorrhage
D. Guillain–Barré syndrome
E. Herpes simplex virus encephalitis
F. Hydrocephalus
G. Meningioma
H. Multiple sclerosis
I. Subarachnoid haemorrhage
J. Viral meningitis

For each scenario below, choose the most likely corresponding option from the list given above.

1. The diagnosis in a patient with diffuse ventricular dilatation on CT scanning of the brain; patient has had ventriculoperitoneal shunt surgery.
2. A possible diagnosis in a 70-year-old woman whose husband complains that she has been getting increasingly forgetful over a period of months.
3. The diagnosis in a 23-year-old man presenting with rapidly developing focal neurological signs several hours after he sustained a head injury in a motorbike accident.
4. A condition that causes episodes of acute central nervous system (CNS) demyelination separated in time and space.
5. The diagnosis in a patient with an infection of the leptomeninges that has caused brain abscess. Lumbar puncture revealed a cloudy cerebrospinal fluid (CSF) with increased protein and decreased glucose.

Nervous system tumours

A. Anaplastic astrocytoma
B. Ependymoma
C. Glioblastoma
D. Medulloblastoma
E. Meningioma
F. Metastatic disease
G. Neuroblastoma
H. Neurofibroma
I. Neuroma
J. Oligodendroglioma
K. Schwannoma

For each scenario below, choose the most likely corresponding option from the list given above.

1. A 38-year-old woman was drunk and fell over, sustaining a head injury with retrograde amnesia. CT of the head showed no intracranial haemorrhage; however, an incidental parietal lobe lesion was detected. Appearances were of a well-circumscribed, dural-based lesion, 2 cm in maximum dimension with no underlying parenchymal infiltration. Flecks of calcium were present. Prognosis for these tumours is generally good.
2. A 9-year-old complains of persistent headache and has been vomiting in the mornings for 3 weeks. On examination he is found to have an ataxic gait and papilloedema. MRI of the head shows a mass within the posterior fossa arising in the midline involving the fourth ventricle.

3. A 35-year-old male presents with lower back pain associated with progressive pain and weakness of his left leg. Imaging shows an intramedullary tumour of the spinal cord.
4. A 40-year-old woman complains of a painful foot. A white fusiform mass is excised from the third metatarsal space. Histologically it is composed of fibrotic tissue admixed with Schwann cells and fibroblasts.
5. A 57-year-old female presents with photophobia, stiff neck, headache and arm weakness. Cytological examination of cerebrospinal fluid (CSF) reveals numerous groups of atypical epithelial cells. Her drug history includes tamoxifen.

Chapter 8 Pathology of the head and neck

Salivary gland tumours

A. Acinic cell carcinoma
B. Adenoid cystic carcinoma
C. Basal cell adenoma
D. Carcinoma ex pleomorphic adenoma
E. Kuttner tumour
F. Mucoepidermoid carcinoma
G. Pleomorphic adenoma
H. Squamous cell carcinoma
I. Warthin tumour

For each scenario below, choose the most likely corresponding option from the list given above.

1. This is the commonest malignant salivary gland neoplasm and is often associated with a t(11;19) translocation. It is the commonest salivary gland neoplasm in the paediatric population.
2. The commonest neoplasm of the salivary glands, usually arising in the parotid gland. It is benign.
3. This is an inflammatory lesion, not neoplastic, associated with autoimmune disease.
4. Associated with middle-aged to elderly smokers and may be bilateral.
5. This is an aggressive, malignant basaloid tumour.

Neck lumps

A. Branchial cyst
B. Carotid body tumour
C. Cervical rib
D. Cystic hygroma
E. Kuttner tumour
F. Lymph node metastasis
G. Lymphoma
H. Mononucleosis
I. Papillary thyroid carcinoma
J. Tonsillitis
K. Thyroglossal duct cyst
L. Zenker diverticulum

For each scenario below, choose the most likely corresponding option from the list given above.

1. A midline mass that moves upwards with tongue protrusion.
2. The parents of a 1-year-old boy notice a lump on his neck. On examination, the lump is nontender and located within the posterior triangle. He is otherwise well.
3. A 50-year-old man presents with pain and tingling in his left arm and the left side of his neck following a fall. He also reports weakness in the left arm. On examination he has a palpable lump at the left base of his neck. He reports that it has 'always been there'.
4. A 20-year-old student returns from university with a painful sore throat and extreme fatigue. On examination, her tonsils are swollen to the point of touching and are coated in a membranous purulent exudate. She has diffuse and tender cervical lymphadenopathy.
5. A 25-year-old female presents with a nontender lump at the angle of the mandible. Her past medical history includes a 'stomach tumour' and a 'cartilage tumour' in her lungs.

Chapter 9 Pathology of the cardiovascular system

Cardiovascular pain

A. Aortic dissection
B. Acute ischaemia
C. Angina pectoris
D. Aneurysm rupture
E. Coronary artery spasm
F. Deep vein thrombosis (DVT)
G. Intermittent claudication
H. Myocardial infarction (MI)
I. Pericarditis
J. Thrombophlebitis
K. Varicose veins

For each scenario below, choose the most likely corresponding option from the list given above.

1. A 60-year-old cachexic male is admitted to hospital for investigation. He is profoundly jaundiced and his liver is enlarged, hard and craggy on palpation. He also has extensive tattoos. He is witnessed by other patients to collapse after exiting the toilet and is found in cardiorespiratory arrest. A crash call is

issued but resuscitation is unsuccessful, and he is pronounced dead.
2. The diagnosis in a patient with sudden onset chest pain, radiating through to the back between the scapulae, and who develops asymmetry of pulses in his arms and legs. Chest X-ray reveals mediastinal widening and a contrast CT shows the 'tennis ball' sign.
3. A 78-year-old woman is awaiting discharge in hospital when she develops sudden-onset severe leg pain whilst sitting in her chair, which is only partially relieved by morphine. On examination no pedal pulses can be felt. She has a history of atrial fibrillation.
4. A 57-year-old man has been complaining of nonspecific abdominal pain for a week. His wife hears a loud crash from upstairs and finds him collapsed on the floor. He was unable to be resuscitated. He had a past medical history of MI, peripheral vascular disease, obesity and diabetes. He was also a heavy smoker.
5. A 66-year-old male smoker presents with sudden-onset crushing central pain that radiates to his left arm.

Chapter 10 Pathology of the respiratory system

Solitary lung lesions

A. Chondroma
B. Congenital pulmonary airway malformation (CPAM)
C. Granulomatosis with polyangiitis (Wegner granulomatosis)
D. Hamartoma
E. Hydatid cyst
F. Lung carcinoma
G. Metastasis
H. Pneumoconiosis
I. Pulmonary abscess
J. Pulmonary haematoma
K. Rheumatoid nodule
L. Sarcoidosis
M. Tuberculosis

For each scenario below, choose the most likely corresponding option from the list given above.

1. A 68-year-old female, non-smoker, has a routine chest X-ray as she feels 'under the weather'. This shows a single round opacity within the upper zone which is described by the radiologist as a 'cannonball lesion'. She has no other symptoms. On examination there is an old nephrectomy scar in the left flank.
2. A 32-year-old female presents with fever, night sweats and weight loss. She has recently visited relatives in India. A chest X-ray shows a small peripheral nodule associated with an enlarged hilar lymph node. She is otherwise well.
3. A 67-year-old man with known chronic obstructive pulmonary disease (COPD) presents with worsening of his chronic cough and reports intermittent blood within his sputum and unintentional weight loss. There is no history of fever. Chest X-ray is difficult to interpret, but there appears to be a central cavitating lesion.
4. A 20-year-old student is found to have a well-circumscribed dense round lesion in the left upper zone on chest X-ray. He has no other symptoms and no previous chest X-ray for comparison. A biopsy is performed which is difficult as the biopsy needle keeps bouncing off the lesion. Histologically the mass is composed of hyaline cartilage.
5. A 45-year-old Afro-Caribbean man presents with shortness of breath and intermittent haemoptysis. He is found to have a coin-like lesion on his chest X-ray. Biopsy shows necrotizing granulomas surrounded by lymphocytes and plasma cells. Special stains for microorganisms are negative. Blood serology shows a positive cANCA with normal angiotensin-converting enzyme (ACE) and calcium. No hilar lymphadenopathy is seen.

Chapter 11 Pathology of the gastrointestinal system

Colitis

A. *Bacillus cereus*
B. *Clostridium difficile*
C. Cytomegalovirus colitis
D. Collagenous colitis
E. Crohn disease
F. *Escherichia coli*
G. *Mycobacterium tuberculosis*
H. Norovirus
I. Schistosomiasis
J. Ulcerative colitis

For each scenario below, choose the most likely corresponding option from the list given above.

1. A 20-year-old student has just returned from his gap year. He has been to South Africa and enjoyed the local food and swimming in lake Malawi. However, he now has bloody diarrhoea and abdominal pain. Stool cultures show 'eggs'.
2. A 32-year-old female experiences sudden-onset nausea and vomiting after having previously been well. Her last meal was a frozen chicken korma containing rice 5 h ago.
3. A 68-year-old male is admitted to hospital for treatment of community-acquired pneumonia. He is given co-amoxiclav (a broad-spectrum penicillin) and

improves over the forthcoming week. However, on the day of his discharge he develops foul-smelling watery diarrhoea and becomes unwell.
4. An 18-year-old female presents with weight loss, abdominal pain and bloody diarrhoea for 1 month. She is also suffering from backache and painful red bumps on her shins. On examination she has a tender mass in the right iliac fossa. There is no history of foreign travel or ill contacts.
5. A 38-year-old Asian man presents with fever, weight loss and night sweats. He has also had bloody diarrhoea and abdominal pain. He denies a cough or any chest symptoms.

Chapter 12 Pathology of the hepatopancreaticobiliary system

Microscopic features of liver disease

A. Ballooning degeneration
B. Congo red
C. Cirrhosis
D. Councilman bodies
E. Fibrosis
F. Macrovesicular steatosis
G. Mallory–Denk bodies
H. Microvesicular steatosis
I. Periodic-acid Schiff diastase-resistant-positive (PASD+) protein globules

For each question below, choose the most likely corresponding option from the list given above.

1. Suggests alcohol as the underlying aetiology of a hepatitis.
2. Characteristic change seen in Reye syndrome.
3. End stage of liver disease.
4. Pathognomonic liver entity seen in patients with α_1-antitrypsin deficiency.
5. Can have a chicken wire appearance in patients with alcoholic liver disease.

Chapter 13 Pathology of the kidney and urinary tract

Glomerular disease

A. Alport syndrome
B. Amyloidosis
C. Benign nephrosclerosis
D. Focal segmental glomerulosclerosis
E. Goodpasture syndrome
F. Membranoproliferative glomerulonephritis
G. Membranous glomerulonephritis
H. Minimal change disease
I. Postinfectious glomerulonephritis
J. Systemic lupus erythematosus (SLE)

For each scenario below, choose the most likely corresponding option from the list given above.

1. The likely diagnosis in a 5-year-old boy who develops facial swelling. Urinalysis reveals heavy proteinuria, but no blood. A kidney biopsy shows no abnormality on light microscopy.
2. The likely diagnosis in a 25-year-old man who is being investigated for renal failure. He is complaining that he is having to change the prescription for his glasses every few weeks to see clearly and that he is struggling to hear some sounds.
3. A 70-year-old woman known to have myeloma is found to have poor renal function. A renal biopsy shows amorphous deposits of pink material, which are positive on Congo red staining and show apple-green birefringence when they are polarized.
4. The diagnosis in a 55-year-old man presenting with haemoptysis and haematuria. A renal biopsy shows crescentic change and IgG deposits in the basement membrane.
5. A 25-year-old woman presents with general malaise, a malar rash and is found to have anti-dsDNA antibodies as well as protein and red cell casts in her urine. A renal biopsy shows glomerular crescents and 'full house' immunofluorescence.

Haematuria

A. Acute pyelonephritis
B. Calcium oxalate stone
C. Cystitis
D. Granulomatosis with polyangiitis
E. Invasive urothelial carcinoma
F. Lupus nephritis
G. Nephrogenic adenoma
H. Renal papillary necrosis
I. Squamous cell carcinoma
J. Uric acid stone

For each scenario below, choose the most likely corresponding option from the list given above.

1. A 45-year-old man presents with dull loin pain and haematuria. Imaging shows a radioopaque mass in the kidney.
2. A 75-year-old woman with diabetes mellitus complains of dysuria, lower abdominal pain and frequency. A midstream urine sample is positive for microscopic haematuria and cultures *Escherichia coli*.

3. A 35-year-old man with a history of renal transplantation is noted to have painless microscopic haematuria at a routine screening. Further investigation shows a slightly raised lesion in the bladder.
4. A 40-year-old woman who recently moved to the UK from Egypt presents to her GP for an annual review. A urine dipstick test is positive for blood. Urine cytology shows atypical keratinizing cells and a Schistosoma ovum.
5. A 52-year-old woman with sickle cell disease and recent acute painful crisis presents with fever, flank pain and haematuria. Urine culture is negative.

Chapter 14 Pathology of the endocrine system

Endocrine neoplasia

A. Adrenal cortical carcinoma
B. Adrenal cortical adenoma
C. Adrenal cortical nodular hyperplasia
D. Neuroendocrine tumour
E. Parathyroid adenoma
F. Parathyroid carcinoma
G. Parathyroid hyperplasia
H. Papillary thyroid carcinoma
I. Phaeochromocytoma
J. Pituitary macroadenoma
K. Pituitary microadenoma
L. Small cell lung carcinoma
M. Thyroid follicular adenoma

For each scenario below, choose the most likely corresponding option from the list given above.

1. A 66-year-old male presents with centripetal weight gain, muscle wasting of his arms and legs, abdominal striae and a 'swollen' face. He has a persistent cough and smokes 30 cigarettes per day. He is not currently taking any medication.
2. A 40-year-old female complains of new-onset abdominal pain. She is also struggling to sleep at night due to thirst and the need to drink. On blood biochemistry, parathyroid hormone (PTH) and calcium are high. A diagnosis of hyperparathyroidism is made. Imaging shows a single enlarged parathyroid gland, which is excised with difficultly. Histological assessment demonstrates a tumour composed of epithelial cells encased in a thick capsule traversed by broad fibrous trabeculae. The tumour invades the capsule and adjacent blood vessels.
3. A 40-year-old woman presents with a thyroid nodule. Fine needle aspiration (FNA) is inconclusive so a diagnostic lobectomy is performed. On macroscopic dissection, a well-circumscribed but unencapsulated white lesion is seen. Histology shows follicular cells arranged around fibrovascular cores with the nuclei appearing optically clear or with grooves.
4. A 50-year-old female presents with bitemporal hemianopia and a mild increase in prolactin.
5. A 58-year-old male undergoes a full body scan as part of a health assessment. He is otherwise fit, well and asymptomatic. The scan shows a single, homogenous 2-cm nodule within the left adrenal gland but is otherwise normal.

Chapter 15 Pathology of the reproductive system

Cervical and uterine pathology

A. Adenomyosis
B. Benign ovarian cyst
C. Cervical cancer
D. Choriocarcinoma
E. Complete mole
F. Ectopic pregnancy
G. Endometrial cancer
H. Endometriosis
I. Fibroids
J. Ovarian cancer

For each scenario below, choose the most likely corresponding option from the list given above.

1. A 56-year-old woman presents with persistent painless bloating. What is the most likely diagnosis?
2. A 36-year-old woman presents to her general practitioner with extremely heavy periods. She is referred to her gynaecologist and an ultrasound scan is performed. She is diagnosed with the commonest uterine tumour.
3. What condition that has the following risk factors: human papilloma virus (HPV) infection, multiple sexual partners and smoking?
4. A 32-year-old woman with a history of molar pregnancy presents with vaginal bleeding. She is diagnosed with a malignant tumour of trophoblastic tissue.
5. A 24-year-old female complains of severe lower abdominal pain that came on very suddenly, and shows signs of cardiovascular collapse and shock. What is the most likely diagnosis?

Chapter 16 Pathology of the musculoskeletal system

Bone lesions

A. Achondroplasia
B. Metastatic disease

C. Osteoarthritis
D. Osteogenesis imperfecta
E. Osteoid osteoma
F. Osteopetrosis
G. Osteoporosis
H. Osteosarcoma
I. Paget disease
J. Rheumatoid arthritis

For each scenario below, choose the most likely corresponding option from the list given above.

1. The most common primary tumour found in bones.
2. The likely diagnosis in a 60-year-old man presenting with bone pain of the femur. On X-ray of the affected bone, alternating areas of increased and decreased bone density are seen. Blood tests are normal with the exception of a highly elevated alkaline phosphatase.
3. A degenerative disease of articular cartilage.
4. The term given for a group of hereditary disorders that result in abnormal type I collagen formation.
5. The majority of these lesions occur around the knee with increasing pain. They characteristically demonstrate 'sunburst' type periosteal reaction.

Muscle weakness

A. Becker muscular dystrophy
B. Botulism
C. Dermatomyositis
D. Duchenne muscular dystrophy
E. Eaton–Lambert syndrome
F. Inclusion body myositis
G. Myasthenia gravis
H. Myotonic muscular dystrophy
I. Neurofibromatosis
J. Polymyositis

Match these characteristic descriptions to the conditions they represent.

1. Proximal muscle weakness that improves on exercise.
2. Proximal muscle weakness that worsens on exercise.
3. Early childhood onset of proximal muscle weakness associated with a high creatinine phosphokinase (CK) and pseudohypertrophy of the calves.
4. Symmetrical weakness and pain of the proximal limb muscles.
5. Late childhood onset of proximal muscle weakness with walking maintained into adulthood.

Chapter 17 Pathology of the blood and immune system

Autoimmune disease

A. Antiphospholipid syndrome
B. Diffuse cutaneous systemic sclerosis
C. Limited cutaneous systemic sclerosis
D. Lupus pernio
E. Rheumatoid disease
F. Sjögren syndrome
G. Systemic lupus erythematosus (SLE)
H. Systemic sclerosis

For each scenario below, choose the option that corresponds best from the list given above.

1. The condition for which positive dsDNA antibodies are most specific.
2. A condition associated with recurrent miscarriages.
3. A condition in which the gold standard diagnosis is by lip biopsy.
4. A condition where antibodies against Fc region of IgG are found in 75% of cases.
5. A condition in which Scl70 (topoisomerase I) is positive.

Haematological disorders

A. Acute myeloid leukaemia
B. Chronic lymphocytic leukaemia
C. Chronic myeloid leukaemia
D. Hairy cell leukaemia
E. Hodgkin lymphoma
F. Idiopathic thrombocytopenic purpura
G. Multiple myeloma
H. Myelofibrosis
I. Non-Hodgkin lymphoma

For each scenario below, choose the option that corresponds best from the list given above.

1. A disorder in which the Philadelphia chromosome abnormality is detected within affected cells.
2. A disease characterized by the development of Reed–Sternberg cells.
3. The likely diagnosis in a 50-year-old male who presents with worsening back pain and persistent tiredness. Bone imaging shows lytic bone lesions and serum electrophoresis reveals an intense gamma-globulin band.
4. This often produces a 'dry tap' on bone marrow aspiration.
5. The likely diagnosis in a 50-year-old male who presents with splenomegaly and pancytopenia. Blood film shows characteristic cells with cytoplasmic projections.

Chapter 18 Pathology of the skin

Skin infections

A. *Bacillus anthraxis*
B. *Borrellia burgdoferi*
C. Herpes simplex virus (HSV)
D. Herpes zoster
E. Human papilloma virus
F. *Leishmania donovonii*
G. *Mycobacterium leprae*
H. *Mycobacterium tuberculosis*
I. *Staphylococcus aureus*
J. *Streptococcus pyogenes*
K. *Treponema pallidum*

For each scenario below, choose the most likely infective organism from the list given above.

1. It causes a characteristic targetoid migratory rash.
2. It is a vesicular rash arising as a localized band in a 65-year-old. It is very painful.
3. These are corkscrew organisms, visible on silver stains, which can persist for years resulting in cardiac and neurological disease.
4. This can be described as paucibacillary or multibacilliary, and may cause a few localized nodules to widespread disfiguring disease.
5. This characteristically causes superficial erythema which is plaque like, most commonly occurring on the face.

SBA answers

Chapter 2 Postmortem pathology

1. B. Although intraoperative deaths and deaths in the immediate postoperative period are indications for coronial referral, an operation 3 months ago is not an automatic cause for referral to the coroner. Unknown causes of death and unnatural deaths, as in the case of morphine overdose or neglect, are always indications for coronial referral. Deaths in anyone who has not seen a doctor within the 2 weeks prior to their demise (even if they have a known terminal illness) also require coronial referral.

2. A. To write a death certificate, a doctor must have treated/attended the patient in the 2 weeks prior to death. Doctors do not need to be present at the time of death, to pronounce the death or view the body to write a death certificate. There is no monetary fee for death certification.

Chapter 3 Inflammation, repair and cell death

1. A. The neutrophil is the predominant cell type in acute inflammation. Acute inflammation is mediated by chemical factors. The duration of acute inflammation is a few hours to a few weeks. Chronic inflammation is characterized by macrophages, lymphocytes and plasma cells (involved in humoral antibody-mediated immunity).

2. B. Vasodilatation resulting in increased blood flow (hyperaemia) is a feature of acute inflammation, not vasoconstriction. Increased vascular permeability also occurs, caused by histamine and nitric oxide, both of which are chemical mediators of inflammation. Oedema (fluid retention), not diuresis, occurs because of transudation of fluid through the blood vessels and into the interstitium.

3. C. Oxygen free radicals are one of the causes of necrosis. Necrosis is an irreversible pathological response to injury. Necrosis does not maintain plasma membrane integrity, with spillage of cell contents into the interstitial tissue inciting a local inflammatory response. It is an energy-independent process, in contrast to apoptosis, which is energy-dependent.

4. C. Apoptosis can be either a pathological or physiological process, and usually involves single cells rather than whole groups. The cells characteristically appear hyperchromatic, fragmented and shrunken (apoptotic bodies). The plasma membrane remains intact, encircling blebs of the cell, which are engulfed by neighbouring cells or macrophages, with no inflammatory response. Endonucleases cleave DNA, which is an energy-dependent process. Proteases cleave proteins. DNA damage is usually the initiating event, not Golgi body disintegration.

5. D. Fat necrosis can be seen after trauma to the breast, usually presenting as a firm, painless, palpable mass which clinically can mimic breast cancer. A history of trauma may not be apparent. Liquefactive necrosis occurs within the central nervous system. Coagulative necrosis is associated with ischaemia so can occur anywhere, especially in solid organs such as kidney, liver and bowel. Caseous necrosis is necrotizing granulomatous inflammation that is classically seen with tuberculosis infection. Fibrinoid necrosis is a special type of necrosis affecting blood vessel walls.

Chapter 4 Cancer

1. B. Anaplasia is the almost complete lack of differentiation of a cancer. It is associated with a poor prognosis and, by definition, an anaplastic cancer is high grade. Dysplasia is the disordered development of cells resulting in an alteration in their size, shape and organization. Metaplasia is the change from one type of differentiated epithelium to another and is an adaptive response to injury. Carcinomas are malignant tumours derived from epithelial cells; benign epithelial are called adenomas. Carcinoma in situ is severely dysplastic epithelium with all the features of malignancy except it has *not invaded* through the basement membrane.

2. A. Tumours originally arise from single cells that proliferate to form a clone of cells. As they develop additional mutations are acquired by different cells such that they are genetically heterogeneous. Lymphomas are all malignant lymphoreticular tumours and melanomas are all malignant melanocytic tumours; neither has a benign counterpart. Transcoelomic spread occurs across a body cavity, i.e., via the pleural, pericardial and peritoneal cavities.

3. E. Malignant cells commonly, but not always, have prominent nucleoli which can be large, multiple and sometimes eosinophilic (pink). Inconspicuous nucleoli are more commonly associated with benign tumours

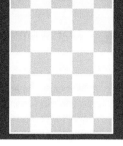

or reactive changes. Variation in cell size and shape (pleomorphism) and nuclear shape (anisonucleosis) are common characteristics of malignant tumours. As there are significant genetic changes in malignant cells the chromatin appearance is altered, commonly becoming hyperchromatic (dark). Malignant tumours have uncontrolled growth and therefore tend to be associated with lots of abnormal mitotic figures, e.g., tripolar mitoses, owing to genomic instability.

4. E. *p53* is the so-called 'guardian of the genome' and triggers cell-cycle arrest and/or apoptosis in response to DNA damage. Tumour suppressor genes encode proteins that negatively regulate cell growth such that growth is controlled, appropriate and the integrity of the genome protected. Mutations in tumour suppressor genes result in a loss of their function. Gain of function is seen in proto-oncogenes. Germline mutations within the DNA mismatch repair genes (*MSH6, MSH2, MLH1, PMS2*) cause Lynch syndrome, whereas mutations in the *APC* tumour suppressor gene causes familial adenomatous polyposis. Viral proteins such as HPV E6 can deregulate tumour suppressor function and hence some viruses are oncogenic.

5. C. *H. pylori* is a bacterium commonly found in the stomach. Its presence increases the risk of gastric MALT lymphomas and gastric adenocarcinomas. Benzene is an aromatic amine found in residual smoke, indoor air (secondary to paint and adhesives) and in crude petroleum. It is a chemical carcinogenic agent associated with development of leukaemia and urothelial carcinomas. EBV is associated with several types of cancer, including nasopharyngeal carcinoma, Burkitt lymphoma and classical Hodgkin lymphoma. MALT lymphomas are not known to be associated with EBV. HPV is another common virus, which has been linked to several cancers, particularly associated with HPV serotypes 16, 18 and 45. Cervical carcinoma, anogenital carcinomas and oral carcinomas are linked to HPV. UV radiation increases the risk of skin cancer: basal cell carcinoma, squamous cell carcinoma and melanoma.

Chapter 5 Infectious disease

1. E. Host cell lysis is a method of release of new viral particles. Budding from the host cell occurs with enveloped viruses. Viruses are neither prokaryotes nor eukaryotes but instead are obligate intracellular parasites. Viral genomes can be either RNA or DNA but not both.

2. D. Bacterial antibiotic resistance is very common and arises from a number of mechanisms, one of which is altering the antibiotic target site. Resistance can be transferred from bacteria to bacteria through extrachromosomal DNA called plasmids via bacterial conjugation, transduction or transformation. Although resistant to many common antibiotics, MRSA is still treatable (e.g., vancomycin).

3. C. *Pneumocystis jirovecii* (PCP) infection classically occurs in immunosuppressed patients (e.g., AIDS) and is characterized clinically by oxygen desaturation on exercise and bilateral ground glass perihilar infiltrates on chest X-ray. Cytologically, the yeasts are seen in fluffy alveolar casts. Silver stains are used for many things but are good at highlighting fungi and yeast, hence options A–C will all be positive with silver stains but the morphology (shape) will be different. Aspergillosis is a filamentous fungus so appears as long hyphae; it does not have an acute presentation. Cryptococcus is usually a neural disease affecting the brain. Both mycobacterial diseases listed are associated with immune suppression, but the clinical features and X-ray appearances are not consistent with them. These organisms are identified using Ziehl–Neelsen stain.

Chapter 6 Molecular pathology

1. C. PCR is the method used to amplify the quantity of DNA in a sample so that it can undergo further investigation. It is performed in a tube where the mixed reactants undergo several thermal cycles enabling polymerases to copy the DNA. The products can be visualized on a gel but this has now been superseded by using fluorescently tagged bases so that they can be read and recorded as a trace. PCR forms the backbone of some DNA sequencing reactions, but it is not sequencing. Restriction enzymes cleave DNA into pieces whereas PCR uses polymerase enzymes to form new strands of DNA.

2. D. RAS is part of the serine/threonine intracellular signalling cascade. It is associated with guanosine triphosphate (GTP) rather than ATP. It does not activate MAPK directly but instead activates RAF, which in turn activates mitogen-activated protein kinase kinase (MEK) and then MAPK. The most common isoforms are N-RAS and K-RAS; the 'B' form does not exist. No drugs to date have been produced that convincingly inhibit RAS, although it remains a potential drug target. Drugs have been targeted against RAF.

Chapter 7 Pathology of the nervous system

1. D. Hydrocephalus is an increase in the volume of CSF resulting in expansion and dilatation of cerebral ventricles. Obstructive noncommunicating

hydrocephalus is the commonest form. A ventricular shunt with one-way valve to the peritoneum can be used in the management. Congenital hydrocephalus, associated with Arnold–Chiari and Dandy–Walker malformations, may be diagnosed antenatally via ultrasound.

2. D. EDH is associated with a posttraumatic lucid interval that can last for several hours. Unlike subdural haemorrhage, EDH occurs between the skull and the dura and forms a crescent-shape on imaging due to limitation by suture lines. EDH is nearly always associated with a linear skull fracture, usually of the temporal bone. The artery usually involved is the middle meningeal artery. Prompt neurosurgery results in a good outcome.

3. C. Neurofibrillary tangles (tau protein) occur within neurones of patients with Alzheimer disease. Another characteristic finding are senile plaques of β-amyloid protein. Only 5% of Alzheimer disease is familial, 95% is sporadic. Alzheimer disease affects 15%, not 50%, of those aged over 80 years of age. Memory loss and emotional lability are frequently seen in Alzheimer disease.

4. C. Oligodendrogliomas are slow-growing tumours, typically occurring within the cerebral hemispheres, especially the temporal lobe. Gliomas are the most common primary CNS tumour, accounting for 50% of cases. Astrocytomas are more common in children than adults and tend to be low grade in children and high grade (i.e., glioblastoma) in adults. Meningiomas commonly compress rather than invade deeper CNS tissue as they are durally based. Metastatic prostatic carcinoma to the brain is extremely rare; it is more common to have metastatic prostate carcinoma of the spine.

5. A. Carpal tunnel syndrome is caused by entrapment of the median nerve resulting in sensory loss over the lateral 3.5 fingers (including thumb) with wasting of the thenar eminence and pollicis brevis. Sensory loss over the medial 2.5 fingers is seen in ulnar nerve palsy and wrist drop is caused by a radial nerve palsy. Trousseau sign is carpal spasm induced by blood pressure cuff inflation in hypocalcaemia. Tinel sign is positive in carpal tunnel syndrome where tapping along the course of the median nerve reproduces ‘pins and needles’ or pain in the distribution of the nerve. The cuboid bone is in the foot.

Chapter 8 Pathology of the head and neck

1. B. Nasopharyngeal carcinoma is usually associated with Epstein–Barr virus, which is endemic to North Africa and South-East Asia. Many cases present with cervical (neck) lymphadenopathy. Although associated with abundant lymphoid stroma, necrotizing granulomatous inflammation is not a feature. This may be seen in a lethal midline granuloma. Bony destruction in the nose is most commonly seen with olfactory neuroblastomas and nasopharyngeal angiofibromas.

2. C. There is a direct relationship between the number of cigarettes smoked and oral cancer risk. The lips are the most common site for squamous cell carcinoma of the oral cavity. The incidence is twice as high in males as in females. Moderate alcohol intake has been shown to decrease the risk of oral cancer. Oral cancer has a 5-year survival rate of about 50%.

3. E. Laryngeal carcinoma. All of the options are valid options; however, in adults a lump in the neck is metastatic carcinoma until proven otherwise, especially with a history of smoking. Squamous cell carcinomas are more common than lymphomas in the head and neck. Carotid body tumours are rare tumours and tend to occur in midlife. Tonsillitis would have other symptoms and tends to occur more frequently within children. Epidermoid cyst is a skin lesion—it is important to establish whether the lump is in the skin or deep to it.

4. B. Persistent hoarse voice for over 3 weeks is a red flag symptom of laryngeal cancer and requires urgent referral to an ENT specialist for assessment. Acute laryngitis is not worrying and is self-limiting; it usually occurs following an upper respiratory tract infection. Squamous cell carcinoma (SCC) is the commonest tumour both of the larynx and tonsils. (Note: tonsils are located in the oropharynx.) Subglottic laryngeal carcinomas have the worst prognosis as they have rich lymphatic drainage and so metastasize early and can invade paratracheal and thyroid tissues. Glottic SCCs have the best prognosis as they arise on the true vocal cords, cause early symptoms of hoarseness and have no lymphatic access. Papillomas are unilateral; singer’s nodules are bilateral.

Chapter 9 Pathology of the cardiovascular system

1. D. Small defects often involve membranous areas; larger defects also involve the muscular wall. Ventricular septal defects cause a left-to-right shunt because of the higher pressure within the left ventricle. The degree of shunting is determined by the size of the defect. Large defects are associated with Eisenmenger syndrome, whereby there is shunt reversal owing to pulmonary hypertension.

The pansystolic murmur of a ventricular septal defect is caused by high-pressure blood on the left side flowing to the right side. Ventricular septal defects are the most common of all congenital heart disease (25%–30%).

2. E. Coarctation of the aorta causes weak femoral pulses with radiofemoral delay. Hypertension is present proximal to the stricture, with normotension or hypotension distal to the stenosis. Coarctation of the aorta is more common in males by a factor of 2:1. It is associated with a bicuspid aortic valve in 50% of cases. Serious complications in severe cases include heart failure and aortic dissection.

3. D. It may be seen as a pathological response to endothelial injury. Atherosclerosis is the accumulation of lipid-rich material in the intima of arteries. It is uncommon in pulmonary arteries and is a sign of pulmonary hypertension. Atherosclerosis is more commonly seen in the aorta. Atherosclerosis is associated with hypercholesterolaemia, hypertension and diabetes mellitus. Macrophages take up lipid within a plaque to produce foam cells.

4. D. Hyaline change in the arterial walls results in hyaline arteriosclerosis. Fibrinoid deposition occurs in malignant hypertension. In benign hypertension, thickening and hypertrophy of the muscular media are seen histologically, and there is thickening of the elastic intima. Benign hypertension is characterized by stable elevation of blood pressure over many years.

5. A. MI results in necrosis of the myocardium following severe ischaemia. MI induces acute inflammatory changes. The infarcted tissue is replaced by a collagenous scar, not new cardiac muscle. Occlusion of the right coronary artery results in an inferior MI. Dressler syndrome is an autoimmune condition characterized by the three Ps—*p*ericarditis, *p*leuritis and *p*yrexia. It is a long-term complication that sometimes occurs following MI, usually around week 2.

6. A. Heart failure is where the heart cannot maintain adequate cardiac output. Left-sided failure is more common than right-sided. The progression of left-sided heart failure is the most common cause of right-sided failure. Heart failure may be a complication of myocardial infarction owing to ventricular remodelling. Heart failure commonly follows severe aortic, mitral or pulmonary valve disease.

7. B. Both stasis and turbulence predispose to thrombosis (one of Virchow triad). Thrombus occurs in flowing blood, a clot occurs in nonflowing blood, with the deep veins of the legs being the most common site (deep vein thrombosis). Portal vein (Budd–Chiari syndrome) and pelvic vein thrombosis can also occur. Antiphospholipid antibody promotes thrombosis, as seen in systemic lupus erythematosus. Factor V Leiden mutation is present within 5% of the population and confers a prothrombotic tendency.

8. D. ARVC has a higher incidence in Italian men and is the underlying cause of 22% of sudden deaths in sport in Italy. Symptoms of presyncope, palpitations and shortness of breath in an otherwise fit young person should alert you to possible cardiomyopathy. Hypertrophic cardiomyopathy presents with similar symptoms and there can be a family history of cardiomyopathy. There is nothing else given within the history to suggest restrictive or dilated cardiomyopathy. Takotsubo cardiomyopathy is rare, linked to intense emotional or physical stress and is seen predominantly in postmenopausal women.

9. D. In AF there is unsynchronized contraction of the atria, which can result in akinetic wall segments and turbulent flow, predisposing to mural thrombus formation. These are prone to fragment and embolize, hence patients with AF are anticoagulated to reduce this risk. Emboli can impact anywhere within the circulation to cause acute ischaemia, e.g., leg, brain. Right-sided hemiplegia results from infarction of the left side of the brain so pathology arising from a right carotid artery stenosis would cause a left hemiplegia. DVTs are within the venous system and embolization results in impaction within the lungs. A berry aneurysm, if it ruptures, will cause a haemorrhagic rather than an ischaemic stroke. An embolus from a mural thrombus within an abdominal aortic aneurysm is possible if the patient has a communication between the systemic and pulmonary circulations, e.g., an atrial septal defect. The embolus can then pass directly from right to left. This is known as a paradoxical embolus.

Chapter 10 Pathology of the respiratory system

1. A. COPD is characterized by chronic bronchitis, emphysema and bronchiolitis. Unlike asthma, it is incompletely reversible by bronchodilators. Like most obstructive lung diseases, lungs are hyperinflated in COPD. It is common in smokers but may occur without smoking in those occupationally exposed to dust or with α-1-antitrypsin deficiency. Emphysema causes permanent airways dilatation and tissue destruction without fibrosis.

2. B. Cigarette smoking is very important in the aetiology. Chronic bronchitis is defined as a productive cough

on most days for 3 months of the year for at least 2 successive years. Hypersecretion is associated with hypertrophy and hyperplasia of the bronchial mucus-secreting cells (increased Reid index). It is characterized by chronic inflammation rather than acute inflammation. Lung function tests show an obstructive pattern.

3. C. Bronchospasm, oedema and mucus plugging are commonly seen. Asthma reverses spontaneously or with bronchodilators. Asthma may be caused by a type I hypersensitivity reaction. α-1-antitrypsin deficiency is associated with COPD development. Bronchial smooth muscle hypertrophy may occur.

4. A. Repeat infections occur in the stagnated secretions with organisms such as *Pseudomonas* spp. CF is the most common autosomal recessive condition in Europe. Mutation results in a defective cystic fibrosis transmembrane regulator (CFTR), resulting in impaired transport of Cl^- ions. Malabsorption occurs owing to reduced pancreatic secretions (mucus plugs in exocrine glands). The most common mutation is the deletion of phenylalanine 508 on chromosome 7.

5. E. Lobar pneumonia occurs in a younger age group without any underlying lung disease and resolves completely. Red and grey hepatization are pathological stages of lobar pneumonia. Bronchopneumonia classically occurs in elderly, debilitated patients, or those with underlying lung damage. Resolution is not complete and various degrees of scarring result. Pneumonia is of bacterial origin in 80%–90% of cases, with Gram-negative bacteria associated with hospital-acquired pneumonia and Gram-positive with community-acquired. Empyema is pus within the pleural cavity and is a complication, not a type, of pneumonia.

6. D. Immunocompromised patients are very susceptible to tuberculosis. Tuberculosis is caused by the organism *Mycobacterium tuberculosis.* Pathogenesis is due to host hypersensitivity reaction to constituents of the bacterial cell wall. Predisposing factors include chronic lung diseases such as silicosis. Necrotizing granulomas which contain Langhans cells are the classic histological finding.

7. A. Adenocarcinoma is the most common subtype of lung cancer, having superseded squamous cell carcinoma as the most common type. Cigarette smoking is a major aetiological factor in the formation of lung cancer. Occupational exposure to asbestos increases risk of lung cancer and mesotheliomas. Metastatic spread is seen in 70% of patients at presentation, with pleural effusions being common owing to involvement of the pleura.

8. D. Peripheral honeycombing describes the appearance of a cut lung surface (or CT scan). Idiopathic pulmonary fibrosis (which presents histologically as usual interstitial pneumonia) is not an infectious condition. It is a restrictive airways disease which causes interstitial fibrosis. Idiopathic pulmonary fibrosis is one of the causes of finger clubbing.

9. B. Idiopathic pulmonary fibrosis is a type of interstitial lung disease which results in restriction of lung expansion. Other examples include the pneumoconioses and sarcoidosis. Restrictive lung diseases often result in a hypoinflated lung. Emphysema, bronchiectasis, asthma and chronic bronchitis are examples of obstructive lung diseases which result in obstruction of airflow, often resulting in lung hyperinflation.

10. D. Thromboembolism from deep leg veins is the most common cause of PE. Other emboli include fat, amniotic fluid, air, foreign bodies and tumour. The thrombus assumes the shape of the vessel in which it is formed, not the vessel in which it impacts. Mural thrombi of the left ventricle will embolize into the systemic circulation, resulting in ischaemia of downstream arterial beds. Ventilation/perfusion mismatching is a cardinal effect of PE, where alveoli are ventilated but not perfused because of vascular blockage. D-dimers can be positive in PE; however, they can also be positive in a variety of other conditions, e.g., after surgery, renal failure, infection. The value of D-dimers is in their negative predictive value (see Common pitfalls: D-Dimers).

11. E. Mesothelioma is a primary malignancy of the pleura and is associated with recurrent pleural effusions. There is a long latency between asbestos exposure and mesothelioma. Haematogenous spread is rare in mesothelioma. Mesothelioma is rapidly progressive, with death usually occurring within 10 months of diagnosis. The incidence has been increasing each year as the population ages and the consequences of asbestos exposure are realized.

Chapter 11 Pathology of the gastrointestinal system

1. E. Dysphagia for solid foods then liquids is seen especially when the middle and upper oesophagus are affected, whereas dysphagia predominantly for liquids is common in achalasia. Two percent of cancers in the UK are in the oesophagus. Squamous cell carcinoma is more common and is associated with heavy smoking and drinking. Oesophageal adenocarcinoma may develop from Barrett metaplasia.

2. A. Oesophageal varices are dilated submucosal veins in the oesophagus. They are commonly associated with cirrhosis of the liver. Rupture causes torrential bleeding and haematemesis. They are associated with portal vein *hypertension*. Variceal banding can be used in the management as a local measure to control bleeding.

3. C. Epithelial damage is mediated by the immune response against *H. pylori.* The gastritis is initially acute, but then becomes chronic. *H. pylori* colonizes the epithelium below a layer of protective mucus. Gastritis is most commonly found at the antrum. Infection often persists for many years.

4. E. Patients with antibodies to *H. pylori* have a higher risk of gastric cancer. The vast majority of gastric tumours are adenocarcinomas. Males are more affected than females. Sixty percent of tumours are found at the pylorus. There is an interesting geographical pattern, with incidence higher in East Asia than Europe.

5. E. Ulcerative colitis (UC) always involves the rectum, with continuous proximal extension for a variable distance, and can involve the whole of the large bowel (pancolitis). Crohn disease (CD) distribution is characterized by discontinuous skip lesions. Ulcerative colitis causes diffuse superficial inflammation that is limited to the mucosa, in contrast to CD, which is transmural, thus enabling fistula formation. Interestingly, smoking is associated with a decreased risk for UC and worsening of disease in CD. Granulomas are characteristically seen in CD.

6. D. Serum screening for anti-endomysial antibodies is a useful aid to diagnosis. Gold standard diagnosis is by duodenal biopsies whilst on a gluten-containing diet. The classic histological triad is subtotal villous atrophy, crypt hyperplasia and increased numbers of intraepithelial lymphocytes. Coeliac disease is caused by an abnormal immune response to gluten that affects the small intestine. HLA-B27 is associated with Crohn disease, whereas coeliac is associated with HLA-DQ2.

7. A. Colorectal carcinoma is thought to develop from adenomas. By the age of 45, 90% of individuals with familial adenomatous polyposis will have developed carcinoma. Colorectal carcinoma is staged using the tumour, node, metastasis (TNM) system; the Dukes system (A–D) is used for historical reasons. Breslow thickness is used to stage melanomas. Left-sided carcinomas cause mechanical obstruction to faeces and so present earlier, whereas caecal tumours present later with anaemia as the caecum can significantly expand to accommodate the growing tumour. The rectosigmoid colon is the most common site of colorectal carcinoma.

8. B. Haemorrhoids classically present with bright red, painless rectal bleeding seen either on the paper or in the toilet. The blood is not mixed in with stool. Perianal haematoma and anal fissures are painful. Perianal haematoma is of acute onset and there is continuous pain not associated with defaecation. Anal fissures are associated with hard stool and constipation, with pain persisting after defaecation and blood that can streak the stool. Rectal carcinoma is highly unlikely in this age group and other symptoms, such as weight loss, obstruction and tenesmus, are likely to be present. Proctalgia fugax is stabbing anal pain. No blood is associated with this.

Chapter 12 Pathology of the hepatopancreaticobiliary system

1. D. Cirrhosis is the nodular appearance of the liver formed by regenerating hepatocytes separated by bands of fibrosis. It is an irreversible condition with many causes. Commoner causes include alcoholic liver disease, hepatitis B and hepatitis C. Less common causes include autoimmune hepatitis, α_1-antitrypsin deficiency, haemochromatosis and Wilson disease. The liver produces many coagulation factors. In a cirrhotic liver, prothrombin time is increased because of reduced synthesis of these factors.

2. C. Complexed ceruloplasmin and copper cannot be secreted, causing accumulation within the liver, saturation of ceruloplasmin and overspill of free copper into the blood. Free copper is deposited in the cornea and the brain, causing Kayser–Fleischer rings and psychiatric/motor disturbances, respectively. Accumulation in the liver eventually results in cirrhosis. Wilson disease is an autosomal recessive condition of the copper transporter gene *ATP7B*. The ultimate definitive diagnosis is the weight of copper in dry liver tissue. Excessive iron absorption is found in haemochromatosis.

3. D. Vaccination for hepatitis B utilizes the surface antigen, HBsAg (Table 12.13). Hepatitis B is a DNA virus whereas hepatitis A and C are RNA viruses transmitted by the faecal–oral (including contaminated water) and blood-borne routes, respectively. Transmission routes for hepatitis B are blood-borne, sexual contact and vertical. Initial infection is subclinical and transient in 65% of cases, compared to hepatitis C where chronic infection develops in 70%–80% of cases. Cirrhosis and HCC are potential complications if hepatitis B infection becomes chronic; however, these are more commonly seen in hepatitis C. Hepatitis A does not progress to a chronic state.

4. C. Males are affected more often than females (8:1). Although HCC is the commonest primary malignant liver neoplasm, the majority of malignant tumours are metastatic (lung, breast, colon, stomach). Predisposing factors include hepatitis B and C, but not hepatitis A, which can cause acute liver failure but not cirrhosis (as it never progresses to a chronic infection). Prognosis is very poor, with a median survival rate of less than 6 months post diagnosis. It is cholangiocarcinoma that arises from the bile duct epithelium, not HCC.

5. E. Progression to cirrhosis invariably occurs in PBC. Drugs are ineffective and individuals eventually need a liver transplant. PBC is much more common in females than in males (10:1), and a strong association with several autoimmune diseases is seen, e.g., rheumatoid arthritis and systemic lupus erythematosus. Unlike PBC, primary sclerosing cholangitis is more common in males and is strongly associated with ulcerative colitis.

6. E. Patients with pancreatic cancer are usually over the age of 60 at presentation, with a higher frequency in males than females. The commonest association is excess alcohol consumption. Sixty percent of adenocarcinomas occur in the head of the pancreas, whereas neuroendocrine tumours of the pancreas are more common in the tail. Lesions are typically adenocarcinomas, not squamous cell carcinomas.

Chapter 13 Pathology of the kidney and urinary tract

1. D. Enlarging cysts replace and compress functioning renal parenchyma. Both kidneys are progressively replaced by cysts. It is an inherited autosomal dominant disease. Associations are with berry aneurysms of the cerebral arteries. Uncontrolled hypertension accelerates the development of renal failure.

2. E. Postinfectious glomerulonephritis may follow a streptococcal throat infection. Minimal change disease is the commonest cause of nephrotic syndrome in children, whereas focal segmental glomerulosclerosis is the commonest cause of nephrotic syndrome in adults. Between 80% and 90% of membranous glomerulonephritis cases are idiopathic. Children with minimal change disease have a good prognosis with corticosteroids. Goodpasture syndrome is indicated by anti–collagen IV antibodies and glomerulonephritis and is an example of a rapidly progressive glomerulonephritis.

3. B. Occasionally renal carcinomas may present with a paraneoplastic syndrome. The kidney is responsible for producing erythropoietin, which stimulates erythrocyte development. It is therefore not surprising that polycythaemia can occur in a neoplastic situation. Haematuria rather than proteinuria is a common presenting symptom; others include flank pain and a flank mass. The most common subtype is clear cell RCC, so-called because the tumour cells classically have optically clear cytoplasm. Papillary and chromophobe carcinomas are less common subtypes. Oncocytomas (benign) have a brown appearance with central scar whereas RCC has a yellow/tan variegated cut surface. Renal vein, not artery, invasion is part of the staging classification for RCC.

4. D. Bladder cancer may obstruct urinary flow as it commonly arises at the base of the trigone and ureteric orifices. Men are affected more often than women (3:1), and almost all cases are urothelial carcinomas; adenocarcinomas and squamous cell carcinomas are rare. Known environmental associations include aniline dyes, rubbers and cigarette smoking. Radical cystectomy is usually performed for lesions that show invasion into the muscularis propria (pT2). Superficial lesions are usually resected or given intravesical BCG therapy.

Chapter 14 Pathology of the endocrine system

1. D. Only about 5% of patients show exophthalmos. Graves disease is much more common in women than men (8:1). Graves disease causes hyperthyroidism, Hashimoto thyroiditis causes hypothyroidism. Ninety-five per cent of Graves individuals are serum positive for TSH-receptor antibodies (TRAbs). Diffuse hypertrophy and hyperplasia of the acinar epithelium are seen with follicles showing scalloped edges to the colloid.

2. B. There is a link between childhood radiation exposure (e.g., Chernobyl) and thyroid cancer. Toxic adenomas are benign tumours that secrete thyroid hormones. Papillary carcinomas tend to develop in younger patients and show a female predominance. Medullary carcinoma is derived from parafollicular C cells that secrete substances like calcitonin and serotonin. In about half of anaplastic carcinoma cases there is a history of multinodular goitre.

3. B. Iatrogenic administration of corticosteroids (e.g., prednisolone) can cause Cushing syndrome. Addison disease results in a hypofunction of the adrenal cortex. Phaeochromocytoma is a tumour of the adrenal chromaffin cells that results in the secretion of catecholamines (adrenaline and noradrenaline). Waterhouse–Friderichsen syndrome

is caused by adrenal gland haemorrhage resulting from *Neisseria* infections. Sheehan syndrome is infarction of the pituitary gland secondary to postpartum blood loss. Pituitary adenomas can secrete adrenocorticotrophic hormone and cause Cushing disease, not syndrome.

4. D. Histologically, destruction of insulin-secreting cells of the islets of Langerhans is observed. Type 1 diabetes mellitus is a disease of childhood/adolescent onset and is characterized by absent or low plasma insulin levels. It is an autoimmune-induced disorder, which may be triggered by a viral infection. Genetic predisposition is seen and there is an association with HLA-DR genotype.

5. B. Insulin resistance is an important first step in the development of type 2 DM. Type 2 DM is almost exclusively a disease of adults, but is increasingly being seen in cases of childhood obesity. It is commonly treated by diet and oral hypoglycaemic agents, although insulin may eventually be required in the later stages. Both macrovascular and microvascular complications occur in all types of diabetes and are a sign of disease progression. Diabetic ketoacidosis is a complication of type 1 DM.

6. C. Phaeochromocytomas are a specific type of paraganglioma arising from the chromaffin cells of the adrenal medulla. The majority are benign, not malignant. The '10% rule' no longer holds true, with nearer 30% being familial (Box 14.10). MEN 2, not MEN 1, is associated with phaeochromocytomas.

Chapter 15 Pathology of the reproductive system

1. B. CIN is a dysplastic (preneoplastic) state. The majority of cervical tumours are squamous cell carcinomas. HPV 6 and 11 are associated with laryngeal papillomatosis. Many HPV serotypes are associated with cervical carcinoma, but the high-risk serotypes include 16, 18, 33 and 45. Cigarette smoking has a positive association with cervical cancer. HIV infection has a positive association with cervical cancer due to its immunosuppressive action.

2. A. Endometriosis is defined as endometrial glands or stroma occurring outside of the uterus. The ovaries are a commonly affected site, others include the fallopian tubes, Pouch of Douglas, uterine ligaments and pelvic wall; however, it can occur almost anywhere. Retrograde menstruation is a common theory of aetiology. Endometriosis is oestrogen dependent and therefore improves after the menopause.

3. A. PID is a disorder of the fallopian tubes, ovaries and peritoneum. Predisposing factors include intrauterine contraceptive devices. *Neisseria gonorrhoeae* and *Chlamydia trachomatis* are common aetiological agents. Initially inflammation is acute; untreated PID may progress to chronic inflammation and scarring which increases the risk of ectopic pregnancies and tubal infertility.

4. B. Mutation of tumour suppressor genes *BRCA1/2* are implicated in some inherited cancers. Carcinoma of the breast is the most common cause of death in women aged 35–55 years. In older age groups, cardiovascular disease is the commonest cause of death. Screening by mammography is available for all women over the age of 50. Tamoxifen is an antioestrogen therapy which is used in oestrogen receptor-positive tumours. Ductal carcinoma is the most common histological subtype.

5. E. The majority of prostate carcinomas have a well-differentiated glandular pattern. It is an adenocarcinoma that commonly metastasizes to bone. Prostate carcinomas usually arise in the peripheral zone whereas benign prostatic hyperplasia is more likely to cause urinary symptoms as it affects the central zone.

6. D. Krukenberg tumour is a metastatic tumour to the ovaries. Whilst it can theoretically be any tumour, it is most commonly associated with signet ring type (diffuse) gastric adenocarcinoma. These diffusely infiltrate the stomach wall resulting in a thickened and rigid appearance ('leather bottle stomach'/linitis plastica). Unintended weight loss is always a red flag symptom and a neoplastic cause must be considered.

   Bilateral lesions of the ovary suggest a metastatic rather than primary lesion. Primary mucinous carcinomas are usually unilateral and cystic which makes this option less likely. There are numerous causes of ascites, however in the context of pelvic mass lesions they are suspicious for a malignant effusion. In Meigs syndrome a combination of pleural effusions and ascites are seen with benign ovarian tumours (commonly fibromas), which are unilateral.

   Polycystic ovarian syndrome, whilst bilateral, produces cystic not solid lesions, and is associated with weight gain not loss. Endometriosis can affect multiple organs but does not produce solid tumours.

7. C. Any PMB must be investigated to exclude a malignant cause. Endometrial serous carcinoma is always high grade and classically presents with peritoneal disease. 'Omental cake' refers to metastatic disease of the omentum. Endometrioid endometrial cancers tend to occur in younger obese women,

related to a hyperoestrogenic state. Pseudomyxoma peritonei is seeding of a mucinous tumour in the peritoneal cavity that produces copious amounts of mucin and commonly occurs from an appendiceal lesion.

Endometriosis is an oestrogen-dependent disease, which regresses after the menopause and would not cause a thickened endometrium. Leiomyoma is a benign tumour of smooth muscle that occurs in the myometrium and does not involve the peritoneal cavity.

Chapter 16 Pathology of the musculoskeletal system

1. E. Osteoporosis is very common, especially in elderly women due to lack of oestrogen, and is a common cause of pathological fractures, e.g., hip and vertebral crush fractures. Microscopically, bony trabeculae are thinned and reduced in number in osteoporosis with thickened trabeculae seen in Paget disease and in association with bone tumours. Plain X-ray changes include decreased bone density, biconcave 'fish' lumbar vertebrae and cortical thinning of tubular bones; however, 30%–50% reduction in density is required before changes on plain X-rays can be seen. The assessment of mineral density is therefore most commonly performed with DEXA scans.

2. D. Rheumatoid arthritis is an autoimmune condition affecting 1% of the UK population, with peak onset between 35 and 45 years, compared with osteoarthritis, which tends to present later (>45 years). A destructive inflammatory pannus is the underlying joint pathology, which can be accompanied by widespread extraarticular manifestations. Rheumatoid factor (RhF) is not specific for rheumatoid arthritis, with approximately 70% of patients having circulating RhF; anti-cyclic citrullinated peptide (CCP) antibody is a more sensitive and specific marker which is positive in 95% of patients.

3. B. Perthes disease is idiopathic avascular necrosis of the femoral head and is typically painless, in contrast to septic arthritis which is exquisitely painful, with refusal to weight bear and a reduced range of motion. Fever and localized signs of inflammation around the hip are usually seen in septic arthritis. Whilst SUFE is a possibility, these tend to present in an older age group (mean age 13 years) and are usually associated with puberty, periods of rapid growth and obesity. Still disease is acute onset juvenile rheumatoid arthritis that presents with fever, rash, stiffness and joint pain within multiple joints. Osgood–Schlatter disease is a traction apophysitis of the tibial tubercule. It presents in 12- to 15-year-olds with anterior knee pain and is usually associated with sport. It is, however, important to remember that pain in the knee is considered as referred pain from the hip unless proven otherwise.

4. B. Human leukocyte antigens (HLA) encode major histocompatibility complex (MHC) proteins which present antigens to T cells. MHC class II proteins encode for the HLA-DR serotype, of which the DR4 is a subgroup. The DR4 serotype is associated with many diseases, including rheumatoid arthritis. Ankylosing spondylitis, psoriatic arthritis and reactive arthritis are associated with HLA-B27, which belongs to MHC class I. Osteoarthritis is not associated with an HLA serogroup.

5. C. In a middle-aged/elderly man with an *isolated* raised ALP, metastatic prostate carcinoma must always be considered and excluded. Symptoms of back pain, leg weakness and buttock (saddle) anaesthesia are red flag symptoms for cauda equina syndrome which is a medical emergency and is a well-recognized complication of metastatic prostate carcinoma. Urinary retention and faecal incontinence are late signs in cauda equina. Urinary retention most commonly occurs with BPH and UTI. 'Off legs' is a common presentation of UTIs/urosepsis within the elderly. Numbness, however, never occurs and the patients will be acutely unwell with more common symptoms of frequency, urgency and pain passing urine (dysuria). Although ALP is included in 'liver function tests', it is important to remember that it also arises from bone. It is unusual to have isolated raised liver enzymes in liver disease, apart from gamma-glutamyl transferase (GGT), which is seen in alcohol consumption. In decompensated liver disease the patient is acutely unwell with global derangement of liver function tests. Alcoholism can cause peripheral neuropathies in a 'glove and stocking' distribution but not saddle anaesthesia.

6. A. Pseudogout presentation is similar to gout but it is due to deposition of calcium pyrophosphate dihydrate crystals (CPPD) in joints, whereas monosodium urate crystals (needle-shaped with strong birefringence, 'flaring' under polarized light, and yellow when parallel) are seen in gout. CPPD crystals can occur in osteoarthritis. No crystals are seen in rheumatoid arthritis or septic arthritis.

7. B. Paget disease of the bone is a metabolic disorder of increased bone turnover; therefore alkaline phosphatase will be raised. Osteoporosis is a loss of the bone substance, not increased turnover, and is not associated with pain. Serum biochemistry is normal and X-rays show normal bone architecture

with reduced density, not focal lesions. Osteomalacia causes global pain and weakness rather than focal bone pain. Characteristic features are Looser zones on X-ray. Whilst this could be a metastatic tumour, given the normal calcium, the X- ray appearances and lack of other symptoms make Paget disease top of the list of differentials.

Chapter 17 Pathology of the blood and immune system

1. E. Amyloidosis, characterized by the β_2-microglobulin protein, may complicate long-term haemodialysis. Although amyloid is composed of different proteins, it is not structureless as it forms fibrils that are arranged in large, nondigestible β-pleated sheets. These accumulate in the extracellular matrix and have systemic effects, especially in the liver, kidneys and tongue. The AA type is seen in reactive systemic amyloidosis; AL is associated with excess immunoglobulin light chain. Congo red classically stains amyloid brick red with apple-green birefringence.

2. B. Neutropenia is part of the autosomal recessive Kostmann syndrome. Agranulocytosis describes severe neutropenia. Neutrophil increase is the most common cause of leucocytosis. Primary leucocytosis occurs in bone marrow disease, e.g., leukaemia, lymphoma. Eosinophilia is commonly seen in allergic reactions.

3. A. Reed–Sternberg cells are seen in Hodgkin lymphoma. Males are affected more often than females. The current staging system used for Hodgkin lymphoma is the Ann Arbor system. Suffix B indicates the presence of systemic symptoms and a worse prognosis. Mixed cellularity with numerous Reed–Sternberg cells has a poor prognosis.

4. E. Extranodal involvement is more common in non-Hodgkin lymphoma. Many non-Hodgkin lymphomas have been linked to immunosuppression. *Helicobacter pylori* infection has been linked to gastric lymphoma. Seventy percent of NHLs are derived from B cells. Chromosomal translocations are a common feature of many lymphomas.

5. E. Lymph nodes can be affected with normal architecture becoming effaced by infiltrating cells. The Philadelphia chromosome occurs in chronic myeloid leukaemia. CLL is the commonest leukaemia in adults. It is indolent and survival of more than 10 years following diagnosis is common. Males are affected more often than females.

6. C. Chronic haemolysis may result in gallstones and jaundice due to free bilirubin. Sickle cell anaemia is caused by a point mutation in the gene encoding the β-globin chain. Mutations involving the α chains cause α thalassemias. It is common in West and East Africa, the Mediterranean and the Middle East. Hyposplenism is seen, as sickled cells congest the microcirculation of the spleen causing occlusion and local infarction, leading to fibrosis and eventually a nonfunctioning spleen (autosplenectomy). Young children (1–2 years) can have sequestration crises with pooling of blood within the spleen causing splenomegaly, haemoglobin drop and hypovolaemic shock. HbS confers protection against malaria by creating a hostile environment for the plasmodium parasite in the red blood cells.

7. D. 'Cold' type autoimmune haemolytic anaemia results in red cell agglutination and 'warm' type results in microspherocytosis, with red cell destruction in the spleen. Haemolytic anaemia is most commonly autoimmune but may be associated with lymphoma. Uncommonly high levels of bilirubin from haemolysis can cause brain damage within neonates (kernicterus). Rhesus-negative newborns cannot develop haemolytic disease of the newborn regardless of their mother's rhesus status, as they lack the rhesus antigen on their red cells.

8. E. Microcytic anaemia is commonly caused by iron deficiency. Women with heavy periods and vegans are particularly at risk of iron deficiency. Blood films characteristically show microcytic hypochromic erythrocytes. Pregnancy and liver disease can be associated with a macrocytosis, whereas renal failure and acute blood loss both produce a normochromic normocytic anaemia. Renal failure causes reduced production of normal red blood cells due to declining levels of erythropoietin and acute blood loss causes haemodilution of normal red blood cells on restoration of the circulating fluid volume.

Chapter 18 Pathology of the skin

1. E. Spongiosis means epidermal oedema. In a spongiotic epidermis, the intercellular bridges between keratinocytes are pronounced because of oedema. A nodule is a raised lesion >1 cm in diameter. A vesicle is a blister <5 mm across. A macule is a flattened lesion measuring <1 cm. A pustule is a small pus-containing blister, often indicating infection.

2. C. Lithium may precipitate or worsen psoriasis. Psoriasis is a chronic, noninfective inflammatory disease. The epidermal proliferation rate is increased 20-fold. Psoriasis

affects extensor surfaces, e.g., elbows and knees, but also the trunk and scalp. Nail involvement is common, with pitting and thickening of the nail.

3. E. Bacterial and viral infections complicate atopic eczema. The incidence of atopic eczema is increasing. Family history is a strong risk factor for the development of atopic eczema. Atopic eczema is caused by a type 1 hypersensitivity reaction. Atopic eczema decreases in incidence with increasing age through childhood.

4. B. Pemphigus is associated with flaccid blisters occurring within the epidermis which burst easily resulting in erosions. It has a higher untreated mortality than pemphigoid. Pemphigoid blisters are subepidermal (therefore deep) and do not burst easily. Dermatitis herpetiformis is an intensely itchy vesicular rash associated with coeliac disease and granular IgA deposition at the dermal papillae. Pemphigus and pemphigoid have IgG deposition.

5. D. Strawberry naevus is an example of a benign capillary angioma. Vascular naevi are vascular malformations present from birth, examples of which include salmon patches and port wine stains. Capillary angiomas have no malignant potential and spontaneously regress over time, only requiring surgical excision if they are troublesome, e.g., if they affect the eye or recurrently bleed.

   Angiosarcomas are rare malignant vascular tumours which uncommonly occur in the skin. Kaposi sarcomas are vascular tumours that are associated with immunosuppressed states, most commonly HIV. Remember that congenital immunodeficiency syndromes do not present until around 3–6 months of age, when maternal immunoglobulins, and therefore protection, begin to wane.

6. B. Repeated exposure to UV radiation may play an aetiological role. Melanoma is a tumour of melanocytes. Familial dysplastic naevus syndrome is a major risk factor. A Breslow thickness (staging of melanoma) of >3.5 mm has a poor prognosis, as do tumours with ulceration and a high mitotic rate. Lentigo maligna melanomas arise in preexisting lentigo maligna.

EMQ answers

Chapter 3 Inflammation, repair and cell death

Chemical mediators of inflammation

1. N. Thromboxane is released from platelets, causing vasoconstriction, in contrast to histamine and serotonin, also released from platelets, which cause vasodilatation. Platelet activating factors are released by endothelial cells and cause platelets to degranulate.
2. E. IL-1 is the interleukin most responsible for causing fever during inflammation.
3. K. Nitric oxide is released by endothelial cells, usually in response to increased sheer pressure, resulting in vascular relaxation and therefore reduced pressure. Platelet activating factor is released from mast cells and neutrophils, histamine from mast cells, serotonin from platelets, and the interleukins from inflammatory cells.
4. D. Interferon is released by T-helper 1 cells, causing macrophage activation.
5. H. IL-6 causes the terminal differentiation of B-cells into plasma cells. IL-4 causes immunoglobulin class switching in B-cells. IL-10 helps to downregulate the inflammatory response. IL-12 stimulates natural killer cells.

Chapter 5 Infectious disease

1. B. Chlamydia. PID can be caused by chronic infection with Chlamydia, which may be subclinical. Multiple sexual partners and unprotected sex are risk factors for sexually transmitted infections. Ectopic pregnancies are associated with PID owing to scarring of the fimbrial end of the Fallopian tube. Pelvic adhesions can distort the normal anatomical relationships within the pelvis, contributing to infertility. The other infections are not associated with PID. *Burkholderia cepacia* causes respiratory tract infection in those with cystic fibrosis.
2. I. Syphilis is caused by *Treponema pallidum*, a spirochaete bacteria, whereas *Trypanosoma brucei* is a parasite causing trypanosomiasis (sleeping sickness) and trichomonas are protozoa that cause vaginal infections in women. *Plasmodium ovale* is one of the causative organisms in malaria and is not sexually transmitted. Syphilis has three stages: the first is genital ulceration which resolves, then cutaneous manifestations (see Chapter 18) and, lastly, tertiary (gummatous) syphilis, which can cause chronic meningoencephalitis with progressive neurological decline (see Chapter 7).
3. F. Human papillomavirus (HPV) is the causative organism of cervical intraepithelial neoplasia and the majority of cervical carcinomas (subtypes 16 and 18). It also causes usual-type vulval intraepithelial neoplasia in women, and is at risk of progressing to vulval squamous cell carcinoma. With the exception of HIV, none of the other organisms listed above have been linked with carcinogenesis, apart from HPV.
4. C. *H. ducreyi* (chancroid) is a rare infection in westernized countries but is still common in Africa and south-west Asia. Differential diagnosis of penile ulceration includes syphilis, herpes and chancroid. Syphilitic ulcers tend to be painless and do not have any preceding lumps and no lymphadenopathy. Herpes ulcers are more numerous and in primary infection can be associated with fever and lymphadenopathy. It is important to ascertain HIV status as the presence of genital ulcers increases the risk of HIV infection. HIV is prevalent in parts of Africa.
5. B. Chlamydia can also cause lymphogranuloma venereum and can affect women as well as men. It is caused by different serotypes (L1–3) of Chlamydia. Frequency is increasing, and it is important to be aware of this infection as it may mimic inflammatory bowel disease (the treatment of each is radically different), and partners may have asymptomatic infections which may lead to infertility in women in the long term. It is commonly seen in men who have sex with men.

Chapter 6 Molecular pathology

Genetic techniques

1. H. NGS—pyrosequencing and Sanger sequencing are not parallel processes. Nanopore sequencing is still in its infancy and is not a parallel process (yet).
2. D. Immunohistochemistry is the work horse of most histopathology departments. Labelled

antibodies are used to detect specific epitopes as markers for different proteins. CISH hybridizes labelled DNA not antibodies to tissues. The remainder of the techniques are not antibody based.

3. B. FISH uses fluorescent probes which can look at the whole karyotype, but is most commonly used to detect chromosomal rearrangements. Karyotype analysis looks at all 23 pairs of chromosomes and can detect large structural abnormalities. It uses a Giemsa stain or fluorescence, but no probes as such are used and it is not as sensitive as FISH.
4. I. The temperature of the reaction mix is altered to allow cyclical DNA melting, primer annealing and extension to amplify the sample DNA; dideoxynucleoside triphosphates (ddNTPs) are used as chain terminators in Sanger sequencing. The quantity and quality of DNA available for testing is important as it can affect the result.
5. K. Sanger sequencing was used to sequence the human genome and, from this, new technologies such as pyrosequencing, NGS etc. were born.

Clinically relevant mutations

1. H. *MLH2* is one of the mismatch repair genes that can be mutated in Lynch syndrome. Others include *MSH6, MSH2* and *PMS2*. Mutations in these genes lead to microsatellite instability and the predisposition to develop a variety of cancers.
2. C. *C-KIT*. Other mutations present in GISTs are *PDGFRA, SDH* and *BRAF*.
3. A. *BCR-ABL*: known as the Philadelphia chromosome; whereby *ABL* (chromosome 9) is translocated to chromosome 22 under control of the B-cell receptor promoter and hence is constitutively switched on. *EWSR-FLI1* is another example of a fusion gene that is characteristically present in Ewing sarcoma.
4. J. RAS is involved in the downstream signalling pathways of EGFR. If *EGFR* is mutated, then blocking its action using drugs will block the divide signal. However, if *RAS* is mutated then the divide signal is occurring further down the pathway and EGFR blockers will have no effect.
5. G. *HER2* can be mutated in breast and gastric cancers. *ER/PR* are commonly mutated in breast cancer too, but are not present within gastric cancers. *BRCA* mutation is associated with inherited breast and ovarian cancer, but not gastric cancers. *p53* is mutated in a wide variety of cancers.

Chapter 7 Pathology of the nervous system

Neural pathology

1. F. Hydrocephalus. An increase in CSF within the brain that may be congenital or acquired. Often treated with ventriculoperitoneal shunt surgery.
2. B. Alzheimer disease. Memory disturbance is a common initial presentation of disease.
3. C. Extradural haemorrhage. This is almost always the result of skull fracture, with decline in neurological function occurring several hours after a posttraumatic lucid interval.
4. H. Multiple sclerosis. Diagnosis requires at least two episodes of CNS demyelination separated in time (i.e., recovery between episodes) and space (i.e., affecting different CNS areas).
5. A. Acute bacterial meningitis. Often presents with fever, headache, petechial rash and neck stiffness. CSF is cloudy because of increased neutrophils.

Nervous system tumours

1. E. Meningioma. These are benign lesions; however, they have the potential to cause significant morbidity/mortality depending on where they occur. Many are asymptomatic. Unlike the other conditions listed, meningiomas are dural-based rather than arising from the brain parenchyma or peripheral nerves.
2. D. Medulloblastoma. The history is that of raised intracranial pressure, which is common in posterior fossa space-occupying lesions. In a child, the differential diagnosis of posterior fossa mass lies between astrocytoma, ependymoma and medulloblastoma. Medulloblastomas are the second commonest posterior fossa tumour in childhood and occur in the midline involving the fourth ventricle. Astrocytomas are the commonest tumours, but are usually low grade in children (pilocytic) rather than anaplastic astrocytomas or glioblastomas. Ependymoma is also a possibility, but these are rarer than medulloblastomas and the rapid onset of symptoms would support an aggressive neoplasm. Oligodendrogliomas and glioblastomas are tumours of adults and preferentially affect the cerebral hemispheres. Neuroblastomas commonly occur in the adrenal glands, with 90% of cases occurring in before 5 years of age.
3. B. Ependymoma. This history is classical for lumbar spinal nerve root compression. Nerve root compression can be caused by a variety of conditions, commonly by degenerative spinal changes or prolapsed intervertebral discs. However, the young age of the patient

and the fact the pain is progressive points to a more sinister cause. Ependymomas can occur within the spine in adults and cause regional symptoms of nerve root compression. They are associated with neurofibromatosis type 2 (NF-2). In older patients, metastatic disease (especially prostate cancer in men) is possible and should be excluded. Intramedullary tumours also include (plexiform) schwannoma of neurofibromatosis. Meningiomas are more common in the skull.

4. I. Neuroma. This is the classical site and appearance of a Morton neuroma. It is not a neoplastic process, but rather a reactive one in response to trauma. Women are more affected than men because of poorly fitting shoes. The remainder of the tumours listed are intracranial neoplasms, apart from schwannomas and neurofibromas, which are found peripherally, and meningiomas and ependymomas, which can occur in the spinal cord.
5. F. Metastatic disease. The symptoms are those of meningitis plus a localizing sign (arm weakness). Meningitis has many causes apart from infection. In this case, the meningitis is due to malignant metastatic meningeal disease, and possibly a space-occupying lesion of the motor cortex. The clues to a neoplastic process are the cytology findings in the CSF and history of tamoxifen. Normally CSF is acellular and should never contain epithelial cells. Tamoxifen is an oestrogen receptor antagonist and is frequently used as an adjuvant treatment for breast cancer. Breast cancer is well known to metastasize to the CNS. Remember that metastatic brain disease is more prevalent than primary brain tumours.

Chapter 8 Pathology of the head and neck

Salivary gland tumours

1. F. Mucoepidermoid carcinoma is the commonest malignant tumour and paediatric tumour of the salivary glands. It is often seen in the minor salivary glands. It is associated with a t(11;19) translocation (*MEC1/MAML2* fusion gene).
2. G. Pleomorphic adenoma is the commonest tumour (benign or malignant) of the salivary glands and is usually in the parotid gland.
3. E. A Kuttner tumour is a nonneoplastic condition arising in the submandibular gland. It is caused by chronic sclerosing sialadenitis forming a mass lesion. This condition is associated with the autoimmune process known as IgG4 disease.
4. I. Warthin tumours are the second commonest salivary gland tumour. They are often bilateral and are usually found in the parotid gland, although minor glands may also contain this tumour. They are strongly associated with smoking.
5. B. Adenoid cystic carcinomas are one of the three main basaloid tumours (also basal cell adenomas and basal cell adenocarcinomas). They are highly aggressive and usually contain perineural invasion.

Neck lumps

1. K. Thyroglossal duct cyst. Thyroid pathology occurs within the midline. Papillary thyroid carcinoma can be asymptomatic, present as a thyroid nodule (moving on swallowing, not tongue protrusion) or can be fixed. A Zenker diverticulum is a pharyngeal pulsion diverticulum found in the anterior triangle. It occurs in older people and is associated with regurgitation of food and gurgling within the neck.
2. D. Cystic hygroma. These occur within the posterior triangle along with cervical ribs and lymph nodes. Branchial cleft cysts occur in the anterior triangle. As the child is 1-year-old, the lump is highly unlikely to be malignant. A reactive lymph node is a possibility; however, there are no symptoms or signs of infection and reactive lymph nodes tend to be tender to touch.
3. C. Cervical rib. The symptoms described are those of thoracic outlet syndrome, which results from compression of the nerves (brachial plexus) and blood vessels of the thoracic outlet. It is important to recognize these as they can be caused by various pathologies such as trauma and tumour growth. Cervical ribs are usually asymptomatic and may only declare themselves following trauma.
4. H. Mononucleosis. The description is that of severe tonsillitis; however, there are specific infectious agents that can cause it. The appearance of a membranous purulent exudate with cervical lymphadenopathy should prompt investigations for mononucleosis (colloquially known as 'the kissing disease'), especially as it commonly occurs in adolescence. It is caused by the Epstein–Barr virus and diagnosis is by the Paul-Bunnell (monospot) test.
5. B. Carotid body tumour. This is a paraganglioma arising from the carotid body. In this scenario it has arisen as part of the Carney triad where 'stomach tumour' refers to a gastrointestinal stromal tumour and 'cartilage tumour' refers

to a pulmonary chondroma; together with a paraganglioma they form the Carney triad. In young people with a history of unusual tumours, always have a low threshold for suspecting an underlying genetic condition or syndrome. Lymph node metastasis and lymphoma are valid differentials, although less likely due to the age. A Kuttner tumour is a fibrotic mass secondary to chronic sclerosing sialadenitis and the history does not fit with this.

Chapter 9 Pathology of the cardiovascular system

Cardiovascular pain

1. F. DVT. Clinically this patient has presented with an advanced malignancy (until proven otherwise) as evidenced by cachexia and a liver that is likely to be full of malignant disease. Tattoos raise the possibility of hepatitis C, which is a risk factor for hepatocellular carcinoma. Any form of malignancy increases the risk of thrombosis. It is a classical scenario whereby patients literally 'drop dead' of massive pulmonary emboli after visiting the toilet. In all of the other scenarios, pain is felt, except for varicose veins, which tend to produce heaviness and aching; they may become painful if thrombophlebitis is present. They carry a small risk of thrombosis; however, massive pulmonary emboli are more likely to arise from the deep veins. DVT can cause acute calf pain and swelling but can be asymptomatic.
2. A. Aortic dissection. This classically causes central chest pain radiating to the back between the scapulae with pulse asymmetry. Chest X-ray may appear normal or show mediastinal widening, aortic knuckle distortion and left-sided pleural effusion. CT angiogram classically shows the tennis ball sign in the aorta, i.e., two lumens (true and false).
3. B. Acute ischaemia. The most likely scenario here is a thromboembolism to the lower leg arising as a result of her atrial fibrillation. Acute ischaemic pain is severe, sudden in onset and unremitting (unless the blood supply is restored). The requirement for morphine is an indicator that the pain is severe, and absence of pedal pulses confirms the arterial occlusion. This is an emergency. Intermittent claudication produces similar intense pain, but it is precipitated by exercise and relieved by rest. Varicose veins and DVTs do not produce severe pain.
4. D. Ruptured aneurysm. The abdominal aorta is the most common site of aneurysm formation. Aneurysms are usually asymptomatic unless they compress adjacent organs or begin to dissect/rupture. When rupture occurs then chances of survival are slim as exsanguination occurs rapidly. His medical history indicates that he is a vasculopath and therefore primed for vascular accidents. Whilst sudden death from an MI is possible, the key here is the subacute abdominal pain. Coronary artery spasm does not usually result in an MI/death and, whilst a DVT can cause sudden death, he has no risk factors for this and there is no mention of leg pain.
5. H. MI. This is a classical presentation of MI with the classical risk factors of male gender and smoking. MIs do not always present with central crushing chest pain. Pain can be perceived in the epigastrium as 'indigestion' or discomfort, especially in those with diabetes.

Chapter 10 Pathology of the respiratory system

Solitary lung lesions

1. G. The lungs are a common site of metastatic disease and metastases are usually multiple; however, solitary lesions are not uncommon. The finding of a nephrectomy scar should sound alarm bells as, whilst nephrectomies are performed for benign conditions, they are commonly performed for malignancy. Renal cell carcinomas can re-present with metastatic disease many years after initial treatment. Classically metastases from renal cell carcinomas are described as cannonball lesions in the lungs, as they are well-circumscribed, dense and look like balls. There is nothing else in the history to suggest an alternative diagnosis. Chondromas are asymptomatic and, whilst a primary lung carcinoma is possible, she is a nonsmoker and the finding of a nephrectomy scar points towards a metastatic condition.
2. M. The lesion described here is a Ghon complex, which is seen in primary TB. Arguably it could represent a malignant lesion; however, the history, including foreign travel to an endemic location, is classical for TB and the age is too young for primary lung cancer. Hydatid disease is a possibility, but hydatid cysts tend to be larger and the clinical history is different. Congenital lesions will not produce fever.
3. F. COPD is highly suggestive of a significant smoking history and, with the presence of a mass lesion and haemoptysis in an older person, malignancy must be excluded. The location of the lesion and cavitation is strongly

suggestive of a squamous cell carcinoma (SCC), especially with a smoking history, as this induces squamous metaplasia/dysplasia which precedes the development of SCC. Differentials of a cavitating lung lesion on X-ray include abscess, TB, malignancy, septic pulmonary emboli, CPAM, sequestration, bronchogenic cyst and granulomatosis with polyangiitis et al.

4. A. Chondromas are usually incidental findings as they tend to be asymptomatic. Characteristically they are difficult to biopsy, likened to 'spearing a ping pong ball' because of their high cartilaginous/calcified content. The relatively young age makes primary or metastatic disease unlikely and favours a congenital benign process. There are no other symptoms to suggest any underlying infections or inflammatory diseases as possible aetiologies.
5. C. Granulomatous conditions of the lungs include granulomatosis polyangiitis with or without eosinophilia, TB, sarcoidosis, rheumatoid nodules and foreign body reactions. Granulomatosis polyangiitis and other small-vessel vasculitides are associated with p and c ANCA positivity. ANCA is not raised in any of the other conditions listed. Sarcoidosis is unlikely as, histologically, the granulomas seen are nonnecrotizing and lack a rim of lymphocytes/plasma cells. Serum ACE and calcium levels are also normal. Primary TB is possible but there is no history of fever, travel, ill contacts and no associated lymphadenopathy.

Chapter 11 Pathology of the gastrointestinal system

Colitis

1. I. Lake Malawi is notoriously infested with schistosomiasis so this history of swimming and colitic symptoms strongly suggests schistosomiasis. This diagnosis is further supported by ova or 'eggs' (from the parasite) present in the stool.
2. A. Reheated rice is classic for *Bacillus cereus* food poisoning; the rapid onset (1–6 h after ingestion) also supports this. *Salmonella* is associated with meat, especially chicken. *E. coli* is associated with undercooked meats, especially minced beef, animal contact or animal faecal-contaminated water. Norovirus is the 'winter vomiting' virus and causes significant vomiting as well as diarrhoea.
3. B. *C. difficile* infection usually occurs following use of broad-spectrum antibiotics, such as co-amoxiclav and ciprofloxacin, because of overgrowth of the commensal *C. difficile*, causing a pseudomembranous colitis. It is usually associated with hospitalized patients but can occur within the community.
4. E. Crohn disease. It is unusual for an infection to persist for 1 month so alternative causes of bloody colitis must be considered, e.g., inflammatory bowel disease. Crohn disease is favoured over ulcerative colitis as it most commonly affects the terminal ileum, resulting in a palpable mass in the right iliac fossa. Crohn disease also has extraintestinal manifestations of which erythema nodosum is one. Tuberculosis is in the differential, but no history of ill contacts or travel makes this less likely.
5. G. Tuberculosis (TB) is most commonly seen in the lungs; however, it is important not to forget extrapulmonary TB; the terminal ileum is a common site. TB is endemic to India and, with the classical history of fever, weight loss and night sweats, must always be excluded.

Chapter 12 Pathology of the hepatopancreaticobiliary system

Microscopic features of liver disease

1. G. Mallory-Denk bodies, also known as Mallory hyaline, when present in hepatitis point to alcohol as the causative agent; however, they are not 100% specific to alcohol. Other features of alcoholic liver disease include fibrosis, macrovesicular steatosis, cirrhosis, ballooning degeneration and councilman bodies (apoptotic hepatocytes). These changes are nonspecific and are seen in a variety of conditions. The key to the diagnosis is a history of alcohol use.
2. H. Microvesicular steatosis. Reye syndrome, sudden severe hepatic impairment, is a feared side effect of high-dose aspirin use in children/adolescents. Other causes of microvesicular steatosis include fatty liver of pregnancy and sodium valproate toxicity.
3. C. Cirrhosis is replacement of the liver parenchyma by bands of collagenous tissue with regenerative parenchymal nodules, giving the liver a shrunken and knobbly appearance. Cirrhosis is the common end stage of chronic liver disease regardless of aetiology and it is irreversible. The functional capacity of the liver is reduced; however, unlike end-stage renal failure, patients may survive for many years with compensated cirrhosis. Fibrosis can have different degrees of severity.

4. I. PASD+ protein globules. These refer to the bright pink staining cytoplasmic accumulations of the mutant α_1-antitrypsin protein in α_1-antitrypsin deficiency in periportal hepatocytes. Patients do develop cirrhosis, fibrosis etc.; however, these are nonspecific features and therefore not pathognomonic.
5. E. Fibrosis, which is perivenular and pericellular in distribution, has the appearance of 'chicken wire', which is visualized with the use of elastic stains, e.g., trichrome. It is seen in alcohol liver disease and other fatty liver diseases.

Chapter 13 Pathology of the kidney and urinary tract

Glomerular disease

1. H. Minimal change disease. This is the most common cause of nephrotic syndrome in children. The glomeruli appear normal on light microscopy and there is no immunoglobulin deposition. Changes (effacement of the podocyte foot processes) are only seen by electron microscopy. Membranous glomerulonephritis also causes proteinuria; however, this is seen in adults and changes are seen on light microscopy and immunofluorescence. Postinfectious glomerulonephritis usually causes haematuria.
2. A. Alport syndrome. A hereditary glomerulonephritis (85% X-linked) that commonly causes the triad of glomerulonephritis, deafness and ocular lesions. Renal failure occurs in the second decade of life in males. Goodpasture syndrome affects the lungs.
3. B: Amyloidosis. Myeloma is a well-recognized cause of amyloidosis owing to excess light-chain production. Nephrosclerosis is possible; however, amyloidosis is more likely in this scenario because of the history of myeloma and the Congo red positivity.
4. E. Goodpasture syndrome. Autoimmune disease targeting type IV collagen in both the kidney and the lung. Lung disease is not seen in the other conditions listed.
5. J. SLE mainly affects women and can present in a variety of ways. There are different types of renal involvement, one of the more significant being crescentic glomerulonephritis. It is important to detect this as it can lead to renal failure within a few weeks. 'Full house' immunofluorescence means that there is positive staining across the board for complement and immunoglobulins, which is characteristic of SLE and not seen in the other conditions. The malar ('butterfly') rash is classical but is not always present. Antibodies against dsDNA are highly suggestive of SLE. In Goodpasture disease the antibodies are directed towards the glomerular basement membrane.

Haematuria

1. B. Calcium oxalate stones are the commonest cause of urolithiasis. Unlike uric acid stones, calcium oxalate stones are radioopaque and can be seen on imaging. Flank pain is caused by distension of the renal pelvis.
2. C. Cystitis is more common in women than in men as women have shorter urethras. Gram-negative organisms like *Escherichia coli* and *Proteus* spp. commonly cause cystitis. It presents with the classic triad of dysuria, lower abdominal pain and frequency. Glycosuria of diabetes aids infection. Although acute pyelonephritis can be considered with this history, fever is a common presenting symptom, and pain is usually in the back.
3. G. Nephrogenic adenomas are benign urothelial lesions which may be found in the renal pelvis, ureters, bladder or urethra. They are often seen in young men and are associated with genitourinary surgery. Histologically, the lesions resemble renal tubular epithelium.
4. I. Squamous cell carcinoma of the bladder is less common than urothelial carcinoma. It is associated with *Schistosoma haematobium* infection, which is endemic to parts of Africa. Atypical keratinizing squamous cells may be seen on urine cytology, though it is rare to see parasitic ova on cytology.
5. H. Renal papillary necrosis occurs secondary to compromise of the medullary vasculature. Causes are often multifactorial. In this case, it is precipitated by both ischaemia associated with sickle cell disease and its treatment using nonsteroidal antiinflammatory drugs (drugs which increase susceptibility for papillary necrosis in patients with previous ischaemic compromise). With this history, acute pyelonephritis should also be considered, but renal papillary necrosis is more likely as urine culture is negative.

Chapter 14 Pathology of the endocrine system

Endocrine neoplasia

1. L. Small cell lung carcinoma can be associated with a paraneoplastic syndrome of ectopic

adrenocorticotrophic hormone (ACTH) production causing Cushing syndrome. Other paraneoplastic syndromes include syndrome of inappropriate antidiuretic hormone (SIADH) and hypercalcaemia. Functioning pituitary tumours can produce ACTH and an adrenal cortical adenoma can produce cortisol; however, the history of a persistent cough and smoking makes lung carcinoma more likely. Pituitary macroadenomas present with visual field defects.

2. F. Malignant parathyroid carcinomas are rare but classically are adherent and difficult to remove at surgery. Calcium concentration is usually very high, causing polydipsia (NB There are a variety of causes of polydipsia, not only diabetes mellitus and insipidus). Parathyroid hyperplasia classically affects all four glands and adenomas have thin delicate capsules with no invasive components.

3. H. Papillary thyroid carcinoma appears white macroscopically and, microscopically, follicular cells are arranged in papillae (which by definition have fibrovascular cores). Nuclei characteristically are grooved and/or optically clear. In contrast, thyroid adenomas are tan and encapsulated and the nuclei lack the features of papillary thyroid carcinoma.

4. J. Large pituitary adenomas can impinge on the optic chiasm causing bitemporal hemianopia. Mild increases in prolactin can occur due to the stalk effect (see Box 14.1). Microadenomas are too small to cause impingement symptoms.

5. B. Most adrenal cortical adenomas are incidental findings when the abdomen is imaged for other reasons or are found at postmortem, as the majority are nonfunctioning. In contrast, most adrenal cortical carcinomas are functional presenting with endocrine sequelae, e.g., Cushing syndrome or virilization in women. Carcinomas tend to be large (>12 cm) and replace most of the adrenal gland whereas adenomas are smaller (<3 cm) and contained within the gland. Adrenal cortical hyperplasia consists of more than one hyperplastic nodule within the cortex of varying sizes. Phaeochromocytomas are centrally located, symptomatic and tend to be larger (>6 cm). A metastatic lesion is important to consider. Common primary sites include lung, colorectal and breast. In this case, the rest of the scan did not show any other abnormalities, and metastatic deposits tend to be bilateral rather than unilateral.

Chapter 15 Pathology of the reproductive system

Cervical and uterine pathology

1: J. Ovarian cancer. Symptoms of ovarian cancer are vague. Endometrial cancer is possible, however this commonly presents as postmenopausal bleeding (PMB) and cervical cancer is likely to cause vaginal bleeding—blood in both situations comes from the vagina. Fibroids can cause bloating symptoms but are more commonly associated with menorrhagia. They are also oestrogen dependent so become less symptomatic after the menopause. Endometriosis is also oestrogen dependent and causes cyclical pain, not bloating.

2: I. Fibroids. These are benign tumours of smooth muscle (leiomyomas). They are very common. Endometriosis and adenomyosis are not tumours but ectopic endometrial stroma outside the uterus and within the myometrium, respectively.

3: C. Cervical cancer. The same risk factors exist for development of the premalignant state, cervical intraepithelial neoplasia. Risk factors for endometrial cancer are obesity, smoking, oral contraceptive pill, early menarche, late menopause, nulliparity. Risk factors for ovarian cancer include smoking, obesity and hormone replacement therapy.

4: D. Choriocarcinoma. This carcinoma is formed of syncytiotrophoblast and cytotrophoblast. The majority arise from molar pregnancies in females. A complete mole has a 1%–3% risk of developing into a choriocarcinoma.

5: F. Ectopic pregnancy. The implantation of a fertilized ovum outside the uterus most commonly in the fallopian tube. Severe haemorrhage occurs from tubal rupture.

Chapter 16 Pathology of the musculoskeletal system

Bone lesions

1. E. Osteoid osteoma is the commonest primary bone tumour, however, the most common tumours found in bone are blood-borne metastases.

2. I. Paget disease is uncontrolled bone resorption and deposition. It is most common in men over the age of 40 years. Metastatic diseases tend to cause an elevated calcium as well as raised alkaline phosphatase.

3. C. Osteoarthritis is a very common disease of articular cartilage degeneration compared with rheumatoid arthritis which is caused by autoimmune destruction.
4. D. Osteogenesis imperfecta comprises group of disorders (also known as 'brittle bone disease') which are characterized by the development of abnormal type I collagen. In achondroplasia, collagen formation is normal but ossification is deranged.
5. H. Osteosarcoma. Classically located around the knee. Sunburst appearance results from elevation of the periosteum with calcification secondary to underlying malignant erosion. Osteoid osteoma is benign and well-circumscribed. Radiologically, it is seen as a rim of sclerotic bone surrounding a radiolucent nidus.

Muscle weakness

1. E. Eaton–Lambert syndrome is important to recognize, as 40% are associated with lung carcinoma.
2. G. Myasthenia gravis; this condition worsens with exercise as the neuromuscular junction naturally fatigues over time; this is compounded by autoantibody-mediated postsynaptic loss of acetylcholine receptors. In comparison, Eaton–Lambert syndrome involves presynaptic blocking of acetylcholine (ACh) release which can be ameliorated by increased release of ACh quanta after repetitive stimulation. Botulism results in acute onset of progressive paralysis affecting all muscle groups and is irreversible. Myotonic muscular dystrophy results in progressive weakness of distal muscle groups and myotonia.
3. D. Duchenne muscular dystrophy (DMD): early onset of symptoms due to an X-linked inherited mutation in the dystrophin gene resulting in loss or production of an ineffective dystrophin protein.
4. J. Polymyositis: The most important feature here is pain with muscle weakness as the muscle is inflamed. Dermatomyositis has additional cutaneous lesions and has a stronger association with cancer. Inclusion body myositis affects proximal and distal muscles in an asymmetric pattern.
5. A. Becker muscular dystrophy is a less severe form of DMD. Mutations are in-frame such that a truncated but functional dystrophin protein is produced, equating to a less severe phenotype and later onset. Neurofibromatosis does not characteristically cause weakness.

Chapter 17 Pathology of the blood and immune system

Autoimmune disease

1. G. SLE. The most specific autoantibody is dsDNA and can be used to monitor disease activity; however, it is not positive in 100% of cases. Lupus pernio is a form of cutaneous sarcoidosis affecting the nose. It is not SLE, but confusion arises due to the misleading name!
2. A. Antiphospholipid syndrome is an important cause of miscarriage owing to prothrombotic state.
3. F. Sjögren syndrome. Lip biopsy is performed to assess minor salivary glands. These show lymphocytic sialoadenitis in Sjögren syndrome.
4. E. Rheumatoid disease. Antibodies against Fc portion of IgG = rheumatoid factor. It is not 100% specific or sensitive for rheumatoid arthritis and is found only in 75% of cases. Anti-CCP antibodies are more sensitive and specific. Rheumatoid factor is also positive in Sjögren syndrome, mixed essential cryoglobulinemia and primary biliary cholangitis.
5. B. Diffuse cutaneous systemic sclerosis. Scl70 is specific but not sensitive for this. Limited cutaneous systemic sclerosis (CREST) tends to be positive for anticentromere antibody.

Haematological disorders

1. C. Chronic myeloid leukaemia is the commonest myeloproliferative disorder. A large proportion of patients show mutation of the BCR-ABL gene, and are consequently able to be treated with imatinib (a tyrosine kinase inhibitor).
2. E. Classical Hodgkin lymphoma has a bimodal age distribution and often presents with unilateral neck lymphadenopathy. Histologically, characteristic Reed–Sternberg cells with 'owl's eye' nuclei are often seen.
3. G. Multiple myeloma is a plasma cell neoplasm of the middle aged and elderly. Patients often have a combination of paraproteinemia, hypercalcemia, renal impairment, anaemia and bone pain. Lytic bone lesions and pathological fractures may occur.
4. H. Myelofibrosis is a myeloproliferative disorder which may arise de novo or develop from other myeloproliferative disorders. Aspiration commonly produces a 'dry tap' due to extensive bone marrow fibrosis. Bone marrow trephine is diagnostic.
5. D. Hairy cell leukaemia is a rare B-cell neoplasm which presents with splenomegaly and pancytopenia. The condition derives its name from the hairy cytoplasmic projections seen on blood film.

Chapter 18 Pathology of the skin

Skin infections

1. B. This is the classic rash of Lyme disease, which is caused by *B. burgdoferi*, a spirocheate transmitted by hard tick bites. None of the other options produce a targetoid rash. Staphylococcal and streptococcal infections may produce migrating erythema.
2. D. This is shingles, which is caused by herpes zoster. The vesicular rash affects a single dermatome so can appear as a band. It is notoriously painful and the pain can persist for months after the rash subsides (postherpetic neuralgia). Herpes simplex virus infection can also be painful but the distribution is not dermatomal, and it commonly affects the lips or genital areas.
3. K. *T. pallidum* is the causative organism of syphilis. The primary chancre is painless and spontaneously resolves. A rash is seen in secondary syphilis. Tertiary syphilis can occur without treatment, causing gumma to form within the central nervous system, heart and other organs. It is the only option that requires a silver stain.
4. G. Leprosy is a mycobacterial infection caused by *M. leprae*. The pauci and multibacillary types refer to the tuberculoid and lepromatous forms. Tuberculosis can have cutaneous involvement (lupus vulgaris), characterized by reddish-brown plaques. Leprosy is the only option with both a protracted course and disfigurement. HSV also has a long course in that the virus is not cleared from the body; however, this is characterized by intermittent attacks and a vesicular rash, and does not cause permanent disfigurement.
5. J. This is a description of erysipelas, which is commonly caused by *S. pyogenes*. It causes a superficial infection affecting the upper dermis. Cellulitis, by contrast, is commonly caused by *S. aureus* and is a deep dermal infection typically affecting the limbs. Both differ from *B. anthraxis* (anthrax), which occurs as a single lesion that evolves to form a black eschar.

Glossary

Abscess A localized collection of pus in a tissue, cavity or confined area; usually associated with infection.

Adenocarcinoma A malignant tumour arising from glandular epithelium.

Adenoma A benign tumour arising from glandular epithelium.

Aetiology The cause of a disease.

Alloimmune An immune response to antigen from members of the same species.

Amyloid Abnormal protein aggregates formed of extracellular fibrils.

Antinuclear antibodies (ANA) Antibodies against different antigens within the nucleus.

Antineutrophil cytoplasmic antibodies (ANCA) Antibodies directed against the cytoplasmic constituents of neutrophils. The pattern of staining can be perinuclear (pANCA) or cytoplasmic (cANCA). ANCA positivity is associated with small vessel vasculitides.

Anaplastic A lack of cellular differentiation which is characteristic of some malignant cells.

Anhidrosis The absence of sweating.

Apoptosis Programmed cell death.

Ascites A collection of extracellular fluid within the peritoneal cavity.

Atelectasis Collapse of lung tissue (partial or complete).

Atrophy Describes the decrease in size (or wasting) of a cell, tissue or organ.

Autoantibody Antibody directed towards self-antigens.

Autocrine Describes the process whereby a cell secretes a substance whose target for action is the secreting cell itself.

Blastema Primitive undifferentiated cells which may form organs/structures.

Bursa A small fluid-filled sac that reduces friction on movement between a tendon and bone, or between bone and skin.

Carcinoma A malignant tumour arising from epithelium.

Caseation A form of necrosis that appears soft and cheese like. It is almost synonymous with tuberculosis.

Chemokine A chemoattractant.

Chimera An organism composed of two genetically different cell types, e.g., following bone marrow transplant the recipient has their own DNA and that of the donors within the bone marrow.

Colic Describes a pain that gradually increases, reaches a peak and then subsides slowly. This pattern may then be repeated.

Complement A group of serum proteins that form an enzyme cascade that is involved in innate immunity.

Congo red Histological stain for amyloid; considered positive if the tissue stains brick red, with apple-green birefringence on polarization.

Consolidation Solidification of an organ into a firm dense mass with fluid, cellular debris or tumour cells.

Contralateral On the opposite side (to a lesion).

Cortex The peripheral area or rind of a tissue or organ.

Crypt A deep pit-like structure found in the wall of the intestine.

Cyst A closed sac-like structure lined by epithelium.

Cytokine Chemical messengers that act over short distances to modulate and regulate cell function.

Dermatitis Inflammation of the skin; it is used interchangeably with eczema.

Diploid A set of paired chromosomes.

Dysphagia Difficulty in swallowing.

Dyspnoea Shortness of breath.

Empyema The accumulation of pus in a cavity of the body.

Endophytic A pattern of inward growth, i.e., growth is into the tissue away from the epithelial surface.

Epistaxis A nosebleed.

Epithelium A layer of cells covering the surface of a tissue which performs various functions.

Erythrocyte sedimentation rate (ESR) A nonspecific marker of inflammation, based on the rate at which red blood cells settle in a column of liquid.

Eviscerate The removal of internal organs, such as at a postmortem examination.

Exophytic A pattern of outward growth, i.e., growth is away from the epithelial surface. Used to describe a tumour that grows outwards from an epithelial surface.

Fistula An abnormal epithelized communication between two epithelial-lined cavities.

Germ cell tumour A tumour derived from germ cells.

Giant cell A multinucleated cell formed from the fusion of many histiocytes.

Giemsa A tinctorial stain that gives cells a two-tone purple and pink appearance.

Gliosis The proliferation of glial cells within the central nervous system in response to injury to produce a scar.

Glossitis Inflammation of the tongue.

Gram stain A crystal violet histological stain used to identify and classify bacteria based on the differential staining of the bacterial cell wall, i.e., Gram positive or Gram negative.

Granulation tissue Connective tissue formed during inflammation which contains numerous capillaries, fibroblasts and plasma cells. It temporarily replaces lost tissue and is the precursor to repair/scar formation.

Granuloma A collection of epithelioid histiocytes, which can be surrounded by a peripheral rim of lymphocytes +/− giant cells.

Haematoxylin and eosin (H&E) An enduring histological stain used routinely on initial examination of all tissues. Eosin stains proteins pink and haematoxylin stains acidic molecules dark blue/purple, e.g., nucleic acids.

Haploid A single set of unpaired chromosomes.

Heterodimer A protein formed of two different types of polypeptides.

Hodgkin disease A lymphoproliferative disorder characterized by the presence of Reed–Sternberg and Hodgkin cells.

Homodimer A protein formed of the same types of polypeptides.

Histiocyte A resident tissue macrophage which has a long lifespan.

Humanized (antibody) A synthetic antibody where the Fc portion is formed from human DNA sequence rather than an animal.

Hybridization The formation of a bond between two molecules, e.g., complementary strands of DNA, antibodies and epitopes.

Hyperhidrosis Excessive sweating.

Hyperplasia An increase in the number of cells within a tissue.

Hypertrophy An increase in the size of cells or organs.

Hypoxemia Low arterial concentration of oxygen.

Hypoxia Oxygen deficiency due to insufficient oxygen to meet demand either globally or focally.

Iatrogenic Caused by medical treatments, interventions or actions.

Idiopathic Where the cause is unknown.

Immunohistochemistry The use of labelled antibodies on histological slides to identify various epitopes within a cell population of interest.

Incidence The number of new cases in a population over a period of time.

Intraepithelial neoplasia Dysplastic changes within an epithelium confined to the epithelium.

Intussusception The telescoping of a segment of bowel into itself, akin to how a telescope collapses.

Ipsilateral On the same side (as a lesion).

Ischaemia A reduction in blood supply to tissues, resulting in reduction in oxygen AND glucose, which are necessary for metabolism.

Karyotype The set of chromosomes for an individual.

Leukaemia A malignancy of haematopoietic cells of the bone marrow.

Lithiasis Calculi (stone) formation.

Lymphoid Relating to cells of the lymphocyte lineage, e.g., T cells and B cells.

Lymphoma A malignancy of lymphoid cells, predominantly arising in lymphoid tissue.

Medulla The inner region of an organ usually underneath the cortex, e.g., renal medulla.

Metachronous Occurring at a different time to the initial event, e.g., a second tumour occurring 3 years after the primary tumour.

Metaplasia The change from one type of mature fully differentiated epithelium to another mature fully differentiated type.

Microbiome The genomes of all of the resident microorganisms that colonize the body.

Microbiota The resident microorganisms that colonize the body.

Mitogen A substance that induces a cell to undergo mitosis.

Mucinous Producing mucin, a glycosylated glycoprotein.

Mucocele A cyst-like swelling containing mucous.

Mucosa The mucous membrane and underlying connective tissue that lines the surface of body cavities or organs.

Myeloid Refers to the myeloid lineage of blood cells, i.e., neutrophils, eosinophils, basophils.

Naevus A circumscribed lesion of the skin or mucous membranes.

Necrosis Cell/tissue death that is energy independent. Necrosis is the unregulated death of cells or tissues in a living organism. It is a pathological process following cellular injury that incites an inflammatory reaction.

Oncogene A gene that has the potential to cause cancer. Mutation is usually required in only one copy of the gene.

Onycholysis Separation or loosening of the nail within the nail bed. It is associated with many conditions e.g., trauma, psoriasis, fungal infection.

Opsonization The coating of a surface, e.g., by antibodies or complement.

Osteoid Bone matrix that has not yet ossified.

Palisaded Arrangement of cells/nuclei to resemble a picket fence.

Paracrine Describes the process whereby a cell secretes a substance that has an action on nearby cells.

Paraneoplastic syndrome Syndromes arising as a result of secreted substances by a tumour, e.g., hypercalcaemia and syndrome of inappropriate antidiuretic hormone (SIADH) secretion.

Paraphimosis The foreskin is retracted behind the glans penis and unable to be returned to the normal anatomical position.

Parenchyma The functional component of a gland or organ (distinct from supportive or connective tissue).

Paroxysmal Describes sudden attacks of a given effect occurring spontaneously in no fixed pattern.

Pathogenic Capable of causing disease.

Pellagra Niacin deficiency causing symptoms of dermatitis, dementia, diarrhoea and death.

Petechiae Pinpoint haemorrhages occuring as small red spots on the skin (1–2 mm).

Phimosis Unretractable foreskin over the glans of the penis.

Plasmid An extrachromosomal small circular double-stranded DNA molecule, which independently replicates. They are found in bacteria and some eukaryotes and usually contain genes that confer a survival advantage.

Portal hypertension Abnormally elevated blood pressure of the portal venous system.

Promoter A region of noncoding DNA that regulates the transcription and expression of a gene.

Pruritus Generalized itchiness.

Pseudocyst A collection of fluid that does not have an epithelial lining.

Pseudopodia A dynamic cytoplasmic-filled projection from a prokaryotic or eukaryotic cell.

Ptosis Drooping of the upper eyelid.

Pyknotic Condensation and clumping of nuclear chromatin and reduction in size of the nucleus; seen in degenerating or apoptotic cells.

Sepsis A systemic inflammatory response syndrome (SIRS) (tachycardia, tachypnoea, pyrexia or hypothermia) secondary to infection.

Serous A fluid of thin, watery consistency that may be secreted by epithelial cells.

Sinus A blind-ending tract leading from a focus of suppurative infection that is not lined by epithelial tissue. Also, an anatomical description relating to a cavity or sac.

Stroma The supporting connective tissue of an organ.

Submucosa The area of connective tissue directly under an epithelial surface.

Super antigen Antigens which cause unregulated T-cell activation and cytokine release independent of the normal signalling pathways.

Suppurative An inflammatory process that produces pus.

Synchronous Existing or occurring at the same time—for example, two malignancies occurring at the same time.

Syrinx A cyst-like cavity within the nervous system, usually within the spinal cord or base of the brain.

Teratoma A tumour arising from germ cells derived from one or more of the germ cell layers, e.g., mesoderm, ectoderm, endoderm.

Transcription factor A molecule that binds to a promoter region of a gene in the regulation of gene expression.

Tumour suppressor gene A gene that reduces the risk of neoplasia developing. Malignancies usually require both copies of the gene to be mutated ('two hit hypothesis').

Ulcer A full thickness defect of epithelium.

Venesection The removal of blood from a vein.

Virulence The ability of a pathogen to cause an infection. The more virulent a pathogen is, the fewer microorganisms required to cause disease (smaller effective dose).

Volvulus A twisting of a loop of small or large bowel on its mesentery.

Xanthoma A benign yellow-coloured lesion, common on the eyelid, formed by an accumulation of fat-containing macrophages. They commonly indicate an underlying lipid disorder such as elevated serum cholesterol levels.

Index

Note: Page numbers followed by *f* indicate figures, *t* indicate tables, and *b* indicate boxes.

A

I

J

K

L

Q

R

S

W

X

Y

Z

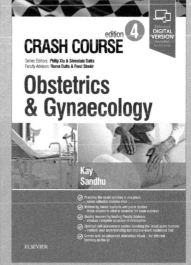

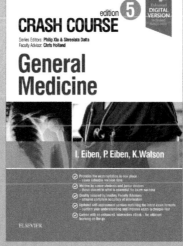

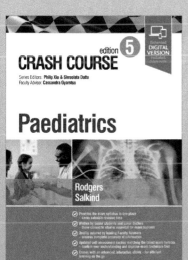

Printed and bound by CPI Group (UK) Ltd, Croydon, CR0 4YY
03/10/2024
01040305-0005